Endocrine Conditions

Takara Stanley • Madhusmita Misra
Editors

Endocrine Conditions in Pediatrics

A Practical Guide

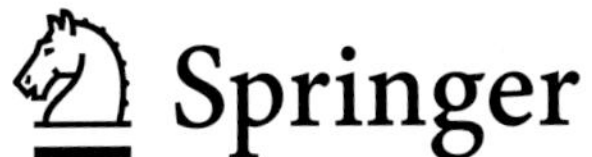

Editors
Takara Stanley
Division of Pediatric Endocrinology
Massachusetts General Hospital and
Harvard Medical School
Boston, MA
USA

Madhusmita Misra
Division of Pediatric Endocrinology
Massachusetts General Hospital and
Harvard Medical School
Boston, MA
USA

ISBN 978-3-030-52214-8 ISBN 978-3-030-52215-5 (eBook)
https://doi.org/10.1007/978-3-030-52215-5

This Springer imprint is published by the registered company Springer Nature Switzerland AG
The registered company address is: Gewerbestrasse 11, 6330 Cham, Switzerland

Preface

The primary intention of this book is to provide easily accessible information to primary care providers about the initial evaluation and management of signs and symptoms that may suggest pediatric endocrine disease. The book is organized by discussion of presenting signs or symptoms with suggested initial evaluation (Part I), followed by a discussion of how to interpret relevant laboratory testing and imaging (Part II), and ending with a discussion of the etiology and management of common pediatric endocrine conditions (Part III). We hope that this organizational structure provides rapid reference to just-in-time information for primary care providers caring for patients with possible endocrine conditions. We also hope that this book will be useful to students and trainees interested in pediatric endocrinology as well as pediatric endocrine fellows.

This book is not intended to provide a comprehensive discussion of all pediatric endocrine pathophysiology, a purpose which multiple excellent textbooks already fulfill. Rather, we hope that this book will provide guidance regarding how to approach symptoms of possible endocrine disease, how to interpret evaluative testing carefully, and how to begin initial management and counsel patients and families regarding what to expect for further management, which may often require referral to pediatric endocrinology. We also hope that, for many patients, this book may facilitate management of benign conditions in the primary care setting, as we know that patients and families are most comfortable and best-served staying in their medical home when possible. Related to that purpose, we hope that Part II will be particularly useful in highlighting limitations of assays and lab-provided reference ranges, as well as situations in which mildly abnormal labs can be repeated before pediatric endocrine referral is required.

We are grateful to our many wonderful colleagues who contributed to this book, and we salute primary care providers who engage daily in the difficult jobs of fielding patient and family concerns, and discerning between normal physiology and possible pathology. We hope that this book will assist in that task.

Boston, MA, USA — Takara Stanley
Boston, MA, USA — Madhusmita Misra

Acknowledgment

To our patients and their families, who give us the privilege of caring for them and learning with them.

Contents

Contributors

Sungeeta Agrawal, MD Division of Pediatric Endocrinology, Floating Hospital for Children at Tufts Medical Center/Tufts University School of Medicine, Boston, MA, USA

Nourah Almutlaq, MD Division of Pediatric Endocrinology, Department of Pediatrics, Riley Hospital for Children at Indiana University Health, Indiana University School of Medicine, Indianapolis, IN, USA

Ambika P. Ashraf, MD Department of Pediatrics, Division of Endocrinology and Diabetes, University of Alabama at Birmingham, Birmingham, AL, USA

Jennifer M. Barker, MD Pediatric Endocrinology, University of Colorado School of Medicine, Aurora, CO, USA

Paul Boepple, MD MassGeneral Hospital for Children, Boston, MA, USA

Sasigarn A. Bowden, MD Division of Endocrinology, Department of Pediatrics, Nationwide Children's Hospital/The Ohio State University College of Medicine, Columbus, OH, USA

Luz E. Castellanos, MD Pediatric Endocrine Division, Massachusetts General Hospital and Harvard Medical School, Boston, MA, USA

Christine E. Cherella, MD Division of Endocrinology, Department of Pediatrics, Boston Children's Hospital, Boston, MA, USA

Hannah Chesser, MD Division of Pediatric Endocrinology and Diabetes, University of California at San Francisco, San Francisco, CA, USA

Anna Chin, MD, MPH Department of Pediatric Endocrinology, Warren Alpert Medical School of Brown University and Hasbro Children's Hospital, Providence, RI, USA

Aluma Chovel-Sella, MD Massachusetts General Hospital, Boston, MA, USA

Julia R. Donner, ScB The Warren Alpert Medical School of Brown University, Providence, RI, USA

Oscar Escobar, MD Division Pediatric Endocrinology, University of Pittsburgh School of Medicine, UPMC Children's Hospital of Pittsburgh, Pittsburgh, PA, USA

Erica A. Eugster, MD Division of Pediatric Endocrinology, Department of Pediatrics, Riley Hospital for Children at Indiana University Health, Indiana University School of Medicine, Indianapolis, IN, USA

Meghan E. Fredette, MD Division of Pediatric Endocrinology, Hasbro Children's Hospital/ Warren Alpert Medical School of Brown University, Providence, RI, USA

Rebecca J. Gordon, MD Division of Endocrinology, Boston Children's Hospital, Harvard Medical School, Boston, MA, USA

Nursen Gurtunca, MD UPMC Children's Hospital of Pittsburgh, Division of Endocrinology and Diabetes, Pittsburgh, PA, USA

Alyssa Halper, MD, MS Massachusetts General Hospital, Boston, MA, USA

Rebecca M. Harris, MD, PhD, MA Department of Pediatrics, Division of Endocrinology, Boston Children's Hospital, Boston, MA, USA

Juanita K. Hodax, MD Pediatric Endocrinology, Seattle Children's Hospital and University of Washington, Seattle, WA, USA

Rabab Jafri, MD Massachusetts General Hospital, Boston, MA, USA

Liya Kerem, MD, MSc Pediatric Endocrinology Unit, Massachusetts General Hospital for Children, Boston, MA, USA

Division of Pediatric Endocrinology, Massachusetts General Hospital, Harvard Medical School, Boston, MA, USA

Brenda Kohn, MD Division of Pediatric Endocrinology and Diabetes, New York University-Langone Medical Center, Hassenfeld Children's Hospital, New York, NY, USA

Charlene Lai, MD The Division of Endocrinology and Diabetes, The Children's Hospital of Philadelphia, Philadelphia, PA, USA

Diva D. De León, MD, MSCE Department of Pediatrics, The Perelman School of Medicine at the University of Pennsylvania, Philadelphia, PA, USA

Lynne L. Levitsky, MD Harvard Medical School, Boston, MA, USA

Massachusetts General Hospital, Boston, MA, USA

Sonali Malhotra, MD Pediatric Endocrinology and Obesity Medicine, Massachusetts General Hospital for Children, Boston, MA, USA

Christine March, MD Division of Pediatric Endocrinology, University of Pittsburgh, UPMC Children's Hospital of Pittsburgh, Pittsburgh, PA, USA

Seth Daniel Marks, MD, MSc Children's Hospital HSC Winnipeg, Pediatrics and Child Health, Winnipeg, MB, Canada

Brynn E. Marks, MD, MSHPEd Division of Endocrinology, Children's National Medical Center, Washington, DC, USA

Dayna McGill, MD Division of Pediatric Endocrinology, Massachusetts General Hospital for Children, Boston, MA, USA

Shilpa Mehta, MD Department of Pediatrics, Division of Pediatric Endocrinology, New York Medical College, Valhalla, NY, USA

Kate Millington, MD Division of Endocrinology, Boston Children's Hospital, Boston, MA, USA

Madhusmita Misra, MD, MPH Division of Pediatric Endocrinology, Massachusetts General Hospital and Harvard Medical School, Boston, MA, USA

Deborah M. Mitchell, MD Massachusetts General Hospital, Harvard Medical School, Boston, MA, USA

Radhika Muzumdar, MD Division of Endocrinology and Diabetes, Department of Pediatrics, UPMC Children's Hospital of Pittsburgh, Pittsburgh, PA, USA

Division of Endocrinology and Diabetes, UPMC Children's Hospital of Pittsburgh, University of Pittsburgh School of Medicine, Pittsburgh, PA, USA

Eliana M. Perez-Garcia, MD Division Pediatric Endocrinology, University of Pittsburgh School of Medicine, UPMC Children's Hospital of Pittsburgh, Pittsburgh, PA, USA

Bianca Pinto, MD Division of Pediatric Endocrinology, University of Pittsburgh, UPMC Children's Hospital Pittsburgh, Pittsburgh, PA, USA

Barbara Pober, MD Department of Pediatrics, Genetics Unit, Massachusetts General Hospital, Boston, MA, USA

Katherine Jane Pundyk, MD, MSc Children's Hospital HSC Winnipeg, Pediatrics and Child Health, Winnipeg, MB, Canada

Nora E. Renthal, MD, PhD Division of Endocrinology, Department of Pediatrics, Boston Children's Hospital, Boston, MA, USA

Danielle Renzi, BS Department of Pediatrics, Genetics Unit, Massachusetts General Hospital, Boston, MA, USA

Cemre Robinson, MD Division of Pediatric Endocrinology and Diabetes, Icahn School of Medicine at Mount Sinai, New York, NY, USA

Mohamed Saleh, MD Division of Endocrinology and Diabetes, Department of Pediatrics, UPMC Children's Hospital of Pittsburgh, Pittsburgh, PA, USA

Eray Savgan-Gurol, MD Pediatric Endocrine Division, Massachusetts General Hospital, Harvard Medical School, Boston, MA, USA

Jessica Schmitt, MD University of Alabama at Birmingham, Birmingham, AL, USA

Monica Serrano-Gonzalez, MD Pediatric Endocrinology and Diabetes Center, Hasbro Children's Hospital, The Warren Alpert Medical School of Brown University, Providence, RI, USA

Nabiha Shahid, MD UPMC Children's Hospital of Pittsburgh, Division of Endocrinology and Diabetes, Pittsburgh, PA, USA

Jordan S. Sherwood, MD Massachusetts General Hospital, Boston, MA, USA

Vibha Singhal, MD Division of Pediatric Endocrinology, Massachusetts General Hospital, Harvard Medical School, Boston, MA, USA

Ambreen Sonawalla, MD Arkansas Children's Hospital, Little Rock, AR, USA

Shylaja Srinivasan, MD Division of Pediatric Endocrinology and Diabetes, University of California at San Francisco, San Francisco, CA, USA

Takara Stanley, MD Division of Pediatric Endocrinology, Massachusetts General Hospital and Harvard Medical School, Boston, MA, USA

Bhuvana Sunil, MD Department of Pediatrics, Division of Endocrinology and Diabetes, University of Alabama at Birmingham, Birmingham, AL, USA

Vidhu V. Thaker, MD Division of Molecular Genetics, Department of Pediatrics, Columbia University Irving Medical Center, New York, NY, USA

Division of Pediatric Endocrinology, Department of Pediatrics, Columbia University Irving Medical Center, New York, NY, USA

Seth Tobolsky, MD Massachusetts General Hospital for Children, Boston, MA, USA

Lisa Swartz Topor, MD, MMSc Department of Pediatric Endocrinology, Warren Alpert Medical School of Brown University and Hasbro Children's Hospital, Providence, RI, USA

Pediatric Endocrinology, The Warren Alpert Medical School of Brown University and Hasbro Children's Hospital, Providence, RI, USA

Taylor M. Triolo, MD Barbara Davis Center for Diabetes, University of Colorado School of Medicine, Aurora, CO, USA

Marwa Tuffaha, MD Pediatric Endocrine Division, Massachusetts General Hospital and Harvard Medical School, Boston, MA, USA

Janaki D. Vakharia, MD Department of Endocrinology, Massachusetts General Hospital, Boston, MA, USA

Pushpa Viswanathan, MD University of Pittsburgh School of Medicine, Department of Endocrinology, UPMC Children's Hospital Pittsburgh, Pittsburgh, PA, USA

Rachel Whooten, MD, MPH Massachusetts General Hospital for Children, Boston, MA, USA

Coleen Williams, PsyD Division of Endocrinology, Boston Children's Hospital, Boston, MA, USA

Selma Witchel, MD Division of Pediatric Endocrinology, University of Pittsburgh, UPMC Children's Hospital of Pittsburgh, Pittsburgh, PA, USA

Soundos Youssef, MD Neuroendocrine Unit, Massachusetts General Hospital, Boston, MA, USA

Jia Zhu, MD Division of Endocrinology, Department of Medicine, Boston Children's Hospital, Boston, MA, USA

Part I

Common Presenting Signs and Symptoms That May Reflect Endocrine Disease

Decreased Growth Velocity and/or Short Stature

1

Oscar Escobar and Eliana M. Perez-Garcia

Abbreviations

ADD	Attention deficit disorder
ADHD	Attention deficit and hyperactivity disorder
BMI	Body mass index
CBC	Complete blood cell count
CDGP	Constitutional delay of growth and puberty
CMP	Complete metabolic panel
CRP	C-reactive protein
ESR	Erythrocyte sedimentation rate
Free T4	Free thyroxine
FSS	Familial short stature
GH	Growth hormone
GV	Growth velocity
HV	Height velocity
IgA	Immunoglobulin A
IGF-1	Insulin-like growth factor 1
IGFBP3	Insulin-like growth factor binding protein 3
MPH	Mid-parental height
MRI	Magnetic resonance imaging
PAH	Predicted adult height
SS	Short stature
TH	Target height
TORCH	Toxoplasma Gondii, other viruses, Rubella, Cytomegalovirus, Herpes
TSH	Thyroid-stimulating hormone
TTG-IgA	Tissue trans glutaminase IgA
XLH	X-linked hypophosphatemia

O. Escobar (✉) · E. M. Perez-Garcia
Division Pediatric Endocrinology, University of Pittsburgh School of Medicine, UPMC Children's Hospital of Pittsburgh, Pittsburgh, PA, USA
e-mail: Oscar.escobar@chp.edu; perezgarciae@upmc.edu

T. Stanley, M. Misra (eds.), *Endocrine Conditions in Pediatrics*, https://doi.org/10.1007/978-3-030-52215-5_1

Introduction

Linear and ponderal growth are important indicators of health in children. Therefore, close attention to growth trajectory is an essential component of the routine evaluation of the child by the primary care provider.

Linear growth is defined as the increment in length/height over time while ponderal growth is defined as the increment of weight over time.

Harmonious growth in both height and weight within reference range for age and sex would represent a normal growth pattern. Deviations from the norm could lead to "worrisome growth patterns".

Conceivable abnormalities of growth include, on one hand, either slow or rapid linear growth, and slow or rapid ponderal growth and, on the other hand, short stature, tall stature, underweight, and overweight/obesity.

Decreased growth velocity and *short stature* are the focus of this chapter. Increased growth velocity and tall stature are covered in Chap. 2, weight gain and obesity in Chap. 19, and weight loss in Chap. 20.

Definitions

Linear growth velocity or, simply, *growth velocity (GV)*, also called *height velocity (HV)*, is defined as the delta of length or height divided by the delta of time between 2 separate measurements. It is expressed in centimeters/year (cm/y).

Decreased growth velocity, frequently referred to as *growth failure*, is a condition where linear growth is suboptimal, and may or may not lead to short stature.

Short stature (SS) is defined as a length or height below 2 standard deviations from the mean for age and sex, which is roughly equivalent to less than the 3rd percentile. Short stature may or may not result from growth failure.

Important Considerations in Assessing Growth

Accuracy of Measurements

Accurate measurements of length and height are crucial for the correct calculation of growth velocity. Inaccurate measurements will lead to erroneous calculation of growth velocity and inappropriate work-up and referrals.

Length

For children 2 years of age or younger, it is recommended to obtain a length measurement in supine position using a measuring table with a fixed headpiece and a movable foot piece. The measurement needs to be performed by 2 people, one of whom holds the head of the child in the Frankfort plane against the fixed head block and the other ensures appropriate extension of lower extremities and neutral position of the ankles at a right angle, and moves the foot block toward the soles of the feet to read the measurement. No shoes should be worn during measurement, and any hair-do that may have an impact on the measurement should be undone.

Height/Stature

For children older than 2 years of age, measurement of standing height (stature) is recommended. This is best performed using a stadiometer with a movable headboard. The child needs to be positioned in such a way that heels, calves, buttocks, upper back, and occiput are in contact with a vertical board (see Fig. 1.1). The head needs to be placed in the Frankfort plane. The movable headboard needs to be perpendicular to the vertical measuring board. A slight up pressure of the mandible allows for correction of the physiologic intervertebral disc compression that occurs throughout the day; however, caution must be exercised to avoid lifting the child from the floor. No shoes should be worn during measurement, and any hair-do that may have an impact on the measurement should be undone.

Frankfort Plane

The Frankfort plane refers to a neutral position of the head in which an imaginary straight line connecting the lower edge of the orbit and the upper border of the external auditory canal is perpendicular to the measuring board (see Fig. 1.2).

Weight

Weight measurements should be made in appropriately calibrated scales (infant/adult) with light clothing or only underwear, and making sure clothing pockets are emptied and shoes are removed.

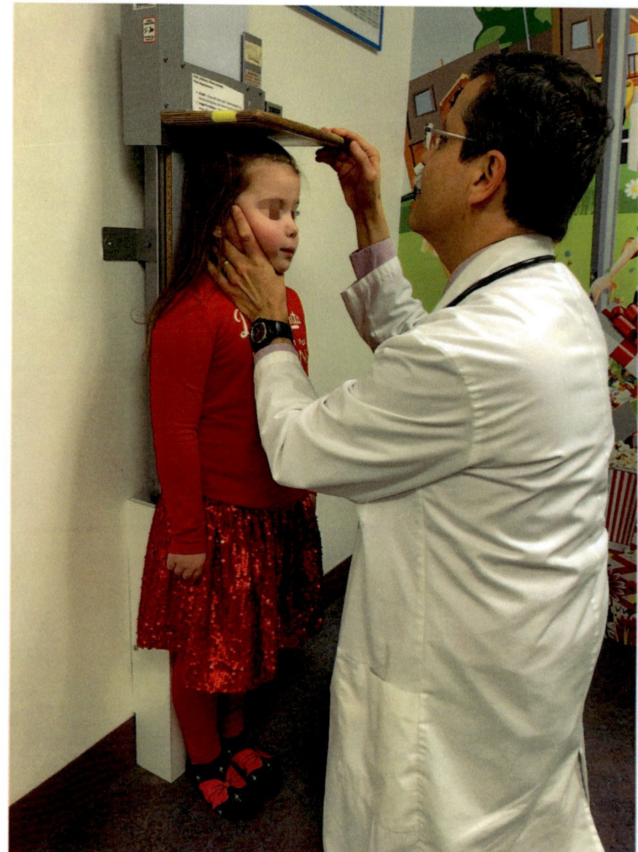

Fig. 1.1 Standing height measurement

Growth Velocity

It is preferable to calculate the growth velocity based on 2 measurements performed ≥6 months apart to avoid the amplification of the inherent error of measurement. The shorter the time between 2 measurements, the greater the multiplication of the measurement error reflected in the GV calculation.

Growth velocity changes throughout the growth process from birth to final closure of growth plates at the end of puberty. On average, prenatal length is acquired at a rate of 1.2 to 1.5 cm/week. In the first year of age, the average growth velocity is approximately 25 cm/year and decreases to approximately 12.5 cm/year by the second year of life, then to approximately 8 cm/year by the third year of life with a persistent but attenuated decline over the next 7 years to the lowest growth velocity (average 5 cm/year) just before puberty starts, the so-called prepubertal dip or physiologic prepubertal deceleration of growth. Following this, the pubertal growth spurt begins, leading to a significant acceleration of GV which reaches a peak of 8.3 cm/year in girls (at around 11.5 years of age and Tanner stage III of pubertal development) and 9.5 cm/year in boys (at around 13.5 years

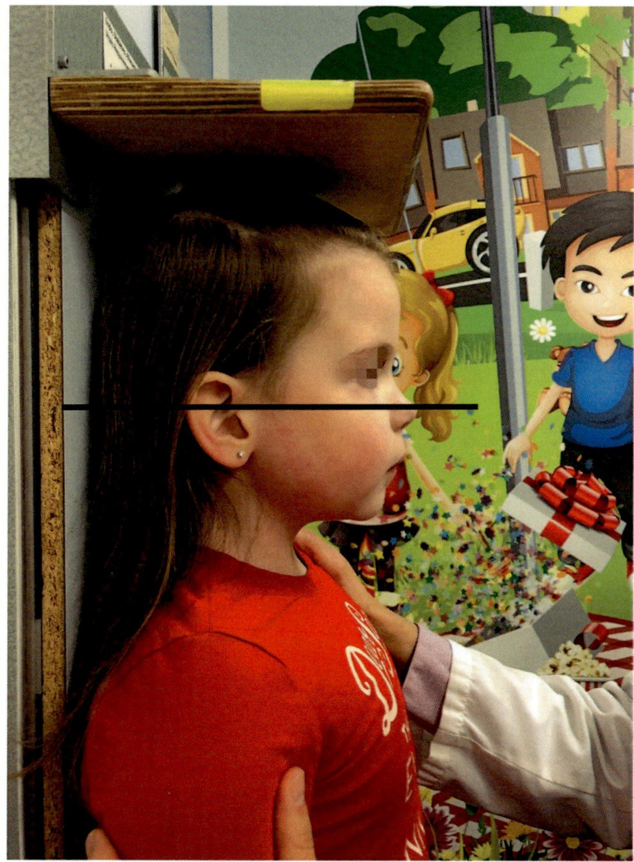

Fig. 1.2 Frankfort plane, indicated by black line. The child's head should be positioned so that the Frankfort plane is perpendicular to the measuring board during the measurement

of age and Tanner stage IV of pubertal development). Variation in the timing of pubertal onset can lead to early or delayed maturation and may have an impact on the age of onset of the growth spurt and the peak growth velocity.

A special mention here is that of children born small for gestational age (SGA). A large proportion (close to 90%) of these children show catch-up growth (increased GV) within the first 2 years of life [1], which brings them to at least the lower percentiles of normal height for age. The remainder fail to demonstrate this, suggesting that there could be an underlying genetic disorder or an endocrine dysfunction.

Tanner and Whitehouse established standards for growth velocity for age and sex with normal variation expressed in percentiles above and below the mean [2] (see Fig. 1.3a, b). Although these growth velocity charts can be used for more precise interpretation, the simple tracking of the plotting of accurate measurements in the height charts should provide the clinician with a visual assessment of the growth pattern to make an interpretation of whether it is normal or abnormal. Standard height charts include several major percentiles (3rd, 5th, 10th, 25th, 50th, 75th, 90th, 95th, and 97th). In general, a downward drift in the length or height measurements that crosses two major percentiles should be regarded as worrisome growth pattern, suggestive of growth failure which requires prompt investigation and consideration of a referral.

Additional Considerations in Determining the Etiology of Altered Growth Patterns

Important considerations in the assessment of growth disorders are: (a) correlation of linear and ponderal growth, (b) attention to body proportions, (c) association of growth with pubertal development, and (d) genetic determination of growth potential (Table 1.1).

Relation of Weight and Height

As mentioned above, the assessment of weight gain trajectory (ponderal growth) gives important clues to the clinician when evaluating a child that displays abnormalities in linear growth. Short stature or growth failure accompanied by normal or increased weight gain should rise the suspicion of an endocrinopathy. On the other hand, the presence of poor ponderal growth in a child with short stature or growth failure should alert the clinician about nutritional problems, chronic illness, or psychosocial causes. Available tools to assess the correlation between linear and ponderal growth include weight-for-height and body mass index (BMI) charts. BMI is calculated by dividing the weight in kilograms by the square of the height in meters.

Proportionate Versus Disproportionate Growth

Assessment of the body proportions provides a diagnostic clue to orient the differential diagnosis. These may include the assessment of the upper and lower "segments," arm span, and sitting heights. Comparison of a child's various anthropometric ratios, as described below, with established norms determines whether short stature is proportionate or disproportionate. In general, disproportionate short stature is associated with skeletal dysplasia or acquired causes, such us spinal radiation, while most other causes of short stature present with proportionate anthropometric measurements.

Normal body proportions suggest a harmonic growth of the spine and extremities. This can be assessed calculating the *upper-to-lower body segment ratio*, as well as comparing the arm span to the standing height. The *lower segment* is measured from the symphysis pubis to the floor on a standing position. The *upper segment* is calculated by subtracting the lower segment measurement from the standing height.

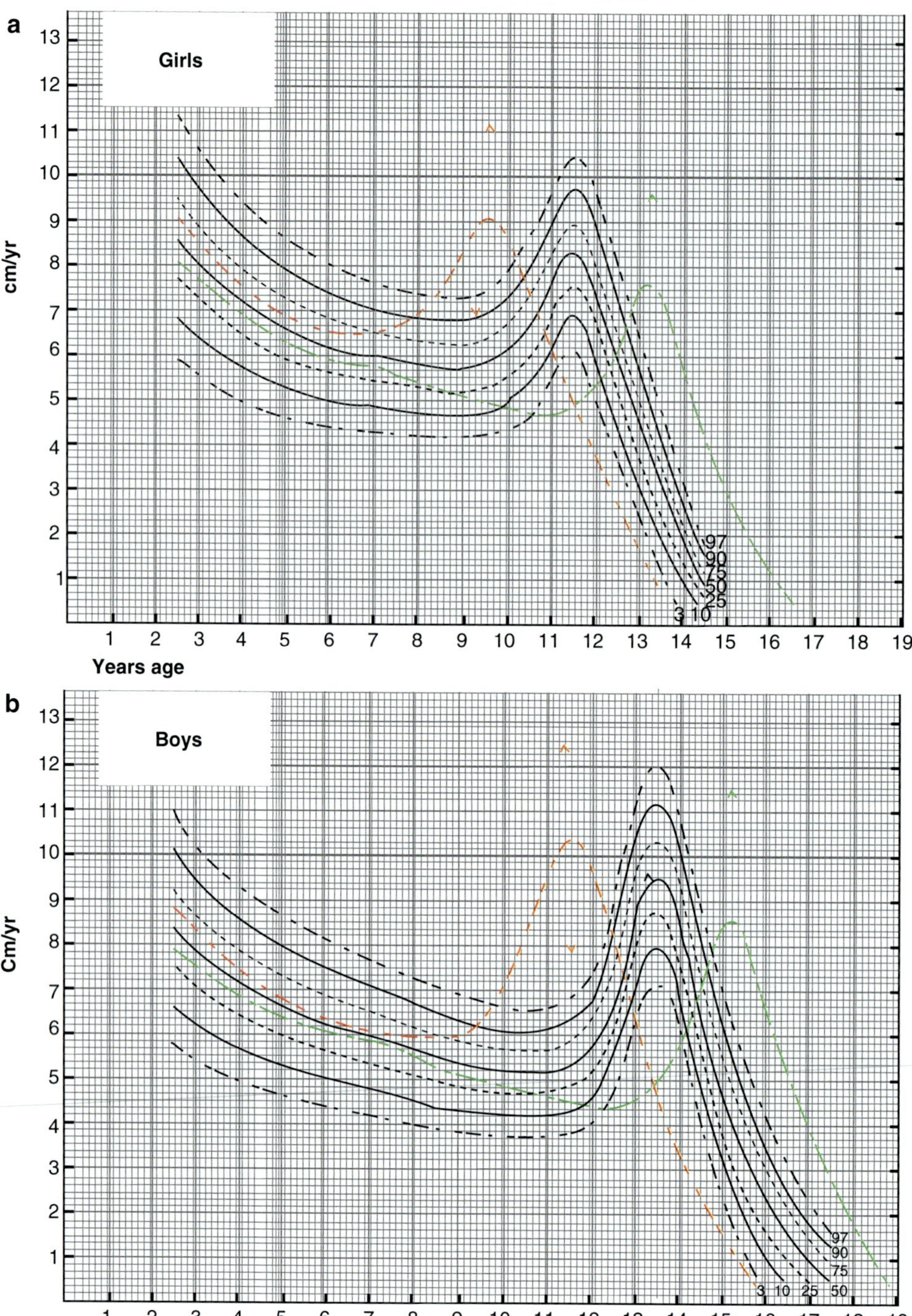

Fig. 1.3 (**a**) Height velocity for age for girls. (Adapted from Tanner and Davies [7]). The black curves indicate percentiles for children with "average" pubertal timing. The red curve indicates 50th percentile for a girl with early pubertal timing, with the red ^'s indicating 97th and 3rd percentiles. The green curve indicates 50th percentile for a girl with late pubertal timing. (**b**) Height velocity for age for boys. (Adapted from Tanner and Davies [7]). The black curves indicate percentiles for children with "average" pubertal timing. The red curve indicates 50th percentile for a boy with early pubertal timing, with the red ^'s indicating 97th and 3rd percentiles. The green curve indicates 50th percentile for a boy with late pubertal timing

The upper-to-lower segment ratio varies with age and is roughly 1.7 at birth, 1.3 at 3 years, 1.1 at 7 years and 1.0 in adults [3].

An increased upper-to-lower segment ratio for the child's age suggests a compromise in the growth of the extremities (as seen in diaphyseal, metaphyseal, or epiphyseal bone dysplasias), while the opposite suggests compromised growth of the spine (as seen in spondylodysplasias and radiation therapy to the spine).

Another way to assess body proportions, which is readily available to the primary care provider, is the comparison of *arm span* to standing height. After 8 years of age, the arm span should be approximately equal to the height in the proportionate body. In fact, in older children in whom height measurement cannot be obtained, arm span could serve as a surrogate measurement of linear growth. When the arm span-to-height ratio is higher than normal, the possibilities of decreased spinal growth vs. long extremities are to be con-

Table 1.1 Differential diagnosis of decreased GV and short stature (Adapted from Argente [5])

Sign/symptom	Differential diagnosis
Normal GV with short stature (normal variants)	Familial short stature (FSS) Constitutional delay of growth and puberty (CDGP)
Decreased GV with normal or increased weight for height	Endocrine disorders Hypothyroidism (primary or central) Growth hormone-IGF-1 axis abnormalities Growth hormone deficiency Growth hormone insensitivity IGF-1 deficiency/decreased bioavailability IGF-1 insensitivity Hypercortisolism Endogenous (Cushing syndrome or disease) Exogenous (iatrogenic)
Decreased GV with low weight for height or poor weight gain	Nutritional Calorie-protein malnutrition Malabsorption Stimulant medications for ADD and ADHD Eating disorders Acquired rickets (Vitamin D deficiency, calcium deficiency) Chronic illnesses [5] Gastrointestinal (e.g., Celiac disease, Crohn's disease, cystic fibrosis, short gut syndrome) Hepatic (e.g., biliary atresia, liver transplant) Cardiac (e.g., cyanotic congenital heart disease) Pulmonary (e.g., cystic fibrosis, asthma, bronchopulmonary dysplasia) Metabolic (e.g., uncontrolled diabetes mellitus, untreated central diabetes insipidus) Hematologic (e.g., chronic severe anemia) Oncologic (e.g., leukemias, bone marrow transplant) Renal (e.g., renal tubular acidosis, chronic kidney disease, nephrogenic diabetes insipidus, hypophosphatemic rickets like X-linked hypophosphatemia [XLH]) Neurologic (e.g., cerebral palsy) Rheumatologic (e.g., juvenile arthritis) Psychosocial short stature Child neglect, child abuse, poverty, domestic violence, orphanages, etc.
Disproportionate short stature	Congenital: Skeletal dysplasias Increased upper-to-lower segment ratio for age (short extremities, epiphyseal/metaphyseal dysplasias) Decreased upper-to-lower segment ratio for age (short trunk, spondylo-dysplasias) Acquired Spinal radiation Skeletal neoplasia
Short stature with dysmorphic features	Genetic syndromes/chromosomal abnormalities Turner syndrome Down syndrome Prader-Willi syndrome Russel-Silver syndrome Noonan syndrome Williams-Beuren syndrome Others

sidered. The opposite would suggest attenuated growth of the extremities.

A more refined way of assessing body proportions, which may not be easily available to the primary care provider, is the measurement of sitting height on a special stadiometer and the calculation of the *sitting height index* (sitting height divided by standing height), for which standardized reference tables have been published [4].

Pubertal Development

As previously discussed, pubertal development is associated with an increase in linear GV, the pubertal growth spurt. It is important to interpret growth velocity in the context of pubertal progression. For example, a child with mid- or late pubertal stage on exam who continues to grow at a prepubertal growth velocity may require assessment for underlying causes of poor growth.

Children with very early onset of puberty have an earlier growth spurt which often leads to relative tall stature for age. If untreated, the rapid pubertal progression is followed by early epiphyseal fusion, often resulting in short adult height.

The absence of an acceleration in linear growth in a child who does not show evidence of pubertal development at the expected age can be perceived as growth failure, when compared to other adolescents of the same age. This can be the hallmark of a physiologic process such as constitutional delay of growth and puberty, in which the growth spurt occurs at a later chronological age, or a pathologic process with complete lack of pubertal development such as, hypogonadotropic hypogonadism (e.g., Kallman syndrome) or hypergonadotropic hypogonadism (e.g., Klinefelter syndrome).

Determination of Genetic Potential

It is estimated that 80–90% of the height of an individual is determined by genetic factors and 10–20% by environmental factors. The *mid-parental height (MPH)*, also called *target height (TH)*, allows the clinician to have an idea of the genetic growth potential and determine whether the child is tracking appropriately. Significant deviations should alert about possible growth abnormalities. The calculation of the MPH can be obtained by using the formula described in Fig. 1.4. MPH should be interpreted with caution if one or both parents had circumstances adversely affecting height, such as malnutrition or severe chronic medical conditions.

For boys TH (cm)= $\frac{[\text{father's height (cm)} + \text{mother's height (cm)}]}{2}$ + 6.5 cm

For girls TH (cm)= $\frac{[\text{father's height (cm)} + \text{mother's height (cm)}]}{2}$ − 6.5 cm

Fig. 1.4 The target height (TH) range can be calculated using the 95% confidence intervals: ±10 centimeters (cm) for boys and ±9 centimeters (cm) for girls (Tanner and Whitehouse [2])

Important Clarifying Questions in the Medical History

When evaluating a child with decreased growth velocity and/or short stature, the clinician needs to obtain a complete history and physical examination. Important aspects to be addressed in the medical history sections are included in Table 1.2.

Important Aspects of the Physical Examination

Besides the anthropometric measurements and calculations discussed in detail above, the clinician should pay particular attention to some physical exam findings that might yield additional clues to direct the diagnosis. Table 1.3 shows a non-exhaustive list of findings by systems.

Considerations for Laboratory Evaluation

The clinician should consider laboratory evaluation for children in whom pathologic short stature or altered growth pattern is suspected, especially if any of the following features is present: decreased GV, presence of symptoms of systemic disease, abnormal physical exam findings, or significant discrepancy between growth trajectory and genetic potential (MPH).

As previously discussed, pathologic etiologies include endocrine and non-endocrine disorders. Therefore, helpful tests would include a complete metabolic panel (*CMP*) to evaluate for electrolyte abnormalities, hepatic and renal function; complete blood cell count (*CBC*) to evaluate for anemia or other cell count abnormalities that could be manifestations of a systemic illness; tissue trans glutaminase IgA (*TTG-IgA*) antibodies and *total IgA* to screen for celiac disease; C-reactive protein (*CRP*) and erythrocyte sedimentation rate (*ESR*) to evaluate for chronic inflammation; thyroid-stimulating hormone (*TSH*) and *free T4* to rule out hypothyroidism; and insulin-like growth factor 1 (*IGF-1*), insulin-like growth factor binding protein 3 (*IGFBP3*) to screen for growth hormone deficiency/insensivity.

Table 1.2 Important aspects to consider in the medical history

History section	Important components
History of present illness	Age at onset of abnormal growth
Review of systems	Decreased energy level, poor appetite Headaches or visual impairment Recurrent ear infections Abnormal bowel habits (constipation, diarrhea), abdominal pain Polyuria, polydipsia, nocturia, enuresis, temperature intolerance Dry skin, hair loss Presence/absence of pubertal signs and age of onset
Birth history	Gestational age Birth weight and birth length Maternal complications during pregnancy Complications in prenatal, perinatal, and postnatal course
Developmental history	Milestones for age Tooth eruption Supportive therapies
Nutritional history	Appetite and source of nutrition Food insecurity
Past medical and surgical history	Chronic illness Medications (e.g., ADHD medications, corticosteroids) Trauma (e.g., skeletal trauma, head injuries) Surgical procedures
Social history	House and family composition Smoking exposure School attendance and performance Favorite activities Recent stressors
Family history	Height of parents (calculate MPH), and siblings Age of onset of puberty of the parents and siblings Presence of short stature in family members Genetic diseases or chronic illnesses in the family History of consanguinity

As Turner syndrome could be the cause of short stature in girls (even in the absence of clinical stigmata), the possibility of performing a Karyotype should be entertained. More specific genetic testing has become available in recent years and should be directed by endocrinology/medical genetics, when indicated.

Additional Evaluation

The evaluation of skeletal maturation is an important aspect of growth assessment. Delayed skeletal maturation in a short child growing at a normal rate would suggest constitutional delay of growth, while familial short stature would be

Table 1.3 Key physical exam findings

Physical exam system	Exam finding	Think of (but not limited to)
General	Obesity	Prader-Willi syndrome
HEENT	Prominent forehead, triangular face	Silver-Russell syndrome
	Microcephaly	Prenatal factors (e.g., TORCH), genetic syndrome (e.g., Seckel syndrome)
	Epicanthal folds	Down syndrome
	Nystagmus	Septo-optic dysplasia
	Ptosis	Noonan syndrome
	Low-set ears	Turner syndrome, Noonan syndrome
	Choanal atresia	Hypopituitarism
	Cleft lip/cleft palate	Hypopituitarism
	High arched palate	Turner Syndrome
	Solitary upper central incisor	Hypopituitarism
	Bifid uvula	Hypopituitarism
Neck	Webbed neck	Turner syndrome, Noonan syndrome
	Goiter	Hypothyroidism
	Rigid cervical spine	Hypopituitarism (LHX3 mutation)
Chest	Wide-spaced nipples	Turner syndrome
	Heart murmurs, abnormal breathing, peripheral edema	Congenital heart disease and associated syndromes
Abdomen	Hepatomegaly	Calorie-protein malnutrition
Genitalia	Micropenis	Hypopituitarism
	Delayed pubertal development for age	Constitutional delay of growth and puberty, hypopituitarism
Musculoskeletal	Leg bowing	XLH or vitamin D deficiency rickets
	Short 4th metacarpals	Turner syndrome, pseudohypoparathyroidism
	Clubbing	Cystic fibrosis, cyanotic heart disease
	Increased upper-to-lower segment ratio	Skeletal dysplasias with short extremities
	Decreased upper-to-lower segment ratio	Skeletal dysplasias with short trunk, effect of spinal radiation
Skin	Dry skin	Hypothyroidism
	Café au lait spots	Silver-Russell syndrome
Lymphatic	Lymphedema	Turner syndrome
Neurologic	Intellectual disability	Down syndrome, Prader Willi syndrome
	Hypotonia	Down syndrome, Prader Willi syndrome
	Hyporeflexia	Hypothyroidism
Psychiatric	Over-affectionate to strangers	Psychosocial dwarfism
	Hyperactivity/inattention	ADHD

more likely if the same child has concordant skeletal maturation and is at a percentile consistent with genetic potential.

Delayed skeletal maturation in a short child with decreased GV may suggest the possibility of endocrine disorders, malnutrition, chronic illness, or even psychosocial causes of growth failure. A concordant skeletal maturation in a short child with decreased GV may suggest dysgenetic conditions.

Skeletal maturation is assessed with an X-ray of the left hand and wrist, referred to as *bone age*. The atlas of Greulich and Pyle is the most frequently used method for interpretation of skeletal maturation in the United States [6].

The pediatric endocrinologist can calculate the *predicted adult height (PAH)* based on the bone age and a concomitant accurate height measurement using one of several methods. The most commonly used method has been proposed by Bayley-Pinneau, as an appendix to the Greulich and Pyle atlas. As a general concept, a PAH that falls within the MPH range is reassuring.

In addition, suspected cases of disproportionate short stature could be further evaluated with a *skeletal survey* that needs expert radiologic interpretation to pinpoint possible skeletal dysplasias.

Brain and pituitary MRI are helpful in the evaluation of children confirmed to have growth hormone (GH) deficiency via formal GH stimulation tests performed by the pediatric endocrinologist. Complete lack of linear growth over ≥1 year in a child who has not completed pubertal development may also be an indication for imaging of the central nervous system.

Next Steps in Diagnosis and Management

The primary care provider should consider referring the child with short stature for further evaluation and management when the child has decreased GV, crossing downward across major percentiles; when the growth trajectory of a child tracks below the genetic potential; when test results show significant abnormalities; when the child has significant short stature without weight deficit; when the child has dysmorphic features or disproportionate anthropometric measurements; or when in doubt. Endocrinology referral is appropriate for children with short stature and proportionately normal weight trajectory, and in children whose decline in growth velocity appears to precede any changes in weight trajectory. Gastroenterology referral may be more appropriate for children whose weight trajectory begins to decline before changes in growth velocity. Obtaining the laboratory evaluation described above in advance of a subspecialist visit can significantly facilitate care. Further details on diagnosis and management of short stature are discussed in Chap. 40 (Part III).

References

1. Rose SR, Vogiatzi MG, Copeland KC. A general pediatric approach to evaluating a short child. Pediatr Rev. 2005;26(11):410–20.
2. Tanner JM, Whitehouse RH. Clinical longitudinal standards for height, weight, height velocity, weight velocity, and stages of puberty. Arch Dis Child. 1976;51:170–9.
3. Hall JG, Froster-Iskenius UG, Allanson JE. Limbs. In: Handbook of normal physical measurements; 1989. p. 221–88.
4. Frisancho A. Anthropometric standards: an interactive nutritional reference of body size and body composition for children and adults. Ann Arbor: University of Michigan Press; 2008.
5. Argente J. Horm Res Paediatr. 2016;85:2–10.
6. Greulich WW, Pyle SI. Radiographic atlas of skeletal development of the hand and wrist. 2nd ed. Stanford: Stanford University Press; 1959.
7. Tanner JM, Davies PSW. Clinical longitudinal standards for height and height velocity for North American children. J Pediatr. 1985;107(3):317–29.

Increased Growth Velocity and/or Tall Stature

2

Pushpa Viswanathan and Bianca Pinto

Normal Growth

A careful measurement of height and growth velocity is a sensitive indicator of health and well-being and therefore an essential part of every well child visit to the primary care physician.

A complete growth evaluation includes an accurate measurement of recumbent length or height, assessment of height based on mid-parental target height and ethnicity, and monitoring of growth velocity. The Centers for Disease Control and Prevention (CDC) recommends using the World Health Organization (WHO) growth charts for children 0–2 years of age and CDC growth charts for children 2 years of age and older [1]. The assessment of body proportions, including upper-to-lower-segment ratio and arm-span-to-height ratio, is described in Chap. 1.

> **Clinical Tool**
> In children 2 years and younger, recumbent length should be measured with an infantometer. In children older than 2 years, a wall-mounted stadiometer should be used to measure height [3].

Growth velocity should be measured using at least two accurately measured heights obtained at least 3–6 months apart. An infant's length at birth is a reflection of the maternal and uterine factors affecting fetal nutrition and insulin availability. Hormones like growth hormone and thyroid hormone only have a modest influence. It is not uncommon to see "genetic channeling," where one might see an upward or downward crossing of percentiles to move toward the child's genetic potential. This is usually seen around 12 months to 24 months of age [2]. Crossing growth percentiles in this age range is therefore normal. The recumbent length of a small baby, who was exposed to an adverse prenatal environment, with tall parents will channel up across percentiles, while a large baby (e.g., infant of a diabetic mother with uncontrolled blood sugars, who was exposed to large amounts of insulin in utero) born to short parents will channel down. After about 36 months, children who are growing normally should then follow a consistent height percentile during pre-pubertal years. Growth velocity changes throughout childhood (Table 2.1). Growth should be interpreted in the context of pubertal status, and providers must ensure that the growth velocity is appropriate for the different growth phases – infancy, childhood, and pubertal growth.

Tall Stature

Tall stature is defined as linear height above the 97th percentile or more than two standard deviations above the mean for age and sex. Concern over tall stature is a relatively rare initial presentation to a primary care office. However, it is not uncommon to see a rapid increase in growth velocity during a well visit. A relative increase in growth velocity can be seen in endocrine conditions such as premature adrenarche,

Table 2.1 Growth velocity during childhood and adolescence

Age range	Growth velocity
Birth – 1 year	~ 25 cm/year
1–2 years	~ 10 cm/year
2–4 years	5–10 cm/year
4 years – Puberty	5–6 cm/year
Puberty – Final height	8–12 cm/year

P. Viswanathan (✉)
University of Pittsburgh School of Medicine, Department of Endocrinology, UPMC Children's Hospital Pittsburgh, Pittsburgh, PA, USA
e-mail: pushpa.viswanathan@chp.edu

B. Pinto
Division of Pediatric Endocrinology, University of Pittsburgh, UPMC Children's Hospital Pittsburgh, Pittsburgh, PA, USA
e-mail: bianca.pinto@chp.edu

T. Stanley, M. Misra (eds.), *Endocrine Conditions in Pediatrics*, https://doi.org/10.1007/978-3-030-52215-5_2

precocious puberty, hyperthyroidism, and growth hormone excess (Table 2.2).

In addition to hormonal disorders that increase the rate of growth and body size, there are overgrowth syndromes that can cause tall stature. These are mainly non-hormonal/genetic conditions. Overgrowth is defined by extreme physical size and stature including tall stature or generalized/localized overgrowth of tissues and/or increased head circumference (macrocephaly). A degree of intellectual disability may be present, as well as associated dysmorphic features, although intelligence may be normal in some overgrowth syndromes.

Table 2.2 Differential diagnosis

	Diagnosis	Clinical features
Normal variant	Familial/constitutional tall stature	Most common cause of tall stature. Due to genetic potential from family history of tall stature. Otherwise healthy child with normal physical exam.
Endocrine/hormonal causes	Exogenous obesity	Second most common cause of tall stature in childhood. Increased linear growth and weight gain from increased nutritional intake.
	Precocious puberty (gonadotropin-dependent or gonadotropin-independent)	Pubertal changes in boys prior to age 9 years or girls prior to age 8 years (see Chap. 10). Accelerated linear growth in childhood secondary to pubertal growth spurt occurring at a young age.
	Androgen insensitivity syndrome (rare)	Phenotypical females with XY karyotype. May present with inguinal hernias in childhood or with amenorrhea at pubertal age. Adult height is usually taller than women without the syndrome, but shorter than typical males.
	Growth hormone excess (rare)	Caused by overproduction of GH, often from a GH-secreting tumor. This may be an isolated finding or in association with conditions like McCune Albright syndrome, Carney complex, tuberous sclerosis, familial isolated pituitary adenoma.
	Hyperthyroidism	Increase in growth rate in uncontrolled hyperthyroidism.
	Estrogen resistance and aromatase deficiency [6, 7] (rare)	Suspect if continued growth well after puberty. Due to resistance at the estrogen receptor level (estrogen resistance) or low level of estradiol (aromatase deficiency). Bony epiphyses remain open into adulthood.
	Familial glucocorticoid deficiency (rare)	Patients with point mutations in the ACTH receptor gene are usually noted to be of tall stature.
	McCune Albright syndrome (rare)	Precocious puberty, café au lait lesions, fibrous dysplasia. Tall stature from any hormone over secretion – estradiol, thyroid, growth hormone.
	Generalized lipodystrophy, XY males with 17 alpha-hydroxylase deficiency inactivating mutations of FGFR3, and others [8] (rare)	Tall stature in these conditions with causes including phenotypic females with a Y chromosome, hyperinsulinemia, or mutations in receptor pathways affecting growth.
Genetic/overgrowth syndromes (non-hormonal)	Klinefelter syndrome (47 XXY)	Relatively common. Clinical manifestations include tall stature, small testes, infertility, gynecomastia, and intellectual disability [9].
	Neurofibromatosis type 1 [10]	Associated with café-au lait spots, neurofibromas, freckling. While many patients have poor growth, tall stature due to GH excess has been reported.
	Fragile X syndrome	Tall stature, large ears, macroorchidism in males [11].
	Beckwith-Wiedemann [12]	Congenital overgrowth disorder. Infants are large at birth with macroglossia, omphalocele, and hypoglycemia. Growth rate may slow down after the first few years. Increased risk of embryonal tumors, such as Wilms' tumor,neuroblastoma, and others.
	Sotos syndrome (cerebral gigantism) (rare)	Born LGA with increased growth rate that continues into childhood. Prominent forehead, prominent ears, down-slanting palpebral fissures, narrow jaw, large hands, high-arched palate. Macrocephaly present at all ages. Abnormal body proportions with arm span exceeding height [12].
	Weaver syndrome (rare)	Excessive growth both prenatally and postnatally. Features resemble Sotos syndrome. Macrocephaly and tall stature.
	Marfan syndrome and other fibrillinopathies [13]	Marfan syndrome is an autosomal dominant disorder of collagen metabolism associated with tall stature with abnormal body proportions due to long extremities, subluxation of lens of the eye, and dilation of the ascending aorta.
	Homocystinuria (rare)	Autosomal recessive disorder similar to Marfan syndrome including tall stature and lens subluxation.
	47, XYY syndrome	Tall stature with possible behavioral problems or intellectual disability.
	Simpson-Golabi-Behmel syndrome (SGBS), Partington, and other syndromes [8] (rare)	Macrocephaly +/– intellectual disability, visceromegaly.

History: Important Clarifying Questions

Age of onset of tall stature

- Intrauterine overgrowth is seen in multiple genetic syndromes including Beckwith-Wiedemann and Sotos syndrome.
- In addition to prenatal overgrowth, rapid growth rate in the first 3–4 years of life is also seen in genetics syndromes such as Sotos and Weaver syndrome.
- Tall stature in later childhood may suggest exogenous obesity or hormonal causes.

Pubertal history

- Age at first signs of puberty including pubic hair, breast development, and testicular development will aid in the diagnosis of precocious/delayed puberty (see Chaps. 10 and 11).

Developmental milestones/academic performance

- May be delayed in various genetic conditions.

Past medical history including prenatal and perinatal history

- Many genetic syndromes are associated with multiple medical conditions. For example, lens dislocation and aortic dilation in Marfan syndrome.
- Birth weight to assess for intrauterine overgrowth; neonatal hypoglycemia from hyperinsulinemia is important to diagnose conditions like Beckwith-Wiedemann syndrome.

Family history

- Calculation of mid-parental height and parental ages of puberty will help make the diagnosis of familial/constitutional tall stature.
- Family history of genetic diagnoses, congenital disorders, endocrinopathies.

Important Aspects of the Physical Exam

Vitals

- Tachycardia and hypertension in hyperthyroidism.

Height and growth velocity

- Is the growth rate normal or too fast? Acceleration unexpected from familial pattern?
- Growth velocity can be estimated from two linear measurements separated by months and calculated as cm/year and compared to the normal velocities for age (Table 2.1).
- *Increased growth velocity and/or tall stature may be the only manifestation of a growth hormone (GH) secreting tumor*. Children might not have acromegalic features [4].

Weight

- Overnutrition is a common cause for linear growth acceleration.
- Weight gain precedes and increases more rapidly than height gain in exogenous obesity. Endocrine causes of excessive weight gain usually lead to deceleration in growth velocity.
- Children with obesity from overnutrition will have increased height velocity and therefore are taller than their lean peers. Skeletal maturation in this group will be advanced with possible early epiphyseal fusion.

Body proportion and dysmorphic features

- Measurement of head circumference, upper-to-lower body segment ratio, and arm span (see Chap. 1) is useful to identify some causes of tall stature such as Marfan syndrome and Klinefelter syndrome.
- Identification of coarse/dysmorphic features like large head and visceromegaly might give clues to the diagnosis of overgrowth syndromes.

Pubertal exam

- Pubertal staging is important in tall stature as this may suggest precocious or delayed puberty.

Thyroid exam

- Goiter in hyperthyroidism.

Visual field evaluation

- May be abnormal in GH-secreting tumor.

Skin/musculoskeletal

- Coarse facial features, large hands, and feet (acromegaloid features) may suggest GH excess
- Birthmarks and neurocutaneous findings may suggest a genetic diagnosis. For example, café au lait spots for McCune Albright syndrome, neurofibromatosis with GH excess, blue nevi for Carney complex [5].

Clinical Key
Peak height velocity is reached 2 years earlier in girls than boys and is dependent on pubertal status.

Height velocity should be correlated with pubertal exam, making breast evaluation in females and testicular evaluation in males a vital component of the pediatric evaluation.

Consideration for Further Evaluation

Baseline evaluation

- Bone age study: X-ray of the left hand and wrist for a child over 3 years of age (see Chap. 36 for interpretation). A normal bone age in a tall child growing in concordance with genetic potential is very reassuring. *Laboratory testing is not routinely required in cases of familial/constitutional tall stature, especially if bone age evaluation is normal.*
- Insulin-like growth factor (IGF)-1, Insulin-like growth factor binding protein 3 (IGFBP-3).
- TSH, Free T4.
- Karyotype: Especially in tall stature associated with absent or markedly delayed puberty, primary amenorrhea, or small testicular volume, to rule out conditions such as androgen insensitivity, 47 XXY (Klinefelter), 47 XXX (Trisomy X), 47 XYY.

Specific investigations based on history and exam findings (Table 2.2)

- Gonadotropins (LH, FSH) and sex hormone levels (testosterone, estradiol) if indicated by pubertal exam findings.
- Serum (and urine) homocysteine is advisable in patients with intellectual disability, central nervous system (CNS) abnormalities, or Marfan-like phenotype.
- Molecular studies for overgrowth syndromes if indicated by exam findings (or referral to genetics).
- Prolactin and other pituitary hormones if GH-secreting tumor suspected.
- Glucose suppression test, performed by Endocrinology, is the gold standard diagnosing GH excess – lack of suppression of GH levels to an oral glucose load using an oral glucose tolerance test.
- MRI of the pituitary if GH excess is suspected.
- Morning serum cortisol level in the rare event of tall stature with features of adrenal insufficiency (fatigue, weight loss, hypoglycemia).

Summary of Approach to Tall Stature

Not all tall stature is pathological; however as tall stature is socially acceptable and often desirable, pathological causes of tall stature and increased growth velocity can often be missed due to a lack of concern and subsequent workup.

Familial/constitutional tall stature is most common and is characterized by a normal history, exam, and growth velocity. There are not early signs of puberty. Parents will also be tall. A thorough family history, therefore, is critical for the diagnosis. Familial/constitutional tall stature is non-pathological, and generally reassurance is appropriate. Acceleration of height in constitutional tall stature is seen as early as the first 3 years of life with height plots crossing up percentiles towards genetic potential. Normal body proportions will be maintained, and pubertal timing will be based on family pattern. Growth after 3 years of age may be parallel to, but above, the 95th or 97th percentiles. Psychosocial concerns with tall stature are important to address and may be more common in females.

Exogenous obesity, caused by a mismatch between caloric intake and caloric expenditure, is a common cause of increased growth velocity in childhood. Usually final height prediction does not exceed mid-parental target height range, as there is proportionate bone age advancement. Exogenous obesity may be associated with premature adrenarche, which may further advance bone age. Healthy weight loss through diet and exercise should be instituted and will prevent further bone age advancement. Increased growth velocity and weight gain from excessive nutritional intake are usually seen later in childhood. If intrauterine or perinatal obesity is identified, it becomes important to rule out overgrowth syndromes that are associated with future risk of tumors and require long-term surveillance. As noted in Table 2.2, findings such as body disproportion with long extremities, delayed development, and intellectual disability are common in multiple genetic syndromes associated with tall stature. More specific findings can help pinpoint particular diagnoses, such as the overgrowth in infancy seen in Beckwith-Wiedemann and Sotos syndrome, lens dislocation and aortic dilation in Marfan syndrome, and neurocutaneous markers including café au lait spots seen in neurofibromatosis and McCune Albright syndrome.

Clinical Key
Children with precocious puberty will be tall during childhood; however if left untreated, these children may become short adults due to premature closure of the growth plates.

Referral to endocrinology is indicated for evaluation for pubertal suppression.

Uncontrolled hyperthyroidism will cause increased growth velocity in children. Identification of symptoms and signs including weight loss, diarrhea, tachycardia, palpitations, and goiter could lead to lab work and timely treatment, leading to normalization of growth without significant bone age advancement. Similarly, with precocious puberty, although children may be tall or relatively tall for familial pattern, there is advanced skeletal maturation with premature fusion of bony epiphyses and final height will usually be compromised in the absence of intervention. To evaluate for growth hormone excess, a high index of suspicion is needed with careful review of systems. Although physical exam may reveal coarse facial features and large hands and feet, rapid growth rate might be the only clue for the primary care provider. This reemphasizes the importance of proper linear measurement of a child with careful attention to growth velocity in primary care offices.

When to Consult Endocrinology?

- Growth velocity significantly higher than expected for age and pubertal status.
- Tall stature with inappropriate pubertal status for age (precocious puberty, premature adrenarche).
- Height prediction corrected for bone age places at a much higher percentile than mid-parental height.
- Detection of abnormal body proportions, dysmorphology with tall stature.
- If a diagnosis of familial/constitutional tall stature cannot be confidently made, labs and bone age should be obtained, and endocrine consult placed.

References

1. Growth Charts - Homepage [Internet]. Centers for Disease Control and Prevention. Centers for Disease Control and Prevention; 2010 [cited 2019Oct14]. Available from: https://www.cdc.gov/growthcharts/index.htm.
2. Smith DW, Truog W, Rogers JE, Greitzer LJ, Skinner AL, Mccann JJ, et al. Shifting linear growth during infancy: illustration of genetic factors in growth from fetal life through infancy. J Pediatr. 1976;89(2):225–30.
3. A health professional's guide to using growth charts. Paediatr Child Health. 2004;9(3):174–6.
4. Bowden S, Sotos J, Stratakis C, Weil R. Successful treatment of an invasive growth hormone-secreting pituitary macroadenoma in an 8 year-old boy. J Pediatr Endocrinol Metab. 2007;20(5):643–7.
5. Correa R, Salpea P, Stratakis CA. Carney complex: an update. Eur J Endocrinol. 2015;173(4):M85.
6. Smith EP, Boyd J, Frank GR, Takahashi H, Cohen RM, Specker B, et al. Estrogen resistance caused by a mutation in the estrogen-receptor gene in a man. N Engl J Med. 1994;331(16):1056–61.
7. Jones ME, Boon WC, Mcinnes K, Maffei L, Carani C, Simpson ER. Recognizing rare disorders: aromatase deficiency. Nat Clin Pract Endocrinol Metab. 2007;3(5):414–21.
8. Sotos JF, Argente J. Overgrowth disorders associated with tall stature. Adv Pediatr. 2008;55(1):213–54.
9. Davis S, Howell S, Wilson R, Tanda T, Ross J, Zeitler P, et al. Advances in the interdisciplinary care of children with Klinefelter syndrome. Adv Pediatr. 2016;63(1):15–46.
10. Cambiaso P, Galassi S, Palmiero M, Mastronuzzi A, Bufalo FD, Capolino R, et al. Growth hormone excess in children with neurofibromatosis type-1 and optic glioma. Am J Med Genet A. 2017;173(9):2353–8.
11. Hersh JH, Saul RA. Health supervision for children with fragile X syndrome. Pediatrics. 2011;127(5):994–1006.
12. Ko JM. Genetic syndromes associated with overgrowth in childhood. Ann Pediatr Endocrinol Metabol. 2013;18(3):101.
13. Hayward C, Brock DJH. Fibrillin-1 mutations in Marfan syndrome and other type-1 fibrillinopathies. Hum Mutat. 1997;10(6):415–23.

3 Skeletal Disease

Nora E. Renthal

Abbreviations

BMD	Bone mineral density
DXA	Dual-energy X-ray absorptiometry
OI	Osteogenesis imperfecta
PTH	Parathyroid hormone
SHOX	Short stature homeobox-containing gene

Introduction

Skeletal disease in children presents as a spectrum of physical findings from overtly misshapen bones, to frequent fractures, to short stature. Skeletal disease can be inherited or acquired. Inherited forms of skeletal disease can be isolated (e.g., achondroplasia or osteogenesis imperfecta) or associated with other syndromic manifestations (e.g., Turner's syndrome or pseudohypoparathyroidism). Examples of acquired bone disease include nutritional rickets, hyperparathyroidism, and drug-induced osteoporosis. Careful evaluation with a history, physical examination, and appropriate lab testing can help to differentiate common acquired pathology, such as hypovitaminosis D, from skeletal disease requiring further evaluation by a pediatric endocrinologist (Tables 3.1 and 3.2).

Table 3.1 Presenting signs concerning for skeletal disease

Children presenting to primary care with fractures
Accidental trauma
Non-accidental trauma
Osteogenesis imperfecta (look for dentinogenesis imperfecta)
Disuse osteoporosis (e.g., cerebral palsy, chronic illness)
Osteotoxic medications (e.g., glucocorticoids, anticonvulsants, methotrexate. radiation)
Children presenting to primary care with short stature
Skeletal dysplasia (look for disproportionate limb growth)
Rickets
Pseudohypoparathyroidism
Turner syndrome
Children presenting to primary care with limb bowing
Hypophosphatasia (look for early loss of deciduous teeth)
Vitamin D deficiency
Dietary calcium or phosphate deficiency (consider in formula or PN-dependent children)
Genetic conditions associated with hypophosphatemia
Skeletal dysplasia
Children presenting to primary care with abnormal serum calcium
Hypoparathyroidism
Pseudohypoparathyroidism
Hyperparathyroidism

Abbreviations: *PN* parenteral nutrition

Pathophysiology and Differential Diangosis

One of the largest organ systems in the human body, the skeleton provides structural support and protection of vital organs but also represents a metabolically active organ system. Bone modeling and remodeling is directed by a symphony of endocrine, paracrine, and autocrine factors [1]. Throughout childhood, bone undergoes both growth and constant remodeling of existing bone [2]. During childhood, modeling is the gradual adjustment of overall shape in response to hormonal and mechanical forces. Remodeling is the continual renewal of bone required to maintain strength and mineral ion homeostasis. Remodeling occurs through the cooperation of osteoclasts and osteoblasts, resulting in bone resorption and subsequent replacement with unmineralized osteoid that is later mineralized [3].

The presentation of skeletal disease is highly diverse. Before exploring endocrine-related causes of skeletal complaints, it is important to consider common alternative causes such as accidental or non-accidental trauma in the case of fractures, and poor nutrition, or malabsorption in the case of hypovitaminosis D.

N. E. Renthal (✉)
Division of Endocrinology, Department of Pediatrics, Boston Children's Hospital, Boston, MA, USA
e-mail: Nora.Renthal@childrens.harvard.edu

T. Stanley, M. Misra (eds.), *Endocrine Conditions in Pediatrics*, https://doi.org/10.1007/978-3-030-52215-5_3

Table 3.2 Physical exam pearls for skeletal disease

Growth trajectory:
Interval weight loss → malabsorption, chronic disease
Decreased growth velocity → rickets, scurvy, skeletal dysplasia, chronic disease
Obesity → pseudohypoparathyroidism
Anthropometric measurements:
Shortening of the long bones → skeletal dysplasia (rhizomelic, mesomelic, campomelic)
Shortening of the fourth/fifth metacarpals/metatarsals → pseudohypoparathyroidism
Other features:
Blue sclerae → osteogenesis imperfecta
Prominence of rib heads at the osteochondral junction (rachitic rosary) → rickets
Widened epiphyses of the long bones → rickets
Madelung deformity → Turner syndrome, SHOX gene deletions/mutations, skeletal dysplasia

Abbreviations: *SHOX* short stature homeobox

Children Presenting to Primary Care with Fractures

Fractures are common in the pediatric population, with an incidence of approximately 50% in boys and 40% in girls [4]. A thorough history will help distinguish a traumatic from a fragility, that is, atraumatic, fracture. In the absence of a significant trauma, such as a motor vehicle collision, vertebral compression and femur fractures are rare in childhood and should prompt further evaluation. A history of "significant fracture" is defined by the International Society for Clinical Densitometry (ISCD) as a vertebral compression fracture at any age, two or more long bone fractures (excluding fingers, toes, and stress fractures) prior to 10 years old, and/or three or more long bone fractures prior to 19 years old [5].

Despite this definition, a history of significant fracture is not diagnostic of skeletal disease, but rather should prompt further questioning depending on the clinical situation. A chronically ill child with multiple risk factors for skeletal fragility may necessitate a more aggressive work-up, including endocrine referral. An otherwise healthy-appearing child should be questioned regarding diet, physical activity, and family history of skeletal fragility. In each case, the pediatrician should ensure that the child's dietary calcium and vitamin D intake are sufficient and that the patient is engaged in weight-bearing activities. Conditions such as malabsorption, low weight eating disorders, and the female athlete triad should be considered. A child with multiple long bone fractures and a family history of the same should be referred to endocrinology for consideration of osteogenesis imperfecta, a group of genetic disorders characterized by impaired collagen gene expression or processing. Any child presenting with repeated soft-tissue injuries and fractures prior to being ambulatory, or fractures that appear inconsistent with the reported history, should raise immediate red flags for non-accidental trauma.

Children Presenting to Primary Care with Limb Bowing

Causes of limb bowing seen in the Endocrine Clinic include metabolic bone disease (rickets, hyper- and hypoparathyroidism) and skeletal dysplasia. By definition, rickets is the result of insufficient mineralization of the growth plate and patients may first be identified due to short stature or growth failure. Most children with rickets manifest bilateral, symmetric lower limb bowing, and radiographs classically demonstrate widened and cupped physes with flared metaphyses, and subjectively diminished bone density [6].

Rickets can be broadly characterized as calcipenic or phosphopenic in etiology [7]. The causes of calcipenic rickets include nutritional vitamin D deficiency and, more rarely, dietary calcium deficiency (e.g., in the case of malabsorption, dependence on parenteral nutrition, or a chronically ill child). The causes of phosphopenic rickets include X-linked hypophosphatemic rickets, other renal phosphate wasting, and very rarely, dietary phosphate deficiency [8]. Hypophosphatasia can also cause bowing of the legs. Much less common, given modern nutritional abundance, are cases of scurvy resulting from vitamin C deficiency (ascorbic acid plays a critical role in the formation of type II collagen). Children with scurvy can present with poor growth, bowing, leg pain, gingivitis, frequent infections, and delayed wound healing. In the United States, scurvy occurs primarily as a sequala of malabsorption or extreme dietary restriction (e.g., mainly described in children with autism or neurological problems), but should be considered in children with delayed wound healing and gingival findings [9]. All children with rickets should be evaluated for disordered intestinal absorption and kidney dysfunction. Suspected rickets should prompt a through dietary history and endocrine referral.

Skeletal dysplasias can also present with bilateral, symmetric bowed legs; however, serum calcium, phosphorous, and PTH are typically normal. A skeletal survey, which includes the skull and spine, is helpful in cases of suspected skeletal dysplasia. Radiographic features of skeletal dysplasia vary. Referral to endocrinology, genetics, and orthopedics is appropriate.

Children Presenting to Primary Care with Short Stature

As in the case of skeletal dysplasia and rickets, skeletal disease can first present as short stature. However, the causes of short stature are many, most of which do not represent intrinsic skeletal disease. If there is proportional short stature with decreased weight-for-height ratio, for example, one should instead consider undernutrition, malnutrition, malabsorption, or a chronic systemic disease. During an evaluation for short stature and poor growth, the provider will want to evaluate the child for signs suggestive of a syndromic etiology. Girls with Turner's syndrome, for example, manifest short stature, short metacarpals, cubitus valgus, Madelung deformity, and mesomelia, as well as skeletal fragility, likely secondary to a combination of haploinsufficiency of the SHOX gene and estrogen deficiency [10].

Children Presenting to Primary Care with Manifestations of Hypocalcemia

Metabolic bone disease resulting from primary disorders of the parathyroid axis is rare in children. When they present, hypoparathyroidism and PTH resistance (i.e., pseudohypoparathyroidism) more frequently manifest as hypocalcemia and hyperphosphatemia, with low or elevated PTH, respectively, rather than skeletal pathology. Instead, symptoms of hypocalcemia in school-age children include muscle weakness and hypotonia, motor retardation, and/or stunted growth. Symptoms of hypocalcemia in infants may not be obvious and most babies are asymptomatic. If a neonate is symptomatic, findings may include irritability, jitteriness and muscular hyperexcitability, poor feeding, lethargy, and seizures.

The most common reason metabolic bone disease will present to primary care is from a secondary disruption of the parathyroid axis, commonly from hypovitaminosis D. Without adequate vitamin D, children suffer from subclinical calcipenia, which in turn drives elevation in PTH, that is, secondary hyperparathyroidism. Over time, with the depletion of calcium stores and/or variation in dietary calcium intake (e.g., reduced milk intake during illness) subclinical calcipenia can become overt and/or emergent. In this instance, the role of the primary care provider is to identify symptoms and obtain laboratory studies confirming hypocalcemia, followed by referral to emergency services for urgent repletion and endocrine specialist consultation. Outpatient endocrine follow-up will be appropriate depending on the identified etiology of metabolic derangement.

Important Aspects of the History

A careful history is essential to assess for common non-endocrine-mediated causes of secondary skeletal disease and to narrow the differential diagnosis. As many causes of skeletal disease will present with short stature or delay of growth, a review of the patient's growth on age- and gender-specific charts is essential, as are correct and complete anthropometric measurements (see Key Components of the Physical Exam).

The primary care physician should also seek to elicit a history of fractures in the patient and patient's family. A significant family history of recurrent fractures at a young age can be suggestive of an underlying inherited condition such as osteogenesis imperfecta. Because sex steroids are an important contributor to bone accrual during puberty, a careful pubertal history should be obtained, including the onset of breast (female) and testicular (male) enlargement, in addition to the onset of pubic hair, and menstrual history in females. A complete dietary history, including several days of dietary recall, is critical to ascertain whether vitamin D, calcium, magnesium, phosphorus (rare), and ascorbic acid (rare) are being omitted from diet. A dietary recall or food record may also reveal restrictive eating patterns and point to a diagnosis of an eating disorder. A detailed history of exercise activity should be obtained to determine whether the female athlete triad is a possibility.

Because dietary vitamin and mineral absorption is critical to skeletal health, the physician could inquire about symptoms related to gastrointestinal malabsorption. One should ascertain the frequency of bowel movements, the quality of the stool, the presence of any blood, mucus, or unusually foul odor. In addition, inquire about constipation, diarrhea, and abdominal pain. A positive symptom during GI screening could indicate gastrointestinal pathology underpinning poor skeletal health. Negative screening, however, does not exclude malabsorption, as parents of older children may not be able to give a complete GI history, and conditions such as celiac disease can manifest in the skeleton (with low bone density) prior to onset of GI symptoms [11, 12].

Lastly, the physician should carefully ascertain any patient drug exposures, current or previous. A full medical history, including history of prematurity and any co-morbid conditions, should be obtained. Medications generally considered toxic to bone and widely used in the pediatric population include glucocorticoids, anticonvulsants, methotrexate, and radiation [13]. Other medications can indirectly impact the skeleton, such as loop diuretics that increase urinary excretion of calcium and exogenous phosphate supplements, which can result in secondary hyperparathyroidism [14]. All such exposures should be investigated as potential contributors to poor bone health of a child with suspected skeletal disease.

Key Components of the Physical Exam

As much as looking at the growth chart is a critical part of the skeletal assessment, so too are anthropometric measurements during the physical exam. To be accurate, standing height should be measured without shoes against a wall, preferably via fixed stadiometer. Similarly, supine length is optimally measured via device with a fixed head plate and moveable foot plate. In addition to vertical height/length, body proportions (arm span and upper to lower segment ratios) should be ascertained. The upper segment to lower segment ratio (US/LS ratio) can be helpful in distinguishing conditions of disproportionate growth, such as skeletal dysplasia. To obtain this ratio, one should measure the lower segment from the top of the symphysis pubis to the plantar surface of the foot. The upper segment is calculated by subtracting the lower segment from the patient's height. Of note, there are ethnic and family differences in the upper-to-lower segment ratio, but in general, we expect that children under 10 years of age will have ratios greater than one, and children older than 10 years of age will have ratios less than one. Conditions with increased US/LS ratio (i.e., relatively short extremities in relation to upper body) include achondroplasia, Turner syndrome, and severe hypothyroidism. Conditions with decreased US/LS ratio (i.e., longer legs relative to upper body) include delayed puberty, spondyloepithelial dysplasia, scoliosis, and Klinefelter syndrome.

One can also assess the patient's arm span relative to height. In general, arm span should be less than height until age 10 years in boys and age 11 years in girls [1, 15]. If arm span is much longer than height, we consider conditions that either inhibit growth of the axial skeleton (spondyloepithelial dysplasia, scoliosis, and spinal radiation) or those that are associated with relatively long limbs (Marfan syndrome, homycystinuria, Klinefelter's, and delayed puberty). These measurements can be incorporated into the overall skeletal examination, which includes evaluation to look for bowing or shortening of the long bones, vertebral defects/scoliosis, rib abnormalities, blue sclerae, and shortening of the fourth/fifth metacarpals/metatarsals. Lastly, because ascertainment of peak bone mineral density is dependent on timely exposure to sex steroids, pubertal Tanner staging should be incorporated into the physical exam. Children with delayed puberty will have low bone mineral density compared to age-appropriate norms [16].

Laboratory and Imaging Evaluation

Laboratory evaluation for skeletal disease will depend on the presenting symptoms and signs prompting the provider's suspicion for pathology; however, a general laboratory work-up includes routine hematologic and biochemical indices, blood urea nitrogen (BUN) and creatinine to assess renal function, erythrocyte sedimentation rate, and screening for celiac and thyroid screening with a TSH. Intact PTH should be measured concurrently with serum calcium, magnesium, and phosphorus, and ideally in the morning after an overnight fast [17, 18]. A measurement of alkaline phosphatase can be useful as a marker of PTH-driven bone turnover, but careful consideration should be taken to interpret with age-appropriate norms. Since alkaline phosphatase is a marker for osteoblastic activity, levels are highest during the rapid growth phases of infancy and puberty [19, 20].

An assessment of urinary calcium excretion can be helpful to identify calcium wasting (high urine calcium) and calcium deficiency (low urine calcium), as well as, more rarely, to differentiate between disorders of the calcium sensing receptor [21]. Be mindful of medications such as diuretics that will confound interpretation of urinary calcium results. A 24-hour urine calcium is more representative in children who are able to collect it. Typically, the patient's first voided morning urine is discarded and all urine for the next 24 hours, including the next morning's first void, is collected. In children who are unable to collect a 24-hour urine sample, a spot urine calcium to creatinine ratio can be informative, particularly when multiple samples are collected and show a similar trend.

Testing for hypovitaminosis D is a critical part of the laboratory evaluation of skeletal disease, as the most common cause of rickets in children. A 25-hydroxy vitamin D level is most informative for the assessment of a child's vitamin D stores [22]. The level of 1,25-dihydroxyvitamin D, or active vitamin D, can be informative if a disorder of vitamin D metabolism is suspected, but is likely best deferred to specialty evaluation, as active vitamin D reflects the hormonal activity of PTH and FGF-23, rather than vitamin D stores. In fact, in vitamin D deficiency, 1,25-dihydroxyvitamin D levels are frequently elevated rather than suppressed [23, 24].

Radiographic evaluation of skeletal disease should be targeted to assess the particular presenting symptoms and signs. Plain radiographs are useful for identifying fractures, skeletal dysplasias, and rickets, and can be performed in any age child. A child older than 4 years of age with a history of fragility fractures should undergo the assessment of bone mineral density (BMD) via dual-energy x-ray absorptiometry (DXA). The preferred sites for pediatric DXA assessment, as recommended by the ISCD, include two sites: (1) postero-anterior lumbar spine and (2) total body in children age 4–7 years or total body-less-head in children 8–15 years of age. In children 16 years and older, postero-anterior lumbar spine and hip are the preferred sites of assessment [5]. Alternative sites, such as distal lateral femur and radius, can be assessed in children with orthopedic hardware or significant contractures preventing proper positioning. Scans of the distal femur, for example, may be preferable in children with impaired mobility [25].

Next Steps in Diagnosis and Management

Initial management for children with skeletal disease and/or impaired bone health will depend on the pathology identified. Patients with hypovitaminosis D in the absence of malabsorption or chronic disease may be managed in primary care, paired with efforts to encourage appropriate weight-bearing exercise and optimize nutrition, especially daily intake of dietary calcium in addition to vitamin D repletion. However, if the patient appears not to improve with therapy, endocrine evaluation is appropriate. Concern for rickets, a disordered parathyroid hormone axis, and/or a clinically significant fracture history merit an endocrine evaluation.

Referral to a Specialist

A child should be referred to an endocrinologist for additional testing and possible therapy if any of the following features is apparent: metabolic bone lab derangement, clinical or radiologic signs of rickets, clinically significant bone fragility, or a BMD z score < −2. If none of these criteria are met and specialist referral is not indicated at present, the primary provider can continue to monitor through routine annual care and careful physical examination, with emphasis on height and pubertal development. If the child experiences additional fractures, referral to a specialist is appropriate.

References

1. Lifshitz F. Pediatric endocrinology. 5th ed. New York: Informa Healthcare; 2007.
2. Clarke B. Normal bone anatomy and physiology. Clin J Am Soc Nephrol. 2008;3(Suppl 3):S131–9.
3. Hilton CMKMJ. Endochondral ossification. In: Primer on the metabolic bone diseases and disorders of mineral metabolism. Wiley, Hoboken, New Jersey. p. 12–9.
4. Danseco ER, Miller TR, Spicer RS. Incidence and costs of 1987-1994 childhood injuries: demographic breakdowns. Pediatrics. 2000;105(2):E27.
5. Weber DR, Boyce A, Gordon C, Hogler W, Kecskemethy HH, Misra M, et al. The utility of DXA assessment at the forearm, proximal femur, and lateral distal femur, and vertebral fracture assessment in the pediatric population: 2019 ISCD official position. J Clin Densitom. 2019;22(4):567–89.
6. Wheeler BJ, Snoddy AME, Munns C, Simm P, Siafarikas A, Jefferies C. A brief history of nutritional rickets. Front Endocrinol (Lausanne). 2019;10:795.
7. Carpenter TO, Shaw NJ, Portale AA, Ward LM, Abrams SA, Pettifor JM. Rickets. Nat Rev Dis Primers. 2017;3:17101.
8. Gonzalez Ballesteros LF, Ma NS, Gordon RJ, Ward L, Backeljauw P, Wasserman H, et al. Unexpected widespread hypophosphatemia and bone disease associated with elemental formula use in infants and children. Bone. 2017;97:287–92.
9. Chalouhi C, Nicolas N, Vegas N, Matczak S, El Jurdi H, Boddaert N, et al. Scurvy: a new old cause of skeletal pain in young children. Front Pediatr. 2020;8:8.
10. Faienza MF, Ventura A, Colucci S, Cavallo L, Grano M, Brunetti G. Bone fragility in Turner syndrome: mechanisms and prevention strategies. Front Endocrinol (Lausanne). 2016;7:34.
11. Turner J, Pellerin G, Mager D. Prevalence of metabolic bone disease in children with celiac disease is independent of symptoms at diagnosis. J Pediatr Gastroenterol Nutr. 2009;49(5):589–93.
12. Shaker JL, Brickner RC, Findling JW, Kelly TM, Rapp R, Rizk G, et al. Hypocalcemia and skeletal disease as presenting features of celiac disease. Arch Intern Med. 1997;157(9):1013–6.
13. Sarinho ESC, Melo V. Glucocorticoid-induced bone disease: mechanisms and importance in pediatric practice. Rev Paul Pediatr. 2017;35(2):207–15.
14. Lee CT, Chen HC, Lai LW, Yong KC, Lien YH. Effects of furosemide on renal calcium handling. Am J Physiol Renal Physiol. 2007;293(4):F1231–7.
15. Barstow C, Rerucha C. Evaluation of short and tall stature in children. Am Fam Physician. 2015;92(1):43–50.
16. Gilsanz V, Chalfant J, Kalkwarf H, Zemel B, Lappe J, Oberfield S, et al. Age at onset of puberty predicts bone mass in young adulthood. J Pediatr. 2011;158(1):100–5, 5 e1-2.
17. el-Hajj Fuleihan G, Klerman EB, Brown EN, Choe Y, Brown EM, Czeisler CA. The parathyroid hormone circadian rhythm is truly endogenous--a general clinical research center study. J Clin Endocrinol Metab. 1997;82(1):281–6.
18. Trivedi H, Szabo A, Zhao S, Cantor T, Raff H. Circadian variation of mineral and bone parameters in end-stage renal disease. J Nephrol. 2015;28(3):351–9.
19. Turan S, Topcu B, Gokce I, Guran T, Atay Z, Omar A, et al. Serum alkaline phosphatase levels in healthy children and evaluation of alkaline phosphatase z-scores in different types of rickets. J Clin Res Pediatr Endocrinol. 2011;3(1):7–11.
20. Schiele F, Henny J, Hitz J, Petitclerc C, Gueguen R, Siest G. Total bone and liver alkaline phosphatases in plasma: biological variations and reference limits. Clin Chem. 1983;29(4):634–41.
21. Manz F, Kehrt R, Lausen B, Merkel A. Urinary calcium excretion in healthy children and adolescents. Pediatr Nephrol. 1999;13(9):894–9.
22. Holick MF, Binkley NC, Bischoff-Ferrari HA, Gordon CM, Hanley DA, Heaney RP, et al. Evaluation, treatment, and prevention of vitamin D deficiency: an Endocrine Society clinical practice guideline. J Clin Endocrinol Metab. 2011;96(7):1911–30.
23. Chesney RW, Zimmerman J, Hamstra A, DeLuca HF, Mazees RB. Vitamin D metabolite concentrations in vitamin D deficiency. Are calcitriol levels normal. Am J Dis Child. 1981;135(11):1025–8.
24. Lund B, Clausen N, Lund B, Andersen E, Sorensen OH. Age-dependent variations in serum 1,25-dihydroxyvitamin D in childhood. Acta Endocrinol. 1980;94(3):426–9.
25. Zemel BS, Stallings VA, Leonard MB, Paulhamus DR, Kecskemethy HH, Harcke HT, et al. Revised pediatric reference data for the lateral distal femur measured by Hologic Discovery/Delphi dual-energy X-ray absorptiometry. J Clin Densitom. 2009;12(2):207–18.

Multiple Fractures

4

Sasigarn A. Bowden

Introduction

Fractures are common in childhood, with up to 40% of girls and 50% of boys experiencing a fracture before 18 years of age [1]. Of those who fracture, 15–20% will have two or more fractures during childhood. The peak incidence of fracture is between 10 and 12 years in girls and 13–14 years in boys [1, 2], corresponding to the period of peak pubertal growth when bone mineral accrual lags behind gains in height. It takes 6–8 months to fully mineralize new bone; therefore, the skeleton is relatively underminealized and transiently vulnerable to fracture during rapid growth in early adolescence [3]. The distal radius/ulna is the most common site of fracture, accounting for approximately 25% of all childhood fractures [4]. Increased participation in competitive sports or engaging in high-speed physical activities in youth during this period may also contribute to a higher risk for childhood fractures [1, 4]. While most activity-related childhood fractures are benign and a normal part of growing up, some children who experience multiple fractures may have underlying bone fragility due to genetic bone disorders or secondary to chronic medical conditions. It is important to identify children with increased susceptibility to fractures who may benefit from therapeutic inventions to reduce fracture risk. This chapter reviews metabolic bone disease as a cause of bone fragility and provides guidance in the assessment of children with multiple fractures.

When to Suspect Bone Fragility?

A history of fracture must always be assessed in the context of the child's developmental stage, medical and social history, and detailed account of the mechanism of injury. For example, when a fracture results from a fall from play equipment, questions should explore the height from which the child fell, whether the child fell on grass or cement, the initial position of the child, the dynamics of the fall, and the final position and location of the child after the fall. A history of previous fractures may require a review of plain radiographs for verification, as parents may confuse sprains that were treated with short-term immobilization (i.e., splinting) for fractures. Fragility or low-impact fractures refer to those that occur following minimal trauma or a fall from standing height or less, and not those that occur from excessive force on normal bone (e.g., a motor vehicle accident or a fall from above ten feet). Distinguishing traumatic fracture from pathological fracture can be challenging, as most recurrent childhood fractures occur as a result of seemingly moderate trauma, during play or sport, or when the degree of trauma is unclear. Long bone fractures of the humerus or femur in the absence of severe trauma may indicate pathologic fractures. In contrast, fractures of the nose, skull, fingers or toes are typically not considered clinically significant for bone fragility.

The 2013 International Society for Clinical Densitometry Position Statement provides a definition for clinically significant fracture and redefines criteria for pediatric osteoporosis (Box 4.1) [5]. Of note, one or more vertebral fractures in the absence of local disease or high-energy trauma, regardless of bone mineral density, are diagnostic for osteoporosis. While pediatric osteoporosis is not associated with increased mortality as it is in adults, it can result in pain, physical disability, deformity, and poor quality of life.

Recurrent fractures in children should prompt a comprehensive systemic and bone health evaluation to diagnose bone fragility or osteoporosis, and also identify the underlying pathology. Clinicians must always keep in mind the possibility of child abuse as a cause of multiple fractures, especially when fractures are noted in children <18 months of age, fractures in various stages of healing, or rib fractures without a history of a major accident (Box 4.2).

S. A. Bowden (✉)
Division of Endocrinology, Department of Pediatrics, Nationwide Children's Hospital/The Ohio State University College of Medicine, Columbus, OH, USA
e-mail: Sasigarn.Bowden@nationwidechildrens.org

T. Stanley, M. Misra (eds.), *Endocrine Conditions in Pediatrics*, https://doi.org/10.1007/978-3-030-52215-5_4

Box 4.1: Definition of pediatric osteoporosis [5]

- $\geq$1 vertebral compression fracture in the absence of local disease or high-energy trauma.
  OR
- In the absence of vertebral compression fractures, presence of both a clinically significant fracture history and bone mineral density *Z*-score of ≤ -2.0[a] at $\geq$1 site.
  - A clinically significant fracture history includes $\geq$1 of the following occurring as a result of mild-to-moderate trauma:
    Two of more long bone fractures by 10 years of age.
    Three of more long bone fractures at any age up to 19 years.

[a]A normal bone mineral density *Z*-score (> -2) does not exclude the possibility of bone fragility.

Box 4.2: Red flags for non-accidental injury in a child with multiple fractures

- Long bone fractures in non-ambulatory children
- Metaphyseal corner (or bucket handle) fractures
- Rib fractures (especially posteromedial)
- Fractures of the sternum, scapula, or spinous processes
- Multiple fractures in various stages of healing
- Vertebral body fractures and subluxations in the absence of high-force trauma
- Digital fractures in children younger than 36 months of age or without a corresponding history
- Displaced physeal fractures
- Complex skull fractures in children younger than 18 months of age, particularly without a corresponding history

Differential Diagnosis of Bone Fragility

Conditions associated with bone fragility or pediatric osteoporosis are extensive, with a broad range of etiologies (Box 4.3). These conditions are divided into two groups: primary osteoporosis from genetic causes, and secondary osteoporosis due to underlying chronic disease. Primary osteoporosis occurs due to an intrinsic skeletal defect of genetic origin such as osteogenesis imperfecta (OI), idiopathic juvenile osteoporosis, Marfan's syndrome, or fibrous dysplasia. OI is the most common cause of primary osteoporosis, with an incidence of 1 in 25,000–40,000 individuals [6]. Patients with severe forms of OI have obvious clinical features such as bone deformities, a triangular-shaped face, blue sclera, and wormian bones of the skull. Milder forms may have near-normal stature without bone deformities. Although OI is a genetic disorder, many patients with OI have a de novo mutation, without any family history.

Box 4.3: Conditions associated with fragility fractures in children[a]

Primary bone disorders

- Osteogenesis imperfecta
- Idiopathic juvenile osteoporosis
- Osteoporosis pseudoglioma syndrome
- Ehlers-Danlos syndrome
- Marfan syndrome
- Homocystiniuria
- Hypophosphatasia
- Fibrous dysplasia
- Osteopetrosis

Secondary bone fragility due to chronic medical conditions

- Immobility (cerebral palsy, Duchenne muscular dystrophy, prolonged immobilization, such as spinal cord injury)
- Chronic inflammation/illnesses (systemic lupus erythematosus, juvenile idiopathic arthritis, inflammatory bowel disease, chronic kidney disease, hematologic disease such as childhood cancers, Thalassemia, post-bone marrow transplant)
- Nutritional deficiencies/malabsorption (celiac disease, biliary atresia, cystic fibrosis, anorexia nervosa, vitamin D deficiency)
- Endocrine disorders (hypogonadism, growth hormone deficiency, hypercortisolemia, hyperthyroidism, diabetes mellitus, Female Athlete Triad, metabolic bone disease of prematurity)
- Drug-induced (glucocorticoids, anticonvulsants, methotrexate, radiation therapy, antiretrovirals)

[a]This list is representative of causes of osteoporosis, but is not exhaustive.

Secondary osteoporosis is a consequence of chronic illnesses, particularly inflammatory conditions, malabsorption, certain endocrine disorders, and decreased mobility. It may also be a consequence of the treatment for chronic disease, especially chronic glucocorticoid treatment or chemotherapy.

Patients with chronic illnesses may have pubertal delay, endocrine dysfunction, vitamin D deficiency, or decreased physical activity, all of which contribute to poor bone health and low bone density. Fractures may be the first sign of sometimes "silent" diseases such as celiac disease. It is important to always screen for celiac disease, as bone fragility can resolve with the implementation of a gluten-free diet [7].

Evaluation and Management of Children with Multiple Fractures

Evaluation of bone health in a child presenting with multiple fractures can be initiated by primary care pediatricians, using the proposed algorithm (Fig. 4.1). In infants and toddlers presenting with fractures, the major differential diagnoses are non-accidental injury (NAI) and OI. Children with OI tend to sustain mid-shaft fractures where the bones are most fragile, whereas metaphyseal corner fractures in non-ambulatory patients are highly specific for NAI [8]. Symmetrical bilateral posterior medial rib fractures are more likely to be NAI and are rarely seen in OI [6]. Red flags for child abuse in young children with multiple fractures [9] are summarized in Box 4.3. When suspecting child abuse, consultation with the child abuse team, geneticist, pediatric radiologist, and bone specialist is essential for timely diagnosis and expedited disposition to protect the child's safety and welfare.

In an otherwise healthy child with no known chronic disease, bone health assessment should be performed when there is a clinically significant fracture history (≥2 long

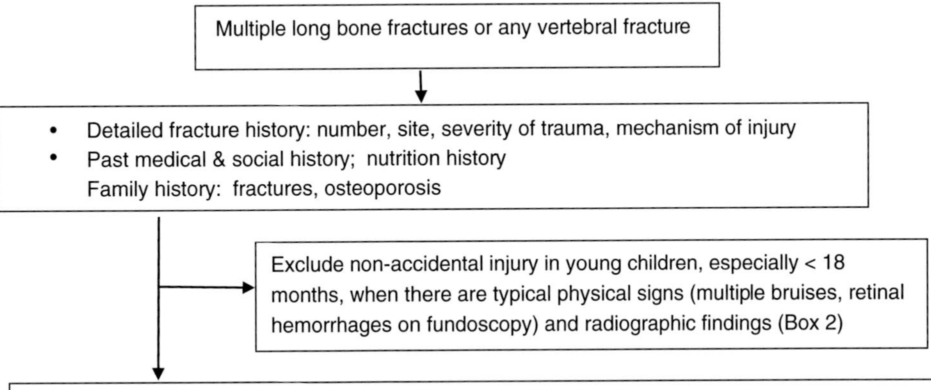

Consideration for further bone fragility assessment

- Recurrent fractures (≥ 2 long bone fractures by age 10 years, ≥ 3 long bone fractures by any age up to 19 years)
- The presence of ≥1 vertebral compression fractures in the absence of local disease or high-energy trauma
- Pathologic fractures (fractures from minimal trauma, or a fall from a standing height or less)
- Underlying conditions associated with secondary osteoporosis (Box 3)

- Review medications: e.g. corticosteroids, anticonvulsants, chemotherapeutic drugs
- Dental history: dentinogenesis imperfecta (OI), premature tooth loss before age 5 years (hypophosphatasia)
- History of eating disorder or excessive exercise, and other relevant history
- Physical examination: blue sclerae (OI), skeletal deformities, joint laxity, growth and pubertal status, mobility/neuromuscular function.
- Laboratory evaluation (Box 4)
- Exclude celiac disease (treatment with gluten-free diet improves bone health)
- Optimize vitamin D and calcium intake
- Encourage weight-bearing exercise (other than in anorexia nervosa)
- Modify environment to reduce risk of injury or prevent fall, if at risk for fragility fractures
- Referral to pediatric bone specialist for:
  - Clinical features suggestive of primary and secondary osteoporosis
  - One or more vertebral compression fractures
  - Pathologic fractures
  - Bone mineral density Z-score < -2

Fig. 4.1 Algorithm for the evaluation of multiple fractures in children

bone fractures by 10 years of age or ≥3 long bone fractures by 19 years of age) [5]. Using these criteria, 18% of children with a significant fracture history were identified as having a mild form of osteogenesis imperfecta in a recent study [10]. First-line laboratory screening (Box 4.4) includes assessment of calcium, phosphorus, magnesium, and alkaline phosphatase levels, vitamin D status, and ruling out hyperparathyroidism, which has catabolic effects on bone. It is important to have age- and gender-specific reference ranges for serum alkaline phosphatase, and low serum alkaline phosphatase should raise concerns of hypophosphatasia. Elevated alkaline phosphatase may reflect vitamin D deficiency or a disease state with high bone turnover, including after fracture. Vitamin D deficiency should be treated, with the goal to maintain 25-hydroxy vitamin D (25OHD) levels above 30 ng/mL, for optimal bone health. Screening for celiac disease must not be missed.

Box 4.4: Laboratory evaluation for bone health

Serum

- Complete blood count
- Comprehensive metabolic profile (includes serum calcium, phosphorus, magnesium, alkaline phosphatase)
- Sedimentation rate +/− C-reactive protein
- 25-hydroxy vitamin D
- Parathyroid hormone
- Celiac screen (tissue transglutaminase antibodies with total immunoglobulin A)
- May obtain additional laboratory studies to exclude endocrine disorders, as clinically indicated (work up for thyroid dysfunction, delayed puberty, or Cushing syndrome).

Urine

- Urine calcium, creatinine

Imaging studies

- Dual-energy x-ray absorptiometry (DXA) scan
- Lateral thoraco-lumbar spine radiograph

Bone radiographs obtained for fractures may reveal diagnostic clues to underlying skeletal pathology (as in primary osteoporosis). For example, ground-glass appearance of long bones is suggestive of fibrous dysplasia (a benign fibro-osseous bone disease characterized by the replacement of bone with fibrous tissue) [11]. Generalized osteosclerosis of bones is pathognomonic for osteopetrosis, a skeletal disorder with high bone mass, resulting in brittle bones [12]. These classic radiographic features should prompt further workup (or referral to a pediatric bone specialist), without the need to meet ISCD criteria of "clinically significant fracture history."

Bone densitometry by dual energy X-ray absorptiometry (DXA) is useful to assess bone mass at baseline and bone accrual over time (see Section "Bone Densitometry"). However, children with fragile bones and increased fracture risk can have normal BMD (BMD *Z*-score greater than −2.0) [5]. Furthermore, many children with primary and secondary osteoporosis and radiographically detected vertebral fractures (loss of at least 20% of vertebral body height) are asymptomatic [13]. It is, therefore, important to screen for vertebral fractures in children with risk factors for osteoporosis by obtaining a lateral spinal radiograph [14]. The presence of vertebral compression fractures allows for the diagnosis of osteoporosis, irrespective of BMD. This would also be an indication for referral to a pediatric bone specialist.

References

1. Clark EM. The epidemiology of fractures in otherwise healthy children. Curr Osteoporos Rep. 2014;12(3):272–8.
2. Naranje SM, Erali RA, Warner WC, Sawyer JR, Kelly DM. Epidemiology of pediatric fractures presenting to emergency departments in the United States. J Pediatr Orthop. 2016;36(4):e45–e8.
3. Faulkner RA, Davison KS, Bailey DA, Mirwald RL, Baxter-Jones AD. Size-corrected BMD decreases during peak linear growth: implications for fracture incidence during adolescence. J Bone Miner Res. 2006;21(12):1864–70.
4. Hedstrom EM, Svensson O, Bergstrom U, Michno P. Epidemiology of fractures in children and adolescents. Acta Orthop. 2010;81(1):148–53.
5. Bishop N, Arundel P, Clark E, Dimitri P, Farr J, Jones G, et al. Fracture prediction and the definition of osteoporosis in children and adolescents: the ISCD 2013 Pediatric Official Positions. J Clin Densitom. 2014;17(2):275–80.
6. Pereira EM, editor. Clinical perspectives on osteogenesis imperfecta versus non-accidental injury. American Journal of Medical Genetics Part C: Seminars in Medical Genetics: Wiley Online Library; 2015.
7. Duerksen D, Pinto-Sanchez MI, Anca A, Schnetzler J, Case S, Zelin J, et al. Management of bone health in patients with celiac disease: practical guide for clinicians. Can Fam Physician. 2018;64(6):433–8.
8. Dwek JR. The radiographic approach to child abuse. Clin Orthop Relat Res. 2011;469(3):776–89.
9. Flaherty EG, Perez-Rossello JM, Levine MA, Hennrikus WL. Abuse AAoPCoC, neglect. Evaluating children with fractures for child physical abuse. Pediatrics. 2014;133(2):e477–e89.

10. Fiscaletti M, Coorey CP, Biggin A, Briody J, Little D, Schindeler A, et al. Diagnosis of recurrent fracture in a pediatric cohort. Calcif Tissue Int. 2018;103(5):529–39.
11. Robinson C, Collins MT, Boyce AM. Fibrous dysplasia/McCune-Albright syndrome: clinical and translational perspectives. Curr Osteoporos Rep. 2016;14(5):178–86.
12. Wu CC, Econs MJ, DiMeglio LA, Insogna KL, Levine MA, Orchard PJ, et al. Diagnosis and management of osteopetrosis: consensus guidelines from the osteopetrosis working group. J Clin Endocrinol Metabol. 2017;102(9):3111–23.
13. Mäkitie O, Doria AS, Henriques F, Cole WG, Compeyrot S, Silverman E, et al. Radiographic vertebral morphology: a diagnostic tool in pediatric osteoporosis. J Pediatr. 2005;146(3):395–401.
14. Ward L, Konji V, Ma J. The management of osteoporosis in children. Osteoporos Int. 2016;27(7):2147–79.

Hypocalcemia

5

Janaki D. Vakharia and Lisa Swartz Topor

Abbreviations

AD	Autosomal dominant
ADH	Autosomal dominant hypocalcemia
AHO	Albright's hereditary osteodystrophy
AIRE	Autoimmune regulator
APECED	Autoimmune polyendocrinopathy-candidiasis-ectodermal dystrophy syndrome
AR	Autosomal recessive
cAMP	Cyclic adenosine monophosphate
CaSR	Calcium-sensing receptor
CHD7	Chromodomain helicase DNAbinding 7
EEG	Electroencephalogram
EKG	Electrocardiogram
FGF23	Fibroblast growth factor 23
GATA3	GATA-binding factor 3
GCM2	Glial cell missing homologue 2
GNAS	Guanine nucleotide–binding protein alpha subunit
HDR	Hypoparathyroidism, sensorineural deafness, and renal disease
HVDRR	Hereditary vitamin D–resistant rickets
MELAS	Mitochondrial encephalomyopathy with lactic acidosis and stroke-like episodes
MTP	Mitochondrial trifunctional protein
PHP	Pseudohypoparathyroidism
PTH	Parathyroid hormone
RANK	Receptor activator of nuclear factor kappa-B ligand

J. D. Vakharia
Department of Endocrinology, Massachusetts General Hospital, Boston, MA, USA

L. S. Topor (✉)
Department of Pediatric Endocrinology, Warren Alpert Medical School of Brown University and Hasbro Children's Hospital, Providence, RI, USA
e-mail: lisa_swartz_topor@brown.edu

Introduction

Low serum calcium levels, or hypocalcemia, can present with neurologic, cardiac, muscular, or bone problems. The differential diagnosis of hypocalcemia is broad, and common causes and evaluation vary based upon the age of the child. This chapter discusses common signs, symptoms, and causes of hypocalcemia in pediatric patients.

Definition

Calcium is the most abundant mineral in the body and is involved in many cellular functions, including muscle contraction, vascular tone regulation, nerve signaling, and hormone secretion. Almost all the calcium in the body is stored in bone and teeth, with only about 1% present in blood, extracellular fluid, muscle, and other tissues.

Calcium Homeostasis

The level of calcium in serum is tightly regulated by parathyroid hormone (PTH), vitamin D, calcitonin, and fibroblast growth factor 23 (FGF23). Calcium is absorbed from the intestinal lumen via active transportation and passive diffusion across the intestinal mucosa. Active transport of calcium into enterocytes is dependent on the action of 1,25-dihydroxyvitamin D [1–4]. Calcium-sensing receptors (CaSRs) on parathyroid chief cells detect acute changes in serum ionized calcium levels, and low serum ionized calcium leads to PTH release [5]. PTH increases serum calcium by (1) activating 1-alpha-hydroxylase [6, 7], thus facilitating conversion of 25-hydroxyvitamin D to 1,25-dihydroxyvitamin D, (2) acting on bone to mobilize readily available calcium stores by increasing bone resorption [8] via increased osteoclast activity [9], and (3) increasing calcium reabsorption in the distal renal tubule [10].

T. Stanley, M. Misra (eds.), *Endocrine Conditions in Pediatrics*, https://doi.org/10.1007/978-3-030-52215-5_5

In addition to promoting intestinal calcium absorption, 1,25-dihydroxyvitamin D increases serum calcium by directly stimulating osteoclast differentiation by increasing receptor activator of nuclear factor kappa-B ligand (RANKL) expression [11], leading to increased bone resorption and decreased bone mineralization [12].

Calcitonin, a peptide secreted by C-cells in the thyroid gland, can quickly decrease serum calcium levels via uncertain mechanisms. In animal studies, calcitonin has been demonstrated to decrease renal tubular reabsorption of calcium and impair osteoclast-mediated bone resorption [13, 14]. FGF23, a protein made by osteocytes, has a primary role in phosphate regulation. However, it also regulates calcium homeostasis through its effects on PTH and 1,25-dihydroxyvitamin D [15].

Inherited or acquired conditions that affect hormones or hormone receptors involved in calcium homeostasis lead to disorders of calcium regulation. In this chapter, we discuss hypocalcemia. Please see Part I Chap. 6 to learn about hypercalcemia.

Signs and Symptoms of Hypocalcemia

Characteristic features of hypocalcemia include neuromuscular, central nervous system, cardiac, and dental/skeletal manifestations. The specific signs and symptoms vary by age and the duration and pace of onset of hypocalcemia.

Neuromuscular Manifestations

Neuromuscular irritability is the hallmark manifestation of hypocalcemia. Low calcium levels lead to increased neuronal excitability [16], resulting in sensory nerve dysfunction and tetany, which can manifest with numbness, tingling, muscle twitching, and spasm. Perioral or peripheral paresthesia may be an initial feature. Hyperventilation leading to respiratory alkalosis can exacerbate paresthesias, as alkaline states decrease ionized calcium levels in the blood [17]. Intercurrent illness can also exacerbate paresthesias or other neurological symptoms. Motor symptoms may be mild, such as intermittent cramping, clumsiness, stiffness, or myalgias. Generalized muscle spasms can occur, and in severe cases can lead to bronchospasm or laryngospasm. Patients with chronic hypocalcemia may have milder neuromuscular symptoms or may be asymptomatic.

Carpopedal spasms are usually painful, brief, and forceful contractions of wrists, fingers, toes, or ankles. The muscle spasms of hypocalcemia can occur spontaneously or may become apparent with repeated muscle use. Trousseau sign is the development of carpal spasm with inflation of a blood pressure cuff on the arm for 3 minutes, which leads to occlusion of the brachial artery and vasa nervosum. Carpal spasm is the forceful adduction of the thumb, flexion of the metacarpophalangeal joints, extension of the interphalangeal joints, and flexion of the wrist. Chvostek sign is characterized as facial muscle twitching evoked by tapping the skin overlying the facial nerve at the angle of the jaw (anterior to the ear). The physical examination section, later in this chapter, has additional information on these signs and other physical exam findings in patients with hypocalcemia.

Central Nervous System and Neuropsychiatric Manifestations

Generalized tonic-clonic seizures, focal seizures, and absence seizures can all result from hypocalcemia. Decreased extracellular calcium leads to effects on neuronal action potentials and enhances excitability [18]. Seizures may occur as the initial manifestation of hypocalcemia, without any other clinical signs. Electroencephalogram (EEG) findings in patients with hypocalcemia and seizure can show a generalized slowing of the background rhythm, increased activity of slow waves, or high-voltage spikes and bursts [19, 20].

Symptoms of delirium, depression, anxiety, psychosis, and cognitive impairment may also occur with hypocalcemia. Symptoms of cognitive impairment, particularly in patients with hypoparathyroidism, are thought to correlate directly with the chronicity of disease and severity of hypocalcemia [21]. Appropriate treatment of hypocalcemia may improve neuropsychiatric manifestations [22].

Long-standing hypocalcemia, particularly when associated with hyperphosphatemia, may lead to basal ganglia calcifications [23, 22, 24]. Reports of papilledema, increased intracranial pressure, and cataracts have also been infrequently described in children with severe hypocalcemia. Papilledema and increased intracranial pressure usually resolve with treatment of hypocalcemia [22, 25].

Cardiac Manifestations

The cardiovascular manifestations of acute hypocalcemia are related to decreased tone of vascular smooth muscle, which can result in hypotension and impaired cardiac contractility. Bradycardia and arrhythmias are also seen in acute hypocalcemia. The hallmark electrocardiogram (EKG) finding of hypocalcemia is QT prolongation. The degree of ST segment prolongation is inversely proportional to the serum calcium level. Other EKG findings include ST-segment elevation and QRS and T-wave abnormalities [26, 27]. Chronic hypocalcemia can lead to myocardial dysfunction, including cardiomyopathy and congestive heart failure. Treatment of hypocalcemia leads to improvement in cardiac function [28, 29].

Skeletal and Dental Manifestations

Chronic hypocalcemia can have adverse effects on bone health. When associated with hypophosphatemia (as can occur with vitamin D deficiency), hypocalcemia can result in rickets, characterized by growth plate abnormalities, or osteomalacia due to impaired mineralization of bone. Hypocalcemia due to hypoparathyroidism is associated with reduced bone remodeling and increased bone density. When hypocalcemia occurs during infancy, enamel hypoplasia, failure of tooth eruption, defective root formation, and dental caries can occur [30, 31].

Causes of Hypocalcemia in Pediatric Patients

This section discusses the broad differential diagnoses of hypocalcemia in pediatric patients, and Table 5.1 summarizes these causes.

Neonatal Hypocalcemia

During pregnancy, calcium is actively transported from the mother to the fetus across the placenta by a transplacental calcium pump regulated by parathyroid hormone–related peptide [32]. In the third trimester and at birth, fetal serum calcium levels are higher than maternal serum calcium levels due to upregulation of the transplacental calcium pump. At birth, placental transfer abruptly ends, and neonatal serum calcium levels decrease to neonatal normal ranges by 24 hours of life. Etiologies of hypocalcemia are typically categorized based on time of onset [33].

Table 5.1 Etiologies of hypocalcemia in pediatric patients

Etiologies of hypocalcemia	
Neonatal hypocalcemia	*Early onset* Prematurity Low birth weight Birth asphyxia Mother with diabetes Mother with preeclampsia
	Late onset Mother with vitamin D deficiency Phototherapy High phosphate load from formula
Associated with high PTH	Vitamin D deficiency
	Vitamin D resistance
	Pseudohypoparathyroidism
Associated with low PTH	Genetic causes (see Table 5.2)
	Congenital hypoparathyroidism
	Autoimmune hypoparathyroidism
	Post-surgical hypoparathyroidism
	Hypomagnesemia
Other etiologies	Hyperphosphatemia
	Hungry bone syndrome
	Tumor lysis syndrome
	Acute pancreatitis
	Citrated blood product or lipid infusion

Early-Onset Neonatal Hypocalcemia

Early-onset neonatal hypocalcemia typically manifests in the first 48–72 hours of life with serum calcium levels below the typical physiologic nadir of calcium. Newborns are commonly asymptomatic, and hypocalcemia may be detected incidentally. However, severe manifestations including tetany and seizure can occur. Early-onset neonatal hypocalcemia is often transient.

Neonatal factors that can lead to symptomatic early-onset hypocalcemia include prematurity, low birth weight, fetal growth restriction, and birth asphyxia. Maternal conditions that predispose newborns to hypocalcemia include preeclampsia, diabetes, vitamin D deficiency, and hyperparathyroidism, and maternal use of anticonvulsant agents. Infants of mothers with diabetes are at risk for hypocalcemia even in the absence of prematurity; the risk of hypocalcemia correlates with severity and duration of maternal diabetes [34]. Hypocalcemia in infants of mothers with diabetes occurs due to lower circulating PTH levels in these infants compared to healthy infants [35].

Neonatal conditions, including sepsis, respiratory distress syndrome, hyperbilirubinemia requiring phototherapy, hypomagnesemia, and renal failure, as well as iatrogenic factors such as blood transfusion, lipid infusion, or bicarbonate infusion (all of which can lower circulating ionized calcium levels), can cause early-onset hypocalcemia.

Late-Onset Neonatal Hypocalcemia

Late-onset neonatal hypocalcemia presents after the third day of life and may be transient or persistent. Newborns with late-onset hypocalcemia are usually symptomatic. Secondary hyperphosphatemia due to high phosphate load from cow milk–based formula or from parenteral nutrition with high phosphorus content can cause hypocalcemia after the first few days of life [36, 33]. Etiologies of early-onset neonatal hypocalcemia, including maternal vitamin D deficiency, hypomagnesemia, renal failure, hyperbilirubinemia requiring phototherapy, blood transfusion, and lipid infusions, can also manifest as late-onset hypocalcemia. Causes of persistent hypocalcemia that present early or late in the neonatal period are discussed in detail based on etiology in the following sections of this chapter.

Hypocalcemia Associated with Low PTH (Hypoparathyroidism)

Hypoparathyroidism is defined as hypocalcemia in the setting of low or inappropriately normal serum PTH and elevated serum phosphate. Hypoparathyroidism may be due to decreased production and/or secretion of PTH (due to genetic, autoimmune, or acquired causes) or defects in the function of calcium-sensing receptor.

Genetic Causes of Hypoparathyroidism

Table 5.2 summarizes the genetic causes of hypoparathyroidism.

DiGeorge Syndrome

In DiGeorge syndrome, hypoplasia of the second and third pharyngeal pouches leads to hypoplasia or absence of the inferior parathyroid glands. DiGeorge syndrome can include hypoparathyroidism, cardiac outflow tract malformations, thymic hypoplasia, facial dysmorphia, developmental delay, and palatal dysfunction. DiGeorge syndrome is most commonly caused by a heterozygous microdeletion of chromosome 22q11.2 (TBX 1 gene), often acquired sporadically or inherited in an autosomal dominant pattern. Deletions at chromosome 10p (NEBL gene) are seen less commonly. About 50% of patients with DiGeorge syndrome will have hypoparathyroidism of varying severity [37].

CHARGE Syndrome

More than half of the patients with CHARGE syndrome have hypocalcemia due to hypoparathyroidism [38]. CHARGE syndrome has clinical overlap with DiGeorge syndrome and is characterized by **c**oloboma (a hole in one or more ocular structures), **h**eart abnormalities, choanal **a**tresia (a congenital nasal airway abnormality), **r**etardation of growth, and **g**enitourinary and/or **e**ar anomalies. CHARGE syndrome is caused by a heterozygous mutation in the chromodomain helicase DNAbinding 7 (CHD7) gene expressed in the pharyngeal ectoderm and may result in defective development of the parathyroid gland [39].

Table 5.2 Genetic causes of hypoparathyroidism causing hypocalcemia

Genetic causes of hypoparathyroidism	
DiGeorge syndrome	AD, heterozygous microdeletion of chromosome 22q11.2 (*TBX1*) (most common) Deletion of chromosome 10p (*NEBL*) Cardiac outflow tract malformations, thymic hypoplasia, facial dysmorphia, developmental delay, and cleft palate
CHARGE syndrome	Heterozygous mutation in chromodomain helicase DNA-binding 7 (*CHD7*) gene Coloboma, heart abnormalities, choanal atresia, growth retardation, and genitourinary and/or ear abnormalities
Autoimmune Polyendocrinopathy-candidiasis-ectodermal dystrophy syndrome (APECED)	AR mutation in the autoimmune regulator (*AIRE*) gene Autoimmune destruction of parathyroid and/or adrenal glands
Hypoparathyroidism, sensorineural deafness and renal disease (HDR) syndrome	AD, heterozygous germline mutation in GATA-binding factor 3 gene
Kenny-Caffey syndrome	*Type 1:* AR mutation in tubulin-specific chaperone E gene (*TBCE*) *Type 2:* AD mutation in family with sequence similarity 111, member A (*FAM111A*) gene Short stature, learning disability, osteosclerosis, immunodeficiencies, and facial dysmorphism
Sanjad-Sakati syndrome	Similar to Kenny-Caffey syndrome without osteosclerosis
Kearns-Sayre syndrome	Mitochondrial disorder with gonadal insufficiency, diabetes mellitus, thyroid disease, hyperaldosteronism, ophthalmoplegia, pigmentary retinopathy, and cardiomyopathy
MELAS	Mitochondrial disorder with encephalomyopathy, lactic acidosis, and stroke-like episodes
Mitochondrial trifunctional protein (MTP) deficiency	Fatty acid oxidative disorder with cardiomyopathy, skeletal myopathy, peripheral neuropathy, liver dysfunction, and pigmentary retinopathy
Autosomal dominant hypocalcemia	*Type 1 (most common):* Gain-of-function mutation in calcium-sensing receptor gene (*CASR*); manifestations including nephrolithiasis and nephrocalcinosis *Type 2:* Gain-of-function mutation in guanine nucleotide-binding protein, alpha-11 (*GNA11*); short stature and less severe renal manifestations
Familial isolated hypoparathyroidism	AR germline mutation in glial cells missing homologue 2 (*GCM2*) gene AD, heterozygous germline mutation in *GCM2* X-linked recessive mutation in Xq27 and 2p25 (almost exclusively in males)

Autoimmune Polyendocrine Syndrome Type 1 or Autoimmune Polyendocrinopathy-Candidiasis-Ectodermal Dystrophy (APECED) Syndrome

APECED syndrome is an autosomal recessive disorder that occurs due to a mutation in the autoimmune regulator (AIRE). Autoimmune destruction of the parathyroid and adrenal glands is the most common endocrinopathy that develops, but other endocrine glands can be involved. Hypoparathyroidism presents most commonly between 4 and 5 years of age. Ectodermal dystrophies, such as hypoplasia of tooth enamel, can also develop [40]. Patients with this disorder often have mucocutaneous candidiasis or other signs of immunodeficiency.

Hypoparathyroidism, Sensorineural Deafness, and Renal Disease (HDR) Syndrome

HDR syndrome is a rare autosomal dominant disorder caused by germline mutations in GATA-binding factor 3 (GATA3). Hypoparathyroidism is due to altered PTH gene expression mediated by GATA3 [41]. The syndrome also manifests with sensorineural hearing loss and renal dysplasia.

Kenny-Caffey Syndrome and Sanjad-Sakati Syndrome

Clinical features of Kenny-Caffey syndrome include congenital hypoparathyroidism in more than 50% of patients, growth failure/short stature, learning disability, osteosclerosis, immunodeficiencies, and facial dysmorphism. Sanjad-Sakati syndrome most typically occurs in Middle Eastern populations, and it has similar features to Kenny-Caffey syndrome, including hypoparathyroidism, except without osteosclerosis [39].

Mitochondrial Disorders

Kearns-Sayre syndrome, mitochondrial encephalomyopathy with lactic acidosis and stroke-like episodes (MELAS) syndrome, and mitochondrial trifunctional protein (MTP) deficiency syndrome can all present with hypoparathyroidism, although the pathophysiology is not understood. Kearns-Sayre syndrome may also present with other endocrine dysfunctions, including gonadal insufficiency, diabetes mellitus, thyroid disease, and hyperaldosteronism, as well as ophthalmoplegia, pigmentary degeneration of the retina, and cardiomyopathy [42]. MTP deficiency syndrome is a fatty acid oxidative disorder that also presents with cardiomyopathy, skeletal myopathy, peripheral neuropathy, liver dysfunction, or pigmentary retinopathy [43].

Autosomal Dominant Hypocalcemia

Autosomal dominant hypocalcemia (ADH) type 1 is caused by a gain-of-function mutation in the calcium-sensing receptor (CaSR), raising the calcium threshold at which PTH is released, and resulting in hypocalcemia without appropriate PTH secretion. Hypocalcemia may be asymptomatic, mild, or severe, and symptoms can be exacerbated by illnesses or fever [44]. Nephrolithiasis and nephrocalcinosis occur due to increased fractional excretion of calcium. Patients with severe activating mutations of CaSR can present with a Bartter-like syndrome (Bartter syndrome type 5) characterized by hypokalemic alkalosis, renal salt wasting, and hyperreninemic hyperaldosteronism [45]. ADH type 2 is less common than ADH type 1 and is caused by a gain-of-function mutation in the guanine nucleotide–binding protein, alpha-11(GNA11) gene. Renal manifestations are typically less severe due to less urinary calcium excretion in ADH type 2. Short stature is also common [46, 39] .

Familial Isolated Hypoparathyroidism

Familial isolated hypoparathyroidism is caused by germline mutations in the PTH gene, leading to impaired PTH biosynthesis and secretion, or the PTH-specific transcription factor gene called glial cells missing homologue 2 (GCM2). Familial isolated hypoparathyroidism can be either autosomal recessive or dominant. X-linked recessive hypoparathyroidism is seen almost exclusively in males and is caused by mutations involving chromosomes Xq27 and 2p25, leading to defects in parathyroid gland development. Patients present with infantile seizures and severe hypocalcemia [39].

Autoimmune Hypoparathyroidism

Autoimmune destruction of the parathyroid gland may present as an isolated process or as a genetic syndrome, such as APECED. Antibody-mediated constitutive activation of CaSR may also result in hypoparathyroidism and hypocalcemia. Patients with autoimmune hypoparathyroidism may present with other autoimmune diseases [47].

Post-surgical Hypoparathyroidism

Pediatric patients with a history of thyroid disease requiring surgical resection, such as with thyroid cancer or Graves disease, are at risk for post-surgical hypoparathyroidism. While most patients with post-surgical hypoparathyroidism have transient disease, about 25% continue with permanent hypoparathyroidism. The risk of post-surgical hypoparathyroidism depends on the extent of the neck surgery and the experience and expertise of the surgeon, with surgeons performing more than 100 anterior neck surgeries per year having the lowest risk [37, 48]. Hypoparathyroidism may be a delayed complication after anterior neck surgery occurring after several years in some cases [49].

Hypomagnesemia

Severe and prolonged hypomagnesemia causes hypocalcemia by impairing PTH secretion. Hypomagnesemia also reduces end-organ responsiveness to PTH. Primary hypomagnesemia is rare and due to genetic mutations. Common causes of secondary hypomagnesemia in children include gastrointestinal losses, decreased intake, or increased urinary excretion. Appropriate magnesium replacement therapy reverses the functional hypoparathyroidism [50].

Congenital Hypoparathyroidism

Congenital hypoparathyroidism can occur when there is agenesis or dysgenesis of the parathyroid gland at birth. Congenital hypoparathyroidism can be idiopathic or part of a genetic disorder and may be transient or permanent.

Hypocalcemia Associated with High PTH

25-Hydroxyvitamin D Deficiency

Vitamin D deficiency is caused by decreased intake or production, impaired intestinal absorption, impaired activation of vitamin D at various stages, increased metabolism of active vitamin D metabolites, or end-organ unresponsiveness to activated vitamin D. Since activated vitamin D is necessary for intestinal absorption of calcium and phosphate, severe vitamin D deficiency can lead to hypocalcemia, especially in the setting of poor dietary calcium intake. Hypocalcemia secondary to severe vitamin D deficiency is associated with an elevated PTH level, and often, hypophosphatemia, due to decreased intestinal absorption and increased urinary excretion of phosphate. Clinical manifestations may include rickets, osteomalacia, growth failure, and seizures.

Decreased Intake or Production of Vitamin D

Infants who are exclusively breast-fed are at risk of developing vitamin D deficiency due to the low concentration of vitamin D in breast milk, especially if the mother has vitamin D deficiency during pregnancy. All breast-fed infants require vitamin D supplementation. Children with limited exposure to sunlight can also have vitamin D deficiency. Individuals with dark skin produce less vitamin D with the same amount of sunlight exposure compared to individuals with fair skin [51]. Intestinal malabsorption of vitamin D is seen in individuals with inflammatory bowel disease, celiac disease, history of bowel resection, or gastrectomy, as well as conditions leading to pancreatic insufficiency such as cystic fibrosis.

Impaired Activation of Vitamin D

Vitamin D3 undergoes 25-hydroxylation in the liver. This hydroxylation process can be impaired in severe liver disease or when mutations exist in the gene encoding vitamin D 25-hydroxylase (*CYP2R1*) [52]. Isoniazid may also impair 25-hydroxylation [53]. 1-hydroxylation of 25-hydroxyvitamin D to 1,25-dihydroxyvitamin D occurs in the kidney by 1-alpha-hydroxylase. Impaired hydroxylation occurs in chronic kidney disease or autosomal recessive 1-alpha-hydroxylase deficiency (previously known as vitamin D–dependent rickets type 1 or pseudovitamin D–deficient rickets) [54, 55].

Increased Metabolism of Vitamin D

Antiepileptic and anti-tuberculosis medications, including phenytoin, phenobarbital, primidone, and rifampin, can activate cytochrome P450 enzymes in the liver and lead to increased metabolism of 25-hydroxyvitamin D and 1,25-dihydroxyvitamin D.

End-Organ Unresponsiveness to Vitamin D

Hereditary vitamin D–resistant rickets (HVDRR) is an autosomal recessive disorder caused by a loss-of-function mutation of the vitamin D receptor gene, which leads to impaired end-organ responsiveness of activated vitamin D. Clinical manifestations include elevated serum 1,25-dihydroxyvitamin D with severe hypocalcemia and rickets, and alopecia totalis in some individuals within the first 2 years of life [56].

Pseudohypoparathyroidism

Pseudohypoparathyroidism (PHP) is characterized by end-organ (primarily bone and kidney) resistance to PTH resulting in hypocalcemia, elevated PTH, and hyperphosphatemia. The PTH receptor is a G-protein-coupled receptor and its signal transduction is mediated by cyclic adenosine monophosphate (cAMP). PHP occurs due to mutations in genes encoding the G-protein or downstream signaling proteins, which leads to impaired cAMP and/or urinary phosphate excretion [57].

Type 1 Pseudohypoparathyroidism

PHP type 1 is caused by mutations or imprinting abnormalities in the guanine nucleotide–binding protein alpha stimulating (GNAS) gene that lead to impairment of urinary cAMP and phosphaturic responses to PTH in the proximal renal tubule.

PHP type 1a is an autosomal dominant disorder characterized by a maternally inherited loss-of-function mutation within GNAS, leading to decreased activity of PTH receptor G-protein and renal tubule resistance to PTH. Patients can have features of Albright's hereditary osteodystrophy (AHO), which includes short stature, subcutaneous ossifications (heterotopic ossifications), reduced mental acuity, round faces, central obesity, dental hypoplasia, and brachydactyly (shortening of the metacarpals and metatarsals, particularly of the third, fourth, and fifth metacarpals and metatarsals). Hormone resistance to thyroid-stimulating hormone, growth hormone–releasing hormone, follicle-stimulating hormone, and luteinizing hormone can also occur. AHO features and consequences of hormone resistance can develop over a variable time frame and are of variable severity [58]. PHP type 1c is phenotypically similar to PHP type 1a but differs, in that the activity of the PTH receptor G-protein is normal [57].

PHP type 1b is an autosomal dominant disorder that can be familial or sporadic (most common), and it is due to maternally inherited imprinting abnormalities of GNAS [58]. Patients with PHP type 1b do not present with features of AHO.

Type 2 Pseudohypoparathyroidism

Patients with PHP type 2 have impaired urinary phosphate excretion due to PTH unresponsiveness. They present with hypocalcemia and hyperphosphatemia without features of AHO. PHP type 2 may be associated with vitamin D deficiency [57].

Other Etiologies of Hypocalcemia

Hungry Bone Syndrome

After resolution of prolonged PTH elevation, excessive deposition of calcium into the bone can occur. This typically occurs immediately after parathyroidectomy for primary hyperparathyroidism and is characterized by hypocalcemia, hypocalciuria, and hypophosphatemia.

Hyperphosphatemia

Acute increases in serum phosphate levels due to intravenous phosphate administration, use of phosphate-containing enemas, rhabdomyolysis, or tumor lysis syndrome can result in profound hypocalcemia due to formation of phosphate-calcium complexes that precipitate in bone or soft tissue. Hyperphosphatemia, through its negative feedback on PTH, also decreases bone resorption and activation of 1,25-dihydroxyvitamin D, contributing to hypocalcemia.

Blood Transfusions

High-volume infusions of citrated blood products result in citrate-calcium complexes that precipitate in plasma and result in low serum ionized calcium levels.

Acute Pancreatitis

Hypocalcemia can occur early in pancreatitis and is thought to be due to the formation of calcium-free fatty acid "soaps," leading to reduced serum ionized calcium levels [59].

The History Can Help Determine the Etiology of Hypocalcemia

A focused history is the essential first step in determining the etiology of hypocalcemia. The age of onset and duration of hypocalcemia can help differentiate between congenital and acquired forms. Prenatal and birth history, such as maternal medical conditions, 25-hydroxyvitamin D status and medications, gestational age, and Apgar score at birth can provide clues to the etiology of neonatal hypocalcemia and direct further evaluation. Associated symptoms, such as signs of cardiac disease, immunodeficiencies, learning disability, neurological symptoms, or symptoms suggestive of other endocrinopathies, can point to syndromic causes of hypocalcemia. Family history of hypocalcemia, autoimmunity, or congenital syndromes may also suggest possible diagnoses. Dietary history, or history suggestive of intestinal malabsorption, such as diarrhea or weight loss, may suggest inadequate intake and stores of calcium and 25-hydroxyvitamin D. Medication lists and the presence of comorbidities, such as epilepsy, cancer (particularly hematologic malignancies with high risk for tumor lysis syndrome), or sickle cell anemia (requiring frequent blood transfusions), are essential components of the history.

Physical Findings of Hypocalcemia

Newborns with hypocalcemia can have nonspecific symptoms and may appear quite ill with hypotension or bradycardia. An EKG should be performed in any patient with an abnormal cardiac exam, if there is clinical concern for hypocalcemia, or if hypocalcemia is detected by laboratory tests.

The neurologic examination can help elicit signs of neuronal irritability. Sensory deficits in hands or feet or signs of spontaneous tetany, including muscle twitching, may be observed. The Chvostek sign is positive in 10–25% of healthy people and absent in up to 30% of patients with hypocalcemia [60, 61]. Therefore, it is neither sensitive nor specific for hypocalcemia. The Trousseau sign may be more specific for hypocalcemia, as it is seen less often in healthy individuals. In some patients, particularly neonates [62], seizures may be the only indication of hypocalcemia. In these patients, EEGs should be performed.

Clues to the underlying etiology include bowing of the legs, which suggests rickets, whereas developmental delay or cardiac anomalies may suggest DiGeorge syndrome. Patients with PHP type 1a/c have short stature, central obesity, and /or shortening of the metacarpals and metatarsals. A surgical scar on the neck may indicate post-surgical hypoparathyroidism. Table 5.3 summarizes common physical findings associated with hypocalcemia in pediatric patients.

Initiating the Laboratory Evaluation

Serum calcium, albumin, ionized calcium, PTH, 25-hydroxyvitamin D, phosphorous, and magnesium levels are the initial blood tests to evaluate for hypocalcemia. These labs will indicate whether hypocalcemia is associated with a

Table 5.3 Clinical features of hypocalcemia and clues to the etiology

Physical exam	Findings of hypocalcemia	Clues to determine the etiology
Vital signs	Hypotension, bradycardia (particularly in neonates)	–
Head, ear, nose and throat	Chvostek sign (evoked facial muscle twitching)	Facial dysmorphia (DiGeorge or CHARGE), ear anomalies, choanal atresia (CHARGE)
Eyes	Papilledema and cataracts (in severe hypocalcemia)	Coloboma (CHARGE)
Mouth	Dental caries, enamel hypoplasia (when hypocalcemic early in life)	Cleft lip/palate (DiGeorge), thrush (APECED)
Neck	–	Surgical scar (post-surgical hypoparathyroidism)
Cardiovascular	Prolonged QT interval on EKG, jugular venous distension, and/or gallop rhythm (in heart failure)	Murmur, sternal scar (DiGeorge or CHARGE)
Respiratory	Respiratory distress (bronchospasm or laryngospasm)	–
Abdomen	–	Epigastric tenderness (pancreatitis)
Extremities	Muscle twitching, muscle spasm of fingers, hands, wrists, ankles, and toes	Bowing of legs (rickets), brachydactyly, short stature (PHP type 1a/c)
Neurologic	Sensory deficit around mouth, hands, feet, seizure activity	Sensorineural hearing loss (HDR syndrome)
Psychiatric	Delirium, depression, anxiety, psychosis, and cognitive impairment	Developmental delay

low (or inappropriately normal) or high PTH. Renal function and liver function tests, 1,25-dihydroxyvitamin D level, as well as urinary calcium and/or phosphate excretion studies may also be helpful. If there is a family history of hypocalcemia, or concerns for genetic syndromes, genetic testing should be considered.

References

1. Myrtle JF, Norman AW. Vitamin D: a cholecalciferol metabolite highly active in promoting -intestinal calcium transport. Science. 1971;171(3966):79–82. https://doi.org/10.1126/science.171.3966.79.
2. Haussler MR, Boyce DW, Littledike ET, Rasmussen H. A rapidly acting metabolite of vitamin D3. Proc Natl Acad Sci U S A. 1971;68(1):177–81. https://doi.org/10.1073/pnas.68.1.177.
3. Omdahl J, Holick M, Suda T, Tanaka Y, DeLuca HF. Biological activity of 1,25-dihydroxycholecalciferol. Biochemistry. 1971;10(15):2935–40. https://doi.org/10.1021/bi00791a022.
4. Holick MF, Schnoes HK, DeLuca HF. Identification of 1,25-dihydroxycholecalciferol, a form of vitamin D3 metabolically active in the intestine. Proc Natl Acad Sci U S A. 1971;68(4):803–4. https://doi.org/10.1073/pnas.68.4.803.
5. Brown EM. Role of the calcium-sensing receptor in extracellular calcium homeostasis. Best Pract Res Clin Endocrinol Metab. 2013;27(3):333–43. https://doi.org/10.1016/j.beem.2013.02.006.
6. Omdahl JL. Interaction of the parathyroid and 1,25-dihydroxyvitamin D3 in the control of renal 25-hydroxyvitamin D3 metabolism. J Biol Chem. 1978;253(23):8474–8.
7. Henry HL, Midgett RJ, Norman AW. Regulation of 25-hydroxyvitamin D3-1-hydroxylase in vivo. J Biol Chem. 1974;249(23):7584–92.
8. Raisz LG. Bone resorption in tissue culture. Factors influencing the response to parathyroid hormone. J Clin Invest. 1965;44:103–16. https://doi.org/10.1172/jci105117.
9. Reynolds JJ, Dingle JT. A sensitive in vitro method for studying the induction and inhibition of bone resorption. Calcif Tissue Res. 1970;4(4):339–49. https://doi.org/10.1007/bf02279136.
10. Bouhtiauy I, Lajeunesse D, Brunette MG. The mechanism of parathyroid hormone action on calcium reabsorption by the distal tubule. Endocrinology. 1991;128(1):251–8. https://doi.org/10.1210/endo-128-1-251.
11. Kitazawa R, Kitazawa S. Vitamin D(3) augments osteoclastogenesis via vitamin D-responsive element of mouse RANKL gene promoter. Biochem Biophys Res Commun. 2002;290(2):650–5. https://doi.org/10.1006/bbrc.2001.6251.
12. Scheven BA, Hamilton NJ. Retinoic acid and 1,25-dihydroxyvitamin D3 stimulate osteoclast formation by different mechanisms. Bone. 1990;11(1):53–9. https://doi.org/10.1016/8756-3282(90)90072-7.
13. Friedman PA, Gesek FA. Cellular calcium transport in renal epithelia: measurement, mechanisms, and regulation. Physiol Rev. 1995;75(3):429–71. https://doi.org/10.1152/physrev.1995.75.3.429.
14. Chambers TJ, McSheehy PM, Thomson BM, Fuller K. The effect of calcium-regulating hormones and prostaglandins on bone resorption by osteoclasts disaggregated from neonatal rabbit bones. Endocrinology. 1985;116(1):234–9. https://doi.org/10.1210/endo-116-1-234.
15. Nabeshima Y. The discovery of alpha-Klotho and FGF23 unveiled new insight into calcium and phosphate homeostasis. Cell Mol Life Sci. 2008;65(20):3218–30. https://doi.org/10.1007/s00018-008-8177-0.
16. Macefield G, Burke D. Paraesthesiae and tetany induced by voluntary hyperventilation. Increased excitability of human cutaneous and motor axons. Brain. 1991;114. (Pt 1B:527–40. https://doi.org/10.1093/brain/114.1.527.
17. Fanconi A, Rose GA. The ionized, complexed, and protein-bound fractions of calcium in plasma; an investigation of patients with various diseases which affect calcium metabolism, with an additional study of the role of calcium ions in the prevention of tetany. Q J Med. 1958;27(108):463–94.
18. Han P, Trinidad BJ, Shi J. Hypocalcemia-induced seizure: demystifying the calcium paradox. ASN Neuro. 2015;7(2) https://doi.org/10.1177/1759091415578050.
19. Nardone R, Brigo F, Trinka E. Acute symptomatic seizures caused by electrolyte disturbances. J Clin Neurol. 2016;12(1):21–33. https://doi.org/10.3988/jcn.2016.12.1.21.
20. Swash M, Rowan AJ. Electroencephalographic criteria of hypocalcemia and hypercalcemia. Arch Neurol. 1972;26(3):218–28. https://doi.org/10.1001/archneur.1972.00490090044003.

21. Aggarwal S, Kailash S, Sagar R, Tripathi M, Sreenivas V, Sharma R, et al. Neuropsychological dysfunction in idiopathic hypoparathyroidism and its relationship with intracranial calcification and serum total calcium. Eur J Endocrinol. 2013;168(6):895–903. https://doi.org/10.1530/eje-12-0946.
22. Sugar O. Central neurological complications of hypoparathyroidism. AMA Arch Neurol Psychiatry. 1953;70(1):86–107. https://doi.org/10.1001/archneurpsyc.1953.02320310092008.
23. Goswami R, Sharma R, Sreenivas V, Gupta N, Ganapathy A, Das S. Prevalence and progression of basal ganglia calcification and its pathogenic mechanism in patients with idiopathic hypoparathyroidism. Clin Endocrinol. 2012;77(2):200–6. https://doi.org/10.1111/j.1365-2265.2012.04353.x.
24. Mitchell DM, Regan S, Cooley MR, Lauter KB, Vrla MC, Becker CB, et al. Long-term follow-up of patients with hypoparathyroidism. J Clin Endocrinol Metab. 2012;97(12):4507–14. https://doi.org/10.1210/jc.2012-1808.
25. Hochman HI, Mejlszenkier JD. Cataracts and pseudotumor cerebri in an infant with vitamin D-deficiency rickets. J Pediatr. 1977;90(2):252–4. https://doi.org/10.1016/s0022-3476(77)80643-4.
26. Reddy CV, Gould L, Gomprecht RF. Unusual electrocardiographic manifestations of hypocalcemia. Angiology. 1974;25(11):764–8. https://doi.org/10.1177/000331977402501105.
27. Lehmann G, Deisenhofer I, Ndrepepa G, Schmitt C. ECG changes in a 25-year-old woman with hypocalcemia due to hypoparathyroidism. Hypocalcemia mimicking acute myocardial infarction. Chest. 2000;118(1):260–2. https://doi.org/10.1378/chest.118.1.260.
28. Wong CK, Lau CP, Cheng CH, Leung WH, Freedman B. Hypocalcemic myocardial dysfunction: short- and long-term improvement with calcium replacement. Am Heart J. 1990;120(2):381–6. https://doi.org/10.1016/0002-8703(90)90083-a.
29. Bashour T, Basha HS, TO C. Hypocalcemic cardiomyopathy. Chest. 1980;78(4):663–5. https://doi.org/10.1378/chest.78.4.663.
30. Cusano NE, Bilezikian JP. Signs and symptoms of hypoparathyroidism. Endocrinol Metab Clin N Am. 2018;47(4):759–70. https://doi.org/10.1016/j.ecl.2018.07.001.
31. Kinirons MJ, Glasgow JF. The chronology of dentinal defects related to medical findings in hypoparathyroidism. J Dent. 1985;13(4):346–9. https://doi.org/10.1016/0300-5712(85)90032-6.
32. Kovacs CS, Lanske B, Hunzelman JL, Guo J, Karaplis AC, Kronenberg HM. Parathyroid hormone-related peptide (PTHrP) regulates fetal-placental calcium transport through a receptor distinct from the PTH/PTHrP receptor. Proc Natl Acad Sci U S A. 1996;93(26):15233–8. https://doi.org/10.1073/pnas.93.26.15233.
33. Wills MR, Bruns DE, Savory J. Disorders of calcium homeostasis in the fetus and neonate. Ann Clin Lab Sci. 1982;12(2):79–88.
34. Tsang RC, Kleinman LI, Sutherland JM, Light IJ. Hypocalcemia in infants of diabetic mothers. Studies in calcium, phosphorus, and magnesium metabolism and parathormone responsiveness. J Pediatr. 1972;80(3):384–95. https://doi.org/10.1016/s0022-3476(72)80494-3.
35. Tsang RC, Chen I, Friedman MA, Gigger M, Steichen J, Koffler H, et al. Parathyroid function in infants of diabetic mothers. J Pediatr. 1975;86(3):399–404. https://doi.org/10.1016/s0022-3476(75)80970-x.
36. Venkataraman PS, Tsang RC, Greer FR, Noguchi A, Laskarzewski P, Steichen JJ. Late infantile tetany and secondary hyperparathyroidism in infants fed humanized cow milk formula. Longitudinal follow-up. Am J Dis Child. 1985;139(7):664–8. https://doi.org/10.1001/archpedi.1985.02140090026018.
37. Gafni RI, Collins MT. Hypoparathyroidism. N Engl J Med. 2019;380(18):1738–47. https://doi.org/10.1056/NEJMcp1800213.
38. Jyonouchi S, McDonald-McGinn DM, Bale S, Zackai EH, Sullivan KE. CHARGE (coloboma, heart defect, atresia choanae, retarded growth and development, genital hypoplasia, ear anomalies/deafness) syndrome and chromosome 22q11.2 deletion syndrome: a comparison of immunologic and nonimmunologic phenotypic features. Pediatrics. 2009;123(5):e871–7. https://doi.org/10.1542/peds.2008-3400.
39. Mannstadt M, Bilezikian JP, Thakker RV, Hannan FM, Clarke BL, Rejnmark L, et al. Hypoparathyroidism. Nat Rev Dis Primers. 2017;3:17055. https://doi.org/10.1038/nrdp.2017.55.
40. Kisand K, Peterson P. Autoimmune polyendocrinopathy candidiasis ectodermal dystrophy. J Clin Immunol. 2015;35(5):463–78. https://doi.org/10.1007/s10875-015-0176-y.
41. Han SI, Tsunekage Y, Kataoka K. Gata3 cooperates with Gcm2 and MafB to activate parathyroid hormone gene expression by interacting with SP1. Mol Cell Endocrinol. 2015;411:113–20. https://doi.org/10.1016/j.mce.2015.04.018.
42. Harvey JN, Barnett D. Endocrine dysfunction in Kearns-Sayre syndrome. Clin Endocrinol. 1992;37(1):97–103. https://doi.org/10.1111/j.1365-2265.1992.tb02289.x.
43. Naiki M, Ochi N, Kato YS, Purevsuren J, Yamada K, Kimura R, et al. Mutations in HADHB, which encodes the beta-subunit of mitochondrial trifunctional protein, cause infantile onset hypoparathyroidism and peripheral polyneuropathy. Am J Med Genet A. 2014;164a(5):1180–7. https://doi.org/10.1002/ajmg.a.36434.
44. Burren CP, Curley A, Christie P, Rodda CP, Thakker RV. A family with autosomal dominant hypocalcaemia with hypercalciuria (ADHH): mutational analysis, phenotypic variability and treatment challenges. J Pediatr Endocrinol Metab. 2005;18(7):689–99. https://doi.org/10.1515/jpem.2005.18.7.689.
45. Watanabe S, Fukumoto S, Chang H, Takeuchi Y, Hasegawa Y, Okazaki R, et al. Association between activating mutations of calcium-sensing receptor and Bartter's syndrome. Lancet. 2002;360(9334):692–4. https://doi.org/10.1016/s0140-6736(02)09842-2.
46. Tenhola S, Voutilainen R, Reyes M, Toiviainen-Salo S, Juppner H, Makitie O. Impaired growth and intracranial calcifications in autosomal dominant hypocalcemia caused by a GNA11 mutation. Eur J Endocrinol. 2016;175(3):211–8. https://doi.org/10.1530/eje-16-0109.
47. Kifor O, McElduff A, LeBoff MS, Moore FD Jr, Butters R, Gao P, et al. Activating antibodies to the calcium-sensing receptor in two patients with autoimmune hypoparathyroidism. J Clin Endocrinol Metab. 2004;89(2):548–56. https://doi.org/10.1210/jc.2003-031054.
48. de Jong M, Nounou H, Rozalen Garcia V, Christakis I, Brain C, Abdel-Aziz TE, et al. Children are at a high risk of hypocalcaemia and hypoparathyroidism after total thyroidectomy. J Pediatr Surg. 2019; https://doi.org/10.1016/j.jpedsurg.2019.06.027.
49. Kamath SD, Rao BS. Delayed post-surgical hypoparathyroidism: the forgotten chameleon! J Clin Diagn Res. 2017;11(2):Od07–od9. https://doi.org/10.7860/jcdr/2017/23609.9260.
50. Agus ZS. Hypomagnesemia. J Am Soc Nephrol. 1999;10(7):1616–22.
51. Holick MF, Chen TC, Lu Z, Sauter E. Vitamin D and skin physiology: a D-lightful story. J Bone Miner Res. 2007;22 Suppl 2:V28–33. https://doi.org/10.1359/jbmr.07s211.
52. Cheng JB, Levine MA, Bell NH, Mangelsdorf DJ, Russell DW. Genetic evidence that the human CYP2R1 enzyme is a key vitamin D 25-hydroxylase. Proc Natl Acad Sci U S A. 2004;101(20):7711–5. https://doi.org/10.1073/pnas.0402490101.
53. Brodie MJ, Boobis AR, Hillyard CJ, Abeyasekera G, Stevenson JC, MacIntyre I, et al. Effect of rifampicin and isoniazid on vitamin D metabolism. Clin Pharmacol Ther. 1982;32(4):525–30. https://doi.org/10.1038/clpt.1982.197.
54. Fraser D, Kooh SW, Kind HP, Holick MF, Tanaka Y, DeLuca HF. Pathogenesis of hereditary vitamin-D-dependent rickets. An inborn error of vitamin D metabolism involving defective conversion of 25-hydroxyvitamin D to 1 alpha,25-dihydroxyvitamin

D. N Engl J Med. 1973;289(16):817–22. https://doi.org/10.1056/nejm197310182891601.
55. Wang JT, Lin CJ, Burridge SM, Fu GK, Labuda M, Portale AA, et al. Genetics of vitamin D 1alpha-hydroxylase deficiency in 17 families. Am J Hum Genet. 1998;63(6):1694–702. https://doi.org/10.1086/302156.
56. Malloy PJ, Pike JW, Feldman D. The vitamin D receptor and the syndrome of hereditary 1,25-dihydroxyvitamin D-resistant rickets. Endocr Rev. 1999;20(2):156–88. https://doi.org/10.1210/edrv.20.2.0359.
57. Clarke BL, Brown EM, Collins MT, Juppner H, Lakatos P, Levine MA, et al. Epidemiology and diagnosis of hypoparathyroidism. J Clin Endocrinol Metab. 2016;101(6):2284–99. https://doi.org/10.1210/jc.2015-3908.
58. review MGC. Pseudohypoparathyroidism: diagnosis and treatment. J Clin Endocrinol Metab. 2011;96(10):3020–30. https://doi.org/10.1210/jc.2011-1048.
59. Stewart AF, Longo W, Kreutter D, Jacob R, Burtis WJ. Hypocalcemia associated with calcium-soap formation in a patient with a pancreatic fistula. N Engl J Med. 1986;315(8):496–8. https://doi.org/10.1056/nejm198608213150806.
60. Hoffman E. The Chvostek sign; a clinical study. Am J Surg. 1958;96(1):33–7. https://doi.org/10.1016/0002-9610(58)90868-7.
61. Fonseca OA, Calverley JR. Neurological manifestations of hypoparathyroidism. Arch Intern Med. 1967;120(2):202–6.
62. Thomas TC, Smith JM, White PC, Adhikari S. Transient neonatal hypocalcemia: presentation and outcomes. Pediatrics. 2012;129(6):e1461–7. https://doi.org/10.1542/peds.2011-2659.

Hypercalcemia

6

Anna Chin and Lisa Swartz Topor

Introduction

Calcium is an essential mineral that directly affects bone stability, muscle contraction, nerve conduction, and membrane voltage potential. Serum calcium concentration is tightly regulated by complex interactions between parathyroid hormone (PTH) via the calcium-sensing receptor (CaSR), 1,25-dihydroxyvitamin D, and calcitonin [1]. These compounds act on multiple organ systems to maintain serum calcium within a narrow range. Please refer to Chapter 5, Hypocalcemia, for a detailed description of calcium homeostasis.

Under normal physiologic conditions, PTH secretion is inversely proportional to the circulating ionized calcium level, which binds to the CaSR in the parathyroid gland [2]. Serum calcium accounts for 0.1–0.2% of extracellular calcium and only 1% of total body calcium. The majority of total body calcium is stored in bone. Ionized calcium is the physiologically active form of serum calcium and accounts for approximately 40% of the total serum calcium. Non-ionized calcium is bound primarily to albumin, with a smaller fraction bound to other anions such as citrate, bicarbonate, and phosphorus. In hypoalbuminemic states, the total calcium level is low due to decreased binding sites, while the ionized calcium level remains unaffected. The formula for calculating total calcium in the setting of low albumin concentration is:

$$\text{Serum calcium}\left(\text{mg / dl}\right) + 0.8\left(4 - \text{serum albumin}\left[\text{mg / dl}\right]\right)^{3}$$

A. Chin · L. S. Topor (✉)
Department of Pediatric Endocrinology, Warren Alpert Medical School of Brown University and Hasbro Children's Hospital, Providence, RI, USA
e-mail: anna_chin1@brown.edu; lisa_swartz_topor@brown.edu

Definition

Hypercalcemia is defined as a serum total or ionized calcium that is above the upper limit of the normal range, which is age dependent. The variation in reference ranges (Table 6.1) is due to changes in normal physiology depending on developmental stage [3].

Pediatric hypercalcemia does not have a formal classification or grading system. Greater elevations in plasma calcium levels are associated with an increased likelihood of experiencing symptoms of hypercalcemia. In the adult population, severity of hypercalcemia is classified as mild (serum calcium concentration <12 mg/dl), moderate (serum calcium concentration 12–14 mg/dl), and severe (serum calcium concentration >14 mg/dl) [4]. Most hypercalcemia in the pediatric population is mild, asymptomatic, and identified incidentally on laboratory evaluation for an unrelated condition [5]. Severe hypercalcemia is rare, occurring in about 1 in 500 children in a general hospital setting, and most frequently seen in neonates due to sepsis [6].

Table 6.1 Age-specific reference ranges for total and ionized serum calcium level

	Total calcium range		Ionized calcium range	
Age range	mg/dl	mmol/L	mg/dl	mmol/L
0–90 days	8.0–11.3	2.0–2.8	Not reported	Not reported
91–180 days	8.9–11.2	2.0–2.8	Not reported	Not reported
181 days – 1 year	9.0–11.3	2.3–2.8	Not reported	Not reported
1–3 years	8.9–11.1	2.2–2.8	4.80–5.52	1.20–1.38
4–11 years	8.7–10.7	2.2–2.7	4.80–5.52	1.20–1.38
12–18 years	8.5–10.7	2.1–2.7	4.80–5.52	1.20–1.38
>19 years	8.5–10.5	2.2–2.6	4.64–5.28	1.16–1.32

Adapted from Stokes et al. [4]

T. Stanley, M. Misra (eds.), *Endocrine Conditions in Pediatrics*, https://doi.org/10.1007/978-3-030-52215-5_6

Signs and Symptom of Hypercalcemia

The range of symptoms of hypercalcemia in the pediatric population will vary based on age and severity of serum calcium elevation. Symptoms may be nonspecific, especially in neonates and infants. Classic signs and symptoms become more prevalent with increasing age among pediatric patients. The well-known mnemonic for signs and symptoms associated with hypercalcemia, "Stones, Bones, Groans, Moans, Thrones, and Psychiatric Overtones" reflects different organ systems affected by calcium excess, as described below:

- *Stones and Thrones*: Excess circulating calcium and deposition of calcium in the kidney parenchyma and tubules can lead to nephrocalcinosis and nephrolithiasis. Stimulation of renal CaSR in the collecting tubule leads to decreased aquaporin-2 expression on the apical membrane, creating a state of vasopressin resistance and polyuria, with subsequent development of polydipsia [7]. Severe cases can result in renal failure [1–3, 5, 6, 8–10].
- *Bones*: Ninety-nine percent of total body calcium is stored in the bone. PTH-dependent hypercalcemia causes increased bone turnover. Subsequent derangements in bone remodeling can lead to increased fragility, pain, and risk of fractures [2, 3, 5, 10, 11]. In primary hyperparathyroidism (PHPT), osteitis fibrosa cystica is a classic finding and should be included in the differential diagnosis when lytic or multilobular cystic changes are identified on radiographic imaging [12].
- *Groans*: Gastrointestinal symptoms associated with hypercalcemia include nonspecific abdominal pain, constipation, nausea, anorexia, vomiting, peptic ulcer disease, and pancreatitis, depending on the etiology of hypercalcemia [2, 3, 5, 10, 13]. Hypercalcemia in the setting of hyperparathyroidism has been associated with increased gastric secretion, leading to stomach and duodenal ulcers [14]. In neonates and infants, failure to thrive may be the only symptom of hypercalcemia [3]. Hypercalcemia reduces neuromuscular excitability and causes atonia in gastrointestinal muscles, which may contribute to pain and constipation [15].
- *Psychiatric undertones*: Calcium plays a significant role in transmembrane migration of potassium and sodium ions. Hypercalcemia may increase electrical resistance of the cell membrane to ion migration and exert a depressive effect on neuronal excitability [16]. It is unclear whether this proposed mechanism accounts for the vague neuropsychiatric symptoms seen in the pediatric population. Symptoms include weakness, hypotonia, lethargy, and, rarely, seizures. In older children and adolescents, symptoms can include fatigue, depression, anorexia, and rarely psychosis [2, 3, 6, 10].
- *Other systemic manifestations*: Cardiovascular system—excess calcium can increase calcium deposition in blood vessels, cardiac myocardium, and cardiac valves [17], leading to hypertension and left ventricular hypertrophy [18]. Hypercalcemia can cause a shortened QT interval, and prolonged PR and QRS intervals, which can lead to arrhythmias [18].

Causes of Hypercalcemia in the Pediatric Patient

Causes of hypercalcemia vary by age and can be categorized into PTH-independent and PTH-dependent categories, and then into genetic versus acquired causes. Table 6.2 summarizes the differential diagnosis of hypercalcemia.

Table 6.2 Differential diagnosis of hypercalcemia

PTH-independent			
	Acquired		
		Neonates and infants	
			Prematurity
			Sepsis
			Enriched formula/ inappropriately supplemented parental nutrition
			Phosphate depletion
			Excessive ingestion of vitamin D
			Vitamin A intoxication
			Subcutaneous fat necrosis (SCFN)
			Congenital hypothyroidism
			Extracorporeal membrane oxygenation (ECMO)
		Children and adolescents	
			Excessive ingestion of vitamin D
			Excessive ingestion of calcium (milk-alkali syndrome)
			Immobilization
			Malignancy
			Hyperthyroidism
			Adrenal insufficiency
			Pheochromocytoma
			Granulomatous disease
	Genetic		Familial hypocalciuric hypercalcemia (FHH)
			Hypophosphatasia
			Williams syndrome
			Blue diaper syndrome

Table 6.2 (continued)

PTH-independent			
			Congenital lactase deficiency
			Bartter syndrome
			IMAGe syndrome
			Jansen metaphyseal chondrodysplasia
PTH-dependent			
	Acquired		
		Neonates and infants	
			Neonatal hyperparathyroidism
		Children and adolescents	
			Parathyroid adenoma
			Parathyroid carcinoma
	Genetic		
			Neonatal severe hyperparathyroidism (NSHPT)
			Familial multiglandular hyperplasia
			Multiple endocrine neoplasias (MEN)
			Hyperparathyroidism-jaw tumor

PTH-Independent Hypercalcemia

These are organized by age for the acquired forms, followed by genetic causes:

- Acquired:
  - Neonates and infancy:

    Prematurity: Most hypercalcemia due to prematurity is transient, owing to immaturity of kidneys, intestines, and parathyroid glands [19]. However, calcium levels require close monitoring and further evaluation to rule out neonatal severe hyperparathyroidism (NSHPT) or other genetic causes based upon duration and degree of hypercalcemia.

    Sepsis and critical illness: Though most commonly associated with hypocalcemia [20], sepsis can also cause hypercalcemia. The mechanism of hypercalcemia is not entirely understood but is possibly related to extrarenal production of $1{,}25(OH)_2D$ by infiltrating macrophages, and/or release of cytokines such as interleukin 6 (IL-6) that increase osteoclastic activity and lead to calcium release [6].

    Enriched formula/inappropriately supplemented parental nutrition: Hypercalcemia due to excessive calcium intake can be seen when term infants are fed high-calcium formula designed for preterm infants, who have higher calcium requirements [21, 22].

    Phosphate depletion: Inadequate consumption of phosphate, malabsorption of phosphate, which can be seen in chronic antacid use, or immature renal function leading to phosphate wasting can lead to hypophosphatemia. Low serum phosphate levels cause suppression of circulating fibroblast growth factor 23 (FGF23), leading to disinhibition of calcitriol production [1] and subsequent hypercalcemia. PTH levels are typically suppressed.

    Excessive ingestion of vitamin D: A "mild" or Lightwood variant of idiopathic infantile hypercalcemia was described in the 1950s when high-dose vitamin D fortification was used. Hypervitaminosis D can also occur in older children due to consumption of milk or other foods with excess fortification or due to excessive vitamin D intake [23]. In this condition, the 25-hydroxyvitamin D level is elevated with variable 1,25-dihydroxyvitamin D levels and suppression of PTH. Hypercalcemia resolves with elimination or correction of excess vitamin D intake [21]

    Vitamin A intoxication: Excessive maternal vitamin A ingestion during pregnancy leading to hypercalcemia is rare. Symptoms of vitamin A intoxication include poor feeding, irritability, bone pain, tender swelling of bone, osteopenia, and hyperostosis of long bone shafts [24].

    Subcutaneous fat necrosis (SCFN): This condition occurs in newborns, typically following perinatal stress (trauma, hypothermia, or fetal distress) [25]. In SCFN, granulomatous infiltrates form in response to inflammation and soft tissue necrosis. Macrophages within these infiltrates produce 1-alpha-hydroxylase, leading to increased production of 1,25-dihydroxyvitamin D and subsequent hypercalcemia. The degree of hypercalcemia is further exacerbated by calcium directly released from necrotic fat tissue and increased prostaglandin E activity [2]. Workup reveals normal 25-hydroxyvitamin D levels, elevated 1,25-dihydroxyvitamin D, and suppressed PTH levels [26]. Treatment is with glucocorticoids and low-calcium formula. Hypercalcemia is typically transient, though the sequelae of hypercalcemia can cause significant morbidity. Skin lesions can persist for months.

    Congenital hypothyroidism: The mechanism of hypercalcemia is unknown and resolves with thyroid replacement [21]. Every state in the United States is mandated to screen for congenital hypothyroidism via newborn screening program.

Extracorporeal membrane oxygenation (ECMO): The mechanism of hypercalcemia is thought to be related to disruption of calcium homeostasis through mechanical factors utilized by ECMO therapy. Use of ECMO can also cause hypocalcemia. Normocalcemia is usually restored once ECMO is discontinued [20].

– Older children:

Excess calcium intake (milk-alkali syndrome): Milk-alkali syndrome is caused by ingestion of large amounts of calcium and base [27] (e.g., excess calcium carbonate intake as treatment of heartburn symptoms) and manifests with hypercalcemia, metabolic alkalosis, and varying degrees of renal failure. PTH level is suppressed.

Vitamin D intoxication: Hypercalcemia may result from excess vitamin D intake, similar to what is seen in neonates and infants.

Immobilization: Acute immobilization results in reduction in osteoblastic activity and increase in osteoclastic activity. Calcium and phosphate are released from the bone, leading to hypercalcemia and hypercalciuria. Patients are at increased risk of decreased bone mineral density, fracture, and nephrolithiasis. Calcium levels normalize with return to mobility and weight-bearing exercise. Bisphosphonate treatment has been used in cases of prolonged immobilization [10].

Malignancy: Hypercalcemia due to malignancy occurs in less than 1% of children with cancer. Pediatric malignancies associated with hypercalcemia include leukemia, lymphoma, myeloma, neuroblastoma, hepatocellular carcinoma, hepatoblastoma, rhabdomyosarcoma, brain cancer, and dysgerminomas. Multiple mechanisms can lead to malignancy-related hypercalcemia. Osteolysis from direct invasion of bone by tumor cells can release calcium directly from bone. Humoral factors from tumor production, including parathyroid-related protein (PTHrP) and 1,25-dihydroxyvitamin D, increase osteoclastic bone resorption. Finally, hypercalcemia can result from direct tumor production of osteoclast-activating factors such as interleukin-1 and 6 (IL-1, IL-6), tumor necrosis factor alpha (TNF-α), and prostaglandins [10].

Hyperthyroidism: Excess triiodothyronine (T3) in hyperthyroidism acts directly on osteoclasts to increase turnover and resorption, leading to hypercalcemia [10, 28]. Hypercalcemia resolves with treatment and normalization of thyroid function.

Adrenal insufficiency: Hypercalcemia is seen in both primary and secondary adrenal insufficiency without a clear underlying etiology. Proposed mechanisms include altered vitamin D synthesis due to glucocorticoid deficiency and/or volume depletion from mineralocorticoid deficiency [10, 28]. Hypercalcemia resolves with glucocorticoid replacement and volume resuscitation [28].

Pheochromocytoma: Hypercalcemia due to pheochromocytoma has been reported in the adult population. One study showed detectable PTHrP levels from tumor extracts [29].

Granulomatous disease: Tuberculosis, sarcoidosis, and certain infectious diseases that activate macrophages are classified as granulomatous diseases. Macrophages undergo a granulomatous reaction in the setting of systemic inflammation, which leads to increased 1,25-hydroxyvitamin D levels and subsequent hypercalcemia [2, 10, 21, 28, 30].

- Genetic:
  - *Familial hypocalciuric hypercalcemia (FHH) (or familial benign hypercalcemia (FBH))*: Inactivating mutations of the calcium-sensing receptor (CaSR) in the parathyroid glands, which play a key role in calcium homeostasis [2, 10, 28], cause FHH. These mutations decrease the sensitivity of parathyroid cells to extracellular calcium, leading to asymptomatic, mild to moderate hypercalcemia. PTH concentrations are typically normal or mildly elevated. The CaSR is also expressed in the kidney, and decreased receptor activity in the distal nephron leads to hypocalciuria [2]. Inheritance is typically in an autosomal dominant fashion and the phenotype is benign. FHH does not require treatment. Homozygous, and rarely paternally inherited heterozygous or de novo heterozygous, mutations of the calcium-sensing receptor (*CASR)* gene can present with neonatal severe hyperparathyroidism, a life-threatening condition causing severe hypercalcemia within the first few weeks of life [2, 10, 28].
  - *Hypophosphatasia (HPP)*: Mutations in the Tissue Nonspecific Alkaline Phosphatase (*ALPL or TNSALP*) gene cause alkaline phosphatase deficiency, leading to impaired bone mineralization. Defective calcium uptake results in hypercalcemia with hypercalciuria and nephrocalcinosis. HPP is classified into six clinical forms, depending on the age at diagnosis and the severity of symptoms. Infantile hypophosphatasia presents before age 6 months and can include craniosynostosis and respiratory complications due to rachitic deformities of the ribs. Workup will show low serum total and bone-specific alkaline phosphatase and elevated levels of urinary phosphoethanolamine. In 2019, a biologic treatment, asfotase alfa (Strensiq), was approved in the United States for pediatric-onset HPP [31].

- *Williams syndrome (or Williams-Beuren syndrome)*: Deletion at chromosome 7q11.23 [10] causes Williams syndrome and occurs in 1 in 10,000 births. Hypercalcemia may present in the neonatal period and usually resolves, although there are reports of its return during adolescence [2, 10, 21, 32]. The etiology of hypercalcemia may be related to increased sensitivity to vitamin D [2, 10, 28]. Dietary calcium restriction may be required [10]. Guidelines for management of Williams syndrome [32] include monitoring serum calcium level at least every 2–3 years or annually if initially elevated at baseline. Urinary calcium-creatinine ratio should be measured every 2 years. Serum calcium should also be measured anytime there are signs and symptoms of hypercalcemia. Other findings in Williams syndrome include small for gestational age, feeding difficulties, developmental delay, nephrocalcinosis, joint hypermobility, congenital heart disease, characteristic craniofacial abnormalities, and loquacious personality [32].
- *Blue diaper syndrome*: This is a rare metabolic disorder caused by a defect in tryptophan metabolism that leads to increased urinary excretion of indole derivatives, giving urine-soaked diapers a blue tint. Findings include hypercalcemia, hypercalciuria, and nephrocalcinosis. The mechanism of hypercalcemia is unknown [2, 33].
- *Congenital lactase deficiency*: Loss of function of the enzyme intestinal protein lactase-phlorizin hydrolase (*LPH*) causes this condition and is inherited in an autosomal recessive fashion. Hypercalcemia may be due to metabolic acidosis or the presence of non-hydrolyzed lactose that promotes calcium absorption [34]. Hypercalcemia usually resolves after initiation of a lactose-free diet, but hypercalciuria and nephrocalcinosis may persist [2].
- *Bartter syndrome (BS)*: Multiple genetic mutations have been described in BS. Hypercalcemia has been described in some infants with homozygous inactivation of the furosemide-sensitive NaK-2Cl-cotransporter (NKCC2) from the Solute Carrier Family 12 member 1 (*SLC12A1*) gene or inwardly rectifying potassium channel (ROMK) from *KCNJ1* gene [2]. Loss-of-function mutation of *SLC12A1* may result in altered threshold of the calcium-sensing receptor in the kidney leading to hypercalcemia [35].
- *IMAGe syndrome*: This is a disorder with findings of *I*UGR, *M*etaphyseal dysplasia, congenital *A*drenal hypoplasia, and *Ge*nital defects [2, 36]. Several modes of inheritance have been proposed, with the strongest evidence supporting a maternally inherited, autosomal dominant variant in the Cyclin-Dependent Kinase Inhibitor 1C (*CDKN1C*) gene [36]. Hypercalcemia can be variable, and it is unclear whether it is related to the syndrome or secondary to adrenal insufficiency [36].
- *Jansen metaphyseal chondrodysplasia*: This condition is caused by heterozygous mutations in the Parathyroid Hormone 1 Receptor (*PTHR1*) gene resulting in constitutively activated PTH/PTHrP receptor. PTH levels are low or undetectable in the setting of hypercalcemia, hypophosphatemia, hypercalciuria, and nephrocalcinosis [10, 37]. Patients have characteristic skeletal abnormalities due to slowed chondrocyte maturation and marked growth plate abnormalities. Growth is typically normal in infancy, and short stature develops later in childhood [10]. Hypercalcemia is persistent, and while no specific treatment is available, use of bisphosphonates and thiazide diuretics may help with bone and renal disease [37].

PTH-Dependent Causes

- Neonates and infants:
  - Acquired:

    Neonatal hyperparathyroidism: Persistent intrauterine hypocalcemia from maternal hypocalcemia stimulates increased production of fetal PTH and leads to hypercalcemia and bone demineralization [10, 38]. This form of neonatal hyperparathyroidism is typically transient with a variable phenotype. Findings can include bone deformities, fractures at birth, and respiratory difficulties if ribs are affected. It is imperative to distinguish this from neonatal severe hyperparathyroidism (NSHPT) with maternal laboratory testing and early analysis of the *CaSR* gene if indicated [10].
  - Genetic:

    Neonatal severe hyperparathyroidism (NSHPT): This condition is caused by homozygous inactivating mutations of the *CaSR* gene (which in the heterozygous form causes FHH) [10, 21, 39]. It is an autosomal-recessive disorder, though cases with paternally inherited heterozygous mutations or apparent de novo heterozygous mutations have been reported [2]. Most infants present in the first few weeks of life but presentation in later childhood has been reported [6]. Findings include severe hypercalcemia, hypophosphatemia, elevated PTH, and skeletal deformities. Treatment includes bisphosphonates, calcimimetics, and, eventually, subtotal parathyroidectomy for cure [2, 10, 21, 39]. Postoperatively, severe hypocalcemia from "hungry bone syndrome" may require large quantities of intravenous calcium [10, 39].

- Older children:
  - Acquired:

    Parathyroid adenoma: Up to 90% of cases of primary hyperparathyroidism (PHPT) in the pediatric population are due to parathyroid adenomas [28]. These adenomas are typically sporadic and often (65% of the time) due to a single parathyroid adenoma. Patients with PHPT are typically symptomatic at presentation but may have end-organ damage. PHPT may also be diagnosed after an incidental finding of hypercalcemia. Imaging typically includes ultrasound and/or a parathyroid scan using 99mTc-sestamibi scintigraphy with single-photon emission computed tomography SPECT/CT (if available) [40].

    Parathyroid carcinoma: This is extremely rare in children, accounting for 1% of cases of primary hyperparathyroidism [28].
  - Genetic:

    Multi-glandular parathyroid hyperplasia: Ten to 15% of primary hyperparathyroidism in the pediatric population is due to multi-glandular hyperplasia and is usually associated with a genetic condition [28]. Findings include inappropriately elevated or normal serum PTH levels, elevated urine calcium-to-creatinine ratio, and nephrocalcinosis in the setting of hypercalcemia. Bone demineralization is less commonly seen in children compared to adults [40]. Surgical excision of abnormal parathyroid tissue is the only definitive cure. This may include resection of a solitary enlarged gland or total four-gland parathyroidectomy with autotransplantation of parathyroid tissue to the neck or forearm [37, 41].

    The most commonly associated genetic syndromes are:

    Familial isolated hyperparathyroidism: This is distinct from MEN1 and 2A, characterized by a positive family history of hyperparathyroidism, adenomatous changes of the parathyroid glands, and absence of other MEN features [42].

    Multiple endocrine neoplasias (MEN) [43]:
    - *Type 1*: This is due to pathogenic Multiple Endocrine Neoplasia type 1 (*MEN1*) variants [41] that follow an autosomal dominant pattern of inheritance, though up to 70% of cases are de novo. It is characterized by hyperplasia of the parathyroid cells as well as pituitary and pancreatic islet cell neoplasms. PHPT is the most common presenting feature and manifests in 95% of patients [41].
    - *Type 2A*: This is due to pathogenic Rearranged During Transfection *(RET)* variants [41] that follow an autosomal dominant inheritance pattern. MEN 2A is characterized by medullary thyroid carcinoma, pheochromocytoma, and hyperparathyroidism. Those with high-risk alleles carry a 20–30% risk for PHPT [41].
    - *Type 4*: This is due to pathogenic Cyclin-Dependent Kinase Inhibitor 1B (*CDKN1B)* variants [41] that follow an autosomal dominant inheritance pattern. Nearly 100% of patients have PHPT.

    Hyperparathyroidism-jaw tumor: This is due to pathogenic Cell Division Cycle 73 (*CDC73)* variants [41] that follow an autosomal dominant inheritance pattern with high, but incomplete, penetrance. It is rare and characterized by ossifying fibromas of the jaw and occasionally parathyroid carcinoma [41].

Evaluation and Assessment of Hypercalcemia

In cases of incidental hypercalcemia without signs or symptoms, a serum calcium concentration should be repeated to confirm hypercalcemia. If calcium levels are persistently elevated, investigation is warranted [10], including a thorough review of the gastrointestinal, renal and urologic, musculoskeletal, neurologic, cardiac, and endocrine systems [44].

A medical history, including recent surgeries, birth history, and maternal history, may provide important information regarding the timing of onset of hypercalcemia. Family history of hypercalcemia, renal stones, parathyroidectomy, or features of multiple endocrine neoplasia syndromes can help narrow the differential diagnosis to acquired versus genetic causes [10]. A medication history should include vitamins, supplements, or complementary alternative medicines.

The physical examination should include a review of vital signs using age-appropriate ranges and a thorough examination with key physical exam findings detailed in Table 6.3. Some of these physical exam findings have specific etiologies.

Laboratory evaluation: Once hypercalcemia has been confirmed, other laboratory studies should include a basic metabolic panel, evaluation of renal function, magnesium, phosphorus, and liver function tests, including alkaline phosphatase, 25-hydroxyvitamin D, 1,25-hydroxyvitamin D, and PTH levels. Urine studies should include urinalysis and spot urine for calcium, phosphorus, and creatinine. Twenty-four-hour urine collections to measure calcium and creatinine may be helpful to determine the degree of calcium excretion.

Depending on lab results, imaging studies may include bone radiographs, renal ultrasound, or parathyroid imaging.

Table 6.3 Physical exam findings in hypercalcemia

	Physical exam findings	Potential etiology
Vital signs	Hypertension	Pheochromocytoma
	Hypotension	Adrenal insufficiency
	Tachycardia	Pheochromocytoma
	Underweight	Williams syndrome
General	Failure to thrive	
	Dysmorphic features	Williams syndrome
	Dehydration	
	Lethargy	
	Irritability	
HEENT	Mucous membranes	
	Exophthalmos	Hyperthyroidism
	Tongue fasciculations	Hyperthyroidism
Neck	Goiter	Hyper- or hypothyroidism
	Lymphadenopathy	Malignancy or granulomatous disease
Cardiovascular	Tachycardia	Hyperthyroidism and pheochromocytoma
	Abnormal heart sounds	
	Arrhythmias	
Abdominal	Tenderness	
	Hypoactive bowel sounds	
Extremities	Edema	
	Weakness	
	Bony tenderness	Hypophosphatasia and phosphate depletion
	Bony deformities	Jansen metaphyseal chondrodysplasia
Neurologic	Hypotonia	
	Hyporeflexia	
	Tremors	
Psychiatric	Psychosis	

Treatment and Management

Severe or symptomatic hypercalcemia warrants urgent treatment, and typically requires hospitalization. Treatment goals are to decrease serum calcium levels by increasing urinary calcium excretion and decreasing bone resorption.

Acute management of hypercalcemia [2, 10, 21, 44] includes aggressive hydration and volume expansion with intravenous normal saline with or without diuretics to increase urinary calcium excretion. Bisphosphonates are used to decrease osteoclastic bone resorption. Use of bisphosphonates requires close electrolyte monitoring as patients will be at risk for hypocalcemia, hypophosphatemia, and hypomagnesemia. Calcitonin can acutely lower serum calcium concentrations and is typically well tolerated. The development of rapid hormone resistance and tachyphylaxis within a few doses are the major disadvantages of calcitonin therapy. Case reports have described use of the calcimimetic cinacalcet in treatment of severe hypercalcemia in children [45, 46], but this is not FDA approved for children. Hemodialysis with a low-calcium dialysate is reserved for life-threatening hypercalcemia resistant to medications [10].

Non-acute management [10, 21, 44] focuses on treating the underlying cause of hypercalcemia. Glucocorticoids have been used in SCFN and granulomatous disease, but chronic use increases risk of impaired linear growth, decreased bone mineralization, and immunosuppression. In Williams syndrome or idiopathic infantile hypercalcemia, a low-calcium formula or reduced calcium diet is typically adequate to maintain normocalcemia. Surgical resection is the only treatment for primary hyperparathyroidism and results in cure. FHH typically does not require treatment.

Referral to Pediatric Endocrinology

Pediatric endocrinology should evaluate any patient with symptomatic or persistent hypercalcemia. Patients with an underlying endocrinopathy may require regular follow-up and long-term treatment. Genetic causes of hypercalcemia may require multidisciplinary management from endocrinology as well as genetics, nephrology, surgery, otolaryngology, orthopedic surgery, or developmental and behavioral pediatrics.

References

1. Ghosh AK, Joshi SR. Disorders of calcium, phosphorus and magnesium metabolism. J Assoc Physicians India. 2008;56:613–21.
2. Lietman SA, Germain-Lee EL, Levine MA. Hypercalcemia in children and adolescents. Curr Opin Pediatr. 2010;22(4):508–15. https://doi.org/10.1097/MOP.0b013e32833b7c23.
3. Stokes VJ, Nielsen MF, Hannan FM, Thakker RV. Hypercalcemic disorders in children. J Bone Miner Res. 2017;32(11):2157–70. https://doi.org/10.1002/jbmr.3296.
4. Bushinsky DA, quintet MRDE. calcium. Lancet. 1998;352(9124):306–11.
5. Auron A, Alon US. Hypercalcemia: a consultant's approach. Pediatr Nephrol. 2018;33(9):1475–88. https://doi.org/10.1007/s00467-017-3788-z. Epub 2017 Sep 6.
6. McNeilly JD, Boal R, Shaikh MG, Ahmed SF. Frequency and aetiology of hypercalcaemia. Arch Dis Child. 2016;101(4):344–7. https://doi.org/10.1136/archdischild-2015-309029. Epub 2016 Feb 22.
7. Clarkson MR, Magee CN, Brenner BM. Mineral bone disease in chronic kidney disease. In: Brenner BM, editor. Pocket companion to Brenner and rector's the kidney. Philadelphia: Elsevier; 2010. p. 616–36.
8. Moe SM. Disorders involving calcium, phosphorus, and magnesium. Prim Care. 2008;35(2):215–vi. https://doi.org/10.1016/j.pop.2008.01.007.
9. Vaidya SR, Aeddula NR. Nephrocalcinosis. [Updated 2019 Jan 7]. In: StatPearls [Internet]. Treasure Island, FL: StatPearls Publishing; 2019.

10. Davies JH, Shaw NJ. Investigation and management of hypercalcaemia in children. Arch Dis Child. 2012;97(6):533–8. https://doi.org/10.1136/archdischild-2011-301284. Epub 2012 Mar 23.
11. Stewart AF. Hyperparathyroidism, humoral hypercalcemia of malignancy, and the anabolic actions of parathyroid hormone and parathyroid hormone-related protein on the skeleton. J Bone Miner Res. 2002;17:758.
12. Misiorowski W, Czajka-Oraniec I, Kochman M, Zgliczyński W, Bilezikian JP. Osteitis fibrosa cystica-a forgotten radiological feature of primary hyperparathyroidism. Endocrine. 2017;58(2):380–5. https://doi.org/10.1007/s12020-017-1414-2.
13. Chang WT, Radin B, McCurdy MT. Calcium, magnesium, and phosphate abnormalities in the emergency department. Emerg Med Clin North Am. 2014;32(2):349–66. https://doi.org/10.1016/j.emc.2013.12.006. Epub 2014 Feb 19.
14. Barreras RF, Donaldson RM Jr. Role of calcium in gastric hypersecretion, parathyroid adenoma and peptic ulcer. N Engl J Med. 1967;276(20):1122–4. https://doi.org/10.1056/NEJM196705182762005.
15. Ragno A, et al. Chronic constipation in hypercalcemic patients with primary hyperparathyroidism. Eur Rev Med Pharmacol Sci. 2012;16(7):884–9.
16. Karpati G, Frame B. Neuropsychiatric disorders in primary hyperparathyroidism. Arch Neurol. 1964;10:387–97. https://doi.org/10.1001/archneur.1964.00460160057005.
17. Brown SJ, Ruppe MD, Tabatabai LS. The parathyroid gland and heart disease. Methodist Debakey Cardiovasc J. 2017;13(2):49–54. https://doi.org/10.14797/mdcj-13-2-49.
18. Walker MD, Silverberg SJ. Cardiovascular aspects of primary hyperparathyroidism. J Endocrinol Invest. 2008;31(10):925–31. https://doi.org/10.1007/BF03346443.
19. Abu Raya B, et al. Transient hypercalcemia in preterm infants: insights into natural history and laboratory evaluation. Glob Pediatr Health. 2014;1:2333794X14560818. . Published 2014 Nov 21. https://doi.org/10.1177/2333794X14560818.
20. Hak EB, et al. Increased parathyroid hormone and decreased calcitriol during neonatal extracorporeal membrane oxygenation. Intensive Care Med. 2005;31(2):264–70. Epub 2005 Feb 1.
21. Rodd C, Goodyer P. Hypercalcemia of the newborn: etiology, evaluation, and management. Pediatr Nephrol. 1999;13(6):542–7. https://doi.org/10.1007/s004670050654.
22. Baker SS, et al. American Academy of Pediatrics Committee on Nutrition: calcium requirements of infants, children, and adolescents. Pediatrics. 1999;104(5 Pt 1):1152–7.
23. Jacobus CH, et al. Hypervitaminosis D associated with drinking milk. N Engl J Med. 1992;326(18):1173–7.
24. Conaway HH, Henning P, Lerner UH. Vitamin a metabolism, action, and role in skeletal homeostasis. Endocr Rev. 2013;34(6):766–97. https://doi.org/10.1210/er.2012-1071. Epub 2013 May 29.
25. Farooque A, et al. Expression of 25-hydroxyvitamin D3-1alpha-hydroxylase in subcutaneous fat necrosis. Br J Dermatol. 2009;160(2):423–5. https://doi.org/10.1111/j.1365-2133.2008.08844.x.
26. Kruse K, Irle U, Uhlig R. Elevated 1,25-dihydroxyvitamin D serum concentrations in infants with subcutaneous fat necrosis. J Pediatr. 1993;122(3):460–3. https://doi.org/10.1016/s0022-3476(05)83441-9.
27. Felsenfeld AJ, Levine BS. Milk alkali syndrome and the dynamics of calcium homeostasis. Clin J Am Soc Nephrol. 2006;1(4):641–54. Epub 2006 Apr 26.
28. Goltzman D, et al. Approach to hypercalcemia. South Dartmouth, MA: MDText.com, Inc.; 2019.
29. Kimura S, et al. A case of pheochromocytoma producing parathyroid hormone-related protein and presenting with hypercalcemia. Clin Endocrinol Metab. 1990;70(6):1559–63.
30. Lagishetty V, et al. 1alpha-hydroxylase and innate immune responses to 25-hydroxyvitamin D in colonic cell lines. J Steroid Biochem Mol Biol. 2010;121(1–2):228–33. https://doi.org/10.1016/j.jsbmb.2010.02.004.
31. Whyte MP. Hypophosphatasia: an overview for 2017. Bone. 2017;102:15–25. https://doi.org/10.1016/j.bone.2017.02.011. Epub 2017 Feb 24.
32. American Academy of Pediatrics Committee on Genetics. Health care supervision for children with Williams syndrome. Pediatrics. 2001;107(5):1192–204.
33. Distelmaier F, et al. Blue diaper syndrome and PCSK1 mutations. Pediatrics. 2018;141(Suppl 5):S501–5. https://doi.org/10.1542/peds.2017-0548.
34. Saarela T, Similä S, Koivisto M. Hypercalcemia and nephrocalcinosis in patients with congenital lactase deficiency. J Pediatr. 1995;127(6):920–3.
35. Wongsaengsak S, et al. A novel SLC12A1 gene mutation associated with hyperparathyroidism, hypercalcemia, nephrogenic diabetes insipidus, and nephrocalcinosis in four patients. Bone. 2017;97:121–5. https://doi.org/10.1016/j.bone.2017.01.011. Epub 2017 Jan 14.
36. Bennett J, Schrier Vergano SA, Deardorff MA. IMAGe syndrome. In: Adam MP, Ardinger HH, Pagon RA, et al., editors. GeneReviews. Seattle: University of Washington; 1993–2019.
37. Saito H, et al. Progression of mineral ion abnormalities in patients with Jansen metaphyseal chondrodysplasia. J Clin Endocrinol Metab. 2018;103(7):2660–9. https://doi.org/10.1210/jc.2018-00332.
38. Glass EJ, Barr DG. Transient neonatal hyperparathyroidism secondary to maternal pseudohypoparathyroidism. Arch Dis Child. 1981;56(7):565–8. https://doi.org/10.1136/adc.56.7.565.
39. Cole DE, et al. Neonatal severe hyperparathyroidism, secondary hyperparathyroidism, and familial hypocalciuric hypercalcemia: multiple different phenotypes associated with an inactivating Alu insertion mutation of the calcium-sensing receptor gene. Am J Med Genet. 1997;71(2):202–10.
40. Huang CB, et al. Primary hyperparathyroidism in children: report of a case and a brief review of the literature. J Formos Med Assoc. 1993;92(12):1095–8.
41. Wasserman JD, Tomlinson GE, Druker H, et al. Multiple endocrine neoplasia and hyperparathyroid-jaw tumor syndromes: clinical features, genetics, and surveillance recommendations in childhood. Clin Cancer Res. 2017;23(13):e123–32. https://doi.org/10.1158/1078-0432.CCR-17-0548.
42. Kollars J, et al. Primary hyperparathyroidism in pediatric patients. Pediatrics. 2005;115(4):974–80.
43. Multiple endocrine neoplasia. Lister Hill National Center for Biomedical Communications U.S. National Library of Medicine National Institutes of Health Department of Health & Human Services. https://ghr.nlm.nih.gov/condition/multiple-endocrine-neoplasia. Published December 10, 2019. Accessed December 20, 2019.
44. Mancilla E, Levine M. Hypocalcemia, hypercalcemia, and hypercalciuria. In: TK MI, American Academy of Pediatrics, editors. American Academy of Pediatrics Textbook of Pediatric Care. 2nd ed. Elk Grove Village: American Academy of Pediatrics; 2017. p. 2170–9.
45. Mogas E, et al. Successful use of cinacalcet to treat parathyroid-related hypercalcemia in two pediatric patients. Endocrinol Diabetes Metab Case Rep. 2018;2018:18–0009. . Published 2018 Jun 6. https://doi.org/10.1530/EDM-18-0009.
46. Fisher MM, Cabrera SM, Imel EA. Successful treatment of neonatal severe hyperparathyroidism with cinacalcet in two patients. Endocrinol Diabetes Metab Case Rep. 2015;2015:150040. https://doi.org/10.1530/EDM-15-0040.

7 Hypophosphatemia

Cemre Robinson

Introduction

Inorganic phosphate (Pi), which is present in every cell of the body, is a critical element in bone mineralization, skeletal development, and cellular signaling. Pi is the second most abundant mineral in the body and an integral component of nucleic acids and energy metabolism. The serum Pi level is maintained within a narrow normal range to allow for optimal cellular function such as generation of ATP, phosphorylation of key enzymes, and skeletal mineralization [1].

Hypophosphatemia is defined as a serum Pi level below the age-appropriate normal range. Normal serum Pi levels in children are considerably higher than those in adults [2–3]. The serum Pi levels peak in the neonatal period, ranging between approximately 6.0 mg/dL and 8.0 mg/dL, then progressively decline until late puberty when they reach the normal adult range, between 2.5 mg/dL and 4.5 mg/dL. Pi levels can fluctuate with age, dietary intake, acid-base status, and the time of the day. Hypophosphatemia can be acute or chronic. Acute hypophosphatemia is most commonly seen in hospitalized infants or children due to redistribution of phosphorus secondary to respiratory alkalosis [1]. Chronic hypophosphatemia is often discovered incidentally, and the diagnosis can be missed in the pediatric population as many children are asymptomatic or, more importantly, a low serum Pi level in a young child might be misinterpreted as normal if adult reference range is used.

Phosphate Homeostasis

Phosphate in the body is predominantly stored in bone [2]. The remaining intracellular "free" phosphate concentration is maintained by sodium-coupled transport proteins [2]. Pi homeostasis is regulated tightly through complex interactions between intestinal absorption, renal Pi excretion, and exchange between intracellular and mineralized bone storage pools [4, 5]. The primary endocrine regulators of bone Pi homeostasis are the fibroblast growth factor 23 (FGF23), parathyroid hormone (PTH), and 1,25-dihydroxyvitamin D (1,25$(OH)_2$D), calcitriol [5].

Pi is abundant in the diet. Approximately 80% of dietary Pi is absorbed in the small intestine by sodium-dependent phosphate cotransporter type IIb (Npt2b), which is regulated by dietary Pi intake and 1,25$(OH)_2$D. The majority of renal Pi reabsorption occurs at the proximal tubule via type IIa sodium-phosphate (Npt2a) and type IIc (Npt2c) cotransporters [6]. At steady state, daily Pi intake is balanced by excretion in the urine and feces [6].

FGF23 is a circulating hormone produced by osteocytes and osteoblasts, which regulates Pi reabsorption at the level of the kidney [5, 7]. High levels of FGF23 cause hypophosphatemia by downregulating Npt2a and Npt2c in the proximal renal tubule, decreasing the renal Pi reabsorption. FGF23 also decreases 1,25D-dependent intestinal Pi absorption, further contributing to hypophosphatemia [8]. Overall, 1,25$(OH)_2$D increases Pi reabsorption in the proximal tubule [9]. PTH, in contrast, causes phosphaturia and decreased renal reabsorption of Pi at the proximal tubule.

Mechanisms of Hypophosphatemia

Mechanisms for hypophosphatemia include decreased intake or absorption, transcellular shifts from extracellular to intracellular space, and excessive renal losses (Table 7.1) [10].

Decreased Supply of Phosphorus

As Pi is present in large amounts in most foods, dietary Pi deficiency is uncommon in most cases. In addition, renal phosphate reabsorption increases as a compensatory mechanism in cases of decreased intake. Instances of

C. Robinson (✉)
Division of Pediatric Endocrinology and Diabetes, Icahn School of Medicine at Mount Sinai, New York, NY, USA
e-mail: cemre.robinson@mssm.edu

T. Stanley, M. Misra (eds.), *Endocrine Conditions in Pediatrics*, https://doi.org/10.1007/978-3-030-52215-5_7

Table 7.1 Etiology of hypophosphatemia in children [10]

Decreased Pi intake and/or absorption	Transcellular shifts	Increased urinary Pi excretion
		FGF23-mediated
Poor dietary intake	Refeeding syndrome	X-linked dominant hypophosphatemic rickets (*PHEX*)
Malnutrition/ starvation	Glucose or insulin infusion	X-linked recessive hypophosphatemic rickets (*CLCN5*)
Chronic diarrhea/ steatorrhea	Respiratory alkalosis	Autosomal dominant hypophosphatemic rickets (*FGF23*)
Malabsorption	Salicylate poisoning	Autosomal recessive hypophosphatemic rickets 1 (*DMP1*)
Medications (antacids with aluminum, magnesium, or calcium)	Catecholamines	Autosomal recessive hypophosphatemic rickets 2 (*ENPP1*)
Vitamin D deficiency	Hyperalimentation (TPN)	*Non-FGF23-mediated*
		Hyperparathyroidism
		Diuretics: Loop diuretics, thiazides, acetazolamide
		Antineoplastic drugs: Cisplatin, ifosfamide
		Antiretroviral agents: Tenofovir, adefovir
		Aminoglycosides
		Hypokalemia
		Hypomagnesemia

Adapted from Root and Diamond [10]

dietary insufficiency include disorders of malabsorption such as short bowel syndrome, children receiving parenteral nutrition, and premature infants who consume breast milk without supplemental Pi [11–13]. In addition, antacids can cause a net Pi loss by binding to both ingested and secreted (intestinal) Pi [14–16] and preventing absorption.

Transcellular Shifts

Refeeding syndrome and respiratory alkalosis are common causes of hypophosphatemia secondary to transcellular shifts [1]. The increased pH of respiratory alkalosis decreases serum Pi concentration through stimulation of phosphofructokinase, which is the rate-limiting step of glycolysis [1]. Glycolysis decreases serum Pi by inducing intracellular phosphorus entry for use in ATP production. In refeeding syndrome, surging insulin stimulates an intracellular shift of Pi, resulting in Pi depletion [17].

Excessive Renal Losses

Increased urinary excretion of Pi, also known as renal Pi wasting, can result from inherited or acquired renal disorders. Hyperphosphaturia can be either an FGF23-mediated or non-FGF23-mediated process (Table 7.1). Inherited disorders of renal Pi wasting generally manifest in infancy. The prototypical disorder of renal Pi wasting is X-linked hypophosphatemic rickets (XLH) [18]. XLH is caused by a loss-of-function mutation in the *PHEX* gene resulting in excess FGF23 and leading to renal Pi wasting and hypophosphatemic rickets. These children usually come to medical attention due to bowing of the extremities. On examination, they typically have rickets, frontal bossing, and short stature. Other inherited forms of hypophosphatemia and their associated gene mutations are listed in Table 7.1 [10].

Acquired renal Pi wasting can result from Fanconi syndrome, nephrotic syndrome, renal tubular insult, oncogenic osteomalacia, or medications such as steroids or loop diuretics [19]. Children with long-standing vitamin D deficiency can develop secondary hyperparathyroidism. Both primary and secondary hyperparathyroidism can cause hypophosphatemia by stimulating increased urinary Pi excretion.

Common Signs and Symptoms and Risk Factors

Most children with hypophosphatemia are asymptomatic, and the symptoms are nonspecific [19]. Presenting complaints for children with hypophosphatemia may include generalized weakness, fatigue, bone pain, and/or bowing of the extremities. The symptoms depend on the duration, severity, and etiology of hypophosphatemia.

Hypophosphatemia can be life threatening in severe conditions such as malnutrition, refeeding syndrome, sepsis, or diabetic ketoacidosis [20–22] as it can cause rhabdomyolysis or myocardial dysfunction [19]. Acutely, children may present with irritability, confusion, altered mental status, seizures, or focal neurologic findings such as numbness [23]. Neonates born prematurely or with very-low-birth weight are prone to metabolic derangements such as hypophosphatemia [24]. Certain medications such as antacids, glucocorticoids, cisplatin, and bisphosphonate use can place children at increased risk for developing hypophosphatemia.

Chronically, the most common symptoms are generalized muscle weakness and fatigue. Hypophosphatemia can lead to chronic bone demineralization and rickets, which is manifested by skeletal deformities such as bowing of the lower extremities [18].

Common causes and cannot-miss causes of hypophosphatemia are depicted below:

Common Causes
- Critical illness
- Prematurity
- Malabsorption
- Medications

Cannot-Miss Causes
- Rickets
- Respiratory or metabolic alkalosis
- Treatment of diabetic ketoacidosis
- Refeeding syndrome

Evaluation

History

The evaluation of a child with hypophosphatemia should include a detailed dietary history with particular attention given to overall nutritional status, the type of elemental formula provided to neonates and infants, and any suggestion of a gastrointestinal or malabsorptive problem. Though uncommon, elemental formula–associated hypophosphatemia has been reported in children whose clinical, biochemical, and radiographic evaluations were consistent with rickets [11, 25, 26] and resolved after a change in formula. Medication history and family history can give clues to the etiology of hypophosphatemia.

Important aspects of the history in a child with hypophosphatemia include the following:
- Prematurity or very-low-birth weight
- Generalized weakness or fatigue
- Chronic diseases such as malabsorption
- Frequent or recurrent bone pain
- History of fractures
- Bowing of the extremities
- Use of certain medications such as antacids

Physical Examination

On physical examination, it is important to pay close attention to the weight, height, body mass index (BMI), and head circumference of the child to assess the overall nutritional status. Skeletal deformities such as frontal bossing, widened wrists, and bowing of the extremities are suggestive of rickets. A complete musculoskeletal exam should assess for hypotonia, which could be related to musculoskeletal disorders. The neurological exam could reveal proximal muscle weakness.

Key Physical Exam Findings
- Decreased subcutaneous adipose tissue
- Hypotonia
- Frontal bossing
- Bowing of the extremities
- Proximal muscle weakness

Laboratory Evaluation

Hypophosphatemia is diagnosed by measuring the serum phosphorus ideally in the fasting state. Age-appropriate pediatric reference ranges should be used in the interpretation of the result. Once the diagnosis of hypophosphatemia is established, the next step is to determine whether this hypophosphatemia is due to excessive renal losses or decreased intake [19] by calculating the tubular reabsorption of phosphate (TRP) according to the formula given below. Then, the established nomogram is used to determine the ratio of tubular maximum reabsorption of phosphate to glomerular filtration rate—(TmP/GFR) [27]. A urine sample should be collected ideally after an overnight fast. The first morning void should be discarded, and the second specimen should be collected and sent for testing. Low TRP values, less than 0.86, suggest renal wasting.

$$\text{TRP} = 1 - (\text{urine phosphate} \times \text{serum creatinine}) / (\text{serum phosphate} \times \text{urine creatinine})$$

In addition to checking serum phosphorus, other pertinent diagnostic studies include serum total and ionized calcium, BUN, creatinine, sodium, potassium, magnesium, intact PTH, alkaline phosphatase, and vitamin D studies, including 25-hydroxyvitamin D (25(OH)D) and $1,25(OH)_2D$ and urine calcium, Pi, creatinine, and pH. These studies aid in the diagnosis of possible vitamin D deficiency and/or secondary hyperparathyroidism as the etiology of the hypophosphatemia. It is also useful to screen for other potential electrolyte abnormalities such as hypokalemia or hypomagnesemia.

25(OH)D is the major circulating form of vitamin D and is the best indicator of vitamin D status. $1,25(OH)_2D$ is the biologically active form of vitamin D. In the presence of hypophosphatemia, $1,25(OH)_2D$ levels are expected to be high because hypophosphatemia stimulates 1α-hydroxylation of calcidiol in the proximal convoluted tubule cells of the kidney and produces calcitriol [28]. However, an inappropriately low or normal 1,25$(OH)_2D$ can be seen in inherited forms of hypophosphatemia mediated by excess levels of FGF23 [18, 29]. Alkaline phosphatase is a surrogate marker for bone healing and is the most useful biomarker for gauging skeletal response to therapy [18].

Pertinent laboratory workup:

- Serum Pi, total and ionized calcium, intact PTH, alkaline phosphatase, BUN, creatinine, sodium, potassium, magnesium, and 25(OH)D and 1,25$(OH)_2D$
- Urine calcium, Pi, creatinine, and pH

Imaging Studies

Radiologic studies, including plain radiographs, are not required for the correct diagnosis, yet should be obtained in those children who present with skeletal symptoms, in order to establish the severity of rickets and to exclude diagnoses of physiologic bowing and other skeletal dysplasias [18]. Standing leg radiographs with particular attention to the growth plates in the knee are particularly helpful. Imaging studies do not differentiate the etiology of rickets, for example, caused by hypophosphatemia versus nutritional vitamin D deficiency. However, baseline plain films serve as a reference point for monitoring progress as the skeleton, and especially growth plates, begin to heal.

Management of Hypophosphatemia

Treatment of hypophosphatemia depends on the underlying etiology. In critically ill patients, correction of hypophosphatemia should be made with parenteral potassium phosphate or sodium phosphate. Mild or stable cases can be corrected with oral replacement [3]. Recommended dosing of phosphorus supplements in children are given below [3]:

Acute hypophosphatemia:

- 5–10 mg/kg/dose IV over 6 hours

Maintenance/replacement:

- *IV:* 15–45 mg/kg over 24 h
- *PO:* 30–90 mg/kg/24 h divided TID or QID

Chronic hypophosphatemia such as inherited hypophosphatemic rickets should be referred to a pediatric endocrinologist. Further studies, including determination of renal Pi excretion, genetic testing when indicated, and other relevant imaging studies, are undertaken by the pediatric endocrinologist. In general, the standard therapy for disorders of FGF23-mediated hypophosphatemia involves multiple daily doses of oral Pi salts and active vitamin D analogs such as calcitriol [18]. Treatment is indicated at least until growth is complete and, in many cases, beyond to ensure proper skeletal healing and development and to enhance linear growth [30]. Close biochemical monitoring is important to assess potential side effects of treatment such as secondary hyperparathyroidism, hypercalciuria, and/or nephrocalcinosis. A novel therapy option, burosumab, which is a human monoclonal antibody against FGF23, has been approved for use in XLH [31]. Burosumab is injected subcutaneously every 2 weeks, and, importantly, Pi supplementation is contraindicated while on this therapy.

Conclusion

Hypophosphatemia can be acute or chronic and results from three main mechanisms, including decreased intake, transcellular shifts, and increased renal excretion. Proper management is differential based on the etiology. Since serum Pi plays a critical role in skeletal mineralization, rickets can be an important clinical manifestation. Further workup and management are undertaken following referral to a pediatric endocrinologist.

References

1. Amanzadeh J, Reilly RF Jr. Hypophosphatemia: an evidence-based approach to its clinical consequences and management. Nat Clin Pract Nephrol. 2006;2(3):136–48.
2. Sharma S, Hashmi MF, Castro D. Hypophosphatemia. In: StatPearls. Treasure Island, FL: StatPearls Publishing LLC; 2019.
3. Kleinman K, McDaniel L, Molloy M, editors. The Harriet Lane Handbook: The Johns Hopkins Hospital, 22nd Edition. Elsevier; 2020. p. 974.
4. Takeda E, Taketani Y, Sawada N, Sato T, Yamamoto H. The regulation and function of phosphate in the human body. BioFactors (Oxford, England). 2004;21(1–4):345–55.
5. Bergwitz C, Juppner H. Phosphate sensing. Adv Chronic Kidney Dis. 2011;18(2):132–44.
6. Blaine J, Chonchol M, Levi M. Renal control of calcium, phosphate, and magnesium homeostasis. Clin J Am Soc Nephrol. 2015;10(7):1257–72.
7. White KE, Larsson TE, Econs MJ. The roles of specific genes implicated as circulating factors involved in normal and disordered phosphate homeostasis: frizzled related protein-4, matrix extracellular phosphoglycoprotein, and fibroblast growth factor 23. Endocr Rev. 2006;27(3):221–41.
8. Clinkenbeard EL, White KE. Systemic control of bone homeostasis by FGF23 signaling. Curr Mol Biol Rep. 2016;2(1):62–71.
9. Kurnik BR, Hruska KA. Mechanism of stimulation of renal phosphate transport by 1,25-dihydroxycholecalciferol. Biochim Biophys Acta. 1985;817(1):42–50.
10. Root AW, FBDJ MD. Disorders of mineral homeostasis in children and adolescents. In: Sperling MA, editor. Pediatric endocrinology. 4th ed. Philadelphia, PA: Elsevier; 2014. p. 734–845.
11. Creo AL, Epp LM, Buchholtz JA, Tebben PJ. Prevalence of metabolic bone disease in tube-fed children receiving elemental formula. Horm Res Paediatr. 2018;90(5):291–8.

12. Leitner M, Burstein B, Agostino H. Prophylactic phosphate supplementation for the inpatient treatment of restrictive eating disorders. J Adolesc Health. 2016;58(6):616–20.
13. Bustos Lozano G, Hidalgo Romero A, Melgar Bonis A, Ureta Velasco N, Orbea Gallardo C, Pallas Alonso C. [Early hypophosphataemia in at risk newborns. Frequency and magnitude]. Anales De Pediatria (Barcelona, Spain : 2003). 2018;88(4):216–22.
14. Lotz M, Zisman E, Bartter FC. Evidence for a phosphorus-depletion syndrome in man. N Engl J Med. 1968;278(8):409–15.
15. Pivnick EK, Kerr NC, Kaufman RA, Jones DP, Chesney RW. Rickets secondary to phosphate depletion. A sequela of antacid use in infancy. Clin Pediatr. 1995;34(2):73–8.
16. Shields HM. Rapid fall of serum phosphorus secondary to antacid therapy. Gastroenterology. 1978;75(6):1137–41.
17. Mehanna HM, Moledina J, Travis J. Refeeding syndrome: what it is, and how to prevent and treat it. BMJ (Clinical research ed). 2008;336(7659):1495–8.
18. Carpenter TO, Imel EA, Holm IA, Jan de Beur SM, Insogna KL. A clinician's guide to X-linked hypophosphatemia. J Bone Miner Res. 2011;26(7):1381–8.
19. Assadi F. Hypophosphatemia: an evidence-based problem-solving approach to clinical cases. Iran J Kidney Dis. 2010;4(3):195–201.
20. Yoshimatsu S, Hossain MI, Islam MM, Chisti MJ, Okada M, Kamoda T, et al. Hypophosphatemia among severely malnourished children with sepsis in Bangladesh. Pediatr Int. 2013;55(1):79–84.
21. Shah SK, Shah L, Bhattarai S, Giri M. Rhabdomyolysis due to severe hypophosphatemia in diabetic ketoacidosis. JNMA. 2015;53(198):137–40.
22. Choi HS, Kwon A, Chae HW, Suh J, Kim DH, Kim HS. Respiratory failure in a diabetic ketoacidosis patient with severe hypophosphatemia. Ann Pediatr Endocrinol Metabol. 2018;23(2):103–6.
23. de Oliveira Iglesias SB, Pons Leite H, de Carvalho WB. Hypophosphatemia-induced seizure in a child with diabetic ketoacidosis. Pediatr Emerg Care. 2009;25(12):859–61.
24. Pajak A, Krolak-Olejnik B, Szafranska A. Early hypophosphatemia in very low birth weight preterm infants. Adv Clin Exp Med. 2018;27(6):841–7.
25. Gonzalez Ballesteros LF, Ma NS, Gordon RJ, Ward L, Backeljauw P, Wasserman H, et al. Unexpected widespread hypophosphatemia and bone disease associated with elemental formula use in infants and children. Bone. 2017;97:287–92.
26. Uday S, Sakka S, Davies JH, Randell T, Arya V, Brain C, et al. Elemental formula associated hypophosphataemic rickets. Clin Nutr (Edinburgh, Scotland). 2019;38(5):2246–50.
27. Walton RJ, Bijvoet OL. Nomogram for derivation of renal threshold phosphate concentration. Lancet (London, England). 1975;2(7929):309–10.
28. Yoshida T, Yoshida N, Monkawa T, Hayashi M, Saruta T. Dietary phosphorus deprivation induces 25-hydroxyvitamin D(3) 1alpha-hydroxylase gene expression. Endocrinology. 2001;142(5):1720–6.
29. Imel EA, Econs MJ. Approach to the hypophosphatemic patient. J Clin Endocrinol Metab. 2012;97(3):696–706.
30. Carpenter TO. The expanding family of hypophosphatemic syndromes. J Bone Miner Metab. 2012;30(1):1–9.
31. Gohil A, Imel EA. FGF23 and associated disorders of phosphate wasting. Pediatr Endocrinol Rev. 2019;17(1):17–34.

8 Hypoglycemia

Katherine Jane Pundyk and Seth Daniel Marks

Definition

Hypoglycemia can be defined by the evidence of clinical manifestations in the presence of glucose levels below normative ranges, or controversially solely by levels below normative ranges. Whipple's triad, defined as the presence of signs and symptoms of hypoglycemia with a documented low glucose value and the resolution of these signs and symptoms with the delivery of glucose, is a classic definition of hypoglycemia [1].

Choosing a glucose level below which defines hypoglycemia can be difficult and controversial, but generally it is now accepted that a blood glucose <2.6 mmol/L (47 mg/dL) in newborns <48–72 hours of age and <3.3 mmol/L (60 mg/dL) in all children >48–72 hours of age is defined as hypoglycemia [2–8].

Hypoglycemia at <48 hours of age is generally considered transitional [2, 8] and may warrant intervention but does not necessarily involve the same diagnostic considerations. This chapter considers hypoglycemia occurring after 48 hours of age.

Signs and Symptoms

Hypoglycemia can lead to neurogenic and neuroglycopenic symptoms. Neurogenic symptoms tend to occur first and are due to autonomic nervous system responses to hypoglycemia. These are then followed by neuroglycopenic symptoms that result from a lack of glucose availability to the brain.

Neurogenic symptoms include trembling, sweating, anxiety, tremor, palpitations, tachycardia, nausea, and hunger. Neuroglycopenic symptoms include lethargy, confusion, irritability, dizziness, loss of consciousness, and seizures [9, 10].

K. J. Pundyk (✉) · S. D. Marks
Children's Hospital HSC Winnipeg, Pediatrics and Child Health, Winnipeg, MB, Canada
e-mail: kpundyk@hsc.mb.ca; smarks@hsc.mb.ca

In neonates the presentation can be slightly different than in older children, and symptoms may include jitteriness, irritability, feeding issues, lethargy, cyanosis, tachypnea, hypothermia, seizures, and apnea.

Laboratory values suggestive of hypoglycemia in the absence of signs or symptoms of hypoglycemia may indicate "true" hypoglycemia or may be due to laboratory variance or other assay-related factors (see Chap. 31).

Differential Diagnosis

Due to the significant possible short- and long-term sequelae of hypoglycemia including seizures, and neurological deficiencies, the diagnosis of hypoglycemia is always an important "cannot-miss" diagnosis regardless of the underlying etiology (Table 8.1).

Important Clarifying Questions in the Medical History

A complete history should be taken including history and timing of the hypoglycemic event(s), birth history, past medical history, and family history (Table 8.2).

A history of recent carbohydrate intake, or, alternatively, duration of fasting time, is important to delineate. In neonates, a feeding history is important in order to calculate glucose requirements. For a neonate, needing >10 mg/kg/min of carbohydrate is considered excessive, suggesting a state of hyperinsulinism. This can be calculated by collecting information on type of nutrition including formula, breast milk, total parenteral nutrition, and intravenous fluids as well as the volume, and frequency of feeds. In older children, details about the timing and the type of food ingested prior to the hypoglycemic episode (carbohydrates, proteins, and fats) can be helpful, as well as the timing the symptoms of hypoglycemia and their resolution in relation to carbohydrate administration (Whipple's Triad). It is also important to

T. Stanley, M. Misra (eds.), *Endocrine Conditions in Pediatrics*, https://doi.org/10.1007/978-3-030-52215-5_8

Table 8.1 Causes of hypoglycemia

Causes
Insulin related:
Persistent hyperinsulinemic hypoglycemia of infancy including genetic hyperinsulinism
Congenital syndromes: e.g., Beckwith-Wiedemann syndrome
Beta cell adenoma, islet cell hyperplasia
Munchausen by proxy with exogenous insulin administration
Fatty acid oxidation disorders:
Acyl-CoA dehydrogenase, medium-chain deficiency
Metabolic diagnoses:
Galactosemia
Hereditary fructose intolerance
Fructose 1-6 diphosphatase deficiency
Glycogen storage disease types 1, 3, 6, 9, 11, 0
Other:
Transient neonatal hypoglycemia[a]
Idiopathic ketotic hypoglycemia[a]
Hypopituitarism: growth hormone deficiency, adrenocorticotropic hormone deficiency
Primary adrenal insufficiency
Ingestion of oral hypoglycemic agents, alcohol, beta blockers, salicylates
Critical illness, stress hyperinsulinism
Dumping syndrome
Hepatic failure
Renal failure

Adapted from a chart in Pediatric Endocrinology A Clinical Handbook 2016 [11], [10]
[a]Common causes

Table 8.2 Clinical pearls for history taking [8, 11–13]

Clinical pearls
Risk factors for neonatal hypoglycemia include:
Maternal diabetes mellitus
Small/large for gestational age
Prematurity
Perinatal asphyxia
Maternal labetalol use
A birth history of hypoglycemia, prolonged jaundice, and micropenis (in males) can be seen in congenital hypopituitarism.

assess if there was a possible ingestion of a substance that can cause hypoglycemia such as oral hypoglycemic agents, alcohol, beta blockers, salicylates, or potential insulin injection. Additionally, children who are critically ill have a higher risk of hypoglycemia.

In neonates or young children, birth history is important, including the presence of neonatal hypoglycemia or jaundice. Prolonged jaundice combined with hypoglycemia can be associated with congenital hypopituitarism. In neonates, risk factors for hypoglycemia include maternal diabetes, maternal labetalol use, infants large or small for gestational age, prematurity, and perinatal asphyxia.

Past medical history should review previous episodes of seizures, loss of consciousness, presence of developmental delay, growth concerns, and prior episodes of hypoglycemia.

A family history of inherited diseases associated with hypoglycemia, or seizures should be sought.

Table 8.3 Laboratory evaluation, performed *during* hypoglycemia unless otherwise indicated

Most important	Glucose – need a serum glucose, not just capillary point of care, to confirm hypoglycemia[a]
Critical sample	Glucose, beta hydroxybutyrate, bicarbonate, lactate, free fatty acids, insulin, growth hormone, cortisol, carnitine, acyl carnitine profile
Also helpful	C-peptide, organic acids[b], pyruvate, ammonia[b]
Consider based on presentation	Free or total thyroxine[b]; toxicology screen for ethanol, salicylates, beta-blockers, sulfonylureas, other anti-hyperglycemics[b]

[a]Please see Chap. 31 for important assay considerations
[b]Hypoglycemia not required at the time of assessment

Physical Examination

Physical examination should include documentation of growth parameters (height, weight, head circumference) with special note of linear growth failure or poor weight gain. Hypopituitarism can be associated with the presence of midline facial defects (cleft lip, cleft palate, single central incisor), optic nerve hypoplasia, micropenis, nystagmus, and/or jaundice. Hepatomegaly may indicate abnormal glycogenesis or glycogen storage disease. Primary adrenal insufficiency may present with hyperpigmentation, weight loss, nausea, and/or abdominal pain. Certain genetic syndromes may have unique physical findings. For example, Beckwith-Wiedemann syndrome presents with hemihypertrophy, macroglossia, and abdominal wall defects.

Investigations

Normal physiological responses to hypoglycemia include an increase in the levels of ketones, growth hormone, cortisol, and catecholamines along with a decrease in insulin (Table 8.3) [14, 15].

Next Steps in Diagnosis and Management

Please refer to Part II for the interpretation of laboratory evaluation. Please refer to Part III for further details on diagnosis and management of hypoglycemia.

References

1. Whipple A. The surgical therapy of hyperinsulinism. J Int Chir. 1938;3:237–76.
2. Thornton PS, Stanley CA, De Leon DD, Harris D, Haymond MW, Hussain K, et al. Recommendations from the Pediatric Endocrine Society for evaluation and management of persistent hypoglycemia in neonates, infants, and children. J Pediatr. 2015;167(2):238–45.

3. Sinclair JC. Approaches to the definition of neonatal hypoglycemia. Acta Paediatr Jpn. 1997;39(Suppl 1):S17–20.
4. Cornblath M, Hawdon JM, Williams AF, Aynsley-Green A, Ward-Platt MP, Schwartz R, et al. Controversies regarding definition of neonatal hypoglycemia: suggested operational thresholds. Pediatrics. 2000;105(5):1141–5.
5. Hoseth E, Joergensen A, Ebbesen F, Moeller M. Blood glucose levels in a population of healthy, breast fed, term infants of appropriate size for gestational age. Arch Dis Child Fetal Neonatal Ed. 2000;83(2):F117–9.
6. Diwakar KK, Sasidhar MV. Plasma glucose levels in term infants who are appropriate size for gestation and exclusively breast fed. Arch Dis Child Fetal Neonatal Ed. 2002;87(1):F46–8.
7. Nicholl R. What is the normal range of blood glucose concentrations in healthy term newborns? Arch Dis Child. 2003;88(3):238–9.
8. Narvey MR, Marks SD. The screening and management of newborns at risk for low blood glucose. Paediatr Child Health. 2019;24(8):536–44.
9. American Diabetes A. 6. Glycemic targets: standards of medical care in diabetes-2019. Diabetes Care. 2019;42(Suppl 1):S61–70.
10. Mukherjee E, Carroll R, Matfin G. Endocrine and metabolic emergencies: hypoglycaemia. Ther Adv Endocrinol Metab. 2011;2(2):81–93.
11. Styne DM. Pediatric endocrinology a clinical handbook. 1st ed. Cham: Springer International Publishing; 2016.
12. Bateman BT, Patorno E, Desai RJ, Seely EW, Mogun H, Maeda A, et al. Late pregnancy beta blocker exposure and risks of neonatal hypoglycemia and bradycardia. Pediatrics. 2016;138(3):e20160731.
13. Ellaway CJ, Silinik M, Cowell CT, Gaskin KJ, Kamath KR, Dorney S, et al. Cholestatic jaundice and congenital hypopituitarism. J Paediatr Child Health. 1995;31(1):51–3.
14. Bougneres PF, Lemmel C, Ferre P, Bier DM. Ketone body transport in the human neonate and infant. J Clin Invest. 1986;77(1):42–8.
15. Chaussain JL, Georges P, Calzada L, Job JC. Glycemic response to 24-hour fast in normal children: III. Influence of age. J Pediatr. 1977;91(5):711–4.

9 Hyperglycemia

Ambreen Sonawalla and Rabab Jafri

Definition

The term is derived from the Greek "hyper" (high), glykys (sweet/sugar), and haima (blood) [1] meaning elevated blood glucose.

History

History should focus on other symptoms related to diabetes mellitus, excluding other possible causes such as acute illness causing secondary hyperglycemia, or medications causing hyperglycemia. Although hyperglycemia from the stress of severe illness exceeds 200 mg/dL in a minority of children in an ICU setting [2], children with glucose >200 mg/dL not receiving high-dose glucocorticoids generally should be suspected of having diabetes mellitus until proven otherwise.

Clinical Key
Children with hyperglycemia and associated nausea, vomiting, headache, Kussmaul respirations (deep labored breathing), ketotic/fruity odor, or altered mental status should be emergently sent to the nearest emergency department, with further work-up deferred to that setting.

Elements of history that are suggestive of diabetes include the classic triad of polyuria, polydipsia, and polyphagia, as well as weight loss or family history of autoimmune disease (for Type 1) or family history of Type 2 diabetes or maturity onset diabetes of the young (MODY) (for Type 2 and MODY, respectively).

Symptoms Associated with Chronic Hyperglycemia

- Polyuria (abnormally large volume of urine accompanied by increased frequency, sometimes manifesting as nocturnal enuresis). This results from serum glucose above the "renal threshold" (180–200 mg/dL).
- Polydipsia (sometimes manifesting as drinking directly from sink faucets, waking up multiple times overnight to drink).
- Fatigue.
- Unintentional weight loss despite polyphagia.
- Frequent infections, especially urinary tract, skin, or fungal infections.
- Mood changes.
- Trouble concentrating.
- Blurred vision.
- Altered mental status (may be caused by hyperosmolarity or cerebral edema).

Important Clarifying Questions

- Is there abdominal pain, nausea, vomiting (suggestive of diabetic ketoacidosis [DKA])?
- Is there a history of recent illness?
- Does the patient have:
  - Cystic fibrosis (cystic fibrosis-related diabetes (CFRD) is present in approximately 2% of children and 20% of adolescents with cystic fibrosis [3])?
  - Chronic pancreatitis?
- What medications is the patient currently on? (See Table 9.1)

A. Sonawalla
Arkansas Children's Hospital, Little Rock, AR, USA

R. Jafri (✉)
Massachusetts General Hospital, Boston, MA, USA
e-mail: jafrir@uthscsa.edu

T. Stanley, M. Misra (eds.), *Endocrine Conditions in Pediatrics*, https://doi.org/10.1007/978-3-030-52215-5_9

Table 9.1 Medications causing hyperglycemia and associated mechanisms

Medication	Mechanism
High-dose glucocorticoids	Increased insulin resistance
Calcineurin Inhibitors (cyclosporine, tacrolimus, sirolimus)	Unclear (beta-cell dysfunction vs. insulin resistance)
Atypical anti-psychotics	Increased insulin resistance [4]
Growth hormone	Increased insulin resistance
Beta-blockers (including inhaled)	Impaired insulin secretion

- Is there a family history of:
  - Diabetes (Type 1, or Type 2 or MODY)?
  - Thyroid disease (hyper- or hypothyroidism)?
  - Celiac disease?
  - Other autoimmune diseases (such as vitiligo, psoriasis, rheumatoid arthritis, multiple sclerosis, inflammatory bowel disease, systemic lupus erythematosus)?

Table 9.2 Differential diagnosis of hyperglycemia and associated symptoms

Symptoms of diabetes mellitus	Other differential diagnoses
Hyperglycemia	Transient stress-induced (Exogenous or endogenous) glucocorticoid-induced Medication-induced (anti psychotics, particularly atypical, such as risperidone, olanzapine; growth hormone; beta blockers; chemotherapy drugs, specifically alkylating agents)
Polydispsia	Behavioral/activity-related Diabetes insipidus (central or nephrogenic)
Polyuria	Excess water or caffeine consumption Urinary tract infection Diabetes insipidus (central or nephrogenic) Hypercalcemia Medication related (e.g., lithium) Renal involvement in systemic illnesses
Weight loss	Dietary, metabolic, infectious, oncologic causes

Physical Exam

Table 9.2 lists other differential diagnoses for signs and symptoms that typically accompany a diagnosis of diabetes. A pertinent history using the clarifying questions above, and a thorough physical exam may help differentiate between these causes.

Pearls of Physical Exam

- Vital signs, including blood pressure
- BMI and weight/BMI trend
- Signs of dehydration
- Respiratory status including evidence of Kussmaul breathing
- Abdominal tenderness
- Acanthosis nigricans: in neck folds, axillae, groin, under breasts
- Cushingoid features: moon facies, buffalo hump, striae
- Presence of skin or yeast infections

Laboratory Evaluation

Initial evaluation includes confirming hyperglycemia and assessing for the presence of ketones, ketoacidosis, and other electrolyte abnormalities.

- Point of care (POC) blood glucose, followed by confirmation with plasma glucose
- Urinalysis or POC urine dipstick for glucose and ketones
- Serum beta hydroxybutyrate to assess ketosis
- Serum electrolytes (Na, K, Cl, HCO3/CO2), calcium, phosphate, magnesium
- If concern for DKA, venous blood gas (venous pH used in diagnosis of DKA)
- Hemoglobin A1c (HbA1c)

Other labs that are often helpful at presentation of diabetes, but do not need to be urgently sent from the primary care setting, include the following:

- Diabetes autoantibodies:
  - Insulin antibodies (anti-insulin), ideally need to be sent before insulin is given.
  - Glutamic acid decarboxylase antibodies (Anti-GAD).
  - Islet tyrosine phosphatase 2 antibodies (Anti-IA2).
  - Zinc transporter protein 8 antibodies (Anti-ZnT8).
- Celiac screen (tissue transglutaminase IgA and total IgA).
- Thyroid screen (TSH, with or without free thyroxine (fT4) or total thyroxine (T4) and anti-thyroid peroxidase antibodies). Please note that illness at presentation may cause abnormalities in TSH, T4, and fT4 due to non-thyroidal illness (i.e., "euthyroid sick" syndrome).
- Serum C-peptide level: may be helpful in differentiating Type 1 vs. Type 2 diabetes after glycemic control has been established.
- An OGTT may be helpful when a fasting plasma glucose and/or HbA1c is non-diagnostic but the suspicion for diabetes is high.

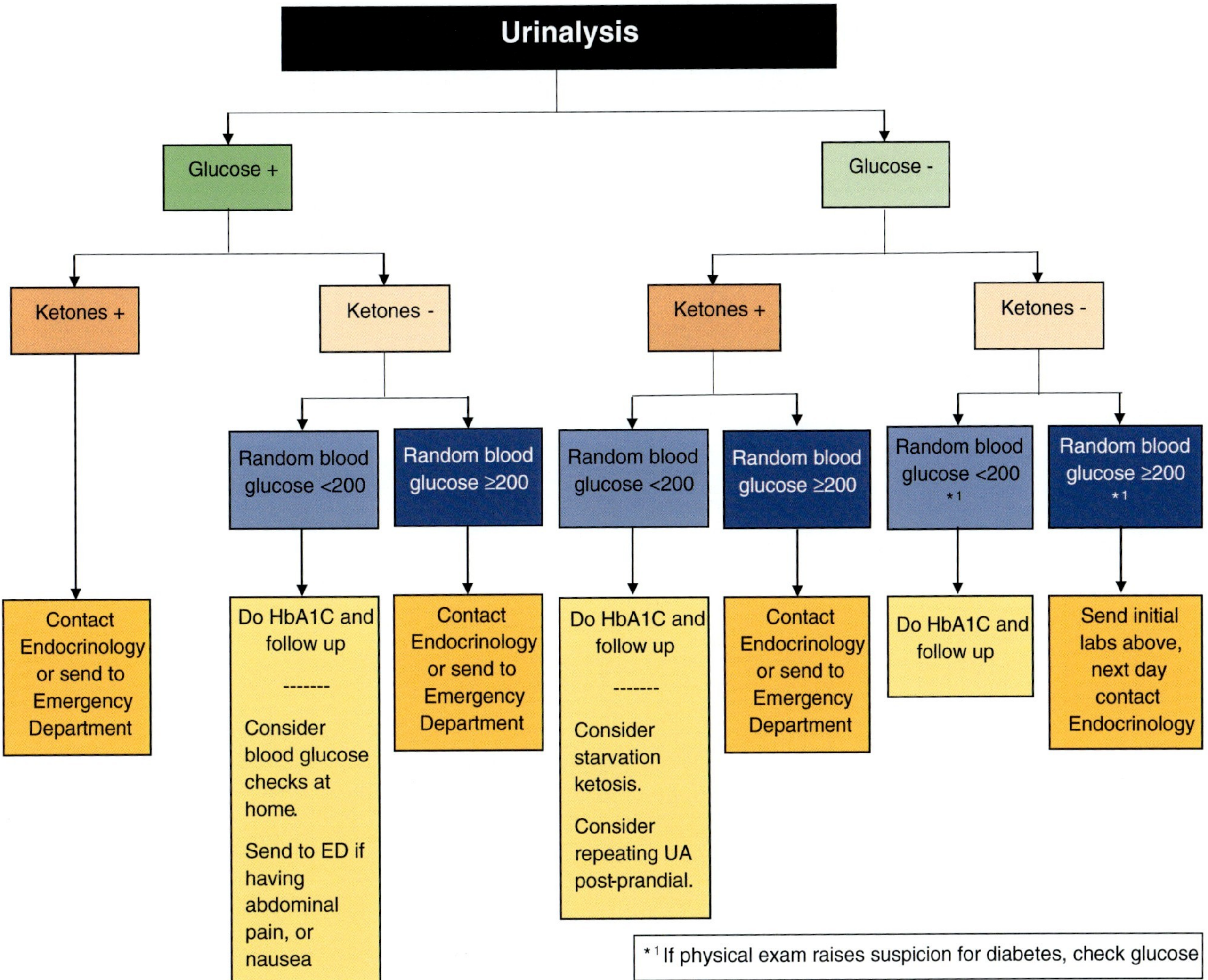

Fig. 9.1 Approach to management of a patient found to have hyperglycemia, glycosuria, or ketonuria. (Used with permission from Dr. Shipra Bansal, University of Arkansas for Medical Sciences)

Next Steps in Diagnosis and Management

Figure 9.1 lists an approach to management based upon initial findings of urinalysis and POC measurements.

- Isolated hyperglycemia or glucosuria in a well-appearing child without any suspicious symptoms and without urine ketones is still likely to indicate diabetes but could also indicate other causes. The initial clinical and laboratory evaluation above should be done, and next-day follow-up can be planned in the primary care setting or as an urgent referral to endocrinology.
- Presence of hyperglycemia with a random blood sugar level of >200 mg/dL or fasting blood sugar of ≥126 mg/dL, in addition to classic symptoms (mentioned in Table 9.1) is highly likely to indicate new-onset diabetes mellitus. Same-day referral to pediatric endocrinology or an emergency department is warranted, particularly if there are ≥trace ketones on urinalysis as same day administration of insulin, directed by an endocrinologist, is critical to prevent DKA.
- If there is concern for *dehydration*, presence of *respiratory or significant abdominal distress*, or presence of *moderate to large ketones* on urinalysis refer to the nearest emergency department for evaluation of diabetic ketoacidosis.

Important Considerations Regarding Patient Counseling

- If the diagnosis is not clear cut, then it is most helpful to leave out the discussion about prognosis until further evaluation is performed.
- If there is a high suspicion of diabetes, discuss briefly what it means and what to expect at the endocrinologist's office.
- Discuss that diabetes is no one's fault.
- Discuss possible adverse events to watch for (such as dehydration, ketonuria), and when to visit the ER, but leave specifics of diagnosis and management for the endocrinologist to discuss.

References

1. Mouri Mi, Badireddy M. Hyperglycemia [Internet]. StatPearls. StatPearls Publishing; 2019 [cited 2019 Aug 18]. Available from: http://www.ncbi.nlm.nih.gov/pubmed/28613650.
2. Faustino EV, Apkon M. Persistent hyperglycemia in critically ill children. J Pediatr. 2005;146(1):30–4.
3. Moran A, Dunitz J, Nathan B, Saeed A, Holme B, Thomas W. Cystic fibrosis-related diabetes: current trends in prevalence, incidence, and mortality. Diabetes Care [Internet]. 2009 [cited 2019 Sep 1];32(9):1626–31. Available from: http://care.diabetesjournals.org/cgi/doi/10.2337/dc09-0586
4. Bergman RN, Ader M. Atypical antipsychotics and glucose homeostasis. J Clin Psychiatry [Internet]. 2005 [cited 2020 Mar 7];66(04):504–14. Available from: http://article.psychiatrist.com/?ContentType=START&ID=10001276.

Early Signs of Pubertal Development

10

Takara Stanley and Madhusmita Misra

Introduction and Definitions

Terms used to describe the onset of puberty are defined in Table 10.1. A critical distinction is between early pubarche versus early breast development/testicular enlargement, as the former usually heralds activation of adrenal androgen synthesis (adrenarche) whereas the latter suggests early activation of gonadal steroid synthesis (gonadarche). Gonadarche and adrenarche have distinct differential diagnoses and are evaluated differently, as discussed below.

Table 10.1 Terms describing the onset of puberty

Terms describing pubertal signs	
Thelarche	Appearance of breast budding
Pubarche	Appearance of pubic hair or axillary hair (Pubic hair usually appears before axillary hair)
Menarche	Onset of menses
Diagnostic terms	
Adrenarche	Onset of synthesis of adrenal androgens, usually heralded by pubarche
Gonadarche	Onset of gonadal steroid (estrogen or testosterone) production, usually heralded by thelarche or testicular enlargement to ≥4 cc
Precocious puberty	Can be a "catch all" term describing early appearance of any pubertal sign; used more commonly by pediatric endocrinologists specifically to refer to early gondarche
Central precocious puberty	Early gonadarche caused by early activation of the hypothalamic-pituitary-gonadal (HPG) axis
Peripheral precocious puberty (or peripheral precocity)	Early peripheral production of or exposure to estrogen or androgen, due to a genetic cause, environmental exposure, or estrogen- or androgen-secreting tumor
Isolated premature thelarche (or benign premature thelarche)	Non-progressive thelarche without any other signs of estrogen exposure and without apparent activation of the HPG axis based on prepubertal gonadotropin levels and/or normal bone age

Definitions of "Early" Puberty

Conventional definitions of precocious puberty are shown in Table 10.2. In addition to these age-based definitions, *rate of progression* of puberty should also be carefully noted by clinicians, as tumors in children of normal pubertal age may present with very rapid pubertal progression. Unfortunately thresholds for "rapid progression" are less well defined than thresholds for precocity. In girls, the median duration from thelarche to menarche is generally 30–36 months [1]; we suggest that time between thelarche and menarche of less than 2 years should prompt additional consideration for evaluation, and a time of less than 18 months should prompt additional evaluation. In boys, the average duration of puberty is 3 years, with a range of normal of 2–5 years [2, 3], such that complete progression through puberty in less than 2 years should also prompt careful consideration.

A second critical point is that there is a clear trend toward earlier pubertal development in girls [5, 6] compared to historical data, with some evidence for the same in boys [7]. Additionally, children with overweight or obesity may enter puberty earlier, and our "conventional" standards did not reflect the racial and ethnic diversity of today's practice settings. Consequently, clinicians may still use traditional definitions of precocious puberty as a guide but should also consider clinical context, including family history, race/ethnicity, and body weight. It may be reasonable to consider a threshold of 7 years for early pubarche in girls who have obesity or girls who are African American or Hispanic, and evidence also suggests that a threshold of 7 years for early thelarche is appropriate for girls with obesity. Although evi-

T. Stanley (✉) · M. Misra
Division of Pediatric Endocrinology, Massachusetts General Hospital and Harvard Medical School, Boston, MA, USA
e-mail: tstanley@mgh.harvard.edu; mmisra@mgh.harvard.edu

T. Stanley, M. Misra (eds.), *Endocrine Conditions in Pediatrics*, https://doi.org/10.1007/978-3-030-52215-5_10

Table 10.2 Conventional definitions of precocious puberty

Females
Thelarche before age 8y.
Pubarche before age 8y.
Although precocious puberty is not generally defined based on menses, since thelarche physiologically precedes menarche, menarche before age 10 years, or menstrual bleeding less than 18 months after the onset of thelarche, would also be concerning for early/rapid pubertal progression.
Males
Testicular volume ≥ 4 cc (corresponding to testicular length along the long axis of ~2.5 cm) before age 9 years.
Pubarche before age 9 years.
In cases of peripheral precocity, testicular enlargement will not occur, and *penile lengthening* along with pubarche may be the first signs. Stretched penile length ≥90th percentile for age should prompt the consideration of precocious puberty. For reference, a stretched penile length of ~8 cm is above the 90th percentile for children up to age 10 years [4].

dence for adjusting thresholds in boys is less clear, boys with overweight or obesity may enter puberty earlier, whereas boys with severe obesity may have hypogonadism.

Differential Diagnosis

A comprehensive differential diagnosis for precocious puberty is presented in Table 10.3. (Please note that endocrine disruptors are not included but may prove to be important in the historical changes in pubertal timing described above.) This chapter focuses on the "cannot miss" and most common diagnoses for children presenting with early puberty, whereas Chap. 43 details the full differential diagnosis. In both sexes, the "cannot miss" diagnoses are tumors: either CNS tumors causing central precocious puberty or peripheral tumors making estrogens or androgens. In contrast, the most common etiologies of early puberty are benign, particularly in girls, as discussed further below.

Children Less Than 3 Years of Age

It is important to recognize that the "mini-puberty of infancy," which lasts through 6–9 months of age in boys and about 12 months in girls, can cause signs of pubertal development. Many girls will develop breast tissue during the first year, and this may take up to 3 years to regress, although careful clinical evaluation should take place for any progressive breast growth after 1 year or for persistent breast tissue at 24–30 months. Similarly, sparse and/or fine pubic hair is relatively common in infancy and is almost always benign [8]. Thus, while *progressive* signs of pubertal development are not expected in infants after 6–9 months of age, clinical observation may be appropriate for stable thelarche or pubic hair if no other concerning signs or symptoms are present.

Table 10.3 Causes of precocious puberty

Central precocious puberty
Idiopathic
Hypothalamic hamartoma
CNS neoplasm
Traumatic brain injury
History of CNS radiation
Neurofibromatosis I
Tuberous sclerosis
Other CNS pathology (e.g., arachnoid cyst, hydrocephalus, history of perinatal hypoxia or CNS infection)
International adoption (unclear mechanism)
Peripheral precocity
Congenital adrenal hyperplasia
McCune Albright syndrome
LH-receptor activating mutation (also called familial male-limited precocious puberty)
Exogenous exposure to estrogen or androgens
Peripheral germ cell tumors
Sex cord-stromal cell tumors
Adrenal tumors
Premature adrenarche
Idiopathic
Congenital adrenal hyperplasia (CAH), including nonclassical CAH
Adrenal tumors
Exogenous exposure to androgens
Other variants
Isolated premature thelarche is often idiopathic or may be caused by exposure to lavender or tea tree oils or other estrogenic compounds
Isolated vaginal bleeding may be caused by vaginal foreign body, functional ovarian cysts (usually self-resolving), or temporary high-level exposure to estrogen for other reasons

CNS central nervous system, *LH* luteinizing hormone

Premature Adrenarche

In children with premature adrenarche, almost all will have idiopathic premature adrenarche. Because of the rare possibility of an androgen producing tumor; however, children with premature adrenarche should be clinically assessed approximately every 6 months initially, with particular attention to rapid progression of signs of hyperandrogenism that would increase suspicion and prompt biochemical testing.

Premature Thelarche or Menarche in Girls

The most common etiologies of early pubertal signs in girls will be isolated/"benign" premature thelarche or idiopathic central precocious puberty. For unknown reasons, there is a much higher prevalence of central precocious puberty in girls than boys, and roughly 90% is idiopathic [9]. In girls presenting at less than age 6 years, pathology is more likely to be present, and careful evaluation is recommended for all girls with precocious puberty because of the possibility of CNS lesions or peripheral estrogen secreting lesions.

Premature Genital Development in Boys

Unlike girls, for whom the etiology of precocious puberty is most commonly benign, over 50% of boys presenting with precocious puberty have identifiable underlying pathology [9]. These various etiologies are detailed in Table 10.3.

Important Clarifying Questions in the History

The primary goals in history taking are as follows:

1. Clarify the exact signs and symptoms to determine if there is adrenarche, gonadarche, or both
2. Clarify the rate of progression of signs and symptoms to determine whether there is rapid progression raising suspicion for pathology
3. Establish an overall clinical context including other medical issues, medication use, and family history to help guide diagnostic evaluation

Querying Signs and Symptoms

The following signs and symptoms of adrenarche and gonadarche should be assessed.

Adrenarchal Signs/Symptoms

- Pubic hair, axillary hair
- Acne
- Body odor, requirement for deodorant

Gonadarchal Signs/Symptoms

- Females: breast development, breast tenderness, vaginal discharge or bleeding
- Males: penile enlargement, morning erections, adrenarchal signs (reflecting testicular production of testosterone)

Signs/Symptoms Concerning for Adrenal Tumor (Query If Adrenarche Present)

- Hyperpigmentation
- Progressive, cystic acne
- Progressive hirsutism

Parental report of a recent growth spurt should raise concern of exposure to sex steroids and should be confirmed on the child's growth chart.

Establishing the onset of each symptom as well as its progression since onset is critical to establishing the level of concern. For example, breast development in an 8-year-old that began 3 months ago and has progressed significantly since is more concerning than breast development in a 7-year-old that began a year ago and has remained stable. Similarly, contemporaneous development of pubic hair, body odor, acne, and hyperpigmentation are much more concerning than appearance of isolated pubic hair.

Querying Medical and Family History

The timing of puberty is highly heritable, so the ages of pubertal development of parents and siblings should be obtained. Females usually recall timing of menarche; males may recall when they began shaving or when they had their growth spurt or stopped growing. The history of precocious puberty in other family members may suggest genetic etiologies such as familial male-limited precocious puberty, whereas relatively early-normal timing in one or more parents may suggest one or more non-pathologic variants in the multiple genes that are increasingly understood to regulate pubertal timing.

Medical history of the child is relevant particularly with regard to any congenital or developmental issues that may predispose to central precocious puberty (see Table 10.3). In addition, children who are adopted internationally and/or children who move from early adversity to improved childhood circumstances may be more likely to have central precocious puberty for unclear reasons. Medications and possible exposures to exogenous androgenic or estrogenic compounds should also be queried. Male family members using topical testosterone may inadvertently expose children to this hormone, leading to precocious pubarche, and lavender and tea tree oil have been implicated in premature thelarche. Finally, a complete review of systems should be used to assess for any possible "red flags" that may suggest CNS pathology or other underlying medical issues.

Key Aspects of the Physical Examination

A complete physical examination should be performed with particular attention to the issues below. Tanner staging should also be performed, as described in Table 10.4. As discussed in Table 10.5, breast tissue must be palpated in girls to distinguish from lipomastia, and testicular sizing via palpation is critical in males to navigate the differential diagnosis. *Testicular sizing* can be accomplished using either an orchidometer to estimate volume or a ruler to measure length (along the long axis of the testis). The scrotal skin should be gently stretched around the testis to ensure that only the testis itself is included in the measurement. *Stretched penile*

Table 10.4 Tanner staging [2, 10]

	Pubic hair	Breast development	Male genitalia
Stage 1	No hair or only vellus hair	No breast budding	Prepubertal in appearance, testes <4cc volume or <2.5cm length
Stage 2	Sparse long, slightly pigmented hair, usually at base of phallus or along the labia	Small amount of breast tissue just under nipple, some areolar enlargement	Testes of ≥4 cc volume or ≥2.5cm length, scrotal skin begins to change in texture
Stage 3	Darker, coarser, and curling hair, spread sparsely over the pubic region	Continued growth of breast tissue, extending beyond nipple	Enlargement in penis, mainly in length. Continued increase in testicular size
Stage 4	Dark, coarse pubic hair covering most of the pubic area without spread to medial thighs	Separation in contour of areola such that areola and nipple form "secondary mound" above breast	Continued enlargement of penis in length and width, continued increase in testicular size
Stage 5	Adult pubic hair covering the pubic area including spread to the medial thighs	Recession of areola so that only nipple is elevated above contour of breast	Adult male genitalia

Table 10.5 Key aspects of the physical examination

Growth Velocity: Increased growth velocity, consistent with a growth spurt, supports a diagnosis of increased exposure to estrogen or androgens. Beware that children presenting with CNS tumors causing early puberty may maintain "normal prepubertal growth velocity" due to the combination of increased estrogen/testosterone with evolving insufficiency of other pituitary hormones (e.g., growth hormone and thyroid-stimulating hormone).
Ophthalmologic Exam: It should include visual fields and fundoscopy when feasible to assess for visual field deficits and/or papilledema that would suggest sellar/suprasellar pathology.
Breast Tissue Versus *Lipomastia:* Palpation of the breasts is critical to determine whether true breast tissue is present, versus adipose tissue in the breast area (so called lipomastia or adipomastia). Breast tissue typically first develops right under the nipple and is firmer than surrounding tissue; it also may be tender. By contrast, lipomastia is often characterized by an absence of tissue just underneath the nipple with adjacent fat tissue.
Pubic Hair Characteristics: "True" pubic hair is coarse, long terminal hair. Early pubic hair (i.e., Tanner Stage 2) may not be as coarse, dark, or curled as typical pubic hair, but it should be distinguishable from vellus hair. Vellus hair in the pubic region is not characterized as pubic hair. Similarly, an increase in the density of hair on the legs or arms is usually familial rather than indicative of increased androgen exposure, although the latter possibility should be considered in extreme cases.
Vaginal Estrogen Exposure: When possible, the vaginal mucosa should be visually inspected to determine if it is pink, indicating estrogen exposure, versus more reddish in color, which is normal for pre-pubertal girls. This can usually be accomplished via a "frog-leg" position with gentle pressure to separate the labia majora.
Pubic Hair Stage Versus *Genital Stage in Boys:* Due to the important distinction between adrenarche and gonadarche with regard to diagnostic evaluation and management, it is critical to perform pubic hair staging, genital staging, and testicular sizing via palpation in boys. Tanner Stage 4 or 5 pubic hair does not indicate progressive gonadal puberty, which instead is characterized by progressive testicular and penile enlargement.

length may also be helpful and is measured by placing a ruler or measuring tape at the base of the pubic ramus, stretching the phallus until there is increased resistance, and measuring to the tip of the glans (excluding excessive foreskin).

Initial Evaluation

After the history and physical exam, the evaluation of early puberty most often starts with a bone age, or a plain radiograph of the left hand (see Chap. 36). Depending on the clinical context, laboratory evaluation (see Table 10.6) may be warranted either concurrent to bone age assessment or if the bone age is advanced. A recommended approach to evaluation is presented according to clinical scenario below.

Premature Pubarche

- Obtain a bone age.
- Obtain adrenal androgens (Table 10.6) if any of the following is present:
  – Bone age advancement (bone age greater than 2 standard deviations above chronological age).
  – Multiple significant signs of androgenization such as pubic hair, acne, hirsutism, or hyperpigmentation.
  – Rapid progression of pubic hair growth and/or other signs of virilization.
- If the initial presentation is relatively benign (e.g., no rapid progression or excessive signs of androgenization) and the bone age is within 2 standard deviations of the chronological age, follow-up in clinic for repeat examination in 6 months to ensure no rapid progression.

Premature Thelarche

- Obtain a bone age.
- Obtain pituitary-gonadal axis labs (Table 10.6) and thyroid studies if any of the following are present:
  – Bone age advancement (bone age greater than 2 standard deviations above chronological age).
  – Additional signs of estrogenization such as pink vaginal mucosa or vaginal discharge/bleeding.
  – Rapid progression of breast tissue growth.

Table 10.6 Recommended laboratory evaluation

Lab	Notes
Adrenal androgens	
DHEA-S	Consider asking for DHEA level if there is a very high suspicion for an adrenal tumor; otherwise DHEA-S will suffice.
Androstenedione	
17-hydroxyprogesterone	To assess for the most common form of congenital adrenal hyperplasia; ideally obtained in the morning (normal morning value is less than 150–200 ng/dL; normal afternoon value not well-defined but should be less than at least 100ng/dL if not lower). Higher values should prompt pediatric endocrine referral.
Pituitary-gonadal axis labs	
LH	Basal value ≥0.3 IU/L indicates central precocious puberty; undetectable values may not be helpful due to the pulsatile nature of LH. However, an undetectable LH in the presence of a robust pubertal estradiol or testosterone level indicates peripheral precocity. Obtain in the morning (before 10 AM) if possible because of higher nocturnal LH pulsatile secretion in early central puberty.
FSH	Values in the pubertal range suggest central precocious puberty (less specific and sensitive than a pubertal LH level), whereas suppressed values in the context of a robust pubertal estradiol or testosterone level indicate peripheral precocity.
Testosterone	Obtain in the morning if possible (before 10 AM), as morning values are highest due to higher nocturnal LH pulsatile secretion in early central puberty.
Estradiol	Request high-sensitivity estradiol assay.
Other useful labs	
TSH and free T4	Profound primary hypothyroidism may cause precocious puberty as high levels of circulating TSH can directly stimulate the FSH receptor (Van Wyk-Grumback syndrome, quite rare).
HCG	May be elevated in germinoma (may not want to test for this until the diagnosis of peripheral precocity is established).
Alpha fetoprotein	May be elevated in germinoma (may not want to test for this until the diagnosis of peripheral precocity is established).

- If labs show precocious puberty (LH ≥ 0.3 U/L or pubertal levels of estradiol) refer to pediatric endocrinology.
- If the initial presentation is relatively benign (e.g., no rapid progression or additional signs of estrogenization) and the bone age is within 2 standard deviations of the chronological age, follow-up in clinic for repeat examination in 6 months to assess progression. If no progression, this is likely isolated/benign premature thelarche. If there is evidence of progression, send labs as above and refer to endocrinology.

Early Signs of Genital Development in Boys

- Obtain a bone age and pituitary-gonadal axis labs (Table 10.6).
- Consider sending "Other useful labs" in Table 10.6.
- If there is unequivocal testicular or penile enlargement before the age of 7–8 years, refer to pediatric endocrinology, as most cases of precocious puberty in boys do have an underlying etiology that may require treatment,

Next Steps in Diagnosis and Management

Whereas isolated premature thelarche and premature adrenarche that is not progressing rapidly can be managed in the primary care setting, children with true precocious puberty and rapidly progressive adrenarche should be referred to pediatric endocrinology. If a timely appointment is not forthcoming and there is concern for either a CNS etiology or a peripheral source of estrogen/testosterone, urgent attention should be requested, and the primary care provider may want to consider initiating the process of obtaining a brain MRI in the case of central precocious puberty or abdominal/pelvic imaging in the case of peripheral precocity.

References

1. Biro FM, Pajak A, Wolff MS, Pinney SM, Windham GC, Galvez MP, et al. Age of Menarche in a longitudinal US Cohort. J Pediatr Adolesc Gynecol. 2018;31(4):339–45.
2. Marshall WA, Tanner JM. Variations in the pattern of pubertal changes in boys. Arch Dis Child. 1970;45(239):13–23.
3. Reiter EO, Lee PA. Have the onset and tempo of puberty changed? Arch Pediatr Adolesc Med. 2001;155(9):988–9.
4. Schonfeld WA. Primary and secondary sexual characteristics. Am J Dis Child. 1943;65:535–42.
5. Aksglaede L, Sorensen K, Petersen JH, Skakkebaek NE, Juul A. Recent decline in age at breast development: the Copenhagen Puberty Study. Pediatrics. 2009;123(5):e932–9.
6. Biro FM, Greenspan LC, Galvez MP, Pinney SM, Teitelbaum S, Windham GC, et al. Onset of breast development in a longitudinal cohort. Pediatrics. 2013;132(6):1019–27.
7. Herman-Giddens ME, Wang L, Koch G. Secondary sexual characteristics in boys: estimates from the national health and nutrition examination survey III, 1988-1994. Arch Pediatr Adolesc Med. 2001;155(9):1022–8.
8. Nebesio TD, Eugster EA. Pubic hair of infancy: endocrinopathy or enigma? Pediatrics. 2006;117(3):951–4.
9. Latronico AC, Brito VN, Carel JC. Causes, diagnosis, and treatment of central precocious puberty. Lancet Diabetes Endocrinol. 2016;4(3):265–74.
10. Marshall WA, Tanner JM. Variations in pattern of pubertal changes in girls. Arch Dis Child. 1969;44(235):291–303.

Delayed or Stalled Pubertal Development

11

Takara Stanley and Madhusmita Misra

Definitions of Delayed or Stalled Puberty

Please refer to Chap. 10, Table 10.1, for the definition of terms used to describe pubertal development. Delayed puberty is defined as a lack of secondary sexual characteristics in girls by age 13 years or in boys by age 14 years. In these definitions, the term "secondary sexual characteristics" refers to signs of activation of the hypothalamic-pituitary-gonadal (HPG) axis, that is, thelarche in girls or testicular enlargement to 4 cc volume or 2.5 cm in length in boys. The development of pubic or axillary hair indicates adrenal androgen production rather than HPG axis activation, so *presence of pubic or axillary hair without other sexual development does not preclude a diagnosis of delayed puberty.*

Clinical Key
Delayed puberty is the lack of breast development in girls by age 13 years or lack of testicular enlargement in boys by age 14 years. Children who start puberty but do not complete pubertal development within 4–5 years should be evaluated for stalled puberty.

Stalled puberty is characterized by a lack of continued pubertal development after thelarche or testicular enlargement to 4 cc volume or 2.5 cm in length. The median duration between thelarche and menarche is 30–36 months in girls [1], and the average time between testicular enlargement to 4 cc and achievement of adult testicular volume is 3 years [2]. Thus, children who have started but not completed puberty within 4–5 years may have an underlying pathology and should undergo evaluation for stalled puberty [2]. Further, in children who have started puberty, a lack of any pubertal progression over 1–2 years is highly suspicious.

Primary amenorrhea is defined as a lack of menarche by age 15 years by some sources and by age 16 years by others. The term "delayed menarche" may also be used to describe lack of menses associated with secondary sexual characteristics that are or are not fully pubertal, with the term "primary amenorrhea" reserved to describe a lack of menses at 16 years in girls with otherwise complete maturation of secondary sexual characteristics.

Differential Diagnosis

As described in Chap. 44, the most common cause of delayed puberty is constitutional delay of growth and puberty (CDGP), a benign entity likely due to variation in one or more of the multiple genes that determine pubertal timing. Children with CDGP usually have a family history of relatively late timing of puberty and are otherwise healthy without concerning signs or symptoms on history or physical examination. However, delayed or stalled puberty may also be the presenting sign of one of many different underlying pathologies, and therefore children with delayed puberty require careful evaluation.

The differential diagnosis, listed in Table 11.1, is conceptually divided into two categories: (1) issues with the testes or ovaries, so-called hypergonadotropic hypogonadism because gonadotropins (luteinizing hormone [LH] and/or follicle-stimulating hormone [FSH]) will be elevated on laboratory testing; (2) issues with hypothalamic and/or pituitary signaling to the gonads, so-called hypogonadotropic hypogonadism because gonadotropins will be low or low-normal on laboratory testing. As described below, when laboratory evaluation is warranted, measuring estradiol or testosterone along with LH and FSH will guide further consideration of

T. Stanley (✉) · M. Misra
Division of Pediatric Endocrinology, Massachusetts General Hospital and Harvard Medical School, Boston, MA, USA
e-mail: tstanley@mgh.harvard.edu; mmisra@mgh.harvard.edu

T. Stanley, M. Misra (eds.), *Endocrine Conditions in Pediatrics*, https://doi.org/10.1007/978-3-030-52215-5_11

Table 11.1 Differential diagnosis of delayed puberty or stalled puberty

Hypergonadotropic hypogonadism (high LH/FSH)	Hypogonadotropic hypogonadism (low or low-normal LH/FSH)
Both sexes Long-term effects of cancer treatment (chemotherapy, particularly alkylating agents, or radiation) Autoimmune: premature ovarian failure or autoimmune orchitis Galactosemia (ovaries more adversely affected than testes) [3] Disorders of sex development causing gonadal dysgenesis or dysfunction, and disorders of sex steroid biosynthesis *Girls* Turner syndrome Fragile X premutation Complete androgen insensitivity syndrome (elevated LH; FSH may be normal) *Boys* Klinefelter syndrome (usually stalled puberty or hypogonadism in young adulthood rather than delayed puberty) Fragile X syndrome Hemochromatosis Testicular regression ("vanishing testis syndrome") Testicular failure due to infection (e.g., mumps) Bilateral testicular trauma or torsion	Constitutional delay of growth and puberty Functional hypogonadotropic hypogonadism Anorexia nervosa Very high levels of physical activity (e.g., cross-country running) Malnutrition Undiagnosed celiac disease Underlying systemic disease, including inflammatory bowel disease, neoplastic disease, chronic renal failure, cystic fibrosis, systemic autoimmune disease Isolated hypogonadotropic hypogonadism Kallmann syndrome (*ANOS1* mutation) Other genetic etiologies Syndromes, including CHARGE syndrome, Prader-Willi syndrome, leptin or leptin receptor deficiencies, X-linked adrenal hypoplasia congenita Congenital or acquired hypopituitarism Pituitary transcription factor defects Septo-optic dysplasia Sellar or suprasellar lesion History of CNS radiation Traumatic brain injury Infiltrative/infections, e.g., hypophysitis, tuberculosis, sarcoidosis Hyperprolactinemia Hypothyroidism Chronic significant opiate use
Eugonadotropic primary amenorrhea	
Müllerian agenesis (Mayer-Rokitansky-Küster-Hauser syndrome)	
Polycystic ovary syndrome	

the differential diagnosis based on whether gonadotropins are high versus low/low-normal.

Important Clarifying Questions in the History

History taking in delayed or stalled puberty is primarily directed at answering the following question: Is this a reassuring situation with family history of delayed puberty and without any concerning signs or symptoms that suggest underlying illness – in which case the most likely diagnosis is constitutional delay of growth and puberty and clinical follow-up is sufficient – or are any of the following present that would suggest the need for laboratory evaluation:

- Delayed puberty without a clear family history of late pubertal timing in at least one parent or sibling
- Stalled puberty
- "Red flags" that may be suggestive of underlying pathology

The following aspects of the history are of particularly relevant:

- Anosmia is suggestive of Kallmann syndrome, as are cleft lip and palate and unilateral renal agenesis [4].
- Habits of nutrition and physical activity are critical to evaluate functional hypogonadotropic hypogonadism. Strenuous athletic activity of 10 or more hours per week may cause functional hypogonadotropic hypogonadism in men [5]. In women, functional hypothalamic amenorrhea may be seen even in those exercising 4–6 hours per week (aerobic weight bearing or endurance training) if dietary intake is insufficient to meet the needs of exercise energy expenditure [6, 7].
- Eating habits and body image should be explored for the possibility of anorexia nervosa or other eating disorders.
- Medical issues in infancy such as lymphedema or hypotonia may suggest syndromic causes such as Turner syndrome or Prader-Willi syndrome, respectively. Similarly, history of cryptorchidism and/or micropenis in infancy increases the likelihood of syndromic/genetic causes.
- History of trauma, treatment for malignancy, or severe infections should be explored for the possibility of CNS or testicular/ovarian sequelae.
- Developmental delay or neuropsychiatric issues may suggest a syndromic cause of delayed puberty.
- Medication use is relevant for substances such as opiates that suppress the HPG axis or atypical anti-psychotics, metaclopromide, and other medications that may cause hyperprolactinemia.
- Extended family history of pubertal timing, characterized by timing of menarche in women and, in men, often ascertained with questions about when they stopped growing or when they began needing to shave.
- Extended family history of infertility, which supports a genetic etiology.
- Complete review of systems to assess for any possible signs or symptoms of underlying illness.

Key Aspects of the Physical Examination

Given the possibility of genetic causes, a full physical examination should take note of any dysmorphic or syndromic features, with particular attention to possible signs of Turner syndrome in girls: webbed neck, wide-spaced nipples, shield chest, wide carrying angle. A careful neurological examination including visual fields and fundoscopic examination should be performed because of the possibility of CNS pathology. If there is question of anosmia, this can be further queried on physical examination either using a commercial testing kit for smell or a readily available substance/object that is strongly scented.

The following auxological features may provide clues to diagnosis:

- Short stature may be consistent with Turner syndrome, Prader-Willi syndrome, hypothyroidism, or growth hormone deficiency (which may be associated with other hormone deficiencies including gonadotropin deficiency from congenital or acquired causes).
- Decreased growth velocity should raise concern for underlying systemic illness, hypothyroidism, or growth hormone deficiency.
- Increased arm-span-to-height-ratio (see Chap. 1) is suggestive of Klinefelter syndrome.

Tanner Staging, described in Chap. 10, Table 10.4, should be performed for breasts in girls, genitalia in boys, and pubic hair in both. In addition to Tanner staging, the following aspects of the pubertal examination are of particular importance:

- *Testicular size* should be measured in boys, using either an orchidometer to assess volume or a ruler to assess testicular length (along the long axis). The scrotal skin should be gently stretched around the testis to ensure that only the testis itself is included in the measurement. A testicular volume of 4 cc or a testicular length of roughly 2.5 cm is indicative of pubertal onset.
- A *stretched penile length* is used to assess for micropenis: Place a ruler or measuring tape at the base of the pubic ramus, stretch the phallus until there is increased resistance, and measure to the tip of the glans (excluding excessive foreskin).
- If there is appearance of breast tissue, *breast palpation* is necessary to discern between true breast tissue versus lipomastia (see Chap. 10, Table 10.5).

Initial Evaluation

CDGP is technically a diagnosis of exclusion, and all children with delayed puberty should be carefully considered for the possibility of underlying pathology. Nonetheless, since CDGP is also the most common cause of delayed puberty, we suggest that clinical observation is sufficient for children with very high suspicion for CDGP based on the following:

- Clear family history of CDGP in at least one parent.
- Well-appearing child of normal height, weight, and growth velocity, with no "red flags" on history or physical examination.
- If performed, bone age is delayed, and adult height prediction based on bone age is consistent with genetic potential.

Even in this case, we recommend clinical evaluation every 6 months (rather than at 1 year well-child visits) to assess for pubertal progression and ensure that concerning signs or symptoms do not develop. CDGP can be difficult to diffierentiate from idiopathic hypogonadotropic hypogonadism (IHH). Of note, adrenarche is typically delayed in CDGP, but not in IHH, although this is not absolute.

For all other children, including all children with stalled puberty, we recommend the first-line laboratory evaluation described in Table 11.2.

Next Steps in Diagnosis and Management

As above, children with a benign presentation and family history of CDGP may be followed in the primary care setting. Otherwise we recommend that all children with delayed or stalled puberty who are not found to have another etiology (e.g., other systemic illness) on initial testing be referred to pediatric endocrinology. *Reasons for urgent referral* include CNS symptoms, growth velocity <4 cm per year (see Chap. 1), hyperprolactinemia, or severe hypothyroidism. Interpretation of the recommended labs above is discussed in Chap. 25 (thyroid studies), 27 (labs related to the HPG axis), 35 (karyotype), and 36 (bone age). Further evaluation and management of delayed puberty is described in Chap. 44.

Table 11.2 Suggested elements of evaluation for delayed or stalled puberty

Test	Notes
First-line evaluation	
Bone age	Delayed bone age, defined as bone age >2 standard deviations below chronological age, is consistent with either CDGP or pathological causes.
Estradiol (girls)	Request high-sensitivity assay.
Testosterone (boys)	Send in the morning (before 10 AM), because of higher nocturnal LH pulsatile secretion in early central puberty.
Luteinizing hormone (LH)	Request sensitive/ultrasensitive assay and send in the morning (before 10 AM) because of higher nocturnal LH pulsatile secretion in early central puberty. An LH $\geq$ 0.3 U/L indicates HPG activation whereas an undetectable level is not definitive because of LH pulsatility.
Follicle Stimulating Hormone (FSH)	Longer half-life, can send any time of day. Elevations in the context of low estradiol/testosterone strongly suggest gonadal failure.
Prolactin	Hyperprolactinemia suppresses GnRH and can cause delayed or stalled puberty. Elevations should prompt further evaluation for CNS pathology after ruling out physiological causes and drug-induced hyperprolactinemia.
Thyroid stimulating hormone (TSH) and free thyroxine (Free T4)	Hypothyroidism can cause delayed or stalled puberty. Central hypothyroidism (low free T4 and low or low-normal TSH) with delayed puberty should prompt further evaluation for CNS pathology.
CBC with differential	To assess for hematologic malignancy or severe anemia (suggestive of underlying systemic disease).
Comprehensive metabolic panel	To assess for underlying systemic disease including liver disease, kidney disease.
Other labs to consider	
Inhibin B	Synthesized by the Sertoli Cells, Inhibin B is a useful adjunct marker of testicular activity in boys. Lower levels suggest testicular failure or hypogonadotropic hypogonadism, whereas low-normal or normal levels are more consistent with CDGP.
Anti-Müllerian hormone (AMH)	AMH is synthesized by the granulosa cells of the ovary (and the Sertoli cells of the testes) and can be a useful adjunctive marker of ovarian reserve in girls for whom there is a question of ovarian failure. Very low/ undetectable values are consistent with ovarian failure.
Karyotype	Karyotype is useful when there is suspicion of Turner or Klinefelter syndrome. Because many girls with Turner syndrome will start puberty and stall, and roughly 10% will have spontaneous menarche, clinicians should have a low threshold for sending karyotype in girls with delayed or stalled puberty.
Insulin-like growth factor-I (IGF-I)	A useful adjunct when there is decreased growth velocity and/or short stature. Reduced levels of IGF-I suggest GH deficiency, which may indicate congenital or acquired CNS pathology.
C-reactive protein and/or erythrocyte sedimentation rate	To assess for systemic inflammation that may suggest underlying illness.
Total IgA and tissue transglutaminase IgA)	To assess for undiagnosed celiac disease.
Magnetic resonance imaging of the brain	This will typically be performed in the pediatric endocrinology setting. A child with delayed puberty who is also found to have hyperprolactinemia, clear growth hormone deficiency, or other pituitary pathology warrants a brain MRI using the pituitary protocol (see Chap. 37).

References

1. Biro FM, Pajak A, Wolff MS, Pinney SM, Windham GC, Galvez MP, et al. Age of Menarche in a longitudinal US Cohort. J Pediatr Adolesc Gynecol. 2018;31(4):339–45.
2. Argente J. Diagnosis of late puberty. Horm Res. 1999;51(Suppl 3):95–100.
3. Rubio-Gozalbo ME, Gubbels CS, Bakker JA, Menheere PP, Wodzig WK, Land JA. Gonadal function in male and female patients with classic galactosemia. Hum Reprod Update. 2010;16(2):177–88.
4. Howard SR, Dunkel L. Delayed puberty-phenotypic diversity, molecular genetic mechanisms, and recent discoveries. Endocr Rev. 2019;40(5):1285–317.
5. Dwyer AA, Chavan NR, Lewkowitz-Shpuntoff H, Plummer L, Hayes FJ, Seminara SB, et al. Functional hypogonadotropic hypogonadism in men: underlying neuroendocrine mechanisms and natural history. J Clin Endocrinol Metab. 2019;104(8):3403–14.
6. Ackerman KE, Slusarz K, Guereca G, Pierce L, Slattery M, Mendes N, et al. Higher ghrelin and lower leptin secretion are associated with lower LH secretion in young amenorrheic athletes compared with eumenorrheic athletes and controls. Am J Physiol Endocrinol Metab. 2012;302(7):E800–6.
7. Rickenlund A, Thoren M, Nybacka A, Frystyk J, Hirschberg AL. Effects of oral contraceptives on diurnal profiles of insulin, insulin-like growth factor binding protein-1, growth hormone and cortisol in endurance athletes with menstrual disturbance. Hum Reprod. 2010;25(1):85–93.

Atypical/Ambiguous/Non-binary Genitalia

12

Seth Tobolsky and Takara Stanley

What Is the Definition of "Atypical/Ambiguous Genitalia"?

Atypical/ambiguous genitalia refers to a condition in which an individual's genitals do not have the appearance of "typical" external male or female genitalia. Although atypical genitalia are generally noted at birth, presentation could occur at any age. There are serious psychosocial dynamics to be considered when defining this topic – the key piece to understand is that *assigned sex at birth and biological sex are different from gender identity,* and that non-binary genitalia are relevant to assigned sex at birth and biological sex. Gender, in contrast, is part of a person's identity and is based on how the person perceives and understands themselves. There is an unfortunate history of the medical community imposing a strict social construct of gender on patients' bodies, and historically physicians have regretfully been a major driving force behind this stigmatizing and alienating practice.

Atypical genitalia usually point to the diagnosis of a disorder of sex development (also referred to as a difference in sex development), or DSD, discussed below. DSDs are defined as "congenital conditions in which development of chromosomal, gonadal, or anatomical sex is atypical [1]." Although atypical genital appearance is a presenting sign of DSD, DSDs can also be present in individuals with normal-appearing genitalia; for example, patients with complete androgen insensitivity syndrome usually have typical female genitalia.

S. Tobolsky (✉)
Massachusetts General Hospital for Children, Boston, MA, USA
e-mail: seth.tobolsky@mgh.harvard.edu

T. Stanley
Division of Pediatric Endocrinology, Massachusetts General Hospital and Harvard Medical School, Boston, MA, USA
e-mail: tstanley@mgh.harvard.edu

What Are the Currently Favored Medical and Layperson Terms for a Condition in Which an Infant's Reproductive Organs Are Non-binary?

Currently, disorders of sex development, or DSDs, is the term the medical community uses [2]. However, recent research from Lurie Children's Hospital suggests that patients in the community tend to identify as "intersex," and that patient engagement and deferral of "corrective" surgery are increased when doctors use the term "intersex" rather than a term containing the word "disorder." "Differences of sex development" rather than "disorders of sex development" is also in use for this reason. Terms such as hermaphroditism and pseudohermaphroditism are inappropriate, as well as clinically inaccurate.

Why Is This Condition Relevant to the Primary Care Practitioner?

Atypical genitalia in a neonate should prompt a clinician to consider congenital disorders and embark on a preliminary endocrine work-up without delay. Clinically, the particular conditions that manifest with atypical genitalia are often difficult to distinguish, and so potentially life-threatening diagnoses must be ruled out first. Congenital adrenal hyperplasia (CAH) is the most common underlying diagnosis and is potentially life threatening if not treated early.

Differential Diagnosis

The differential diagnosis of DSD is shown in Table 12.1. The differential, informed by the karyotype, is generally considered in three categories: 46,XX DSDs, 46,XY DSDs, and sex chromosome DSDs, in which karyotype is some-

T. Stanley, M. Misra (eds.), *Endocrine Conditions in Pediatrics*, https://doi.org/10.1007/978-3-030-52215-5_12

Table 12.1 Categories of disorders underlying atypical genitalia/disorders of sex development

Category	*46,XX DSDs* (more virilized than typical female)	*46,XY DSDs* (less virilized than typical male)	*Sex chromosome DSDs*
Most common cause	Congenital adrenal hyperplasia* due to 21-hydroxylase (*CYP21A2*) deficiency	Androgen insensitivity syndrome	Mixed gonadal dysgenesis
"Cannot-miss" causes	Congenital adrenal hyperplasia due to 21-hydroxylase (*CYP21A2*) deficiency, 3-beta-hydroxysteroid dehydrogenase Type 2 (*HSD3B2*) deficiency, or P450 oxidoreductase (*POR*) deficiency (includes deficiencies of 21-hydroxylase, 17-alpha hydroxylase and aromatase), all of which can cause salt-wasting crisis Androgen-secreting tumor in mother during pregnancy. These tumors can be malignant and life-threatening to the mother Glucocorticoid resistance from mutations in the glucocorticoid receptor	Congenital adrenal hyperplasia due to lipoid hyperplasia (*STAR*), P450 side-chain cleavage enzyme deficiency (*CYP11A1*), 3-beta-hydroxysteroid dehydrogenase type 2 (*HSD3B2*) deficiency, or P450 oxidoreductase (*POR*) deficiency (includes deficiencies of 21-hydroxylase, 17-alpha hydroxylase, and aromatase), all of which can cause salt-wasting crisis	
Other causes	Congenital adrenal hyperplasia due to 11-beta-hydroxylase deficiency (*CYP11B1*) 17-beta-hydroxysteroid dehydrogenase type 3 deficiency (*HSD17B3)* XX testicular or ovo-testicular DSD Maternal exogenous androgen or synthetic progestogen exposure during pregnancy Aromatase deficiency (may cause maternal virilization during pregnancy because of lack of placental aromatase) .	Congenital adrenal hyperplasia due to17-alpha-hydroxylase/17,20-lyase (*CYP17A1)* deficiency or P450 oxidoreductase (*POR*) deficiency 17-beta-hydroxysteroid dehydrogenase type 3 deficiency (*HSD17B3)* 5-alpha-reductase deficiency (5 types, all with different phenotypes, typically develop typical external male genitalia during puberty) Smith-Lemli-Opitz syndrome (sterol delta-7-reductase deficiency) LH receptor defects (Leydig cell hypoplasia) Androgen receptor defects XY gonadal dysgenesis and XY ovarian DSD Testicular regression syndrome Endocrine disrupters	Other mosaicism such as 45,X/47,XXY; 46,XX/47XXY Chimerism, i.e., 46,XX/46,XY (results from fusion of two zygotes)

N.B., Only types of CAH that are expected to cause atypical genitalia are included above. CAH is described further in Chap. 49

Table 12.2 Clarifying questions and their relevance

Question	Relevance
Was the mother exposed to androgens or synthetic progestogens during pregnancy?	Use of androgens or certain other synthetic steroid medications can cause fetal virilization.
Was there maternal virilization during pregnancy?	Maternal tumors, typically ovarian or adrenal tumors, including luteomas, can produce androgens and cause fetal virilization. Aromatase deficiency in a 46,XX fetus creates high levels of fetal testosterone that overwhelm placental aromatase and can cause maternal virilization; placental aromatase may also be deficient.
Is there parental consanguinity?	If present, raises suspicion for autosomal recessive disorders, including CAH and disorders of testosterone biosynthesis
Is there any family history of unexpected infant death?	If present, raises suspicion for CAH.
Is there any family history of infertility, premature menopause, or atypical genitalia?	Can raise suspicion for various genetic etiologies.

thing other than 46,XX or 46,XY. Infants with mild abnormalities, such as distal hypospadias with otherwise normal male genitalia and bilaterally descended testes, will not necessarily need karyotype testing but should undergo a thorough examination with the consideration of possible syndromic or endocrine causes.

Clarifying Questions in the Medical History

Because some causes of atypical genitalia are heritable and others are related to maternal exposures or conditions, certain questions, shown in Table 12.2, are important to elucidate possible etiology.

Pertinent Physical Exam

A comprehensive examination, including a systematic genital examination as described in Table 12.3, is key to inform the differential diagnosis.

Table 12.3 Systematic approach to the genital examination

Symmetry/asymmetry of the exam	This can provide clues to the etiology of genital ambiguity. Asymmetry may suggest mixed gonadal dysgenesis or another sex chromosome DSD.
Clitoris, penis, or phallic structure	"Phallic structure" or "clitorophallic structure" is used to describe an intermediate organ that is not clearly a penis or clitoris. Length and width should be measured: For "Stretched" penile or phallic length, place base of ruler at the pubic ramus and stretch the phallus until increased resistance to measure length. For clitoral length and width, use gentle pressure to isolate the gland itself and ensure excess skin and subcutaneous tissue are not measured. If relevant, describe the shape of the phallus/penis – whether there is curvature and/or tethering.
Orifices	Penis should have a single urethral opening at the tip of the glans penis. If the urethral opening is not at the tip, describe if it is on the glans but not at the tip, on the distal shaft, mid-shaft, proximal shaft, scrotum, or perineum. Female anatomy should have separate urethral and vaginal openings; a single opening is referred to as a urogenital opening.
Labia, scrotum, or labioscrotal folds	Scrotum or labia minora and labia majora should be inspected. In utero, the labia fuse from posterior to anterior to differentiate into a fused scrotum. For intermediate structures, describe where there is fusion (e.g., posterior fusion of labia, or bifid scrotum) and also rugation and pigmentation.
Gonads	Note if gonads are palpable, and their location: in the scrotum, labioscrotal folds, or inguinal canal. (Retractile testes can often be "milked" into the scrotum from the inguinal canal.)
Anogenital distance [3] (Can reflect prenatal androgen exposure [↑androgen causes ↑distance] but not universally used [2])	Measure from the center of the anus to either the base of the scrotal structure or the base of the posterior fourchette If phallic structure, also measure from the center of the anus to the anterior base of the penis (where the penile tissue meets the pubic bone). If clitoral structure, also measure from the center of the anus to the anterior tip of the clitoral hood.

Clinical Examination Pearls

- Stretched penile length <2.0 cm is abnormal for any gestational age, and <2.5 cm is abnormal for a term infant.
- Clitoral length >1.0 cm is abnormal.
- Pre-term infants often have prominence of the labia minora and clitoris that does not necessarily indicate pathology as long as the remainder of the examination is normal and prominence resolves on follow-up examinations.
- Careful examination for other congenital anomalies may suggest syndromic diagnoses.
- Hyperpigmentation of the genitalia and/or other areas should further raise suspicion for CAH or rarely glucocorticoid resistance.

DSDs and their corresponding physical exam findings are generally characterized along a *spectrum of virilization*, that is, *to what extent is the patient virilized*? At one end, there is the "normal" female phenotype, defined as having typical internal and external female genitalia – for our purposes, "0% virilized." On the other end, there is the "normal" male phenotype, defined as having typical internal and external male genitalia – "100% virilized." The Prader Scale is commonly used to describe virilization of infants; although originally developed to describe the degree of virilization of infants with 46,XX karyotype and CAH, it is often used in other instances. The Quigley Scale [4], less commonly used, characterizes undervirilization in individuals with 46,XY karyotype and androgen insensitivity. These scales are described in Table 12.4.

Table 12.4 Prader Scale and Quigley Scale

Prader Scale to describe virilization [5] *Prader 1* – Mild clitoromegaly, otherwise typical female external genitalia *Prader 2* – Clitoromegaly and posterior labial fusion *Prader 3* – Clitoromegaly, labioscrotal fusion with single perineal urogenital opening *Prader 4* – Clitorophallic structure with urogenital/urethral opening at the base *Prader 5* – Typical male external genitalia without palpable gonads
Quigley Scale to describe undervirilization in androgen insensitivity syndrome [4] *Grade 1* – Typical male phenotype *Grade 2* – Unequivocally male phenotype with mildly defective masculinization, e.g., isolated hypospadias *Grade 3* – Predominantly male phenotype with perineal hypospadias, microphallus, and cryptorchidism and/or bifid scrotum *Grade 4* – Genitalia with intermediate phenotype: clitorophallic structure, single perineal orifice of urogenital sinus, labioscrotal folds with or without posterior fusion. *Grade 5* – Unequivocally female phenotype with limited androgenization evidenced by mild clitoromegaly and/or mild posterior labial fusion *Grade 6* – Typical female phenotype with the emergence of pubic and/or axillary hair during puberty *Grade 7* – Typical female phenotype with the absence of pubic or axillary hair during puberty

Clinical Key: Hypospadias and Microphallus

An infant with isolated glandular/distal hypospadias OR isolated microphallus does not necessarily require further evaluation for DSD if the remainder of the examination is normal, including normal scrotum with bilaterally descended testes. Infants with hypospadias should not be circumcised, however, and will benefit from urology consultation, whereas infants with microphallus will benefit from an endocrine consultation. Testosterone and gonadotropins are helpful between 2 weeks to 4–6 months of life, after which they are not clinically useful. For this reason, early referral to endocrinology for microphallus is warranted to ensure timely evaluation.

Initial Labs and Imaging

Initial laboratory evaluation and imaging (Table 12.5) should be tailored based on findings on history and physical examination. The most urgent issue is to assess for CAH; in this regard, three important principles are as follows:

- If there are no palpable gonads, the external genitalia are symmetrically ambiguous, and a uterus +/− potential ovaries are present on ultrasound, the most likely diagnosis is 21-hydroxylase CAH.
- Electrolyte derangements (hyponatremia and hyperkalemia) from salt-losing forms of CAH (i.e., forms with mineralocorticoid deficiency) are not typically present at birth. These usually manifest within the first 1–2 weeks of life. Infants in whom CAH is suspected should have serial electrolyte measurements through the first few weeks of life or until the diagnosis is definitively excluded.
- In a child with the suspicion for CAH, an ACTH stimulation test using a supraphysiologic dose of exogenous ACTH (250 mcg/m^2) may be required. If the patient is hemodynamically unstable or has concerning electrolyte derangements, do not delay or pause glucocorticoids for the purpose of diagnostic testing.

Specific information on interpretation of these laboratory studies can be found in Chap. 27.

Next Steps in Diagnosis and Management

In addition to sending initial labs, it is important to have a discussion with the child's parents about what to expect.

Table 12.5 Labs and imaging

Diagnostic goal	Testing	Notes
Establish chromosomal sex	Karyotype	Call lab to expedite testing. Can perform FISH for SRY if more expeditious, but may be misleading in 46,XY with SRY mutation/deletion or 46,XX with SRY translocation
Identify gonads and other structures	Abdominal/ pelvic ultrasound	Failure to identify uterus and/or gonads on ultrasound does not completely exclude their presence. MRI may provide more definitive information, but risks of sedation must be weighed.
Assess for salt-wasting	Electrolytes 17-OHP PRA Aldosterone Cortisol ACTH	Electrolytes and 17-OHP first line. Serum 17-OHP unreliable before 36 hours of life [2]. If electrolytes suggest salt-wasting, also send PRA and aldosterone. Random ACTH and cortisol can be sent initially in infants (or 8 AM labs for older children), but ACTH stimulation test may be required.
Assess for hypoglycemia	Glucose	Should be sent with electrolytes, as both adrenal insufficiency and panhypopituitarism can present with hypoglycemia.
Assess gonadal function	Testosterone Estradiol AMH	In males, testosterone is low between day 2 of life and ~2 weeks of life, after which it rises with the mini-puberty of infancy. Use age-specific norms. AMH at male levels indicates presence of testicular tissue.
Assess gonadal and pituitary function	LH and FSH	Use age-specific ranges; mini-puberty in males until ~6 months of age, and in girls until ~12 months. Elevated in primary gonadal dysfunction, disorders of testosterone biosynthesis, LH receptor mutations.

Abbreviations 17-OHP 17-hydroxprogesterone, *ACTH* adrenocorticotrophic hormone, *AMH* anti-Müllerian hormone, *MRI* magnetic resonance imaging, *PRA* plasma renin activity, *SRY* sex-determining region of the Y chromosome

Care and empathy from the initial physicians involved are fundamental to successfully supporting families through reframing assigned sex and gender and making informed decisions. As the child grows older, their input into gender identity should be highly valued and considered. Multidisciplinary care should also be established from the outset to whatever degree this is feasible. Additionally, multiple patient support groups are available for vetted educational materials as well as support and connection for parents and extended families [2]. A comprehensive list is available in the 2016 DSD Consensus Statement [2].

Despite advances in molecular genetic diagnostics, the cause of genital ambiguity may not always be possible to identify, especially in infants with the 46,XY karyotype. This means that *we begin by ruling out cannot-miss diagnoses, such as CAH, before proceeding further down the diagnostic chain*. This is an important expectation to set for parents as well – although an exact diagnosis is not always forthcoming, the team will be able to provide information and support for decision making and management to ensure that the best is done for the child.

Please refer to Chap. 46 for further discussion of diagnosis and management of DSD, as well as Chap. 49 for more detailed discussion of CAH.

References

1. Hughes IA, Houk C, Ahmed SF, Lee PA, Group LC, Group EC. Consensus statement on management of intersex disorders. Arch Dis Child. 2006;91(7):554–63.
2. Lee PA, Nordenstrom A, Houk CP, Ahmed SF, Auchus R, Baratz A, et al. Global disorders of sex development update since 2006: perceptions, approach and care. Horm Res Paediatr. 2016;85(3):158–80.
3. Sathyanarayana S, Grady R, Redmon JB, Ivicek K, Barrett E, Janssen S, et al. Anogenital distance and penile width measurements in The Infant Development and the Environment Study (TIDES): methods and predictors. J Pediatr Urol. 2015;11(2):76 e1–6.
4. Quigley CA, De Bellis A, Marschke KB, el-Awady MK, Wilson EM, French FS. Androgen receptor defects: historical, clinical, and molecular perspectives. Endocr Rev. 1995;16(3):271–321.
5. White PC, Speiser PW. Congenital adrenal hyperplasia due to 21-hydroxylase deficiency. Endocr Rev. 2000;21(3):245–91.

13 Common Breast Complaints [Gynecomastia, Breast Asymmetry, Galactorrhea]

Nabiha Shahid and Nursen Gurtunca

Gynecomastia

Gynecomastia is derived from the Greek word "Gyne" meaning women and "mastos" meaning breasts. The term "gynecomastia" is used to define "women like breasts noted in males." It should not be used to describe enlargement of breasts in females, which is "thelarche." Gynecomastia is very common. It is seen in 70% of adolescent males and in 50% of males at autopsy [1]. Most cases of gynecomastia are benign, such as those seen in the newborn period, puberty, and aging. Occasionally, gynecomastia is associated with an underlying systemic or endocrine disease. Gynecomastia can be a cause of psychosocial distress in adolescence. Appropriate evaluation and counseling are recommended.

Appearance of enlarged breasts in males could be due to glandular breast tissue with fat deposition or adipose tissue alone. The terms "pseudogynecomastia," "adipomastia," and "lipomastia" are used to describe the appearance of enlarged breasts due to adipose tissue only. Glandular breast tissue has a firm, globular consistency and can be distinguished from the surrounding softer adipose tissue. Histologically glandular breast tissue in gynecomastia is comprised of mammary ductules in a fibroconnective stroma [2]. Initially, there is a proliferation of ductules without terminal acini in loose fibroconnective tissue; overtime there is progressive fibrosis [3]. Stromal fibrosis, once present, is permanent and will not completely regress with time. Glandular breast tissue in both males and females contains hormonal receptors including estrogen receptor, androgen receptor, progesterone receptor, prolactin receptor, insulin-like growth factor-1 receptor, luteinizing hormone (LH) receptor, human chorionic gonadotropin (hCG) receptor, and leptin receptor [1]. It is believed that the hormones and growth factors for these receptors have endocrine as well as paracrine effect on breast development. Although most of the studies on the effect of hormones and growth factors have been carried out using female breast tissues, male breast tissue is believed to respond to endocrine and paracrine stimulation in a similar fashion [1].

Estrogens stimulate whereas androgens inhibit the proliferation of breast tissue. The role of other hormone receptors in male breast tissue is not well understood. Gynecomastia develops when there is absolute or relative deficiency of androgen or androgenic action, or when there is excess of estrogen or estrogenic action. Decreased androgen levels such as in hypogonadism, as well as decreased androgen activity due to absent or defective androgen receptor in breast tissue, may result in gynecomastia. Although the absolute levels of androgens and estrogens may be normal, the relative ratio of androgens to estrogens plays a role in the development of pubertal gynecomastia.

Pearls

- Gynecomastia means female-like breasts noted in males.
- Gynecomastia is seen in 70% of adolescent males, and most cases regress after puberty.
- Gynecomastia in peri-pubertal males is almost always benign.
- It is important to differentiate true gynecomastia from lipomastia seen in overweight individuals.

N. Shahid · N. Gurtunca (✉)
UPMC Children's Hospital of Pittsburgh, Division of Endocrinology and Diabetes, Pittsburgh, PA, USA
e-mail: Nabiha.shahid@upmc.edu; Nursen.Gurtunca@chp.edu

T. Stanley, M. Misra (eds.), *Endocrine Conditions in Pediatrics*, https://doi.org/10.1007/978-3-030-52215-5_13

Causes (Table 13.1)

Table 13.1 Causes of gynecomastia

Benign causes	
Physiological neonatal gynecomastia	
Physiological peripubertal gynecomastia	
Phytoestrogen-induced gynecomastia	
Structural lesions [cysts, fibroadenoma]	
Non-benign causes	
Decreased androgen production	Primary (testicular) hypogonadism Secondary (central) hypogonadism
Decreased androgen effects or biosynthesis	Androgen insensitivity syndrome 5 alpha reductase deficiency 17 beta hydroxysteroid dehydrogenase deficiency
Increased estrogen production	Adrenal or testicular tumors hCG-secreting tumors Familial aromatase excess syndrome
Other	Obesity Malnutrition Liver disease Hyperthyroidism Breast cancer [very rare]
Drug-induced gynecomastia	
Antiandrogens	Bicalutamide, flutamide, finasteride, spironolactone
Antibiotics/antifungals	Isoniazid, ketoconazole, metronidazole
Antihypertensive agents	Amlodipine, diltiazem, nifedipine, verapamil, captopril, enalapril
Anti-acid agents	Cimetidine, ranitidine, omeprazole
Hormones	Anabolic steroids, estrogens, hCG, growth hormone, GnRH agonists
Illicit drugs	Alcohol, marijuana, methadone
Psychiatric drugs	Psychotropic agents, tricyclic antidepressants
Other	Antiretroviral agents, digitalis, fibrates, methotrexate, statins

History and Physical Examination

In cases of gynecomastia, it is important to differentiate between benign and non-benign causes. Important clues to seek in history should include the time of gynecomastia development, duration, associated pain, redness, and discharge from the nipples. A detailed medication history or other substances used such as plant-derived oils, skin care products, or anabolic steroids even if used by family members should be obtained. Recent drastic changes in weight with other co-existent medical problems or recovery from any chronic illness can provide additional clues. Family history and consanguinity can be helpful in suggesting a familial hormonal disorders or even benign familial pubertal gynecomastia.

Physical examination for all patients should start with accurate measurements of weight, height, body proportions including the BMI, upper and lower body proportions (see Chap. 1). Examination of breasts should focus on determining if it is true gynecomastia or "lipomastia." There is firm glandular tissue under the nipple with true gynecomastia whereas there is no palpable tissue under the nipple with lipomastia, giving the impression of a "donut" with hollow center. Manipulation of breast to rule out galactorrhea may be necessary. Complete pubertal staging including the Tanner staging for secondary sexual characteristics, external genitalia, penile development, and testicular size should be performed. Fundoscopic examination to rule out raised intracranial pressure and examination of visual fields for defects from hypothalamic/pituitary tumors is an integral part of the physical examination.

Pearl

- On physical exam, gynecomastia is characterized by firm glandular tissue under the nipple, whereas lipomastia is characterized by lack of palpable tissue right under the nipple, giving the impression of a "donut" with a hollow center surrounded by adipose tissue.

Diagnostic Evaluation (Table 13.2)

In most adolescents with pubertal gynecomastia, no laboratory or radiographic imaging is recommended. Reassurance with observation is recommended if history and physical examination are otherwise normal. Obtaining a morning serum level of testosterone (preferably bioavailable/free testosterone, or total testosterone with sex hormone binding globulin), LH, FSH, estradiol [E2], estrone [E1], prolactin levels, and routine liver, kidney, and thyroid function tests are reasonable if pathology is suspected clinically based on any other signs or symptoms on history and physical [1]. Estradiol and hCG should be measured if estrogen-secreting

Table 13.2 Initial laboratory workup for gynecomastia with suspected pathological cause

Gonadotropins [FSH and LH]
Early morning testosterone
Estradiol [E2], estrone [E1]
Prolactin
Thyroid functions [TSH, Free T4]
Liver function tests
Kidney functions tests
hCG
Karyotype if suspicion for Klinefelter syndrome

tumors, hCG-secreting tumors, or germ cell tumors are suspected. Higher E2/Testosterone ratio is often seen in boys with true gynecomastia compared to boys with pseudogynecomastia. It is the higher E2/testosterone ratio that is more important than the absolute values of estrogen in gynecomastia [4]. E1 is a less potent form of estrogen and levels might be high in boys with gynecomastia and pseudogynecomastia [4]. Karyotype may be indicated if there is clinical suspicion for a chromosomal abnormality such as Klinefelter syndrome. Routine breast imaging (e.g., ultrasound) and mammography are not indicated unless a structural lesion is palpable on physical examination. However, ultrasound or mammography can be performed if a discrete mass is palpated, and abdominal CT or testicular US might be indicated if adrenal or testicular cancer is clinically suspected. Brain imaging may be considered if central nervous system involvement is suspected.

Management

The management of gynecomastia varies on a case-by-case basis. We will discuss a few common causes of gynecomastia and their management.

Physiological Neonatal Gynecomastia Palpable breast tissue is common in neonates due to the transfer of maternal estrogen through the placenta. It can be associated with milk secretion, popularly known as "witch's milk." Stagnation of milk and superadded infection can result in complications such as mastitis and breast abscess which may warrant surgical intervention. Minimal manipulation is recommended to prevent further stimulation of breast tissue and the introduction of infection. Gynecomastia is usually self-remitting as effects of maternal estrogen wear off. No intervention is warranted except in cases of mastitis, abscess, or palpation of a suspicious mass.

Physiological Peripubertal Gynecomastia This is mostly seen among boys in their early stages of puberty. The breast tissue resembles breast budding in pubertal females. The most likely explanation is relative estrogen excess due to variable amounts of aromatization of adrenal and testicular androgens to estrogen in peripheral tissues, particularly adipose tissue and liver, while the testosterone levels are not yet robust. This usually resolves spontaneously over 1–2 years. However, it might persist longer in obese boys or never completely resolve due to the higher estrogen levels from aromatization in peripheral fat tissue and permanent glandular breast tissue formation. In a pubertal adolescent male with gynecomastia, reassurance and observation with clinic follow-up every 3–6 months is recommended if the history and physical examination are otherwise normal. If the patient is overweight, weight loss should be recommended. If these strategies fail and the patient is psychologically bothered by gynecomastia, then the option of plastic surgery can be offered to the family. However, if the gynecomastia is progressive and associated with symptoms of breast tenderness further evaluation as mentioned above should be undertaken [1].

Phytoestrogen-Stimulated Gynecomastia Phytoestrogens are plant products that exert estrogenic effect through binding the estrogen receptors. Lavender oil and tea tree oil used in skin and hair products may cause gynecomastia in prepubertal boys. Breast enlargement resolves after discontinuation of the use [5].

Drug-Induced Gynecomastia Androgen abuse should be suspected in athletes and bodybuilders with gynecomastia. Young men with gynecomastia who use illicit drugs such as marijuana, methadone, and anabolic steroids should be counselled against the use of these drugs.

Pearls for Evaluation

- Physiological peripubertal gynecomastia is the most commonly encountered cause of gynecomastia.
- Detailed medication history and exposure to compounds like phytoestrogens found in lavender and tea tree oil must be ruled out before workup for other non-benign causes is sought.

Pearls for Management

- Once the diagnosis of benign peripubertal gynecomastia has been confirmed, appropriate counselling of the patient and family is crucial.
- One should keep in mind and address the psychological distress associated with gynecomastia especially in young boys.

Decreased Androgen Production Both testicular hypogonadism and central hypogonadism can cause gynecomastia mediated through unopposed effects of estrogen. In primary hypogonadism (testicular failure), low testosterone production leads to increased production of LH from the pituitary, which in turn increases the aromatase activity and hence the estrogen to androgen ratio which results in gynecomastia. This is commonly seen in conditions like Klinefelter syndrome or following treatment for orchitis and testicular tumors [5]. Similarly, in central hypogonadism as seen in Kallman syndrome, hypogonadotropic hypogonadism (HH) secondary to head trauma, brain surgery, hypothalamic/pituitary tumors, prolactinoma, pituitary adenomas or cranial irradiation, androgen production decreases, which results in unopposed estrogen effects on breast tissue, leading to gynecomastia. Excessive weight gain or weight loss can also result in HH and altered estrogen androgen ratio. Iron overload as seen in chronic blood transfusion or other genetic conditions may also cause HH. Chronic illness and/or inflammation can result in functional hypogonadism and altered estrogen testosterone ratio. True cases of hypogonadism can benefit from exogenous testosterone therapy to reverse gynecomastia. However, if hypogonadism is secondary to chronic inflammation or illness, addressing those conditions prior to starting testosterone therapy is recommended.

Decreased Androgen Effect or Synthesis Conditions such as androgen insensitivity syndrome, 5 alpha reductase deficiency and 17 beta hydroxysteroid dehydrogenase deficiency can cause gynecomastia mediated through increased aromatization of androgens to estrogen. In androgen insensitivity syndrome, deficient androgen receptor results in accumulation of excess androgens that are aromatized to estrogens, stimulating glandular tissue unopposed by androgens and resulting in gynecomastia. There is accumulation of testosterone due to enzymatic defects in 5 alpha reductase deficiency and 17 beta hydroxysteroid dehydrogenase deficiency. This results in high levels of estrogens from aromatization of testosterone and presents with gynecomastia [6]. Gynecomastia secondary to increased aromatization can be managed with aromatase inhibitors.

Increased Estrogen Production This can be seen in adrenal or testicular tumors, hCG-secreting tumors, or familial aromatase excess syndrome [1]. Phenotypic males with disorders of sex development due to gonadal dysgenesis with ovotestes may present with gynecomastia at the time of puberty [7]. Typically, there is rapid breast development with tenderness when large amounts of estrogens are secreted by hCG-secreting germ cell tumors or feminizing adrenocortical tumors. Resection of the tumor resolves the gynecomastia. Aromatase excess syndrome may be treated with aromatase inhibitors.

Other Causes Other conditions such as obesity can cause appearance of prominent breast tissue. Mostly, this is associated with a homogeneous non-glandular fat tissue on palpation. However increased aromatase activity in excessive adipose tissue may cause a relative increase in estrogen systemically as well as locally in the breast, and this may result in true gynecomastia. The true glandular tissue that forms may not regress after weight loss. Referral to plastic surgery may be considered. Malnutrition can lead to gynecomastia through hypothalamic pituitary dysfunction and resultant decreased testosterone levels. "Refeeding gynecomastia" is seen in young men who resume a regular diet following poor nutrition. This is a self-limiting condition that resolves spontaneously within 2 years after resuming normal diet [1]. Liver disease and hyperthyroidism can also cause gynecomastia through alteration of estrogen/testosterone metabolism and their binding proteins. Treatment of underlying disease usually results in regression of gynecomastia.

Structural Lesions Structural lesions such as fibroadenoma, galactocele, hematoma, or ductal ectasia can also rarely present as gynecomastia or breast asymmetry. Careful physical exam should be performed, and if suspicious for any structural lesion, then breast imaging such as ultrasound can be considered. Breast cancer in the pediatric and adolescent population is very rare. Metastatic disease or hematological malignancy is a more common etiology of a malignant breast mass than breast carcinoma in children and adolescents [8].

Medical Therapy for Gynecomastia Many cases of gynecomastia do not require pharmacological management as they resolve on their own. Pharmacological treatment is most likely to be beneficial in the early proliferative phase of gynecomastia (first 1–2 years), as over time, fibrosis ensues and that cannot be reversed with medical therapy. The medical therapy is aimed at reversing the imbalance of androgens and estrogens. If gynecomastia is secondary to a drug or supplement exposure, the use should be discontinued, and patient should be seen within a few weeks to months, as the breast tissue is expected to regress over this period. If for some reason the medication cannot be discontinued, or the breast tissue does not regress, then medical therapy for gynecomastia can be tried.

There are 3 different categories of medical treatment options available; however, it is worth mentioning that there are not many randomized clinical trials on the use of these drugs in children and adolescent populations.

1. *Testosterone therapy:* Androgens are reserved only for gynecomastia caused by hypogonadism/low testosterone levels to suppress the unopposed effects of estrogen. If given in conditions with normal testosterone levels, aromatization might lead to worsening of gynecomastia. Testosterone should not be used for gynecomastia in boys with otherwise normal pubertal development.
2. *Aromatase inhibitors* [such as letrozole], as the name suggests, block aromatization and hence peripheral conversion of androgens to estrogen.
3. *SERMS* [selective estrogen receptor modulators such as tamoxifen] exert inhibitory effects on the breast tissue and oppose estrogen's effects. It has been used in gynecomastia of puberty with partial response in the majority of boys (90%). Complete response is seen only in <10% [6].

Surgical Therapy for Gynecomastia Referral for surgical treatment should be considered in cases that are long lasting, do not regress spontaneously or following failed medical therapy, and are bothersome for the patient. The extent and type of surgery depends on the amount of breast tissue versus adipose tissue in the breast. The most commonly used surgical approach is the nipple sparing subcutaneous mastectomy [8]. The most frequent surgical complications are numbness of the nipple and adherence of the areola to the pectoral muscle [9].

One other practical caution that needs to be given with benign gynecomastia is not to try to "squeeze" or "rub it away." This may introduce infection and repeated mechanical stimulation can even cause worsening of the gynecomastia [10].

Breast Asymmetry

Breast asymmetry (Fig. 13.1) is a finding rather than a diagnosis and encompasses mild-to-moderate differences in breast shape, size, and position [11]. It is common in pubertal adolescent girls and is mostly seen due to the fluctuating response of the developing breast tissue to the hormonal environment during puberty [12]. Any time an adolescent is being evaluated for breast asymmetry, it is important to evaluate for other causes such as a breast mass and/or abscess. Breast asymmetry can be due to Poland syndrome which is a congenital malformation affecting the chest wall, shoulder, arm, and hand [11]. If no underlying cause is found and the patient is not being affected psychologically, then watchful waiting until complete breast development is reasonable. In many instances where the asymmetry is the result of hormonal fluctuations, it may resolve as breast development is completed. However, if it fails to resolve and if the patient is suffering from poor emotional well-being and lower self-esteem, then surgical referral for augmentation or reduction mammoplasty can be considered. Non-surgical options such as padded bras and prosthetic inserts can be recommended to achieve symmetry.

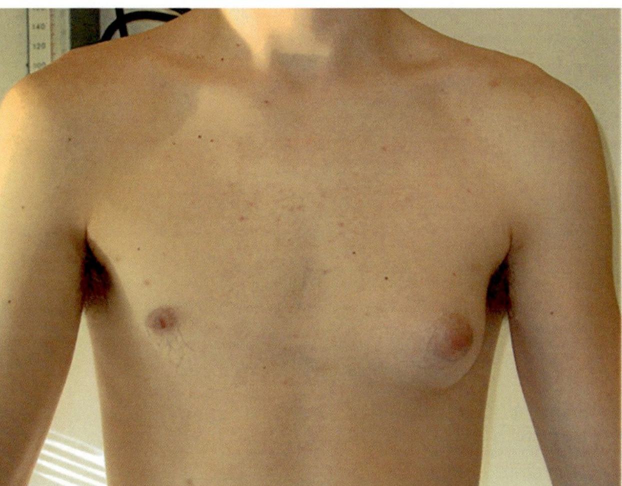

Fig. 13.1 Asymmetric pubertal gynecomastia. (Courtesy of Oscar Escobar M.D, Division of Pediatric Endocrine and Diabetes, UPMC Children's Hospital of Pittsburgh)

Galactorrhea

Galactorrhea is a Greek word derived from "Galakt" meaning milk and "rhoia" meaning flux or flow. Galactorrhea is defined as milk production outside the context of pregnancy or breastfeeding (one year after pregnancy or cessation of breastfeeding) [13]. Galactorrhea can occur in males as well. The key hormone involved in milk production is prolactin, synthesized and secreted from the lactotrophs in the anterior pituitary. There are various stimulatory signals for lactotrophs originating in the hypothalamus such as vasoactive intestinal polypeptide [VIP] or thyrotropin-releasing hormone [TRH] which also stimulates the thyrotropes in the anterior pituitary to secrete thyroid-stimulating hormone [TSH]. Estrogens also directly stimulate the pituitary lactotrophs and prolactin secretion. One important inhibitory signal for lactotrophs is the neurotransmitter dopamine.

Causes of Galactorrhea [13]

Causes of galactorrhea are listed in Table 13.3.

History and Physical Examination

In all patients presenting with galactorrhea a detailed history needs to be taken including menstrual and pregnancy history in post-pubertal adolescent girls and a detailed medication history. Additional questions in history should be focused

Table 13.3 Causes of galactorrhea

Physiological	Pregnancy Nipple stimulation Neonatal due to the transfer of maternal hormones
Pathological	
Central lesions	Prolactinoma Other pituitary macroadenoma Craniopharyngioma Meningioma Germinoma
Local lesions	Herpes zoster Burns Trauma Mammoplasty Breast cancer [rare]
Systemic disease	Hypothyroidism, chronic renal failure
Medications	Antipsychotics such as risperidone Gastrointestinal motility promoting agents, e.g., metoclopramide Antihypertensive medications such as verapamil, methyldopa,
Idiopathic	

toward ruling out the above-mentioned causes of galactorrhea such as symptoms related to hypothyroidism, mass effects of a prolactinoma, or pituitary adenoma such as headache or visual changes.

Physical examination should be directed toward breast examination and a detailed systemic examination to rule out the above-mentioned causes. Manipulation of the breast to confirm galactorrhea should be attempted. It should be kept in mind that breast and nipple stimulation during examination can transiently increase prolactin levels to a mild degree; therefore, prolactin levels should not be checked right after breast examination. Secretions from a Montgomery gland (sebaceous glands on the areola) that can be self-limiting, and transient should not be confused with galactorrhea [14]. Visual field examination and fundoscopic examination are also recommended for evaluating the possibility of CNS lesions causing elevated prolactin.

Diagnostic Evaluation

If galactorrhea is confirmed, and medication-induced galactorrhea is unlikely, then laboratory evaluation should include a prolactin level. An elevated prolactin level should be confirmed at least once. Of note, prolactin level is high in the newborn period (90–100 ng/dl) and should not be considered pathological in a newborn with galactorrhea. Pregnancy testing should also be considered in girls of reproductive age. In addition, thyroid-stimulating hormone and creatinine should be checked to rule out secondary causes of hyperprolactinemia. If hypogonadism is suspected clinically, then evaluation of early morning estradiol, testosterone levels with FSH and LH can also be obtained.

Please see Chap. 33 for considerations in interpretation of prolactin levels.

If no cause of hyperprolactinemia is found by history, physical examination, and above-mentioned laboratory evaluation, then an intracranial lesion might be suspected and referral to endocrinology and/or a brain MRI with contrast and with pituitary cuts (see Chap. 37) is indicated (Table 13.4).

Management

Normo-prolactinemic Galactorrhea In a patient with galactorrhea without elevated prolactin level, no further treatment is needed, and watchful waiting is recommended unless the galactorrhea is bothersome in which case a dopamine agonist can be trialed. Such patients should be advised not to continue checking for galactorrhea as nipple manipulation stimulates prolactin production and delays the resolution of galactorrhea.

Hyper-prolactinemic Galactorrhea With elevated prolactin levels, tumors such as craniopharyngioma, meningioma, or germinoma should be ruled out as they can cause galactorrhea by interfering with the inhibitory action of neurotransmitter dopamine from the hypothalamus. If clinically suspected, formal visual field evaluation and brain imaging is needed. Infiltrative lesions of hypothalamus such as histiocytosis and sarcoidosis are rare but can cause galactorrhea. Pituitary lesions are more commonly associated with galactorrhea with the most common being pituitary adenoma/prolactinoma. Please see Chap. 56 for further discussion of sellar and suprasellar masses that may cause hyperprolactinemia.

Hypothyroidism can result in galactorrhea with elevated prolactin levels, as elevated TRH in hypothyroidism is a stimulatory signal for lactotrophs of the anterior pituitary gland. Also, in renal insufficiency hyperprolactinemia can result secondary to decreased renal clearance of prolactin. Hyperprolactinemia may also be found in patients with severe liver disease.

Medication-Induced Hyperprolactinemia Multiple medications as listed above have been implicated in galactorrhea, with most of them causing hyperprolactinemia through decreased dopaminergic inhibition of the pituitary lactotrophs. Drugs with anti-dopaminergic effects include antipsychotics (risperidone) and gastrointestinal motility promoting agents such as metoclopramide. Some of the antihypertensive medications such as verapamil, methyldopa, can also cause galactorrhea. If hyperprolactinemia is medication induced, then discontinuing or replacing the causative medication is recommended.

Medical Management If no other secondary cause of hyperprolactinemia such as hypothyroidism, renal insufficiency or medication is found then referral to endocrinology is needed to consider treatment with dopamine agonist. Commonly used dopamine agonists are bromocriptine and cabergoline. Bromocriptine is usually taken daily and has more adverse side effects than cabergoline, which is taken once or twice weekly and is usually much better tolerated.

If the cause of galactorrhea is a hypothalamic or pituitary lesion other than a prolactinoma, then the patient should be referred to neurosurgery. Prolactinomas usually respond well to medical management and surgery or radiation therapy is rarely needed (see also Chap. 56).

Table 13.4 Suggested initial laboratory evaluation for galactorrhea

Prolactin
Serum or urine hCG in girls
Thyroid-stimulating hormone and free T4
Creatinine

Pearls

- Detailed medication history is essential prior to the evaluation of other causes of non-physiological galactorrhea.
- Endocrine referral can then be considered for further evaluation of galactorrhea.
- Most cases of prolactinomas are managed medically and surgery or radiation therapy is rarely needed.

References

1. Narula HS, Carlson HE. Gynaecomastia–pathophysiology, diagnosis and treatment. Nat Rev Endocrinol. 2014;10(11):684–98.
2. Nicolis GL, Modlinger RS, Gabrilove JL. A study of the histopathology of human gynecomastia. J Clin Endocrinol Metab. 1971;32(2):173–8.
3. Barros AC, Sampaio MD. Gynecomastia: physiopathology, evaluation and treatment. Sao Paulo Med J. 2012;130(3):187–97.
4. Reinehr T, Kulle A, Barth A, Ackermann J, Lass N, Holterhus P-M. Sex hormone profile in pubertal boys with gynecomastia and pseudogynecomastia. J Clin Endocrinol Metab. 2020;105(4):dgaa044.
5. Henley DV, Lipson N, Korach KS, Bloch CA. Prepubertal gynecomastia linked to lavender and tea tree oils. N Engl J Med. 2007;356(5):479–85.
6. Kanakis GA, Nordkap L, Bang AK, Calogero AE, Bártfai G, Corona G, et al. EAA clinical practice guidelines-gynecomastia evaluation and management. Andrology. 2019;7(6):778–93.
7. Alonso G, Pasqualini T, Busaniche J, Ruiz E, Chemes H. True hermaphroditism in a phenotypic male without ambiguous genitalia: an unusual presentation at puberty. Horm Res. 2007;68(5):261–4.
8. Lee EJ, Chang Y-W, Oh JH, Hwang J, Hong SS, Kim H-J. Breast lesions in children and adolescents: diagnosis and management. Korean J Radiol. 2018;19(5):978–91.
9. Rahmani S, Turton P, Shaaban A, Dall B. Overview of gynecomastia in the modern era and the Leeds Gynaecomastia Investigation algorithm. Breast J. 2011;17(3):246–55.
10. Spyropoulou G-A, Karamatsoukis S, Foroglou P. Unilateral pseudogynecomastia: an occupational hazard in manual metal-pressing factories? Aesthet Plast Surg. 2011;35(2):270–3.
11. Nuzzi LC, Cerrato FE, Webb ML, Faulkner HR, Walsh EM, DiVasta AD, et al. Psychological impact of breast asymmetry on adolescents: a prospective cohort study. Plast Reconstr Surg. 2014;134(6):1116–23.
12. De Silva NK. Breast development and disorders in the adolescent female. Best Pract Res Clin Obstet Gynaecol. 2018 Apr;48:40–50.
13. Huang W, Molitch ME. Evaluation and management of galactorrhea. Am Fam Physician. 2012;85(11):1073–80.
14. Watkins F, Giacomantonio M, Salisbury S. Nipple discharge and breast lump related to Montgomery's tubercles in adolescent females. J Pediatr Surg. 1988;23(8):718–20.

14 Acne, Hirsutism, and Other Signs of Increased Androgens

Christine March and Selma Witchel

Introduction and Definitions

C_{19} steroids and Adrenal Hormone Disease

The adrenal cortex produces three classes of steroid hormones: glucocorticoids, mineralocorticoids, and androgens/androgen precursors [1]. These hormones can be classified by the number of carbon molecules they contain. Androgens contain 19 carbons and are, therefore, termed C_{19} steroids. These steroids are initially produced through the enzymatic activity of 17,20 lyase, which cleaves the bond between carbon atoms 17 and 20 of pregnenolone or progesterone. Additional enzymes process C_{19} steroids into different androgens, or they can be aromatized and converted into C_{18} estrogens. The C_{19} androgens include dehydroepiandrosterone (DHEA), DHEAS, androstenedione, and testosterone. These hormones vary in their potency in terms of androgen activity. In females, either excessive adrenal or ovarian C_{19} androgen production can lead to clinical disorders. Hence, multiple pathways leading to hyperandrogenemic disorders exist.

Hirsutism

Hirsutism is defined by excessive terminal hair growth in a male-pattern distribution, including on the face, chest, abdomen, upper arms, back, and inner thighs [2]. Hirsutism must be distinguished from hypertrichosis. The terminal hair growth observed with hirsutism involves coarse, rigid, pigmented hair in androgen-dependent body areas [3]. Hypertrichosis is characterized by increased fine, vellus hair in multiple body areas in either men or women. Hypertrichosis can be familial or caused by various endocrine/metabolic disorders (e.g., thyroid disturbance, Cushing's syndrome, or anorexia nervosa) or medications (e.g., diazoxide, minoxidil, phenytoin, or cyclosporine) [4]. Several studies estimate that hirsutism affects approximately 10% of adult women in most populations [5]. Though many women may pursue cosmetic treatments alone, an evaluation to assess for an underlying endocrine disorder is often warranted [2].

Key Point: Hirsutism vs Hypertrichosis

- *Hirsutism*: increased coarse, terminal hair growth in androgen-dependent areas (upper lip, chin, chest, upper and lower abdomen, upper and lower back, upper arms, and inner thighs)
- *Hypertrichosis*: increased fine, vellus hair growth over the body in both androgen-independent and androgen-dependent regions

The diagnosis of hirsutism is subjective; several different scoring metrics have been defined. The modified Ferriman-Gallwey (mFG) score is the most commonly utilized method (Fig. 14.1) [6, 7]. This scoring system assesses terminal hair growth at nine androgen-dependent areas on the female body. Attention to ethnic and racial differences needs to be considered because the number of hair follicles per unit area of skin is lower among Asian individuals compared with white and black women [8]. Review of available data suggests that mFG scores ≥4–6 are consistent with hirsutism [9].

C. March (✉) · S. Witchel
Division of Pediatric Endocrinology, University of Pittsburgh, UPMC Children's Hospital of Pittsburgh, Pittsburgh, PA, USA
e-mail: Christine.eklund@chp.edu; witchelsf@upmc.edu

T. Stanley, M. Misra (eds.), *Endocrine Conditions in Pediatrics*, https://doi.org/10.1007/978-3-030-52215-5_14

Other Signs of Androgen Excess

Additional features of hyperandrogenism can include acne vulgaris, androgenic alopecia, irregular menses, anovulation, and, in adults, infertility [5, 10]. Acne vulgaris is common in teenage years due to increased production of C_{19} sex steroids during puberty. The exact prevalence of acne in women with hyperandrogenism is unknown, though it is reported in 15–25% of women with polycystic ovary syndrome (PCOS) [11]. No standardized scoring metrics exist to grade acne severity [12]. However, acne that is extensive, persistent, and unresponsive to topical medications or presents later in life may be suggestive of androgen excess [10]. Androgenic alopecia, a rare finding in adolescents, refers to a decreased hair density typically at the crown of the head [10, 12].

Hyperandrogenism can also affect hypothalamic-pituitary-ovarian (HPO) axis function. Disrupted HPO axis function manifests as irregular menses, oligo-anovulation, infertility, and primary or secondary amenorrhea. Acne and irregular menses are typical during early adolescence; this confounds distinguishing normal variation from clinically significant hyperandrogenic disorders [13]. Typically, irregular menses which persist beyond two years after menarche warrant an evaluation.

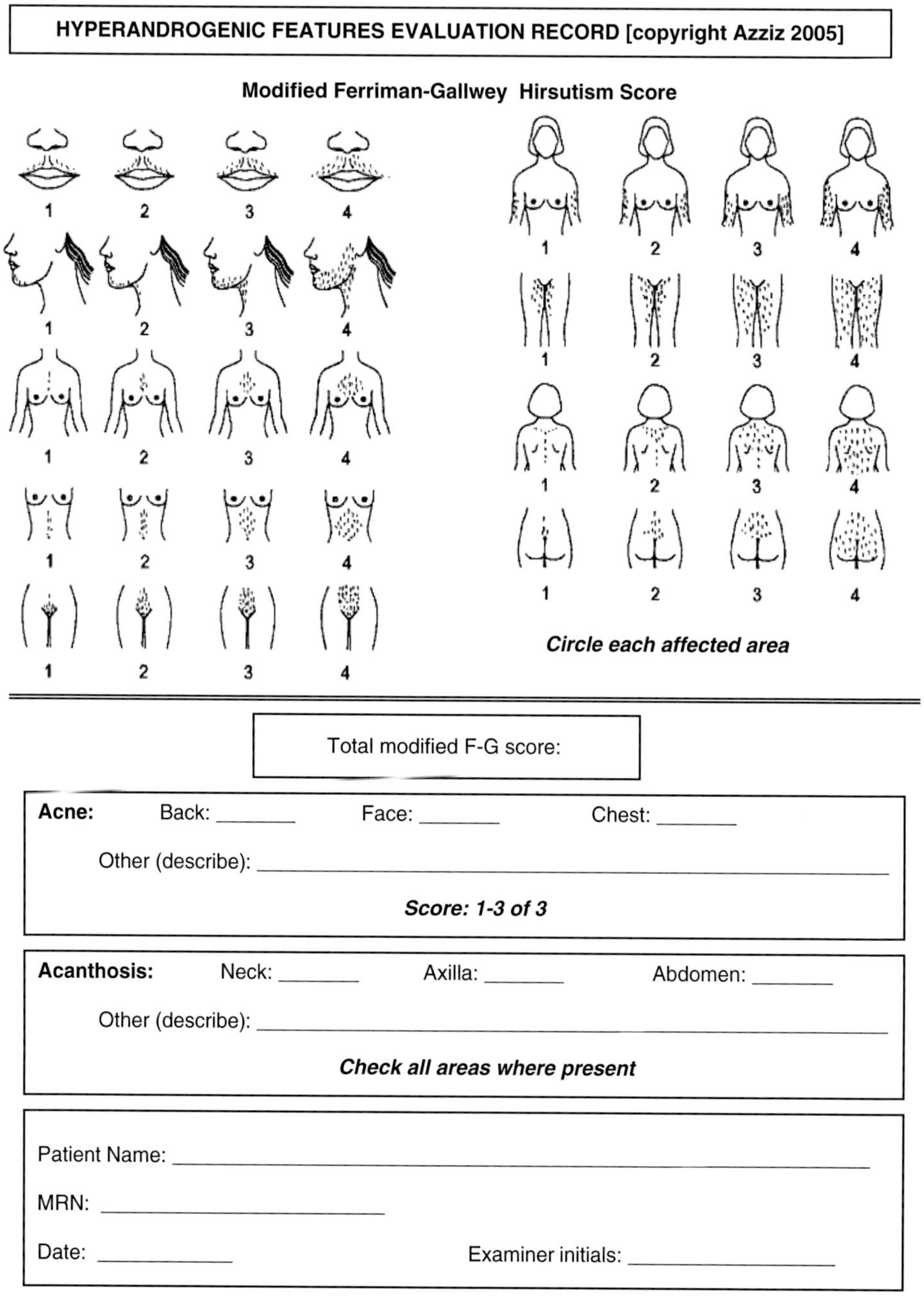

HYPERANDROGENIC FEATURES EVALUATION RECORD [copyright Azziz 2005]

Modified Ferriman-Gallwey Hirsutism Score

1 2 3 4

1 2 3 4

1 2 3 4

1 2 3 4

1 2 3 4

1 2 3 4

1 2 3 4

1 2 3 4

1 2 3 4

Circle each affected area

Total modified F-G score:

Acne: Back: _______ Face: _______ Chest: _______

Other (describe): ____________________

Score: 1-3 of 3

Acanthosis: Neck: _______ Axilla: _______ Abdomen: _______

Other (describe): ____________________

Check all areas where present

Patient Name: ____________________

MRN: ____________________

Date: ____________ Examiner initials: ____________

Fig. 14.1 Modified Ferriman-Gallwey Scoring. Nine body areas (upper lip, chin, chest, arm, upper abdomen, lower abdomen, upper back, lower back, and thighs) are scored from 1 (minimal terminal hairs present) to 4 (equivalent to a hairy man). If no terminal hairs are observed in the body area being examined, the score is zero (left blank). Clinically, terminal hair can be distinguished from vellus hairs primarily by their length (i.e., greater than 0.5 cm) and the fact that they are usually pigmented. (reprinted with permission of R. Azziz, copyright 2005)

Fig. 14.1 (continued)

INSTRUCTIONS FOR COMPLETING FORM

1) Modified Ferriman-Ga llwey Hirsutism Score:

- Nine b ody areas a re assessed, incl uding the uppe r lip, chin, ch est, upper ba ck, lowe r back, upp er a rm, uppe r and lowe r abd omen, and thig hs.
- A sco re of 0 to 4 is assig ned to each a rea examined, based on the den sity of terminal hairs. A sco re of 0 repre sents the ab sence of termin al hairs, a score of 1 minimal terminal hair g rowth, a sco re of 2 mild terminal h air gro wth, a score of 3 moderate hair gro wth and a score of 4 sever e termina l hair growth (i.e. like that of a hairy man).
- Each bo dy area on the form is circle d accord ingly, leaving those a reas with a score of zero blan k.
- Terminal hairs can be generally identifie d beca use they are coarse, pigme nted, and generally grea ter than 1 cm in length (if not cut or trimme d).
- The scor es are summed up to for the 'Total mod ified F-G score'

(Based on Hatch R, Ro senfield RL, Kim MH, Tre dway D. Hirsutism : Implications, etiolog y, and managem ent. Am J Obstet Gyn ecol 198 1;140:81 5-830).

2) Ac ne:

- Acne is score d according t o wheth er it is grade 1 (mil d), 2 (mo dera te), or 3 (sev ere).
- Mild acn e is chara cterized by the presen ce of few to several pa pules and p ustules, but no nodul es.
- Mode rate a cne by the presence of several to many papule s and p ustules, along with a few to seve ral nodule s.
- Severe a cne by the presen ce of nume rous or exten sive papule s and pu stules, as well as many nodul es

(Based on Po chi PE, Shalita AR, Strauss JS, We bster SB, Cunliffe WJ, Katz HI, et al. Report of the Con sensus Conferen ce on Acne Classificati on. Wa shin gton, D.C., March 24 and 2 5, 1990. J Am Acad Derm atol 1991;24:495-500).

3) Aca nthos is nigricans:

- All area s dem onstrating a cantho sis ni gricans shoul d be ch ecke d and indi cated.
- No sco re is u sed to de note severity.

Question: Can Boys Present with Androgen Excess?

Yes! Boys can also develop androgen excess, though this is not always clinically obvious. Symptoms may include early pubic hair development, phallic enlargement, and/or severe acne. The differential diagnosis includes disorders of steroidogenesis, androgen-secreting tumors, precocious puberty, hCG-secreting tumors, or exogenous exposures. For boys, signs of puberty before age 9 years warrant prompt referral to pediatric endocrinology.

Differential Diagnosis

Table 14.1 lists the differential diagnosis in adolescents. Depending on specific diagnostic criteria, PCOS affects between 8% and 15% of women of reproductive age. The diagnosis of PCOS in adult women requires two of three characteristics of PCOS: irregular menses, clinical/biochemical hyperandrogenism, or polycystic ovary morphology on ultrasound and exclusion of other etiologies [9]. The similarities between normal features of adolescence and clinical findings typical of PCOS confound diagnosing PCOS in early

Table 14.1 Differential diagnosis for hirsutism

Common causes
Polycystic ovary syndrome
Familial idiopathic hirsutism
Physiological hyperandrogenism of puberty
Can't miss diagnoses
Non-classic congenital adrenal hyperplasia
Androgen-secreting tumors
Exposure to anabolic steroids or testosterone
Disorders of sex development
Glucocorticoid resistance
PAPSS2 deficiency

adolescence [14]. For example, polycystic ovarian morphology can be physiologically normal in adolescent girls. Hence, ovarian ultrasound imaging is generally not useful in this age group (see also Chap. 45). For adolescent girls who are within two years of menarche, consideration should be given to using a diagnosis of "at-risk" for PCOS, treating their symptoms, and following longitudinally to assess for persistent symptoms [9, 13]. Potential factors contributing to the increased C_{19} androgen secretion in PCOS include altered steroidogenesis, insulin resistance/hyperinsulinemia, and neuroendocrine factors. The increased C_{19} androgens can disrupt gonadotropin secretion, resulting in growth of multiple ovarian follicles with subsequent failure to select a dominant follicle, anovulation, and follicular atresia [13].

The congenital adrenal hyperplasias (CAH) are a group of autosomal recessive disorders characterized by alterations in steroidogenesis. These disorders range in severity from classical to the milder, non-classic, forms. The classical forms, salt-losing and simple virilizing, typically present in the neonatal period. The most common form of CAH is 21-hydroxylase deficiency due to mutations in the 21-hydroxylase (*CYP21A2*) gene [15]. Other forms of CAH associated with hyperandrogenism include 11-beta hydroxylase (*CYP11B1*), 3-beta hydroxysteroid dehydrogenase (*HSD3B2*), and aromatase (*CYP19A1*) deficiencies.

Late-onset or non-classic congenital adrenal hyperplasia (NCCAH) may present with premature pubarche and or adolescent hyperandrogenemia with minimal signs of androgen excess. The prevalence of NCCAH among American Caucasians is estimated to be 1 in 200 [16]. Consideration of NCCAH is important as excessive production of sex steroids can accelerate bone age advancement; some individuals may have impaired cortisol secretion during stress (e.g., significant illness) requiring replacement.

Androgen-secreting adrenal or ovarian tumors are rare. Nevertheless, clinical manifestations of androgen-secreting tumors may be insidious. Adrenal tumors tend to be hormonally active with the specific clinical features reflecting the pattern of excessive adrenal hormone secretion. Androgen-secreting tumors can be either adrenal, testicular, or ovarian in origin and often present with rapid pubertal progression or virilization [17].

Cushing syndrome refers to glucocorticoid excess. The most common etiology of Cushing syndrome is exogenous glucocorticoid treatment. Other causes of Cushing syndrome include excessive pituitary ACTH secretion (Cushing disease) and adrenal cortical tumors. These rare disorders are associated with progressive virilization. Most adrenal tumors are adenomas [18].

Rare genetic disorders include *PAPSS2* and apparent cortisone reductase deficiencies. Mutations in the *PAPSS2* gene disrupt DHEA sulfotransferase activity, leading to decreased DHEAS synthesis, low DHEAS concentrations, and increased C_{19} steroid production [19]. Bone and cartilage malformations may be present due to under-sulfation of the extracellular matrix. Apparent cortisone reductase deficiency, due to loss of function mutations in the hexose-6-phosphate dehydrogenase (*H6PD*) gene, can be associated with hyperandrogenism. The *H6PD* mutations impair peripheral conversion of cortisone to cortisol, resulting in increased cortisol clearance, impaired hypothalamic-pituitary negative feedback inhibition, and increased ACTH secretion [20].

Disorders of sex development such as 5-alpha reductase and 17-hydroxysteroid dehydrogenase type 3 deficiencies interfere with the development of the external genitalia such that affected XY infants may be considered to be female at birth. These disorders are due to *SRD5A2* and *HSD17B3* mutations, respectively. With the onset of puberty, increased C_{19} androgen secretion leads to virilization [21].

Providers must also consider the possibility that adolescents may be using off-label testosterone or anabolic steroids as hormone therapy for gender dysphoria. Testosterone gels, lotions, and creams used by adult males in the household can also contribute to virilization in children if accidentally exposed. The presence of these substances must be ascertained, and extra care should be taken to minimize any potential exposure. If all other diagnoses are ruled out, hirsutism is often termed idiopathic and may be hereditary in nature.

Clinical Evaluation of Hyperandrogenism

History & Physical

Key history and physical exam features are displayed in Table 14.2. This history should assess for personal or family history of hyperandrogenism, symptoms of associated conditions, including PCOS, or unexplained infertility. Clinicians need to be sensitive as hirsutism can be distressing for many women [10]. Providers should ask about the presence of unwanted hair growth in androgen-dependent areas, acne, and hair loss. Providers should inquire about cosmetic treatments such as shaving, waxing, or laser removal; in some instances, patients may perform hair removal immediately prior to office visits. Additional questions should ask about the start and tempo of pubertal development and frequency of menstrual cycles. Rapid virilization increases the suspicion for androgen secreting tumors. Inquiry regarding a family history of infertility, hirsutism, type 2 diabetes, hypertension, dyslipidemia, and metabolic syndrome is important due to the association of these disorders with PCOS.

Table 14.2 Pearls for history & physical

History pearls
Onset and progression of hirsutism and acne
Age and sequence of thelarche, pubarche, and menarche
Topical/cosmetic treatments for hirsutism or acne
Frequency and duration of menstrual cycles
Exposure to testosterone-containing medications/substances/gels
Family history of disorders of hirsutism, irregular menses, infertility, PCOS, or early infant deaths
Family history of metabolic disorders including type 2 diabetes, fatty liver disease, or hyperlipidemia
Physical exam pearls
Body mass index, blood pressure
Coarse hair in androgen-dependent areas (mFG scoring), acne
Clitoromegaly
Signs of insulin resistance including acanthosis nigricans or skin tags

Physical examination assesses for hirsutism and acne; rarely, providers may appreciate androgenic alopecia. Linear growth velocity in prepubertal children should be noted. An external genital exam should be completed to assess for pubic hair, clitoromegaly, and presence of posterior labial fusion. Lastly, acanthosis nigricans and skin tags suggest hyperinsulinemia and insulin resistance, which often occur in PCOS.

Laboratory Studies

Following clinical evaluation, serum hormone concentrations can be obtained. Patients do not need to meet a certain number of clinical criteria to merit evaluation, as some patients will present with isolated symptoms such as just acne [5, 22]. Whether the presenting complaint is hirsutism or acne, the evaluation is similar (Fig. 14.2). When irregular

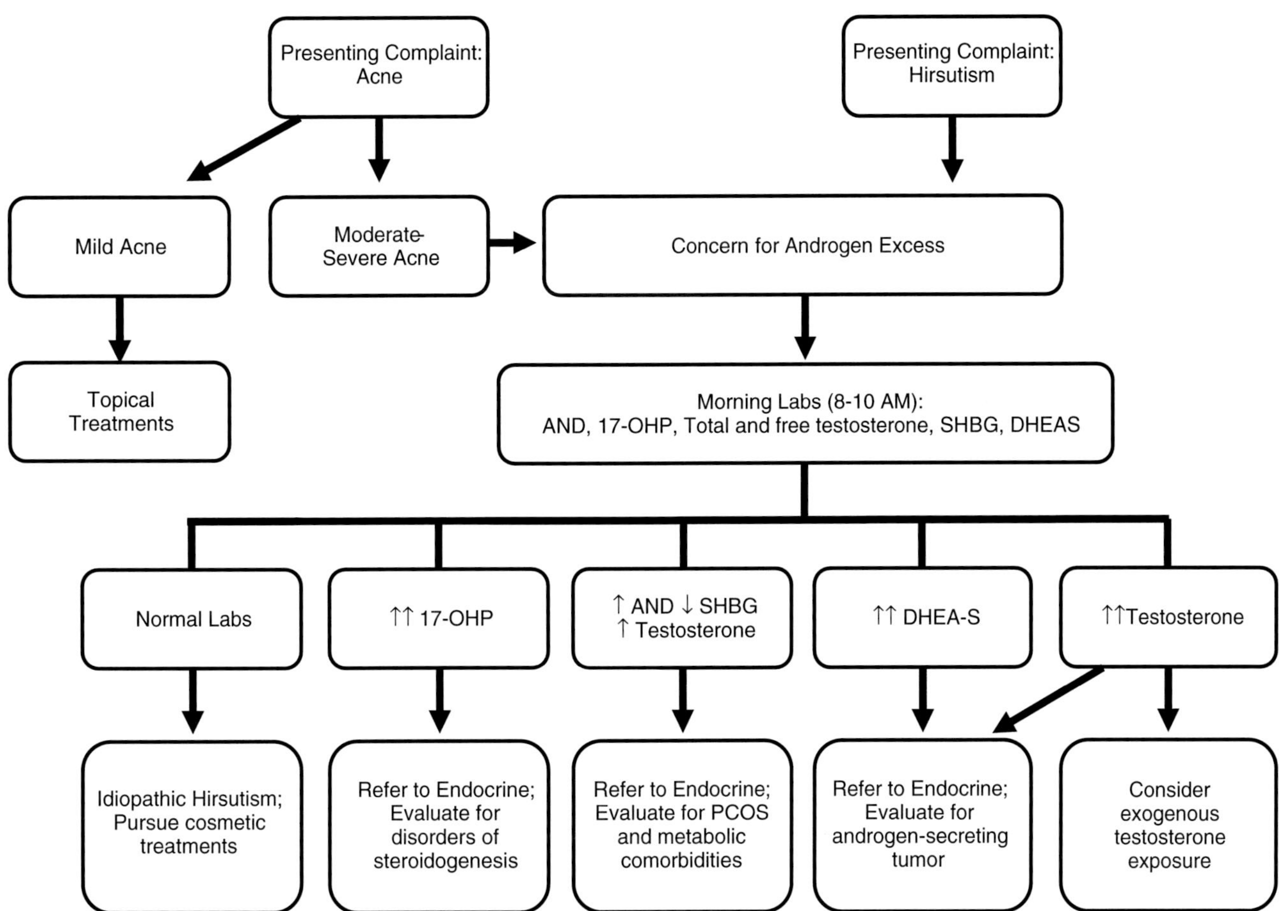

Fig. 14.2 Evaluation for disorders associated with androgen excess. This figure depicts the predominant hormone findings to direct the differential diagnosis. This algorithm directs the initial laboratory evaluation for hyperandrogenism. *Abbreviations:* AND androstenedione, 17-OHP 17-hydroxyprogesterone, SHBG sex hormone–binding globulin, DHEAS dehydroepiandrosterone sulfate

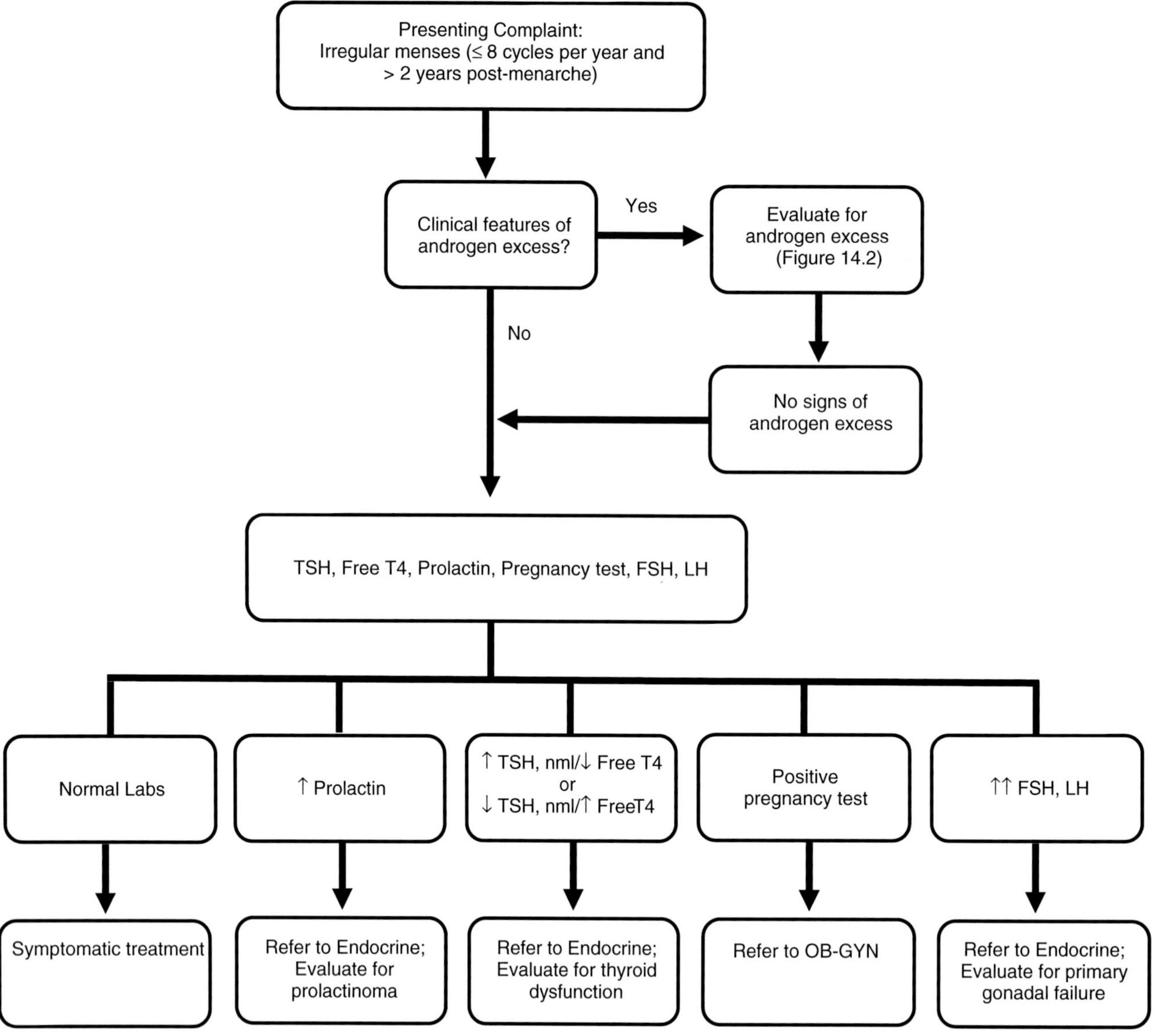

Fig. 14.3 Evaluation when primary complaint is irregular menses. This figure depicts the algorithm for the evaluation of irregular menses and primary amenorrhea. *Abbreviations:* TSH thyroid-stimulating hormone, Free T4 free thyroxine, FSH follicle-stimulating hormone, LH luteinizing hormone

menses or amenorrhea is the presenting complaint, the evaluation should also consider additional possibilities, including pregnancy, abnormal thyroid function, or hyperprolactinemia (Fig. 14.3).

Adrenal cortical hormones, i.e., 17-hydroxyprogesterone and cortisol, tend to peak in the morning due to the ACTH surge and diurnal glucocorticoid variation. The ideal time for measurement is between 8 and 10 AM to capture any supraphysiologic elevations in 17-hydroxyprogesterone, in particular when assessing for NCCAH [22]. In addition, androstenedione, DHEAS, and total testosterone can be measured; sex hormone–binding globulin (SHBG) determination may be helpful as low SHBG is associated with hyperandrogenism and hyperinsulinemia. A morning 17-hydroxyprogesterone concentration greater than 200 ng/dl warrants referral and evaluation for NCCAH [23]. However, a morning 17-hydroxyprogesterone concentration less than 200 ng/dl does not eliminate the possibility of NCCAH.

Androgens are steroid molecules and require high-quality assays for accurate measurements. This is especially true for testosterone, which is best measured with high-quality radioimmunoassay or mass spectrometry with liquid or gas chromatography [12]. Due to limitations of current assays, direct free testosterone assays should be avoided. Rather, total testosterone and sex hormone–binding globulin should be measured. These concentrations can be used to determine the values for calculated free testosterone, free androgen index, or bioavailable testosterone, all of which help ascertain a diagnosis of hyperandrogenism. Due to the variability in total testosterone assays between laboratories, using a cut-point of greater than three times the upper reference range value has been suggested for androgen-secreting ovarian tumors [24]. Hormone determinations may help to distinguish between adrenal and ovarian sources of androgens and screen for NCCAH. Further evaluation depends upon the findings.

Considerations for Imaging Studies

The utility of imaging studies depends upon laboratory evaluation and suspected diagnosis. Though commonly performed in adults, a pelvic ultrasound is rarely indicated for adolescent girls being evaluated for PCOS. Polycystic ovary morphology on ultrasound is found in up to 30–40% of healthy adolescent girls and is not predictive of PCOS. Rather, the clinical and biochemical features are more important in assisting with this diagnosis. Imaging is helpful when evaluating for a tumor. Rapidly progressing symptoms and/or total testosterone levels greater than 150 ng/dL or DHEAS greater than 700 mcg/dL should prompt an evaluation for a neoplastic lesion of the ovaries and adrenal glands, respectively. Ultrasound may be sufficient to screen for ovarian tumors; however, CT or MRI should be used to assess the adrenal glands to improve tumor detection [22].

Key Points in Clinical Evaluation

- Direct free testosterone assays are generally unreliable in women unless they utilize equilibrium dialysis. Total testosterone and sex hormone–binding globulin should be sent and used to calculate free testosterone, free androgen index, or bioavailable testosterone.
- Pelvic ultrasound is rarely indicated in adolescents being evaluated for PCOS.
- Total testosterone >150 ng/dL or DHEAS >700 mcg/dL should prompt an evaluation for a neoplastic lesion of the ovaries and adrenal glands, respectively.

Pathophysiology of Hirsutism and Acne

The pathophysiology, diagnosis, and treatment of hirsutism and acne are discussed below. Please see Chaps. 45, 46, 49, and 50 for additional discussion of the evaluation and management for specific endocrine conditions associated with hyperandrogenism.

Androgen excess contributes to hirsutism and acne through direct effects of androgens on the hair follicle and pilosebaceous subunit (PSU). The PSU consists of a hair follicle, sebaceous gland, and arrector pili muscle [2]. Androgens appear to contribute to the conversion of vellus hair to terminal hair through two mechanisms. First, androgens can have a direct action by stimulating androgen receptors located in the PSU within the dermal papilla, which is responsible for determining the size and color of the hair follicle through local signaling factors. Second, the hair follicle contains all the necessary enzymes to synthesize and metabolize androgens, including 5α-reductase, which converts testosterone to the more potent dihydrotestosterone (DHT). Acting through androgen receptors, testosterone and DHT promote terminal hair growth and prolong the growth phase of the hair cycle, leading to longer and thicker hair [25]. Thus, local production of androgens can contribute to hirsutism even if circulating hormones are not elevated [12]. Hirsutism reflects the outcome of circulating androgen concentrations, local androgen concentrations, and hair follicle androgen sensitivity.

Androgens appear to have different effects on hair follicles in different areas of the body, helping to explain the simultaneous effects of hirsutism and alopecia [26]. Sebaceous glands in acne-prone areas such as the face express 5α-reductase. DHT also contributes to increased sebum production and altered epithelial cell desquamation, leading to comedone formation. Proliferation of *Propionibacterium acnes* in the comedone can subsequently lead to the papules and pustules typically seen in acne vulgaris [10]. Despite the absence of hirsutism, biochemical hyperandrogenism may still be present among patients with other features of androgen excess.

Key Point: Pathophysiology of Hirsutism and Acne

- Increased circulating androgens stimulate the androgen receptor in the PSU.
- Local production of androgens occurs through the enzymatic steroid pathway in the PSU.

Making the Diagnosis

Hirsutism, acne, and irregular menses are clinical signs associated with androgen excess (Table 14.3). Clinical history, physical examination, and relevant laboratory studies help to distinguish the underlying etiology. Idiopathic hirsutism is a diagnosis of exclusion and may be considered in patients who have hirsutism with normal androgen concentrations.

The exact pathophysiology of this condition is unknown but may be related to exaggerated 5α-reductase activity, increased responsiveness of androgen receptors, or altered androgen metabolism in the PSU [25].

Initial Management

Hirsutism

Hirsutism is frequently distressing for patients. Management depends upon the underlying cause and presence or absence of elevated circulating androgens; treatment for specific diseases associated with hirsutism is addressed in other chapters. Both cosmetic and pharmacologic treatments for hirsutism exist; the relative merits of each need to be discussed with the patient. Mild hirsutism may be satisfactorily treated with cosmetic approaches alone. Moderate–severe hirsutism will likely benefit from pharmacologic intervention in addition to cosmetic treatment. The goal of pharmacologic therapies is to decrease production of new terminal hair; these therapies are unlikely to impact terminal hair growth that is already present. Cosmetic treatments are used to remove existing terminal hairs [2].

Cosmetic treatments may be temporary or semi-permanent. Temporary methods include plucking, bleaching, shaving, waxing, or depilation and may be appropriate for mild hair growth. There is a common misconception that shaving can increase both hair growth and hair thickness. Rather, shaving creates a blunt end to the hair, which can make it more noticeable. More permanent methods include electrolysis and laser hair removal. Electrolysis destroys the dermal papilla and, thus, permanently treats the terminal hair in that area. If correctly performed, it is unlikely to result in significant adverse effects such as scarring, though transient discomfort may occur. Laser hair removal destroys the hair through selective absorption of the wavelength by the melanin pigment in the hair follicle. As a result, this works best in women with fairer complexions and darkly colored hair.

Pharmacologic therapies include both topical and systemic options (Table 14.4). Among potential topical treatments, 13.9% eflornithine cream blocks an enzymatic conversion that is critical to hair growth. Continuous use is associated with significant reduction in facial hair growth, but use is not recommended in other areas, and the medication is very expensive. Combined oral contraceptive pills (OCPs) suppress ovarian androgen synthesis and increase concentrations of sex hormone–binding globulin, which in turn reduces circulating levels of free testosterone. Many

Table 14.3 Diagnosis of hyperandrogenism

Clinical features	*Biochemical features*
Hirsutism Acne vulgaris Androgenic alopecia Irregular menses or amenorrhea	Total testosterone greater than adult female normative values Elevated DHEAS and/or androstenedione for pubertal stage Low SHBG

Table 14.4 Pharmacologic treatment for hirsutism or acne

Medication	Mechanism	Common side effects	Treatment considerations
Topical eflornithine	Irreversible inhibitor of L-ornithine decarboxylase	Acne Rash	Approved for unwanted facial hair only
Combined oral contraceptives	Inhibits ovarian androgen synthesis Increases SHBG	Bloating Nausea Headache Mood change Thrombogenic effect Increased blood pressure	Will also regulate periods Must screen for contraindications
Spironolactone	Androgen receptor blocker	Menstrual irregularity Breast tenderness GI upset	Must be prescribed with contraception Dose 25–100 mg daily
Flutamide	Androgen receptor blocker	GI upset Rare severe liver toxicity	Must be prescribed with contraception Not recommended for acne Dose 250 mg daily
Finasteride	5α-reductase inhibitor	Decreased libido Depression	Must be prescribed with contraception Not recommended for acne Dose 5 mg daily

small studies have found symptomatic improvement in hirsutism for women taking OCPs. Providers must obtain a thorough family history to screen for potential contraindications, including a personal or family history of blood clots, strokes, and migraine with aura.

Antiandrogen medications include androgen receptor blockers and 5α-reductase inhibitors, including flutamide, finasteride, or spironolactone. These have all demonstrated efficacy compared with placebo in randomized controlled trials, particularly in combination with OCPs. Flutamide is associated with severe liver toxicity and is less commonly used compared with spironolactone or finasteride. Patients must be counseled that use of any of these antiandrogen medications remains off-label; written consent should be provided prior to prescribing. Antiandrogen medications cannot be used in women who are pregnant or planning to become pregnant given the potential teratogenic effects to a developing male fetus. Any prescription of these therapies should be given in combination with an OCP or other form of effective contraception, such as an intrauterine device. Metformin is often used as a treatment for PCOS; however, it is ineffective in treating the dermatologic symptoms.

Acne

Similar to hirsutism, acne is a symptom which can be treated, but the underlying cause should also be addressed if possible. Topical therapies are typically first line and include topical retinoids or benzoyl peroxide with or without topical antibiotics [27]. Patients who fail topical therapy despite adequate adherence and have evidence of hyperandrogenism would be candidates for hormonal therapy. In this case, clinicians can trial OCPs with or without spironolactone.

Indications to Refer

If an endocrine disorder is suspected, referral to a pediatric endocrinologist is indicated. In the event of an elevated morning 17-hydroxyprogesterone, the patient will likely need to undergo additional evaluation through an ACTH stimulation test. Concerns for adrenal or ovarian tumors warrant referral to complete the evaluation with additional laboratory tests and dedicated imaging. A pediatric endocrinologist can also assist with the evaluation of metabolic comorbidities associated with PCOS, including type 2 diabetes. In all cases, ongoing management and counseling for these conditions typically require specialized care from a pediatric endocrinologist.

Key Points: Important Points in Counseling Patients

- Cosmetic and pharmacologic treatments for hirsutism are chronic and not curative
- Shaving does not increase the growth or thickness of hair
- The effects of hormone treatments may not be evident for several months
- Hormonal treatments may halt new terminal hair growth, but will not affect terminal hair that is already present

References

1. Rege J, Turcu AF, Else T, Auchus RJ, Rainey WE. Steroid biomarkers in human adrenal disease. J Steroid Biochem Mol Biol. 2019;190:273–80.
2. Escobar-Morreale HF, Carmina E, Dewailly D, Gambineri A, Kelestimur F, Moghetti P, et al. Epidemiology, diagnosis and management of hirsutism: a consensus statement by the Androgen Excess and Polycystic Ovary Syndrome Society. Hum Reprod Update. 2012;18(2):146–70.
3. Rosenfield RL. Clinical practice. Hirsutism. N Engl J Med. 2005;353(24):2578–88.
4. Deplewski D, Rosenfield RL. Role of hormones in pilosebaceous unit development. Endocr Rev. 2000;21(4):363–92.
5. Azziz R, Sanchez LA, Knochenhauer ES, Moran C, Lazenby J, Stephens KC, et al. Androgen excess in women: experience with over 1000 consecutive patients. J Clin Endocrinol Metab. 2004;89(2):453–62.
6. Ferriman D, Gallwey JD. Clinical assessment of body hair growth in women. J Clin Endocrinol Metab. 1961;21:1440–7.
7. Hatch R, Rosenfield RL, Kim MH, Tredway D. Hirsutism: implications, etiology, and management. Am J Obstet Gynecol. 1981;140(7):815–30.
8. Yildiz BO, Bolour S, Woods K, Moore A, Azziz R. Visually scoring hirsutism. Hum Reprod Update. 2010;16(1):51–64.
9. Teede HJ, Misso ML, Costello MF, Dokras A, Laven J, Moran L, et al. Recommendations from the international evidence-based guideline for the assessment and management of polycystic ovary syndrome. Hum Reprod. 2018;33(9):1602–18.
10. Essah PA, Wickham EP 3rd, Nunley JR, Nestler JE. Dermatology of androgen-related disorders. Clin Dermatol. 2006;24(4):289–98.
11. Azziz R, Carmina E, Chen Z, Dunaif A, Laven JS, Legro RS, et al. Polycystic ovary syndrome. Nat Rev Dis Primers. 2016;2:16057.
12. Lizneva D, Gavrilova-Jordan L, Walker W, Azziz R. Androgen excess: investigations and management. Best Pract Res Clin Obstet Gynaecol. 2016;37:98–118.
13. Witchel SF, Oberfield SE, Pena AS. Polycystic ovary syndrome: pathophysiology, presentation, and treatment with emphasis on adolescent girls. J Endocr Soc. 2019;3(8):1545–73.
14. Witchel SF, Burghard AC, Tao RH, Oberfield SE. The diagnosis and treatment of PCOS in adolescents: an update. Curr Opin Pediatr. 2019;31(4):562–9.
15. Witchel SF. Congenital adrenal hyperplasia. J Pediatr Adolesc Gynecol. 2017;30(5):520–34.

16. Hannah-Shmouni F, Morissette R, Sinaii N, Elman M, Prezant TR, Chen W, et al. Revisiting the prevalence of nonclassic congenital adrenal hyperplasia in US Ashkenazi Jews and Caucasians. Genet Med. 2017;19(11):1276–9.
17. Arhan E, Cetinkaya E, Aycan Z, Aslan AT, Yucel H, Vidinlisan S. A very rare cause of virilization in childhood: ovarian Leydig cell tumor. J Pediatr Endocrinol Metab. 2008;21(2):181–3.
18. Lodish MB, Keil MF, Stratakis CA. Cushing's syndrome in pediatrics: an update. Endocrinol Metab Clin N Am. 2018;47(2):451–62.
19. Baranowski ES, Arlt W, Idkowiak J. Monogenic disorders of adrenal steroidogenesis. Horm Res Paediatr. 2018;89(5):292–310.
20. White PC. Alterations of cortisol metabolism in human disorders. Horm Res Paediatr. 2018;89(5):320–30.
21. Phelan N, Williams EL, Cardamone S, Lee M, Creighton SM, Rumsby G, et al. Screening for mutations in 17beta-hydroxysteroid dehydrogenase and androgen receptor in women presenting with partially virilised 46,XY disorders of sex development. Eur J Endocrinol. 2015;172(6):745–51.
22. Screening and management of the hyperandrogenic adolescent: ACOG Committee Opinion, Number 789. Obstet Gynecol. 2019;134(4):e106–e14.
23. Armengaud JB, Charkaluk ML, Trivin C, Tardy V, Breart G, Brauner R, et al. Precocious pubarche: distinguishing late-onset congenital adrenal hyperplasia from premature adrenarche. J Clin Endocrinol Metab. 2009;94(8):2835–40.
24. Glintborg D, Altinok ML, Petersen KR, Ravn P. Total testosterone levels are often more than three times elevated in patients with androgen-secreting tumours. BMJ Case Rep. 2015;2015:bcr2014204797.
25. Azziz R, Carmina E, Sawaya ME. Idiopathic hirsutism. Endocr Rev. 2000;21(4):347–62.
26. Randall VA. Androgens and hair growth. Dermatol Ther. 2008;21(5):314–28.
27. Nguyen HL, Tollefson MM. Endocrine disorders and hormonal therapy for adolescent acne. Curr Opin Pediatr. 2017;29(4):455–65.

Irregular Menses

15

Meghan E. Fredette

Abbreviations

ACOG	American College of Obstetricians and Gynecologists
AUB	Abnormal uterine bleeding
FIGO	International Federation of Gynecology and Obstetrics
FSH	Follicle-stimulating hormone
HMB	Heavy menstrual bleeding
IMB	Intermenstrual bleeding
IUD	Intrauterine device
LH	Luteinizing hormone
NAAT	Nucleic acid amplification testing
OCP	Oral contraceptive pill
PBAC	Pictorial Bleeding Assessment Chart
TSH	Thyroid-stimulating hormone

Introduction and Definition of Terms

Abnormal uterine bleeding (AUB) is defined by the International Federation of Gynecology and Obstetrics (FIGO) classification system as bleeding from the uterine corpus that is abnormal in duration, volume, frequency, and/or regularity [1]. Heavy menstrual bleeding (HMB) refers to heavy menstrual flow as described by the patient. Intermenstrual bleeding (IMB) describes bleeding that occurs between regular menses. Terms such as menorrhagia, metrorrhagia, menometrorrhagia, oligomenorrhea, and dysfunctional uterine bleeding are no longer recommended in the FIGO system [2, 3]. Acute AUB is defined as an episode of heavy bleeding of sufficient quantity to require immediate intervention to minimize or prevent further blood loss, as determined by the clinician. Chronic AUB is defined as AUB that has been present for the majority of the preceding 6 months. Acute AUB may present with or without a history of chronic AUB [1, 4].

According to FIGO classifications for adult reproductive-aged women, normal uterine bleeding is defined as menstrual bleeding of ≤8 days duration, occurring every 24–38 days, with normal flow (defined by subject as not interfering with quality of life) with shortest to longest menstrual cycle variation of 9 days or less [1]. Normal menstrual cycles in an adolescent occur every 21–45 days, with duration <8 days with "normal" flow, which is patient defined [5]. The frequency of menstrual cycles decreases with increasing post-menarchal age [6]. Secondary amenorrhea is defined as absent menstrual cycles for 3 or more months in an individual with previously established menstrual cycles [7].

AUB is a common condition, affecting up to 30% of reproductive-aged women, and has been associated with significant health care costs and decreased quality of life [8]. AUB in adolescents is more common in the first 1–2 years after achieving menarche due to immaturity of the hypothalamic-pituitary-ovarian axis, which results in anovulatory cycles. This menstrual irregularity most often normalizes by the third year after menarche, when 60–80% of cycles are 21–34 days long [5]; however in this interval, significant AUB, such as secondary amenorrhea or HMB, may occur, requiring evaluation.

Differential Diagnosis

The etiologies of AUB in reproductive-aged adult women who are not pregnant are vast and have been categorized by the 2011 FIGO classification system according to the acronym PALM-COEIN [9]. This classification system has been endorsed by the American College of Obstetricians and Gynecologists (ACOG) [10]. PALM represents structural etiologies that cause AUB, which include Polyps, Adenomyosis,

M. E. Fredette (✉)
Division of Pediatric Endocrinology, Hasbro Children's Hospital/Warren Alpert Medical School of Brown University, Providence, RI, USA
e-mail: meghan_fredette@brown.edu

T. Stanley, M. Misra (eds.), *Endocrine Conditions in Pediatrics*, https://doi.org/10.1007/978-3-030-52215-5_15

Leiomyomas (fibroid or myoma), Malignancy, and hyperplasia. Structural etiologies of AUB, especially adenomyosis, are rare in adolescent women [11]. COEIN describes the medical etiologies causing AUB including coagulopathy, ovulatory dysfunction, endometrial, iatrogenic, and not otherwise classified. Of the possible medical etiologies, ovulatory dysfunction is most common in the adolescent female [10]. Bleeding disorders are found in approximately 20% of adolescent women who present for evaluation of HBM, and are even higher in women who require hospitalization [12]. Von Willebrand disease is the most common coagulopathy found in women with HMB, and is a disorder resulting in inadequate quantity or function of Von Willebrand factor, which is a critical protein in platelet adhesion, as well as protection against coagulation factor degradation [13].

Table 15.1 reviews the differential diagnosis of AUB in the non-pregnant adolescent and young adult. It is important to note that pregnancy must be ruled out in any person presenting with AUB, as complications of pregnancy or termination procedures (abortion or threatened abortion, ectopic pregnancy, gestational trophoblastic disease) can present with AUB. Non-uterine bleeding should also be ruled out including perianal, perineal, vulvar, vaginal, urinary tract, or cervical etiologies of bleeding. Potential etiologies of vaginal bleeding include vaginal or perineal trauma, retained foreign body, cervicitis, vaginitis, vaginal or cervical carcinoma/sarcoma, or cervical hemangioma and could be confused for AUB in the adolescent or young adult female [5, 14–17].

Table 15.1 Differential diagnosis of AUB in the non-pregnant adolescent/young adult female

Coagulopathy
Von Willebrand's disease
Thrombocytopenia
Platelet disorders
Other bleeding disorders (factor deficiencies)
Acquired bleeding disorders (hepatic failure, malignancy, sepsis, vitamin K deficiency)
Ovulatory dysfunction
Immaturity of the HPA axis*
Functional hypothalamic amenorrhea (eating disorder, malnutrition, excessive weight loss, excessive stress, severe systemic illness)
Pituitary or hypothalamic conditions (genetic, idiopathic, and acquired causes of hypogonadotropic hypogonadism and multiple pituitary insufficiencies)
Hyperprolactinemia
Thyroid dysfunction (hypo- or hyperthyroidism)
Cushing's syndrome
Hyperandrogenemia (polycystic ovary syndrome, non-classic congenital adrenal hyperplasia, androgen-secreting tumors)
Primary ovarian insufficiency (Turner syndrome, autoimmune oophoritis, chemotherapy (particularly with alkylating agents), radiotherapy)
Endometrial
Infection (endometritis, pelvic inflammatory disease)
Iatrogenic/medications
Hormonal contraceptives/intrauterine devices
Anti-coagulation therapies/platelet inhibitors
Structural
Polyp
Leiomyoma
Malignancy

*Most common etiology in adolescent women

Table 15.2 Cannot-miss diagnoses presenting with irregular bleeding

Pregnancy
Sexually transmitted infection
Sexual trauma/abuse
Coagulopathy
Anemia secondary to HMB

Table 15.2 details the "cannot-miss" diagnoses for an adolescent presenting with irregular menses, and includes pregnancy and sexually transmitted infections. Sexual abuse and trauma should also be assessed and ruled out. Individuals with HMB since menarche or other concerning bleeding history should be evaluated for coagulopathy, and anemia should not be missed.

Important Clarifying Questions

The history is best obtained with at least a portion provided when the adolescent is alone with the provider, to ensure confidentiality and encourage disclosure of key information in the menstrual and sexual history.

A complete menstrual history is key to determining whether there is a pattern of AUB [18]. This includes the timing of menarche, duration of bleeding during menses, volume of flow (pad/tampon changes per day, +/− large clots >1 inch in diameter, soaking through clothes/bedsheets, and subjective response to volume), frequency of menses, and regularity of cycles. The timing of the onset of AUB should be assessed as well as potential exacerbating or triggering factors (e.g., the onset of amenorrhea during the athletic season or with the development of an eating disorder). Menstrual cycle length is counted from the first day of the menstrual period to the first day of the next menses. A menstrual calendar is key to assessing menstrual cycles, and several smart phone applications have been designed for this purpose.

A full medical history should be obtained and include information regarding chronic medical illnesses and the use of medications (including over-the-counter medications, vitamins, and herbal agents). A history of radiation therapy or chemotherapy should be obtained. A full sexual history should also be obtained including the use of contraceptives, the type of contraception, and adherence to contraceptive methods. Further, information should be sought regarding the use of condoms, the number of partners, the history of sexually transmitted infections, the history of post-coital bleeding, and the history of prior pregnancies or abortions.

A bleeding history should be obtained in individuals with HMB including easy bruising, gum bleeding, epistaxis, as well as postoperative, post-partum, or dental bleeding. The Pictorial Bleeding Assessment Chart (PBAC) uses a pictorial chart describing the degree to which pads/tampons are soiled as well as the number of pads/tampons used per day on each day of the menstrual cycle [19], and can be helpful in quantifying the amount of bleeding. The PBAC is scored by multiplying the number of pads/tampons per day by a value describing the degree of soiling, with a total score of >100 indicating HMB (correlates with blood loss >80 ml per cycle).

The review of systems should include a history of weight loss or gain, new striae, muscle weakness, hirsutism, worsening acne, changes in voice, galactorrhea, abdominal pain, fever, vaginal discharge, pelvic pain, heat or cold intolerance, fatigue, changes in hair skin or nails, changes in vision, headache, and neck pain or swelling. The patient should be asked about orthostatic symptoms such as dizziness with standing, or history of syncope.

The family history should focus on menstrual disorders, autoimmune disorders, obesity, type 2 diabetes, hypercholesterolemia, hypertension, infertility, as well as bleeding disorders. The social history should include questions related to social stressors, school performance, school attendance, activity level, athletic competition, exercise patterns, and any history of drug or alcohol abuse. The patient should be asked about social embarrassment due to AUB, such as bleeding through clothing or onto furniture/sheets, as well as questions about avoidance of social plans, or cancelling activities in relation to their AUB.

It can be helpful to assess for contraindications to oral contraceptive pills (OCPs) during the initial history, given that OCPs are a common treatment for AUB. Contraindications to estrogen-containing OCP in the adolescents include a history of uncontrolled hypertension, prior or current deep vein thrombosis or pulmonary embolism, complex valvular heart disease, active hepatic dysfunction, known complications of diabetes mellitus such as retinopathy or nephropathy, complicated solid organ transplant, migraine with aura, as well as disorders associated with increased clotting risk [12, 20].

Physical Examination

The physical examination should begin with vital signs including orthostatic vital signs in patients who report HMB. An accurate height and weight should be obtained with calculation of the body mass index. General examination should assess nutritional status and fat distribution. Skin examination should evaluate for acne, acanthosis nigricans, and hirsutism. The degree of hirsutism can be quantified using the Ferriman-Gallwey scoring system, which scores nine regions of the body according to the degree of hirsutism (graded as 1–4) with a score of ≥8 being considered abnormal [21]. Skin should also be assessed for violaceous striae, as well as pallor, bruising, or petechia. The conjunctiva should be assessed for pallor. Breasts should be examined for galactorrhea and Tanner staging performed for both breasts and pubic hair. The thyroid gland should be palpated for a goiter, or nodules. If a goiter is present, the patient should be assessed for fine tremor of the outstretched hands and tongue, and signs of proptosis such as lid lag. Reflexes should be assessed for hypo- or hyperreflexia. In the setting of a severe anemia, a flow murmur may be present. The abdomen should be palpated for masses such as a gravid uterus or hepatomegaly. A genitourinary examination should assess for signs of hyperandrogenemia such as clitoromegaly, and for the evidence of obvious trauma. Patients that are not sexually active do not require an internal pelvic examination. Patients that are sexually active should have a pelvic and bimanual examination to assess for trauma, foreign body, palpable uterine masses, or infection. A speculum examination is often not required. Table 15.3 details physical examination findings that suggest specific diagnoses in the evaluation of AUB.

Table 15.3 Physical examination findings and suggested diagnoses in adolescent/young adult women with AUB

Clinical examination finding	Diagnoses to consider
Vital signs	
Fever	Sexually transmitted infection
Obesity (BMI >95th percentile)	PCOS
Rapid weight gain	Cushing's syndrome
Short stature	Consider Turner syndrome (POI), long-standing hypothyroidism, pituitary hormone deficiencies, non-classic congenital adrenal hyperplasia, hypercortisolemia
Tachycardia +/− hypertension	Hyperthyroidism
Tachycardia, orthostatic hypotension	Acute AUB requiring admission (coagulopathy, pregnancy complication, severe eating disorder)
Bradycardia	Functional hypothalamic amenorrhea
Underweight (BMI <5th percentile)	Functional hypothalamic amenorrhea

(continued)

Table 15.3 (continued)

Clinical examination finding	Diagnoses to consider
Skin	
Acanthosis nigricans, skin tags	PCOS
Acne, hirsutism, androgenic alopecia	Hyperandrogenemia (PCOS, androgen-secreting tumor, non-classic congenital adrenal hyperplasia, certain cases of Cushing's syndrome)
Bruising, petechiae	Coagulopathy
Dry skin, thin hair	Hypothyroidism
Facial flushing	Cushing's syndrome
Violaceous striae	Cushing's syndrome
Pallor	Anemia
Head and Neck	
Conjunctival pallor	Anemia
Dorsocervical fat pad	Cushing's syndrome
Goiter	Hypo- or hyperthyroidism
Lid lag or proptosis, prominent stare	Hyperthyroidism due to Graves' disease
Low hair line, webbed neck	Turner syndrome (POI)
Round face	Cushing's syndrome
Visual field defect	Pituitary tumor
Voice deepening	Hyperandrogenemia
Chest	
Flow murmur	Anemia
Galactorrhea	Prolactinoma
Abdomen	
Hepatomegaly	Liver dysfunction (coagulopathy, systemic illness)
Uterine mass	Pregnancy, large uterine fibroid
Pelvis	
Clitoromegaly	Hyperandrogenemia
Vaginal discharge, ulcers	Sexually transmitted infection
Neurologic	
Hypo- or hyperreflexia	Hypo- or hyperthyroidism
Fine tremor of outstretched hands	Hyperthyroidism

Considerations for Laboratory Evaluation

All women with irregular menses should have a sensitive screening test to evaluate for pregnancy, regardless of their reported sexual history. Testing for sexually transmitted infections using urine nucleic acid amplification testing (NAAT) for *Chlamydia trachomatis* and *Neisseria gonorrhea* should be considered in most adolescent women, given the high prevalence of such infections. It is also important to obtain a screening complete blood count with differential in all women to assess for anemia, thrombocytopenia or leucocytosis. A serum ferritin should be obtained if there is a history of HMB to evaluate for iron deficiency, as a normal physical examination does not rule out anemia. Blood type and screen is indicated if the patient appears hemodynamically unstable and there is consideration for admission [12].

A screening thyroid-stimulating hormone (TSH) can be sent as part of the initial evaluation of adolescents presenting with AUB to rule out primary hyperthyroidism or hypothyroidism. A screening prolactin level may also be obtained, especially when there is a history of headache, galactorrhea, or anti-psychotic use. Further evaluation for disorders of ovulatory dysfunction will depend on the clinical context. Screening for disorders of hyperandrogenemia such as an androgen-secreting tumor, polycystic ovarian syndrome (PCOS), and non-classic congenital adrenal hyperplasia includes serum levels of total and free testosterone, DHEAS and first morning (8 AM) 17-hydroxyprogesterone. Screening for ovarian, pituitary, or hypothalamic disorders such as primary ovarian insufficiency, pituitary insufficiency, or hypothalamic amenorrhea will include an LH, FSH, and estradiol level. If a patient has Cushingoid features such as a round face, dorsocervical fat pad, central obesity, violaceous striae, hypertension, or type 2 diabetes, and there is high suspicion for Cushing's syndrome, evaluation includes the assessment of at least two of the three of the following: 24 hour urinary free cortisol, midnight salivary cortisol, and a low-dose dexamethasone suppression test. This should be guided by a pediatric endocrinologist.

Clinical screening tools have been developed to determine which patients with HMB will benefit from further evaluation for coagulopathy [22]. This screen is considered positive if the individual reports (i) heavy menstrual periods since menarche, OR (ii) one or more of the following: postpartum hemorrhage, surgery-related bleeding, bleeding after dental procedure, OR (iii) two or more of the following: bruising >5 cm >1 time per month, epistaxis >1 time per month, frequent gum bleeding, or family history of bleeding symptoms. The initial screening evaluation for coagulopathy should include prothrombin time, activated partial thromboplastin time, fibrinogen, and Von Willebrand factor activity and antigen, as well as factor VIII activity [12].

Additional Evaluation

Since structural etiologies of AUB are rare in adolescents, pelvic imaging is less useful and routine ultrasonography is not recommended as part of the initial workup of AUB [11]. If there is clinical concern based on the history or physical examination, and imaging is indicated, transabdominal ultrasound is usually more appropriate and acceptable to adolescent patients than the transvaginal approach. Adolescents who are not responsive to initial medical therapy may benefit from imaging to expand their workup.

Management

The initial step in the management of an adolescent with AUB is to accurately assess her hemodynamic status. If she is hemodynamically unstable, she will require inpatient admission for urgent triage and management. In clinically stable patients, management involves the assessment of the underlying cause as described. Bleeding in pregnancy should be managed by an obstetrician-gynecologist. Sexually transmitted infections are treated as per Centers for Disease Control and Prevention 2015 guidelines [23]. In adolescents, most causes of AUB are managed successfully with medical treatment. In those with HMB, treatment goals are to stop HMB, establish regular menses, and treat any anemia (hemoglobin <12 g/dl or iron deficiency (ferritin <12 g/dl)) [12].

A patient with acute AUB with signs of hemodynamic instability should be hospitalized for immediate medical stabilization, which may include volume expansion, iron replacement, and hormonal therapy. The patient should be assessed for contraindications to estrogen therapy. Transfusion is rarely indicated and is reserved for severe hemodynamic instability and anemia.

If there is HMB, but the patient is otherwise hemodynamically stable, without severe anemia, and not experiencing active profuse heavy bleeding, they can be managed as an outpatient using high-dose OCPs or a progestin-only taper. The typical management includes starting monophasic pills containing 30–50 micrograms of ethinyl estradiol given every 6–8 hours until cessation of bleeding, followed by a tapering of the dose as tolerated with close clinical follow-up. If estrogens are contraindicated, progestin therapy with oral medroxyprogesterone acetate (20 mg three times daily for 7 days) may be initiated followed by a progestin taper after cessation of bleeding [12]. An anti-emetic is often required due to nausea/vomiting with high-dose estrogen. If there is no improvement in HMB in 24 hours, inpatient admission should be considered. If bleeding does not stop with these traditional measures, anti-fibrinolytics such as tranexamic acid may be used. Procedural management is reserved for failure of medical therapy. Invasive procedures such as hysterectomy, uterine artery embolization, and endometrial ablation are not considered acceptable in adolescents except in life-threatening situations due to their effects on fertility. Fertility-sparing options include intrauterine balloon tamponade and suction evacuation or suction curettage [12]. After the correction of acute HMB, maintenance hormonal therapy typically consists of continuous OCPs (active pills only) until any anemia resolves. Chronic treatments for AUB can include oral and injectable progestin medications, a progesterone-releasing intrauterine device (IUD), and OCPs.

A high TSH level indicates primary hypothyroidism, and management of this condition is detailed in Chap. 41 (Hypothyroidism). A suppressed or low TSH may indicate primary hyperthyroidism (discussed in Chap. 42: Hyperthyroidism). A patient with irregular menstrual periods and clinical or biochemical evidence of hyperandrogenemia may have PCOS. However, alternate etiologies mimicking this disorder should be ruled out as applicable. A first-morning 17-hydroxyprogesterone of <200 ng/dl is reassuring against non-classic congenital adrenal hyperplasia and a DHEAS level of <700–800 mcg/dl and testosterone level <150 ng/dl are reassuring against an androgen-secreting tumor [24, 25]. Further management of adrenal disorders is described in Chap. 49 (Adrenal Insufficiency). Comprehensive management of PCOS is detailed in Chap. 45 (PCOS), cortisol excess in Chap. 50 (Cushing's Syndrome), and pituitary disorders and hyperprolactinemia in Chap. 56 (Pituitary and Suprasellar Lesions). Primary ovarian insufficiency is diagnosed when LH and FSH levels are elevated to the menopausal range with low estradiol on at least 2 samples, separated by at least 1 month [26]. Etiologies include Turner syndrome (gonadal dysgenesis), Fragile X premutation, autoimmune etiology, or gonadotoxicity from chemotherapy or radiation. The management of POI and functional hypothalamic amenorrhea is discussed in Chap. 44 (Delayed Puberty). A structural etiology of AUB such as fibroid or polyp should be evaluated by an adolescent gynecologist. If screening labs for coagulopathy are abnormal, if iron deficiency or anemia is not resolving with standard treatments, or if there is a family history of coagulopathy, a hematology consultation is recommended.

References

1. Munro MG, Critchley HOD, Fraser IS, Committee FMD. The two FIGO systems for normal and abnormal uterine bleeding symptoms and classification of causes of abnormal uterine bleeding in the reproductive years: 2018 revisions. Int J Gynaecol Obstet. 2018;143(3):393–408.
2. Fraser IS, Critchley HO, Munro MG, Broder M. Can we achieve international agreement on terminologies and definitions used to describe abnormalities of menstrual bleeding? Hum Reprod. 2007;22(3):635–43.
3. Fraser IS, Critchley HO, Munro MG, Broder M, Writing Group for this Menstrual Agreement Process. A process designed to lead to international agreement on terminologies and definitions used to describe abnormalities of menstrual bleeding. Fertil Steril. 2007;87(3):466–76.
4. Munro MG. Practical aspects of the two FIGO systems for management of abnormal uterine bleeding in the reproductive years. Best Pract Res Clin Obstet Gynaecol. 2017;40:3–22.
5. American Academy of Pediatrics Committee on Adolescence; American College of Obstetricians and Gynecologists Committee on Adolescent Health Care, Diaz A, Laufer MR, Breech LL. Menstruation in girls and adolescents: using the menstrual cycle as a vital sign. Pediatrics. 2006;118(5):2245–50.
6. Flug D, Largo RH, Prader A. Menstrual patterns in adolescent Swiss girls: a longitudinal study. Ann Hum Biol. 1984;11(6):495–508.
7. Practice Committee of American Society for Reproductive Medicine. Current evaluation of amenorrhea. Fertil Steril. 2004;82(Suppl 1):S33–9.
8. Liu Z, Doan QV, Blumenthal P, Dubois RW. A systematic review evaluating health-related quality of life, work impairment, and health-care costs and utilization in abnormal uterine bleeding. Value Health. 2007;10(3):183–94.
9. Munro MG, Critchley HO, Broder MS, Fraser IS, FIGO Working Group on Menstrual Disorders. FIGO classification system (PALM-COEIN) for causes of abnormal uterine bleeding in nongravid women of reproductive age. Int J Gynaecol Obstet. 2011;113(1):3–13.
10. Committee on Practice Bulletins—Gynecology. Practice bulletin no. 128: diagnosis of abnormal uterine bleeding in reproductive-aged women. Obstet Gynecol. 2012;120(1):197–206.
11. Pecchioli Y, Oyewumi L, Allen LM, Kives S. The utility of routine ultrasound in the diagnosis and management of adolescents with abnormal uterine bleeding. J Pediatr Adolesc Gynecol. 2017;30(2):239–42.
12. Screening and Management of Bleeding Disorders in Adolescents With Heavy Menstrual Bleeding. ACOG COMMITTEE OPINION, Number 785. Obstet Gynecol. 2019;134(3):e71–83.
13. Committee on Adolescent Health C, Committee on Gynecologic P. Committee Opinion No.580: von Willebrand disease in women. Obstet Gynecol. 2013;122(6):1368–73.
14. Bennett AR, Gray SH. What to do when she's bleeding through: the recognition, evaluation, and management of abnormal uterine bleeding in adolescents. Curr Opin Pediatr. 2014;26(4):413–9.
15. Gray SH. Menstrual disorders. Pediatr Rev. 2013;34(1):6–17; quiz 8.
16. Wilkinson JP, Kadir RA. Management of abnormal uterine bleeding in adolescents. J Pediatr Adolesc Gynecol. 2010;23(6 Suppl):S22–30.
17. Deligeoroglou E, Karountzos V, Creatsas G. Abnormal uterine bleeding and dysfunctional uterine bleeding in pediatric and adolescent gynecology. Gynecol Endocrinol. 2013;29(1):74–8.
18. Matteson KA, Munro MG, Fraser IS. The structured menstrual history: developing a tool to facilitate diagnosis and aid in symptom management. Semin Reprod Med. 2011;29(5):423–35.
19. Higham JM, O'Brien PM, Shaw RW. Assessment of menstrual blood loss using a pictorial chart. Br J Obstet Gynaecol. 1990;97(8):734–9.
20. Ott MA, Sucato GS. Contraception for adolescents. Pediatrics. 2014;134(4):e1244–56.
21. Hatch R, Rosenfield RL, Kim MH, Tredway D. Hirsutism: implications, etiology, and management. Am J Obstet Gynecol. 1981;140(7):815–30.
22. Kouides PA, Conard J, Peyvandi F, Lukes A, Kadir R. Hemostasis and menstruation: appropriate investigation for underlying disorders of hemostasis in women with excessive menstrual bleeding. Fertil Steril. 2005;84(5):1345–51.
23. Workowski KA. Centers for disease control and prevention sexually transmitted diseases treatment guidelines. Clin Infect Dis. 2015;61(Suppl 8):S759–62.
24. Carmina E, Rosato F, Janni A, Rizzo M, Longo RA. Extensive clinical experience: relative prevalence of different androgen excess disorders in 950 women referred because of clinical hyperandrogenism. J Clin Endocrinol Metab. 2006;91(1):2–6.
25. Speiser PW, Azziz R, Baskin LS, Ghizzoni L, Hensle TW, Merke DP, et al. Congenital adrenal hyperplasia due to steroid 21-hydroxylase deficiency: an Endocrine Society clinical practice guideline. J Clin Endocrinol Metab. 2010;95(9):4133–60.
26. American College of Obstetricians and Gynecologists. Committee opinion no. 605: primary ovarian insufficiency in adolescents and young women. Obstet Gynecol. 2014;124(1):193–7.

Hypertension

16

Vidhu V. Thaker

Introduction

Hypertension (HTN) is an important modifiable risk factor for cardiovascular morbidity and mortality, and HTN in youth is associated with persistence in adulthood and long-term negative health effects [1, 2]. The American Academy of Pediatrics (AAP) Clinical Practice Guideline (CPG) for screening and management of high blood pressure (BP) in children and adolescents released in 2017 updated the thresholds and percentile references for BP calculated from a healthy weight population [3]. Based on the new reference ranges, the prevalence of HTN in youth assessed in the National Health and Nutrition Examination Survey (NHANES) cohort from 2013 to 2016 was 4.2% or about 1.3 million youth aged 12–19 years, with higher prevalence in children with obesity and diabetes [4]. In more practical terms, in a classroom of 30 youth, one would have HTN, and about 3 more would have elevated BP. While the prevalence of HTN in youth is lower than that seen in adults, early detection is vital as approximately half of the children with HTN may have secondary causes amenable to therapy or heralding another medical condition requiring attention [5].

Definition

Hypertension is defined as systolic or diastolic BP ≥95th percentile, while elevated BP is defined as BP between 90 and 95th percentile for age, gender, and height. For children 13 years and older, the reference ranges for BP align with that for adults (Table 16.1).

The detailed reference tables for the classification of BP and simplified tables suitable for use in the clinic are available with the AAP 2017 CPG [3]. A number of smart phone apps incorporating the BP reference ranges from the AAP 2017 CPG are available as well as web-based calculators to determine the BP percentile for individual patient at the point of clinical care or a dataset [6, 7]. Masked hypertension is defined as normal office BP but elevated over 24 hours measured by Ambulatory Blood Pressure Monitoring (ABPM), and white-coat hypertension is defined as elevated office BP but normal 24 hours ABPM.

Table 16.1 Criteria for diagnosis of elevated BP and hypertension in children

	For children aged 1–13 years	For children ≥13 years
Normal BP	<90th percentile	Systolic <120 mm Hg Diastolic <80 mm Hg
Elevated BP	90–95th percentile*	Systolic 120–129 mm Hg Diastolic <80 mm Hg
Stage 1 HTN	≥95th percentile – <95th percentile +12 mm Hg*	Systolic 130–139 mm Hg Diastolic 80–89 mm Hg
Stage 2 HTN	≥95th percentile +12 mm Hg*	≥140/90 mm Hg

*For these categories, consider the definition for children ≥13 years if this is lower

Measurement of Blood Pressure in Children

The accurate measurement of BP is critical to the diagnosis of elevated BP or HTN in youth. The child should be seated in a quiet room for 3–5 min prior to measurement with back supported and feet uncrossed. As far as possible, BP should be measured in the right arm supported at the heart level, for consistency and comparison with standard tables (exceptions being some congenital anomalies of the aortic arch). An appropriate BP cuff is the key to the accurate measurement of BP. The length of the bladder of the cuff should be 80–100% of the circumference of the arm and the width at least 40% [3, 8]. When this is difficult to determine, the mid-

V. V. Thaker (✉)
Division of Molecular Genetics, Department of Pediatrics, Columbia University Irving Medical Center, New York, NY, USA

Division of Pediatric Endocrinology, Department of Pediatrics, Columbia University Irving Medical Center, New York, NY, USA
e-mail: vvt2114@cumc.columbia.edu

T. Stanley, M. Misra (eds.), *Endocrine Conditions in Pediatrics*, https://doi.org/10.1007/978-3-030-52215-5_16

arm circumference can be measured at the mid-point between the spine of the acromion and the olecranon process of the ulna. For the interested reader, details can be found in the AAP 2017 CPG [3] and the tools to support reducing diagnostic errors in pediatric elevated BP including a video demonstrating appropriate technique for the measurement of BP on the AAP Project-REDDE website [9].

Per the guidelines of 2017 AAP CPG, BP should be measured annually in children and adolescents ≥3 years of age [3]. For specific conditions more commonly associated with elevated BP, such as obesity, diabetes, renal disease, history of aortic arch obstruction or children who are taking medications known to increase BP, a measurement should be done at every encounter. The initial BP measurement may be oscillometric on a calibrated machine that has been validated for use in pediatric population. If the initial BP is elevated (≥90th percentile), providers should perform 2 additional oscillometric or auscultatory BP measurements at the same visit and average them. BP measurements can change during the visit and typically the repeat BP measurements are lower. If the BP measurements are elevated at the encounter, repeat measurements are advised based on the stage of the BP:

(a) For elevated BP, repeat measurements can be done in 6 months with interim lifestyle management intervention.
(b) For children with Stage 1 HTN, 2nd measurement is advised within 1–2 weeks and 3rd in 3 months.
(c) For children with Stage 2 HTN, 2nd measurement and referral to specialty care are recommended within a week [3].

Physical examination of all children with elevated BP and/or HTN should include height, weight, calculated BMI, and their percentiles. Detailed physical examination can be guided by history and may provide clues to the causes of HTN. The physical findings pertinent for endocrine-related causes will be summarized here and detailed findings for each cause of HTN can be found in Table 14 of the 2017 AAP CPG on management of HTN in children [3].

Hypertension is more common in children with certain common conditions such as obesity, sleep-disordered breathing, chronic kidney disease, and those born preterm. This review will cover the conditions most pertinent from an endocrine perspective.

Children with Obesity

The prevalence of hypertension ranges from 3.8% to 24.8% in youth with overweight and obesity, with a graded increase with increasing adiposity [10–16]. With the revised BP reference standards, 2.6% of the youth in the United States, or nearly 800,000 youth, were reclassified as having hypertension, of whom roughly half have obesity [4, 17]. Obesity is associated with a lack of circadian variability of BP [18], with the absence of the expected nocturnal BP dip in up to 50% of the children who have obesity [19–21].

For children with obesity, it is especially important to use the appropriate size cuff for the measurement of BP. Increased BMI has been associated with increased mid-arm circumference in youth between 3 and 19 years of age. In the 2011–16 NHANES survey, >20% children between the ages of 6–11 years needed an adult or larger cuff size; nearly 35% of adolescents ages 12–19 years required a larger adult cuff and at least 3.7% required an extra-large adults cuff based on the mid-arm circumference [22]. An inappropriate small size BP measurement cuff can result in a falsely higher reading, or conversely lower reading with a larger cuff. Thus, the availability of a variety of cuff sizes and the accurate measurement of mid-arm circumference to determine the right BP measurement cuff is critical to the diagnosis of elevated BP. Adults with obesity have been noted to have conical upper arm shape that may also influence the accurate measurement of BP [23, 24], but similar data is not known in children. Ambulatory Blood Pressure Monitoring (ABPM) is a valuable tool in the diagnosis of HTN in children with obesity due to the discrepancy between casual and ambulatory BP [25] and the possibility of masked hypertension that may not be obvious at the clinical visit but nevertheless is associated with adverse long-term cardiovascular outcomes. If the BP is consistently elevated at 2 visits, at least 6 months apart, consider consultation with a sub-specialist for further management.

Clinical Key
Many children with obesity will need an adult, large adult, or extra-large adult cuff for the appropriate measurement of blood pressure.

Children with Diabetes

Premature cardiovascular disease is the leading cause of mortality and morbidity in individuals with Type 1 diabetes (T1D) [26, 27]. The prevalence of HTN ranges from 4% to 16% in individuals with T1D; higher in children <12 years of age, not significantly different between males and females, but higher in Asian Pacific Islander and American Indian children [28–30]. Similar to the children with obesity, it has been noted that individuals with T1D may have a higher prevalence of masked HTN and loss of the normal nocturnal dip of the BP, and each of these is associated with higher prevalence of diabetic kidney disease [31]. HTN is frequently underdiagnosed and undertreated in individuals with T1D, and associated with overall higher prevalence of morbidities, making it imperative to check BP for all children with T1D at every clinical encounter and refer to an appropriate sub-specialist if needed.

Hypertension Associated with Endocrine Disease

A small proportion of children (0.05–6%) will have HTN secondary to hormonal excess (Table 16.2). While rare and often seen earlier in life, such a diagnosis provides a unique treatment opportunity for surgical cure or to achieve a dramatic response with pharmacologic therapy. Many of such conditions are associated with disorders of the adrenal gland and may have an identifiable molecular etiology.

Screening Tests

If persistent elevated BP or HTN is detected on repeat examinations, for all patients, consideration may be given for urinalysis, chemistry panel including electrolytes, blood

Table 16.2 Endocrine conditions associated with HTN

Endocrine disorder	Clinical features	Workup and notes
Catecholamine excess		
Pheochromocytoma/ Paraganglioma	HTN Palpitations, headache, sweating Abdominal mass Incidental finding Family screening	Diagnostic test: fractionated plasma* and/or urine metanephrines/ normetanephrines. Associated genetic mutations: *VHL* (49%), *SDHB* (15%) and *SDHD* (10%), de novo or AD
Mineralocorticoid excess		
Consider if: Early onset HTN, abnormal potassium levels, family h/o HTN, or refractory HTN Screening test: Aldosterone renin ratio (ARR) = plasma aldosterone concentration (PAC)/plasma renin activity (PRA), preferably obtained between 8 and 10 am		
Congenital adrenal hyperplasia (CAH) 11β –hydroxylase deficiency	HTN Hypokalemia Acne, hirsutism, virilization in girls, Pseudo precocious puberty in boys	Elevated levels of deoxycorticosterone (DOC), 11-deoxycortisol, androstenedione, testosterone, and dehydroepiandrosterone acetate. More common in Moroccan Jews. Genetic mutation: *CYP11B1*, AR
CAH 17-α hydroxylase deficiency	HTN Hypokalemia Undervirilized male or sexual infantilism in female	Elevated DOC and corticosterone Low aldosterone and renin Rare, seen in Dutch Mennonites Genetic mutation: *CYP17*, AR
Familial hyperaldosteronism, Type 1–4	Often severe HTN Young subjects Family history of strokes	Persistent hyperaldosteronism Known genetic mutations: *CYP11B1/CYP11B2, KCNJ5, CACNA1D*, AD.
Apparent mineralocorticoid excess	HTN Hypokalemia Low birth weight Failure to thrive Polyuria, polydipsia	Mimicked by licorice toxicity Genetic mutation: *HSD11B2*, AR
Glucorticoid abnormality		
Cushing's syndrome, Adrenocortical carcinoma, iatrogenic excess	HTN Moon facies Violaceous abdominal striae Central weakness	Measurement of ACTH and cortisol in blood 24-hour urinary cortisol measurement Salivary cortisol, midnight cortisol
Primary glucocorticoid resistance	HTN Ambiguos genitalia Precocious puberty Androgen excess Menstrual abnormalities in women	Excessive DOC and corticosterone production Caused due to loss of function of glucocorticoid receptor Known genetic mutation: *NR3C1*
Other hormonal conditions		
Hyperthyroidism	Tachycardia HTN Tremors Enlarged thyroid Orbital protuberance	TSH, Total T3 and free T4 levels May test for antibodies based on results Initial treatment with beta blockers Resolves with the treatment of hyperthyroidism
Hyperparathyroidism	Hypercalcemia Other signs of hyperparathyroidism	Resolves with the treatment of hyperparathyroidism

Key: AD Autosomal dominant, *AR* Autosomal recessive
*Influenced by posture, specialized medical center preferred. See also Chap. 34.

Table 16.3 Suggested evaluation for persistent elevated BP or HTN

Laboratory evaluation
All patients
Urinalysis
Electrolytes, blood urea nitrogen, creatinine
Lipid profile: fasting or non-fasting
Renal ultrasonography in those <6 years or if abnormal or urinalysis or renal function
In the presence of obesity
HbA1c or suspicion of diabetes
Fasting lipid panel (for dyslipidemia)
Liver enzymes (for fatty liver)
Optional
Thyroid function tests
Drug screen if clinical suspicion
Sleep study (with symptoms or h/o apnea)

urea nitrogen, and creatinine. Renal imaging may be considered for children <6 years of age with abnormal urinalysis or renal function. Lipid profile (fasting or non-fasting) can be considered in all children, while Hemoglobin A1c may be limited to children with obesity. Based on other clinical findings, individual patients may be good candidates for thyroid function tests, sleep study (with history of loud snoring), or drug screen with a suspicion for drug induced HTN (Table 16.3).

Treatment

The goal of the treatment of HTN for both primary and secondary HTN is to achieve a BP level that reduces the risk of target organ damage in childhood and prevents long-term adverse cardiovascular outcomes in adulthood. The 2017 AAP CPG recommends maintaining the BP <90th percentile for age, height, and sex or <120/80 mm Hg, whichever is lower [3].

Lifestyle Management: Diet

The Dietary Approach to Stop Hypertension (DASH) approach focuses on including a diet high in fruits, vegetables, low-fat milk products, whole grains, fish, poultry, nuts, and lean red meats with the limited intake of sugar and sweets along with lower sodium intake [32].

Lifestyle Management: Physical Activity

Observational data have shown that moderate-to-vigorous aerobic physical activity or weight training lasting for 40 min at least 3–5 days/week improves systolic BP [33–35].

Pharmacologic Intervention

Pharmacological treatment of HTN in children and adolescents should be considered in individuals who have persistent HTN despite lifestyle management. Choice of drug may be guided by the suspected etiology. Initial treatment is often considered with drugs belonging to the following classes: angiotensin converting enzyme (ACE) inhibitors, angiotensin receptor blockers (ARB), long-acting calcium channel blockers or a thiazide diuretic. While children with diabetes may benefit from ACE inhibitor or ARBs, individuals of African American heritage may not respond as well to these requiring either higher doses or alternate therapies. Pharmacologic management of HTN in children may be considered in primary care in partnership with a specialty care provider.

References

1. Chen X, Wang Y. Tracking of blood pressure from childhood to adulthood: a systematic review and meta-regression analysis. Circulation. 2008;117(25):3171–80.
2. Juhola J, Magnussen CG, Berenson GS, Venn A, Burns TL, Sabin MA, et al. Combined effects of child and adult elevated blood pressure on subclinical atherosclerosis: the International Childhood Cardiovascular Cohort Consortium. Circulation. 2013;128(3):217–24.
3. Flynn JT, Kaelber DC, Baker-Smith CM, Blowey D, Carroll AE, Daniels SR, et al. Clinical practice guideline for screening and management of high blood pressure in children and adolescents. Pediatrics. 2017;140(3):e20171904.
4. Jackson SL, Zhang Z, Wiltz JL, Loustalot F, Ritchey MD, Goodman AB, et al. Hypertension among youths — United States, 2001–2016. Morb Mortal Wkly Rep. 2018;67:758–62.
5. Gupta-Malhotra M, Banker A, Shete S, Hashmi SS, Tyson JE, Barratt MS, et al. Essential hypertension vs. secondary hypertension among children. Am J Hypertens. 2015;28(1):73–80.
6. MDCalc. AAP Pediatric Hypertension Guidelines: mdcalc.com; 2018 [Web based application to calculate SBP and DBP percentiles for children 1–11 years of age.]. Available from: https://www.mdcalc.com/aap-pediatric-hypertension-guidelines.
7. Sharma A. AAP 2017: Mobile 2018 [Web based application to calculate SBP and SBP percentile for children aged 2–18 years based on 2017 AAP CPG]. Available from: https://apps.cpeggcep.net/BPz_cpeg_dde/.
8. Pickering TG, Hall JE, Appel LJ, Falkner BE, Graves J, Hill MN, et al. Recommendations for blood pressure measurement in humans and experimental animals: part 1: blood pressure measurement in humans: a statement for professionals from the Subcommittee of Professional and Public Education of the American Heart Association Council on High Blood Pressure Research. Circulation. 2005;111(5):697–716.
9. American Academy of Pediatrics: Pediatric Elevated Blood Pressure. 2018 [Quality improvement and professional development tools from American Academy of Pediatrics.]. Available from: https://www.aap.org/en-us/professional-resources/quality-improvement/Project-RedDE/Pages/Blood-Pressure.aspx.
10. Zhang T, Zhang H, Li S, Li Y, Liu Y, Fernandez C, et al. Impact of adiposity on incident hypertension is modified by insulin resistance

in adults: longitudinal observation from the Bogalusa heart study. Hypertension. 2016;67(1):56–62.
11. Sorof JM, Lai D, Turner J, Poffenbarger T, Portman RJ. Overweight, ethnicity, and the prevalence of hypertension in school-aged children. Pediatrics. 2004;113(3 Pt 1):475–82.
12. Sorof J, Daniels S. Obesity hypertension in children: a problem of epidemic proportions. Hypertension. 2002;40(4):441–7.
13. Skinner AC, Perrin EM, Moss LA, Skelton JA. Cardiometabolic risks and severity of obesity in children and young adults. N Engl J Med. 2015;373(14):1307–17.
14. Lurbe E, Invitti C, Torro I, Maronati A, Aguilar F, Sartorio A, et al. The impact of the degree of obesity on the discrepancies between office and ambulatory blood pressure values in youth. J Hypertens. 2006;24(8):1557–64.
15. Koebnick C, Black MH, Wu J, Martinez MP, Smith N, Kuizon B, et al. High blood pressure in overweight and obese youth: implications for screening. J Clin Hypertens (Greenwich). 2013;15(11):793–805.
16. Falkner B, Gidding SS, Ramirez-Garnica G, Wiltrout SA, West D, Rappaport EB. The relationship of body mass index and blood pressure in primary care pediatric patients. J Pediatr. 2006;148(2):195–200.
17. Sharma AK, Metzger DL, Rodd CJ. Prevalence and severity of high blood pressure among children based on the 2017 American Academy of Pediatrics Guidelines. JAMA Pediatr. 2018;172(6):557–65.
18. Torok K, Palfi A, Szelenyi Z, Molnar D. Circadian variability of blood pressure in obese children. Nutr Metab Cardiovasc Dis. 2008;18(6):429–35.
19. Westerstahl M, Marcus C. Association between nocturnal blood pressure dipping and insulin metabolism in obese adolescents. Int J Obes. 2010;34(3):472–7.
20. Westerstahl M, Hedvall Kallerman P, Hagman E, Ek AE, Rossner SM, Marcus C. Nocturnal blood pressure non-dipping is prevalent in severely obese, prepubertal and early pubertal children. Acta Paediatrica. 2014;103(2):225–30.
21. Framme J, Dangardt F, Marild S, Osika W, Wahrborg P, Friberg P. 24-h Systolic blood pressure and heart rate recordings in lean and obese adolescents. Clin Physiol Funct Imaging. 2006;26(4):235–9.
22. Ostchega Y, Hughes JP, Nwankwo T, Zhang G. Mean mid-arm circumference and blood pressure cuff sizes for US children, adolescents and adults: National Health and Nutrition Examination Survey, 2011–2016. Blood Press Monit. 2018;23(6):305–11.
23. Palatini P, Benetti E, Fania C, Malipiero G, Saladini F. Rectangular cuffs may overestimate blood pressure in individuals with large conical arms. J Hypertens. 2012;30(3):530–6.
24. Bonso E, Saladini F, Zanier A, Benetti E, Dorigatti F, Palatini P. Accuracy of a single rigid conical cuff with standard-size bladder coupled to an automatic oscillometric device over a wide range of arm circumferences. Hypertens Res. 2010;33(11):1186–91.
25. Renda R. Comparison of ambulatory blood pressure monitoring and office blood pressure measurements in obese children and adolescents. Acta Clin Belg. 2018;73(2):126–31.
26. Sarwar N, Gao P, Seshasai SR, Gobin R, Kaptoge S, Di Angelantonio E, et al. Diabetes mellitus, fasting blood glucose concentration, and risk of vascular disease: a collaborative meta-analysis of 102 prospective studies. Lancet. 2010;375(9733):2215–22.
27. Laing SP, Swerdlow AJ, Slater SD, Burden AC, Morris A, Waugh NR, et al. Mortality from heart disease in a cohort of 23,000 patients with insulin-treated diabetes. Diabetologia. 2003;46(6):760–5.
28. Schwab KO, Doerfer J, Hecker W, Grulich-Henn J, Wiemann D, Kordonouri O, et al. Spectrum and prevalence of atherogenic risk factors in 27,358 children, adolescents, and young adults with type 1 diabetes: cross-sectional data from the German diabetes documentation and quality management system (DPV). Diabetes Care. 2006;29(2):218–25.
29. Rodriguez BL, Dabelea D, Liese AD, Fujimoto W, Waitzfelder B, Liu L, et al. Prevalence and correlates of elevated blood pressure in youth with diabetes mellitus: the SEARCH for diabetes in youth study. J Pediatr. 2010;157(2):245–51. e1.
30. Margeirsdottir HD, Larsen JR, Brunborg C, Overby NC, Dahl-Jorgensen K, Norwegian Study Group for Childhood Diabetes. High prevalence of cardiovascular risk factors in children and adolescents with type 1 diabetes: a population-based study. Diabetologia. 2008;51(4):554–61.
31. Lithovius R, Gordin D, Forsblom C, Saraheimo M, Harjutsalo V, Groop PH. Ambulatory blood pressure and arterial stiffness in individuals with type 1 diabetes. Diabetologia. 2018;61(9):1935–45.
32. He FJ, MacGregor GA. Importance of salt in determining blood pressure in children: meta-analysis of controlled trials. Hypertension. 2006;48(5):861–9.
33. Torrance B, McGuire KA, Lewanczuk R, McGavock J. Overweight, physical activity and high blood pressure in children: a review of the literature. Vasc Health Risk Manag. 2007;3(1):139–49.
34. Farpour-Lambert NJ, Aggoun Y, Marchand LM, Martin XE, Herrmann FR, Beghetti M. Physical activity reduces systemic blood pressure and improves early markers of atherosclerosis in pre-pubertal obese children. J Am Coll Cardiol. 2009;54(25):2396–406.
35. Chen HH, Chen YL, Huang CY, Lee SD, Chen SC, Kuo CH. Effects of one-year swimming training on blood pressure and insulin sensitivity in mild hypertensive young patients. Chin J Physiol. 2010;53(3):185–9.

Initial Evaluation of Polydipsia and Polyuria

17

Brynn E. Marks

Introduction

Increased thirst, or polydipsia, and increased urination, also called polyuria, can be common complaints in a general pediatric office. These symptoms are intuitively linked, as increased urine output triggers increased thirst to avoid dehydration. Conversely, depending on the underlying cause increased fluid intake can trigger increased urine output to prevent hyponatremia. Careful evaluation with a history, physical examination, and appropriate laboratory testing can help to narrow the differential diagnosis and guide appropriate management including, when necessary, referral to a pediatric endocrinologist.

Polydipsia and polyuria are defined as more than 2 L/m^2/day of fluid intake and output, respectively, in pediatric patients or more than 3 liters per day in adults [1]. Body surface area is measured as meters squared and can be calculated using the following equation based on the patient's height (centimeters) and weight (kilograms): $\sqrt{}$(height × weight)/3600) [2]. When the patient's length is not available, the BSA can be estimated using the weight in kilograms alone: ((4 × weight) + 7)/(90 + weight) [3].

Pathophysiology and Differential Diagnosis

For the purposes of further exploring these chief complaints, we will take a perspective focused on polyuria. Polyuria can occur due to water diuresis or osmotic diuresis. In water diuresis, there is an inability to concentrate the urine, leading to the production of large volumes of dilute urine. By contrast, with osmotic diuresis the presence of a solute in the renal tubules pulls water down its concentration gradient causing decreased reabsorption of water with the production of more concentrated urine.

Before exploring endocrine-related causes of these complaints, it is important to consider alternative causes such as dehydration, primary or secondary enuresis, urinary tract infections, behavioral etiologies often linked to excessive intake of sugar sweetened beverages, and substances such as diuretics, alcohol, and caffeine. Additionally, pollakiuria, or benign idiopathic urinary frequency, should be considered in a previously toilet-trained toddler or young school age child who has urinary frequency, often voiding small amounts several times per hour without any signs or symptoms of infection [4].

Osmotic Diuresis-Glycosuria, Urea Diuresis, Sodium Diuresis

The most common cause of polydipsia and polyuria in the pediatric population is osmotic diuresis resulting from glycosuria. In the kidney glucose is filtered at glomerulus and subsequently reabsorbed in the proximal convoluted tubule [5]. When the plasma glucose concentration exceeds the renal threshold of approximately 180 mg/dL, the renal tubules are unable to reabsorb all of the glucose in the lumen, resulting in glycosuria and subsequent polyuria. Glycosuria may be the result of new onset diabetes mellitus, either type 1 (T1D) or type 2 (T2D), or poorly controlled pre-existing diabetes mellitus. Although T1D and T2D predominate, less common forms of diabetes including cystic fibrosis-related diabetes (CFRD), steroid induced diabetes, post-transplant diabetes, and maturity onset diabetes of the young (MODY) should be considered depending on the clinical scenario. Finally, transient stress-induced hyperglycemia, due to either life-threatening or non-life-threatening illness, may also be seen [6]. (See Chap. 8 for the discussion of the initial evaluation of hyperglycemia.) Stress-induced hyperglycemia self-resolves over time, but is poorly understood, and clinicians

B. E. Marks (✉)
Division of Endocrinology, Children's National Medical Center, Washington, DC, USA

George Washington University School of Medicine and Health Sciences, Washington, DC, USA
e-mail: bmarks@childrensnational.org

T. Stanley, M. Misra (eds.), *Endocrine Conditions in Pediatrics*, https://doi.org/10.1007/978-3-030-52215-5_17

must meticulously exclude other diagnoses due to the risks associated with untreated diabetes mellitus.

Glycosuria may also be seen in patients with normal plasma glucose levels due to renal tubular defects in glucose reabsorption. Patients with isolated renal glycosuria have a lower renal glucose threshold at which the renal tubules are unable to absorb all glucose from the renal lumen, resulting in glycosuria at normal plasma glucose levels. Generalized proximal renal tubular dysfunction, also called Fanconi syndrome, results in an inability to reabsorb phosphate, glucose, amino acids, proteins, and bicarbonate, leading to renal tubular acidosis [7].

Other more rare causes of osmotic diuresis leading to polyuria include increased urea and sodium loads [1]. The presence of high concentrations of these solutes in the renal lumen also pulls water down its concentration gradient, resulting in polyuria. Increased urea loads may be seen in patients on high protein diets, those with tissue catabolism due to glucocorticoid therapy or severe illness, urea therapy for the treatment of syndrome of inappropriate antidiuretic hormone secretion (SIADH), and those with resolving acute kidney injury. High sodium loads, resulting from intravenous saline administration, may also lead to polyuria which can be commonly seen after surgical procedures.

Water Diuresis-Central and Nephrogenic Diabetes Insipidus, Primary Polydipsia

Polyuria may also occur due to increased urinary water losses resulting from an inability to appropriately concentrate urine. Urine concentration is typically tightly regulated to maintain plasma osmolality and sodium levels [1]. When intravascular volume is low and sodium levels begin to rise, thirst increases, and the posterior pituitary releases vasopressin, also known as antidiuretic hormone. Vasopressin acts on the kidney to increase water retention, thereby increasing urine concentration. Abnormalities in thirst, vasopressin production, or response to vasopressin can result in increased water diuresis, leading to polydipsia and polyuria.

Patients with central diabetes insipidus (DI) do not produce vasopressin and as a result are unable to concentrate their urine. Increased urinary output leads to increased thirst in order to maintain hydration. Central DI may result from: brain tumors or infiltrative disease, structural brain abnormalities such as Optic Nerve Hypoplasia Syndrome, neurosurgery, or trauma. Germinomas, large craniopharyngiomas, and optic gliomas are the tumors most commonly associated with central DI. Patients with nephrogenic DI produce vasopressin, but have a resistance to its actions at the level of the kidney and therefore are unable to concentrate urine in the renal tubules [1]. Because these patients have vasopressin resistance rather than a complete deficiency, nephrogenic DI typically has a milder presentation than central DI. Nephrogenic DI may result from genetic etiologies, medications, hypercalcemia, hypokalemia, and underlying renal disease. Please see Table 17.1 for additional information.

Table 17.1 Differential diagnosis for polyuria and polydipsia

Osmotic diuresis	Water diuresis
Glycosuria A. Hyperglycemia 1. Type 1 diabetes mellitus 2. Type 2 diabetes mellitus 3. Other types of diabetes mellitus 4. Stress-induced hyperglycemia B. Euglycemia with renal defects 1. Isolated renal glycosuria 2. Fanconi syndrome	Central diabetes insipidus A. Brain tumor 1. Germinoma 2. Craniopharyngioma 3. Optic Glioma B. Infiltrative disease C. Structural brain abnormalities D. Neurosurgery E. Trauma
Sodium diuresis A. High sodium intake 1. Intravenous saline	Nephrogenic diabetes insipidus A. Genetic etiologies B. Medication related 1. Lithium 2. Cidofovir, foscarnet, amphotericin B, demeclocycline, ifosfamide, ofloxacin C. Electrolyte abnormalities 1. Hypercalcemia 2. Hypokalemia D. Underlying renal disease 1. Sickle cell disease 2. Ureteral obstruction 3. Polycystic kidney disease 4. Sjogren's syndrome
Urea diuresis A. Resolution of acute kidney injury B. Urea therapy for SIADH C. High protein intake D. Tissue catabolism 1. Glucocorticoid therapy 2. Severe illness	Primary polydipsia

Finally, patients with primary polydipsia, also known as psychogenic polydipsia, have a primary increase in fluid intake without an apparent cause. To avoid water intoxication and hyponatremia, these patients produce large quantities of dilute urine. Primary polydipsia often co-occurs with psychiatric illness and may be exacerbated by medications associated with dry mouth.

Important Aspects of the History

A careful history is essential to narrow the differential diagnosis. Most importantly, the parent and child should be questioned to quantify the volume or fluid being consumed and voided to confirm true polyuria and polydipsia (>2 L/m^2/day). Information about the size of the glasses the child is drinking from and attempts to measure the urine are essential for differentiating normal patterns from true polydipsia and polyuria. Additional questions should focus on the frequency of drinking and voiding, differentiating between daytime and nighttime occurrences, and types of beverages the child chooses. The color of the urine can be helpful in ascertaining whether the child is producing dilute, clear or concentrated, dark urine. With suspicion for central DI, the patient should be queried about changes in vision, problems with coordination, and signs of increased intracranial pressure, such as headaches and vomiting that could suggest the presence of a brain tumor. The duration of symptoms, intercurrent illnesses, comorbid conditions including psychiatric ones, interval weight loss, preceding traumas, and systemic symptoms should also be clarified. The provider should inquire about medication history, focusing on glucocorticoids and lithium which may predispose a child to osmotic diuresis or water diuresis (see Table 17.1 for other pertinent medications).

Finally, a family history should be elicited. If there is suspicion for DM, the provider should inquire about the types of diabetes and age of onset for effected family members. T2D has a stronger genetic association than T1D, though familial patterns may be seen in either case. First-degree relatives with autoimmune disease including thyroid disease, vitiligo, and celiac disease can also be seen in children with T1D.

Key Components of the Physical Exam

The physical exam should begin with the consideration of interval growth parameters. Weight loss could be secondary to dehydration in the case of diabetes insipidus and catabolism in the case of diabetes mellitus. If the patient was previously obese or remains obese despite weight loss, the posterior neck and axillae should be assessed for acanthosis nigricans, which is indicative of insulin resistance commonly seen in T2D. Decreased growth velocity is typically not seen in new onset diabetes mellitus, but could suggest growth hormone or deficiency or hypothyroidism if there is suspicion for a brain tumor associated with DI. Signs of dehydration, including tachycardia, hypotension, sluggish capillary refill, and dry mucous membranes, can be seen in both diabetes mellitus and insipidus. Attention should be paid to the pubertal status, as T2D is very rarely seen in prepubertal children. Perineal candidiasis can be seen in T1D or T2D. The neurological status should also be assessed if there is concern for a brain tumor or suspicion for diabetic ketoacidosis. Papilledema and bitemporal hemianopsia can suggest the presence of a brain tumor. Please see Table 17.2 for a summary of the physician examination pearls and Table 17.3 for features to help distinguish diabetes insipidus from primary polydipsia.

Table 17.2 Physical exam pearls for polyuria and polydipsia

Growth parameters: Interval weight loss ➔ diabetes mellitus or insipidus Obesity ➔ Type 2 diabetes mellitus Decreased growth velocity ➔ concern for growth hormone deficiency or hypothyroidism in a patient with suspicion for a brain tumor associated with diabetes insipidus
Vital Signs: Tachycardia, hypotension, delayed capillary refill ➔ diabetes mellitus or insipidus
Dermatologic: Acanthosis nigricans ➔ Type 2 diabetes mellitus
Pubertal status: Prepubertal ➔ Type 2 diabetes is rarely seen in prepubertal patients Perineal candidiasis ➔ diabetes mellitus
Neurological exam: Altered mental status ➔ diabetic ketoacidosis Papilledema, bitemporal hemianopsia ➔ brain tumor associated with diabetes insipidus

Table 17.3 Distinguishing diabetes insipidus from primary polydypsia

	Diabetes insipidus	*Primary polydipsia*
History	Preference for water over any other beverage Polydipsia and polyuria throughout the day and night, awakening from sleep to drink and urinate	No specific beverage preference Unlikely to have polyuria and polydipsia overnight
Physical	Poor weight gain or weight loss May exhibit signs of dehydration (tachycardia, hypotension, delayed capillary refill, dry mucous membranes) Midline defects can be seen in central DI (single central incisor, cleft lip or palate, high arched palate)	No significant weight abnormalities No evidence of dehydration
Laboratory	Serum sodium is usually normal or high Dilute urine	Serum sodium may be low-normal or low Variable urine concentration

Laboratory Evaluation and Next Steps in Diagnosis and Management

Laboratory evaluation, diagnosis, and management of polydipsia and polyuria will vary drastically depending on the underlying cause. As diabetes mellitus and diabetes insipidus are the most likely endocrine etiologies for these complaints, the next steps for both of these conditions will be addressed separately below. If the diagnosis is unclear, studies for both diabetes insipidus and diabetes mellitus should be pursued (see Table 17.4).

Table 17.4 Elements of the initial laboratory evaluation for polyuria and polydypsia

Laboratory	Comments
Blood glucose	Finger-stick or laboratory value appropriate for initial assessment (see Chap. 9).
Urinalysis with glucose, ketones, and specific gravity	Positive ketones of moderate or greater in the context of hyperglycemia should prompt emergent referral to a pediatric endocrinologist or an emergency department.
Serum electrolytes, blood urea nitrogen, creatinine, osmolality, and calcium *AND* Urine sodium and osmolality	Serum and urine studies should be obtained concurrently and may be most helpful after a period of fluid restriction.* *Urine osmolality >600 mOsm/L with normal serum sodium generally excludes a diagnosis of DI* *Urine osmolality <300 mOsm/L with elevated serum sodium suggests DI.*

*In older children, asking the child not to drink after bed and obtaining next-morning testing before any fluid consumption can be helpful. Such testing risks hypernatremia, however, and should not be performed if there is high suspicion for DI or in younger children who cannot adequately communicate symptoms or severity of thirst. In such cases, a shorter period of supervised water deprivation may be warranted

Diabetes Mellitus

Hyperglycemia is the most common cause of polydipsia and polyuria in pediatric patients. Obtaining a point of care glucose in the office can be very helpful in determining the next steps in management. The patient's hands should be washed and dried before checking the glucose level as contaminants and residual water can lead to spuriously high and low values. Information about when the child last ate or drank caloric beverages will guide the interpretation of these values. A point of care glucose testing should be accompanied by urinalysis to assess for glycosuria and *must be* supplemented with an assessment of ketone levels. The presence of moderate ketones or greater in the urine of patients with diabetes is a medical emergency requiring urgent attention. If there is access to a point of care ketone monitor, it can be used to measure beta-hydroxybutyrate (βOHB), a type of ketone, with a finger-stick. Please see Chap. 9 for more information regarding the initial evaluation of hyperglycemia.

Although glycosuria can be a helpful diagnostic clue, the absence of glycosuria only indicates a blood glucose level below the renal threshold of approximately 180 mg/dL and does not completely exclude hyperglycemia, particularly if the sample is collected in the morning when the patient is fasting. Please see Chap. 30 for additional information about the interpretation of laboratory studies related to glucose metabolism and diabetes.

Suspected Type 1 Diabetes

Additional laboratory studies to assess for diabetes may also be considered depending on the clinical scenario. If the patient has ketones of moderate or greater or if there is suspicion for T1D (see below), additional laboratory studies are best deferred until the patient is evaluated in an emergency department. Laboratory studies in the emergency department typically include a venous blood gas, basic metabolic panel, βOHB level, hemoglobin A1c, and often pancreatic autoantibodies (GAD65, insulin, IA-2, and Zinc-transporter 8). Please see Chap. 8 for additional information about pertinent labs and Chap. 52 for additional information about the diagnosis and management of type 1 diabetes. If the patient is hyperglycemic with small ketones or less, obtaining a basic metabolic panel, βOHB level, hemoglobin A1c, and pancreatic antibodies may help to guide the next steps in management.

Suspected Type 2 Diabetes

If there is no significant ketosis and there is a suspicion for type 2 diabetes based on exam and history, it is prudent to discuss the next steps in management with your local pediatric endocrinologist. Severe hyperglycemia with random glucose values ≥250 mg/dL or hemoglobin A1c values ≥8.5% or the presence of ketosis are indications for insulin therapy in pediatric type 2 diabetes [8]. Patients with milder hyperglycemia may be managed with diet and lifestyle changes, oral therapies such as metformin, and glucagon-like peptide-1 agonists (GLP1), a non-insulin injectable therapy [9]. Please see Chap. 53 for additional information about the diagnosis and management of insulin resistance and type 2 diabetes.

Diabetes Insipidus and Primary Polydipsia

Urine concentration varies markedly depending on hydration status and serum sodium levels, ranging from 50 mOsm/kg to 1200 mOsm/kg. As such, laboratory studies to assess for diabetes insipidus must include paired urine and serum sodium and osmolality levels. In the face of hypernatremia, urine should be maximally concentrated to preserve hydration. Conversely, in the presence of hyponatremia urine should be maximally dilute to excrete excess water. The presence of hypernatremia with inappropriately dilute urine is indicative of diabetes insipidus while hyponatremia with dilute urine is suggestive of primary polydipsia.

A point of care urinalysis in the office can provide some useful clues, but should be followed up with laboratory studies including basic metabolic panel, calcium level, serum osmolality, serum vasopressin level, urine sodium, and urine osmolality. It should also be noted that the absence of serum sodium abnormalities does not exclude diabetes insipidus as patients with free access to water may compensate for increased urinary losses with excessive fluid intake. These studies may not be useful unless the patient has been fasting for some period which can be unsafe in the home setting depending on the child's age and underlying diagnosis. Water deprivation tests are typically done in the hospital setting. Please see Chap. 28 for information about laboratory studies involving electrolytes and vasopressin levels.

Central Versus Nephrogenic Diabetes Insipidus

Differentiating central from nephrogenic DI is critical as it determines the next steps in evaluation and management. This is best done with administration of desmopressin, a synthetic form of vasopressin, during a water deprivation test performed by a pediatric endocrinologist. If urine concentration increases after desmopressin is administered and a diagnosis of central diabetes insipidus is confirmed, the patient needs evaluation with a brain MRI including thin cuts of the pituitary to rule out structural abnormalities and masses (see Chaps. 37 and 56). If the urine concentration does not increase after desmopressin is administered, the patient has nephrogenic diabetes insipidus. Pediatric nephrologists often manage nephrogenic diabetes insipidus rather than pediatric endocrinologists. Please see Chap. 55 for additional information about the diagnosis and management of diabetes insipidus.

Conclusions

The differential diagnosis for polydipsia and polyuria includes both endocrine and non-endocrine causes. Careful attention to the history to confirm an intake or output >2 L/m^2/day, physical examination, and basic laboratory assessment can help to narrow the differential diagnosis and guide appropriate initial management until referral to a pediatric endocrinologist. While there are many causes of polydipsia and polyuria, hyperglycemia due to diabetes mellitus remains the most common explanation for these complaints in a pediatric population.

References

1. Muglia LJ, Srivatsa AMJ. Disorders of the posterior pituitary. In: Sperling MA, editor. Pediatric endocrinology. 4th ed. Philadelphia: Elsevier; 2014. p. 405–43.
2. Mosteller RD. Simplified calculation of body surface area. N Engl J Med. 1987;317:1098.
3. Coulthard MG. Surface area is best estimated from weight alone: pocket calculators and nomograms are unnecessary. Arch Dis Child. 1994;71:281.
4. Walker J, Rickwood AMK. Daytime urinary frequency in children Training of surgical registrars : a regional audit. BMJ. 1988;297(6646):455.
5. Mather A, Pollock C. Glucose handling by the kidney. Kidney Int Suppl. 2011;79(120):S1–6. https://doi.org/10.1038/ki.2010.509.
6. Fattorusso V, Nugnes R, Cassertano A, Valerio G, Mozzillo E, Franzese A. Non-diabetic hyperglycemia in the pediatric age: why, how, and when to treat? Curr Diab Rep. 2018;18(12):140.
7. Haque SK, Ariceta G, Batlle D. Proximal renal tubular acidosis: a not so rare disorder of multiple etiologies. Nephrol Dial Transplant. 2012;27(12):4273–87.
8. Care D, Suppl SS. 13. Children and adolescents: standards of medical care in diabetesd2019. Diabetes Care. 2019;42(January):S148–64.
9. Tamborlane WV, Barrientos-Pérez M, Fainberg U, Frimer-Larsen H, Hafez M, Hale PM, et al. Liraglutide in children and adolescents with type 2 diabetes. N Engl J Med. 2019;381(7):637–46.

18 Acanthosis Nigricans

Mohamed Saleh and Radhika Muzumdar

Introduction

Acanthosis nigricans (AN) was first described in 1890 in Paul Gerson Unna's eminent International Atlas of Rare Skin Diseases [1]. It is a common condition characterized by velvety hyperpigmented skin lesions, especially in the intertriginous areas such as the neck and axillae. AN may also appear in other skin regions such as the inframammary, abdominal, antecubital, inguinal skin folds, and the anogenital regions [2]. Clinical recognition of AN is essential because it is associated with a variety of systemic and metabolic disorders, many of which are characterized by insulin resistance. Obesity and diabetes mellitus are frequently associated with AN, and this association was first reported in 1947 [3]. Rarely, AN can be a sign of internal malignancy.

In the pediatric population, AN first appears as hyperpigmentation in the back of the neck or axillae. Initially, AN may be mistaken as dirty skin areas that are difficult to be cleaned [2]. As the lesions progress, the skin becomes thicker and demonstrates accentuation of dermatoglyphics (skin lines) and papillomatous projections. Acrochordons (skin tags) may be present within or around affected areas. AN typically develops in a symmetrical distribution. Unilateral cases of AN may represent a variant of epidermal nevus [4]. Hyperpigmentation plaques localized to knuckles of the hands, elbows, knees, or feet have been described as acral AN [5].

M. Saleh
Division of Endocrinology and Diabetes, Department of Pediatrics, UPMC Children's Hospital of Pittsburgh, Pittsburgh, PA, USA
e-mail: Mohamed.saleh@chp.edu

R. Muzumdar (✉)
Division of Endocrinology and Diabetes, Department of Pediatrics, UPMC Children's Hospital of Pittsburgh, Pittsburgh, PA, USA

Division of Endocrinology and Diabetes, UPMC Children's Hospital of Pittsburgh, University of Pittsburgh School of Medicine, Pittsburgh, PA, USA
e-mail: Radhika.muzumdar@chp.edu

Pathophysiology of AN

The pathogenesis of AN is not fully understood. The activation of the following tyrosine kinase receptors have been proposed as potential causative factors:

1. Insulin-like growth factor receptor-1 (IGF1R): High insulin levels associated with obesity and insulin resistance can directly stimulate IGF-1 receptors, leading to keratinocyte and dermal fibroblast proliferation. Stimulation of IGF-1 receptor could also be the result of increased free IGF-1 resulting from the suppression of IGF-binding protein 1 and 2 by insulin [6].
2. Fibroblast growth factor receptor (FGFR): Activating mutations in FGFR3 have been linked to several inherited syndromes that present with AN including Crouzon syndrome, severe achondroplasia with developmental delay and AN (SADDAN), thanatophoric dwarfism, and hypochondroplasia [7, 8].
3. Epidermal growth factor receptor (EGFR): EGFR stimulation by TGF-α appears to be the mechanism for malignancy-associated AN [9].

Common causes of acanthosis nigricans: Obesity-related insulin resistance, and PCOS.
Causes of acanthosis nigricans that cannot be missed: Diabetes mellitus and hidden malignancy.

Different classifications of AN have been proposed, based on etiology, localization, and severity and textures of skin lesions [10]. The most accepted classification uses etiology and localization to classify AN into obesity-associated, benign, syndromic, malignant, unilateral, acral, and drug-induced [2] (Table 18.1).

Obesity, Endocrine, and Metabolic Disorders Obesity and diabetes mellitus are the most common medical disorders

T. Stanley, M. Misra (eds.), *Endocrine Conditions in Pediatrics*, https://doi.org/10.1007/978-3-030-52215-5_18

Table 18.1 Differential diagnosis of AN in children

Endocrine disorders	Obesity/insulin resistance Type 2 diabetes mellitus PCOS Cushing disease Acromegaly
Genetic syndromes	Genetic syndromes associated with insulin resistance: Type A insulin resistance Type B insulin resistance Leprechaunism Rabson-Mendenhall syndrome Lipodystrophy Down syndrome Alstrom syndrome Genetic syndromes not associated with insulin resistance: Crouzon syndrome Thanatophoric dysplasia Costello syndrome Fibroblast growth factor receptor 3 mutation (i.e., achondroplasia) Other rare genetic syndromes
Drug-induced	Nicotinic acid Steroids Testosterone Oral combined contraceptive pills (OCPs) Aripiprazole
Malignancy	Gastrointestinal adenocarcinoma Wilms tumor Osteogenic carcinoma
Congenital	Benign AN
Idiopathic	Acral AN
Unilateral AN	Epidermal nevus

associated with AN in pediatrics and adults [11, 12]. AN is one of the earliest physical findings in children with obesity and insulin resistance and is often first evident around or after puberty. However, it may occur at any age [13]. Complete resolution of the skin lesions may occur with weight loss. Polycystic ovarian syndrome (PCOS), which is associated with insulin resistance and hyperinsulinemia, is associated with AN [14]. Acromegaly and Cushing disease, endocrine conditions associated with obesity and/or insulin resistance, are also associated with AN [15].

Genetic Syndromes Multiple genetic disorders causing insulin resistance are associated with AN. The Type A insulin resistance syndrome, an insulin receptor defect disorder, is characterized by severe insulin resistance and AN in the absence of obesity [13]. It commonly affects African female adolescents and women, who exhibit severe lesions early in childhood. Affected females also have hyperandrogenism, possibly as a secondary manifestation of hyperinsulinemia, as insulin can suppress sex hormone–binding globulin (SHBG) and lead to increased free androgens [16]. The Type B insulin resistance syndrome occurs secondary to serum autoantibodies against the insulin receptor, leading to impairment of insulin receptor function. It is uncommon in children and typically affects black females [16]. Periocular AN is a distinguishing feature in Type B insulin resistance [17]. Type B insulin resistance is usually associated with hyperandrogenism in girls and women of reproductive age [17]. Patients with Type B insulin resistance may also have other autoimmune diseases such as systemic lupus erythematosus, progressive systemic sclerosis, Sjogren's syndrome, Hashimoto's thyroiditis, and autoimmune thrombocytopenia [18].

Other genetic syndromes that may present with AN and insulin resistance include Down syndrome, leprechaunism, Rabson-Mendenhall syndrome, congenital generalized lipodystrophy (Berardinelli-Seip syndrome), familial partial lipodystrophy, and Alstrom syndrome [19]. Additionally, there are genetic syndromes that are not characterized by insulin resistance but may also present with AN, including Cutis gyrata syndrome, Crouzon syndrome with AN, thanatophoric dysplasia, Costello syndrome, and severe achondroplasia with developmental delay and AN [19, 20].

Malignant AN A paraneoplastic form of AN is most frequently diagnosed in older, non-obese patients [21], and it is rarely diagnosed in the pediatric population [16]. Malignant AN is characterized by rapid onset and extensive distribution. Lesions occur in atypical sites (e.g., mucous membranes, palms, or soles). Additional paraneoplastic findings may include rapid growth or inflammation of seborrheic keratoses (the sign of Leser-Trélat) or velvety to rugose thickening of the palmar skin (tripe palm) [16, 22]. Gastric adenocarcinoma is the underlying etiology in approximately two-thirds of adult patients with malignant AN. In pediatrics, it has also been reported with Wilms tumor and osteogenic carcinoma [23–27].

Drug-induced AN AN due to drug exposure is uncommon. It occurs with medications that promote obesity or hyperinsulinemia such as systemic nicotinic acid [28], glucocorticoids [16], injected insulin (due to repeated insulin injection in the same sites) [29], oral contraceptives [30], protease inhibitors [31], testosterone [10], and aripiprazole [32].

Benign AN is usually congenital and less frequently develops during childhood or adolescence. Inheritance of benign AN is possibly autosomal dominant with a variable penetrance [2].

Unilateral AN may represent a unilateral epidermal nevus or be a precursor to bilateral AN [33].

Acral AN is common in patients of sub-Saharan African descent [34]. Acral AN is localized to elbows, knees, and most commonly in the knuckles of the hands and feet, and occurs in the absence of any other findings in an otherwise healthy child [16, 34]. The etiology of acral AN remains unknown, and it is a diagnosis of exclusion.

Clarifying Questions in the Medical History

1. Onset and progression of AN: Onset of AN in infancy or early childhood suggests the possibility of a syndromic or familial disorder, and less frequently malignancy. A rapid, progressive course may indicate paramalignant AN.
2. Symptoms suggestive of diabetes mellitus: Polyuria, polydipsia, and nocturia, particularly in obese patients, suggest hyperglycemia. Prediabetes and diabetes can also occur in non-obese patients with insulin resistance, such as Type A insulin resistance and lipodystrophy. History of unintentional weight loss, yeast infections, and recurrent infections are also suggestive of new-onset diabetes.
3. Symptoms indicating hyperandrogenism: Oligomenorrhea, amenorrhea, hirsutism, and acne may occur with PCOS, and in hyperandrogenism associated with Type A and Type B insulin resistance.
4. Family history: Family history of AN, particularly in non-obese patients, may suggest benign AN.
5. Medication history: Drugs such as glucocorticoids, nicotinic acid and OCPs could be associated with AN.

Physical Examination

In patients with AN, a complete physical examination is essential to define the underlying cause, and associated disorders such as hypertension, metabolic syndrome, and hyperandrogenism.

General examination should include:

- Body mass index (BMI): BMI >85th percentile for age and sex is suggestive of hyperinsulinism.
- Blood pressure measurement: Obese patients with AN should have an accurate measurement of blood pressure to rule out hypertension associated with metabolic syndrome. (Please see Chap. 16 for discussion of hypertension.)
- Body habitus: Increased waist circumference or abdominal obesity is often associated with insulin resistance. A paucity of subcutaneous fat in the face and extremities may suggest lipodystrophy.
- Signs of hyperandrogenism: The presence of hirsutism and/or acne indicates insulin resistance–associated hyperandrogenism.
- Dysmorphic features: Presence of dysmorphic features may suggest syndromic AN, e.g., Down syndrome and Alström syndrome.
- Height, sitting height, and arm span (see Chap. 1): AN associated with asymmetrical short stature may suggest an FGFR3 mutation.
- Abdominal exam: Palpable mass detected on an abdominal exam, particularly in infants and children, may suggest paramalignant AN.

Local examination of the skin lesion should include morphology and distribution. Typically, AN presents with thickened, velvety to verrucous, grey brown hyperpigmented plaques on the skin. AN in skinfolds may become macerated and inflamed secondary to bacterial colonization or yeast infection. The back and the sides of the neck and axillae are the most common sites of involvement. However, it may occur in other skin folds, including inframammary and abdominal areas. Unilateral AN is suggestive of an epidermal nevus. Extensive AN and its presence in atypical sites such as palms and mucous membranes may suggest malignancy. AN localized to elbows, knees, and knuckles in the absence of any other finding is suggestive of acral AN.

Diagnostic Workup

AN is considered a risk factor for diabetes. The recent ADA position statement recommends that risk-based screening for dysglycemia in pediatrics should be considered in overweight (BMI ≥85th percentile) or obese (BMI ≥95th percentile) children who have one or more additional risk factors for diabetes. These screening criteria are only applied to pubertal children or children older than 10 years, whichever comes first [35]. Given that AN is considered a risk factor, obese/overweight children who have AN should be screened for dysglycemia. This should include fasting glucose and/or hemoglobin A1c. Fasting insulin can also be considered as an assessment of insulin resistance, but mild elevation in fasting insulin in the context of normoglycemia is often seen in non-obese peri-pubertal children who have physiologic insulin resistance of puberty. If there is a high suspicion for dysglycemia, despite normal hemoglobin A1c, an oral glucose tolerance test (OGTT) should be considered. Lipid panel and liver enzymes may be warranted to evaluate for dyslipidemia and nonalcoholic fatty liver disease associated with obesity and insulin resistance. In females with clinical evidence of hyperandrogenism, the primary care physician should obtain total testosterone, sex hormone–binding globulin (SHBG), and dehydroepiandrosterone sulfate (DHEAS), and may want to consider anti-Mullerian hormone (AMH), luteinizing hormone (LH), follicle stimulation hormone (FSH), and free testosterone if a reliable assay is available (see Chap. 14).

The possibility of an occult malignancy should always be considered in infants, nonobese children with new-onset AN, and rapidly progressive AN. However, the recommendations for appropriate cancer evaluation in such patients is lacking. These patients should be evaluated with a thorough review of symptoms, a complete physical examination, and age-appropriate cancer screening, i.e., abdominal ultrasound. Because many of the associated tumors involve the gastrointestinal tract, referral to gastroenterology may be indicated.

Clinical Key
Mid to late stages of puberty are marked by a physiologic worsening of insulin resistance, such that many obese teens with AN will have worsening AN during mid/late puberty with stabilization or improvement following the completion of pubertal development.

Interpretation of Endocrine Laboratory Values in Patients with AN

The laboratory diagnostic criteria for diabetes and prediabetes are the same for children and adults (Table 18.2). It is important to know that several studies have doubted the validity of hemoglobin A1c for the screening of prediabetes and diabetes in pediatrics because of its poor sensitivity that may result in underestimation [36].

For the screening of nonalcoholic fatty liver disease (NAFLD), transaminases levels are a relatively sensitive clinical tool but are not specific. Thus, other causes of chronic liver disease, such as viral hepatitis, should be ruled out [37]. Also, some patients with NAFLD may have completely normal ALT levels [38].

Dyslipidemia is a common metabolic feature in obese children [39], and it is determined based on the following parameters: HDL <40 mg/dl, LDL ≥130 mg/dl, triglycerides (TG) ≥130 mg/dl, total cholesterol (TC) ≥200 mg/dl [40].

In overweight/obese female adolescents with AN and irregular menses, an elevation of serum testosterone and/or free testosterone and low SHBG is highly suggestive of PCOS. Most patients with PCOS have serum testosterone concentrations of less than 150 ng/dL. A total testosterone of higher than 150 ng/dL increases the likelihood of a virilizing ovarian or adrenal neoplasm [41]. Slightly elevated LH and slightly low FSH with increased LH:FSH ratio are characteristic of typical PCOS. Also, mild elevation in AMH is consistent with polycystic ovary syndrome [42]. DHEAS is a marker for adrenal hyperandrogenism and has minimal diurnal variation. Although the most common cause of DHEAS elevation is the functional adrenal hyperandrogenism of PCOS [43], the main reason for measuring DHEAS levels is to identify a rare virilizing adrenal disorder, such as cortisone reductase deficiency [44] or an adrenal tumor. In adrenal tumors, DHEAS levels are often, but not necessarily, markedly elevated (>700 mcg/dL) [43]. An 8 AM 17-hydroxyprogesterone (17OHP) level is a useful screening test to rule out nonclassical congenital adrenal hyperplasia.

Table 18.2 ADA criteria for diagnosis of prediabetes and diabetes [35]

Prediabetes	A1C 5.7% to <6.5%. Impaired fasting glucose: fasting glucose ≥100 but <126 mg/dL. Impaired glucose tolerance: 2-h plasma glucose ≥140 but <200 mg/dL during an OGTT. The test should be performed as described by the World Health Organization, using a glucose load containing the equivalent of 1.75 g/kg (max 75 g) anhydrous glucose dissolved in water.
Diabetes	Diagnosis of diabetes is established if any of the following criteria is present and verified on repeat testing: A1C ≥6.5%. Fasting serum glucose ≥126 mg/dL. 2-h serum glucose ≥200 mg/dL during an OGTT. Patient with classic symptoms of hyperglycemia or hyperglycemic crisis with a random plasma glucose >200 mg/dL.
Other supportive findings	Family history of Type 2 diabetes. History suggestive of hyperglycemia such as polyuria, polydipsia and nocturia. History of weight loss. History of recurrent infections, yeast infections, and poor wound healing.

Treatment

Primary care physicians should refer the patient urgently to a pediatric endocrinologist if the diagnosis of diabetes is established. Likewise, the patient should be referred for an endocrine evaluation if the diagnosis of PCOS is suspected. AN alone, without any other risk factor for diabetes, evidence of dysglycemia/dyslipidemia, or evidence of hyperandrogenism, does not necessarily require pediatric endocrine referral.

The therapeutic approach for AN involves treatment of the underlying cause:

Obesity Weight loss and exercise improve insulin sensitivity and therefore decrease insulin levels. This leads to improvement in obesity-associated AN [45].

Insulin Resistance Medications that improve insulin sensitivity, such as metformin, may ameliorate AN but are not standard of care solely for that purpose [46].

PCOS In addition to lifestyle modification, combined OCPs are the first-line endocrine treatment for patients with dermatologic or menstrual abnormalities [47, 48]. Combined OCPs with antiandrogenic progestins in low doses, i.e., drospirenone, may provide an additional benefit [49]. Progestin monotherapy is an alternative to combined OCPs for the control of menstrual irregularities in the event of contraindications for combined OCPs [50]. OCPs reduce hyperpigmentation and improve clinical signs of hyperandrogenism by lowering the concentration of free circulating androgens [51].

Drug-Induced AN In drug-induced AN, cessation of the offending medication often results in regression of AN [52].

Malignancy-Associated AN Improvement or resolution of AN has been reported in patients following successful treatment of the associated malignancy [21].

Other Interventions Other medications have been associated with the improvement of AN, such as octreotide in obese adolescents [53], and dietary fish oil in lipodystrophy associated with diabetes mellitus [54].

Skin-Directed Therapy Topical treatment may help in localized lesions. Few case reports have shown that topical retinoic acid, a keratinolytic agent, may improve AN [55]. Other local therapies that have been tried for the treatment of AN include topical urea, salicylic acid, glycolic acid peels, and laser therapy [2, 56, 57].

References

1. Pollitzer S. Acanthosis nigricans: a symptom of a disorder of the abdominal sympathetic. JAMA. 1909;53:1369–73.
2. Sinha S, Schwartz RA. Juvenile acanthosis nigricans. J Am Acad Dermatol. 2007;57(3):502–8.
3. Robinson SS, Tasker S. Acanthosis nigricans juvenilis associated with obesity; report of a case, with observations on endocrine dysfunction in benign acanthosis nigricans. Arch Dermatol Syphilol. 1947;55(6):749–60.
4. Jeong JS, Lee JY, Yoon TY. Unilateral nevoid acanthosis nigricans with a submammary location. Ann Dermatol. 2011;23(1):95–7.
5. Schwartz RA, Janniger CK. Childhood acanthosis nigricans. Cutis. 1995;55(6):337–41.
6. Higgins SP, Freemark M, Prose NS. Acanthosis nigricans: a practical approach to evaluation and management. Dermatol Online J. 2008;14(9):2.
7. Berk DR, Spector EB, Bayliss SJ. Familial acanthosis nigricans due to K650T FGFR3 mutation. Arch Dermatol. 2007;143(9):1153–6.
8. Hirai H, et al. Acanthosis nigricans in a Japanese boy with hypochondroplasia due to a K650T mutation in FGFR3. Clin Pediatr Endocrinol. 2017;26(4):223–8.
9. Koyama S, et al. Transforming growth factor-alpha (TGF alpha)-producing gastric carcinoma with acanthosis nigricans: an endocrine effect of TGF alpha in the pathogenesis of cutaneous paraneoplastic syndrome and epithelial hyperplasia of the esophagus. J Gastroenterol. 1997;32(1):71–7.
10. Karadag AS, et al. Acanthosis nigricans and the metabolic syndrome. Clin Dermatol. 2018;36(1):48–53.
11. Rafalson L, Eysaman J, Quattrin T. Screening obese students for acanthosis nigricans and other diabetes risk factors in the urban school-based health center. Clin Pediatr (Phila). 2011;50(8):747–52.
12. Hud JA Jr, et al. Prevalence and significance of acanthosis nigricans in an adult obese population. Arch Dermatol. 1992;128(7):941–4.
13. Friedman CI, Richards S, Kim MH. Familial acanthosis nigricans. A longitudinal study. J Reprod Med. 1987;32(7):531–6.
14. Schmidt TH, et al. Cutaneous findings and systemic associations in women with polycystic ovary syndrome. JAMA Dermatol. 2016;152(4):391–8.
15. Jabbour SA. Cutaneous manifestations of endocrine disorders: a guide for dermatologists. Am J Clin Dermatol. 2003;4(5):315–31.
16. Schwartz RA. Acanthosis nigricans. J Am Acad Dermatol. 1994;31(1):1–19; quiz 20–2.
17. Arioglu E, et al. Clinical course of the syndrome of autoantibodies to the insulin receptor (type B insulin resistance): a 28-year perspective. Medicine (Baltimore). 2002;81(2):87–100.
18. Baird JS, et al. Systemic lupus erythematosus with acanthosis nigricans, hyperpigmentation, and insulin receptor antibody. Lupus. 1997;6(3):275–8.
19. Torley D, Bellus GA, Munro CS. Genes, growth factors and acanthosis nigricans. Br J Dermatol. 2002;147(6):1096–101.
20. Munoz-Perez MA, Camacho F. Acanthosis nigricans: a new cutaneous sign in severe atopic dermatitis and Down syndrome. J Eur Acad Dermatol Venereol. 2001;15(4):325–7.
21. Krawczyk M, Mykala-Ciesla J, Kolodziej-Jaskula A. Acanthosis nigricans as a paraneoplastic syndrome. Case reports and review of literature. Pol Arch Med Wewn. 2009;119(3):180–3.
22. Pentenero M, et al. Oral acanthosis nigricans, tripe palms and sign of leser-trelat in a patient with gastric adenocarcinoma. Int J Dermatol. 2004;43(7):530–2.
23. Anderson SH, Hudson-Peacock M, Muller AF. Malignant acanthosis nigricans: potential role of chemotherapy. Br J Dermatol. 1999;141(4):714–6.
24. Skiljevic DS, et al. Generalized acanthosis nigricans in early childhood. Pediatr Dermatol. 2001;18(3):213–6.
25. Birns J, et al. Acanthosis nigricans associated with acute myeloid leukaemia. Eur J Intern Med. 2004;15(7):473.
26. Garrott TC. Malignant acanthosis nigricans associated with osteogenic sarcoma. Arch Dermatol. 1972;106(3):384–5.
27. Bhargava P, et al. Malignant acanthosis nigricans in a 2 year old child with Wilm's Tumour. Indian J Dermatol Venereol Leprol. 1998;64(1):29–30.
28. Stals H, et al. Acanthosis nigricans caused by nicotinic acid: case report and review of the literature. Dermatology. 1994;189(2):203–6.
29. Fleming MG, Simon SI. Cutaneous insulin reaction resembling acanthosis nigricans. Arch Dermatol. 1986;122(9):1054–6.
30. Skouby SO. Update on the metabolic effects of oral contraceptives. J Obstet Gynaecol (Lahore). 1986;6(Suppl 2):S104–9.
31. Mellor-Pita S, et al. Acanthosis nigricans: a new manifestation of insulin resistance in patients receiving treatment with protease inhibitors. Clin Infect Dis. 2002;34(5):716–7.
32. Manu P, et al. Acanthosis nigricans during treatment with aripiprazole. Am J Ther. 2014;21(3):e90–3.
33. Krishnaram AS. Unilateral nevoid acanthosis nigricans. Int J Dermatol. 1991;30(6):452–3.
34. Schwartz RA. Acral acanthosis nigricans (acral acanthotic anomaly). J Am Acad Dermatol. 2007;56(2):349–50.
35. Arslanian S, et al. Evaluation and Management of Youth-Onset Type 2 diabetes: a position statement by the American Diabetes Association. Diabetes Care. 2018;41(12):2648–68.
36. Buse JB, et al. Diabetes screening with hemoglobin A(1c) versus fasting plasma glucose in a multiethnic middle-school cohort. Diabetes Care. 2013;36(2):429–35.

37. Chan WK, et al. Limited utility of plasma M30 in discriminating non-alcoholic steatohepatitis from steatosis--a comparison with routine biochemical markers. PLoS One. 2014;9(9):e105903.
38. Kohli R, et al. Pediatric nonalcoholic fatty liver disease: a report from the expert committee on nonalcoholic fatty liver disease (ECON). J Pediatr. 2016;172:9–13.
39. Cook S, Kavey RE. Dyslipidemia and pediatric obesity. Pediatr Clin N Am. 2011;58(6):1363–73, ix.
40. Expert Panel on Integrated Guidelines for Cardiovascular Health. Expert panel on integrated guidelines for cardiovascular health and risk reduction in children and adolescents: summary report. Pediatrics. 2011;128(Suppl 5):S213–56.
41. Sharma A, et al. Diagnostic thresholds for androgen-producing tumors or pathologic hyperandrogenism in women by use of Total testosterone concentrations measured by liquid chromatography-tandem mass spectrometry. Clin Chem. 2018;64(11):1636–45.
42. Rosenfield RL, et al. Antimullerian hormone levels are independently related to ovarian hyperandrogenism and polycystic ovaries. Fertil Steril. 2012;98(1):242–9.
43. Elhassan YS, et al. Causes, patterns, and severity of androgen excess in 1205 consecutively recruited women. J Clin Endocrinol Metab. 2018;103(3):1214–23.
44. Lavery GG, et al. Steroid biomarkers and genetic studies reveal inactivating mutations in hexose-6-phosphate dehydrogenase in patients with cortisone reductase deficiency. J Clin Endocrinol Metab. 2008;93(10):3827–32.
45. Bellot-Rojas P, et al. Comparison of metformin versus rosiglitazone in patients with acanthosis nigricans: a pilot study. J Drugs Dermatol. 2006;5(9):884–9.
46. Romo A, Benavides S. Treatment options in insulin resistance obesity-related acanthosis nigricans. Ann Pharmacother. 2008;42(7):1090–4.
47. Legro RS, et al. Diagnosis and treatment of polycystic ovary syndrome: an Endocrine Society clinical practice guideline. J Clin Endocrinol Metab. 2013;98(12):4565–92.
48. Martin KA, et al. Evaluation and treatment of hirsutism in premenopausal women: an Endocrine Society Clinical Practice Guideline. J Clin Endocrinol Metab. 2018;103(4):1233–57.
49. Cremer M, Phan-Weston S, Jacobs A. Recent innovations in oral contraception. Semin Reprod Med. 2010;28(2):140–6.
50. Bagis T, et al. The effects of short-term medroxyprogesterone acetate and micronized progesterone on glucose metabolism and lipid profiles in patients with polycystic ovary syndrome: a prospective randomized study. J Clin Endocrinol Metab. 2002;87(10):4536–40.
51. Tercedor J, et al. Effect of ketoconazole in the hyperandrogenism, insulin resistance and acanthosis nigricans (HAIR-AN) syndrome. J Am Acad Dermatol. 1992;27(5 Pt 1):786.
52. Coates P, Shuttleworth D, Rees A. Resolution of nicotinic acid-induced acanthosis nigricans by substitution of an analogue (acipimox) in a patient with type V hyperlipidaemia. Br J Dermatol. 1992;126(4):412–4.
53. Lunetta M, et al. Long-term octreotide treatment reduced hyperinsulinemia, excess body weight and skin lesions in severe obesity with acanthosis nigricans. J Endocrinol Investig. 1996;19(10):699–703.
54. Sherertz EF. Improved acanthosis nigricans with lipodystrophic diabetes during dietary fish oil supplementation. Arch Dermatol. 1988;124(7):1094–6.
55. Darmstadt GL, Yokel BK, Horn TD. Treatment of acanthosis nigricans with tretinoin. Arch Dermatol. 1991;127(8):1139–40.
56. Ichiyama S, et al. Effective treatment by glycolic acid peeling for cutaneous manifestation of familial generalized acanthosis nigricans caused by FGFR3 mutation. J Eur Acad Dermatol Venereol. 2016;30(3):442–5.
57. Rosenbach A, Ram R. Treatment of acanthosis nigricans of the axillae using a long-pulsed (5-msec) alexandrite laser. Dermatol Surg. 2004;30(8):1158–60.

Weight Gain and/or Obesity

19

Sonali Malhotra

Definition of Overweight and Obesity

Weight gain leading to overweight or obesity simply means accumulation of excess adipose tissue or fat. Due to the limited availability of methods that accurately quantify fat, body mass index (BMI) has been reliably used for clinical evaluation of children older than 2 years [7]. In 2000, the National Center for Health Statistics and the Centers for Disease Control and Prevention (CDC) published BMI reference standards for children between 2 and 20 years of age. The BMI of children can be plotted on these charts and categorized to assess the severity of obesity [9]. In more recent years, to better categorize severe obesity, the "percent of the 95th percentile BMI" is also used. This is the patient's BMI divided by the BMI value at the 95th percentile for the patient's age and sex. (For example, if the 95th percentile BMI value is 25 kg/m^2, and the patient's BMI is 30 kg/m^2, the patient's BMI would be 120% of the 95th percentile.)

Assessment and Classification of Obesity

BMI is obtained by dividing body weight (in kilograms) by height (in meters squared) [(weight [kg]/height [m]^2 = BMI]). It is largely a decent tool to assess adiposity in pediatric population [5]. Some of the limitations of using BMI are that it may not be accurate in adolescents with a high muscle mass and may provide an overestimation of adiposity in highly muscular individuals, or an underestimation of adiposity in individuals with very low muscle mass. For younger children (less than 2 years), weight for length is used to assess for overweight and obesity.

Obesity in children and adolescents is defined using BMI-percentile for age and sex. A BMI ≥95th percentile but <120% of the 95th percentile is Class I obesity. "Severe obesity" is defined as BMI ≥120% of the 95th percentile for age and sex (Class II or higher; BMI >35 kg/m^2) [12]. BMI ≥140% of the 95th percentile for age and sex, or absolute BMI >40 kg/m^2, is defined as Class III severe obesity. This particular terminology was introduced by [4], based on the argument that the use of extreme percentiles (e.g., >99th percentile) from CDC data did not sufficiently differentiate between varying degrees of pediatric obesity [4]. Other indices such as waist circumference and waist-to-hip ratio can also be used to assess obesity, particularly abdominal adiposity [3].

Differential Diagnosis

There are a multitude of conditions which can present with weight gain leading to obesity. The first clear distinction which needs to be made is the onset of weight gain (Table 19.1). A thorough history, with plotting of the time points of weight gain and temporal association of the preceding events, helps the physician in obtaining evaluation for the underlying cause. A careful physical examination (Table 19.2) helps in narrowing down the differential diagnosis.

Important Clarifying Questions

- The age of onset of weight gain.
- If early onset, assessing for hunger levels (hyperphagia), satiety, and food-seeking behaviors.
- Weight gain velocity from one time point to another.
- Any associated developmental delays, or dysmorphic features.
- Other organ system involvement such as congenital midline defects, neurologic deficit, visual or hearing deficits, kidney involvement.
- History of intracranial irradiation, trauma, or surgery.

S. Malhotra (✉)
Pediatric Endocrinology and Obesity Medicine, Massachusetts General Hospital for Children, Boston, MA, USA
e-mail: smalhotra1@mgh.harvard.edu

T. Stanley, M. Misra (eds.), *Endocrine Conditions in Pediatrics*, https://doi.org/10.1007/978-3-030-52215-5_19

Table 19.1 Differential diagnosis

Causes of relatively new-onset weight gain	Causes of early-onset weight gain
Endocrine Glucocorticoid excess (Cushing syndrome) Hypothyroidism Growth hormone deficiency Pseudohypoparathyroidism Neurologic Intracranial insult (tumor, trauma, recent surgery, pituitary resection) Intracranial irradiation Psychological Depression Disordered eating patterns Bulimia nervosa Binge eating disorder (BED) Night eating syndrome Emotionally triggered eating Sleep-related eating disorder (SRED) Drug-induced weight gain Sulfonylureas Insulin Corticosteroids First-generation antipsychotics Tricyclic antidepressants Progestin-only contraceptives First-generation antihistamines β and/or α blockers Others Hypothalamic obesity (mostly seen after craniopharyngioma resection) ROHHAD/ROHHADNET: rapid-onset obesity with hypothalamic dysfunction, hypoventilation, and autonomic dysregulation; ROHHADNET: rapid-onset obesity with hypothalamic dysfunction, hypo- ventilation, and autonomic dysregulation with neural crest tumors	Monogenic obesity Primary disorders of the leptin signaling pathway. [6] Melanocortin 4 receptor mutations Leptin deficiency Leptin receptor deficiency Proopiomelanocortin (POMC) deficiency Proprotein convertase 1 Carboxypeptidase E (*CPE*) Brain-derived neurotrophic factor (*BDNF*) TrkB receptor (*NTRK2*) mutations Associated with the leptin melanocortin pathway Single-minded homologue 1 (*SIM1*) *MRAP2* *GNAS* *RAI1* *SH2B1* *MAGEL2* Syndromic obesity: Prader-Willi syndrome Bardet-Biedl syndrome Alström syndrome Carpenter syndrome Cohen syndrome Smith-Magenis syndrome WAGR 16p11.2 microdeletion syndrome
Polygenic obesity (multiple genes involved, and effect enhanced in the obesogenic environment)	

- Detailed medication history with temporal association of weight gain and trajectory of weight gain.
- Linear growth and growth velocity.
- Associated symptoms of headaches or visual disturbances which can point toward CNS pathology. Difficulty climbing stairs (proximal muscle weakness), which may suggest hypercortisolism. Cold intolerance, constipation, hair loss, menstrual irregularity in a female patient can provide important clues toward hypothyroidism as the underlying cause.

Table 19.2 Important aspects of the physical examination

Growth charts:
Weight gain with poor linear growth: hypercortisolism, growth hormone deficiency, and hypothyroidism
Tall stature (more than the familial norms), increased fat and lean mass, and accelerated linear growth: MC4R mutations
Congenital midline defects with the history of intracranial radiation or surgery: hypothalamic dysfunction
Red hair with orange skin: POMC mutations
Nystagmus, visual disturbances, hearing loss, hypogonadism: Bardet Biedl syndrome
Microcephaly: Cohen syndrome
Fundus exam: Blurred disc margins may be associated with idiopathic intracranial hypertension
Enlarged tonsils: Suggestive of obstructive sleep apnea
Enamel erosion could be a sign of bulimia with self-induced vomiting
Thick purplish striae, interscapular fat pad, ecchymoses: Cushing syndrome
Acanthosis nigricans: Signs of insulin resistance and diabetes
Hirsutism and acne: PCOS
Musculoskeletal:
Polydactyly (Bardet Biedl syndrome), small hands and feet (PWS)
A limited range of motion at the hip, gait abnormality: Slipped capital femoral epiphysis or Blount disease (bowing of the lower legs)
Genitourinary:
Micropenis, undescended testicles, and scrotal hypoplasia: Prader-Willi Syndrome
Stalled or absent or delayed puberty may indicate hypothalamic-pituitary tumors, Prader-Willi syndrome, Bardet-Biedl syndrome, leptin deficiency, or leptin receptor deficiency
Development:
Developmental delays and intellectual deficits: syndromic causes of obesity

- Assessment of microenvironment factors:
  - Diet (quality, quantity, and timing of food).
  - Physical activity.
  - Sleep history. Is there a problem with sleep? When and how does the sleep take place? Any signs and symptoms of sleep related phenomenon? Snoring, frequent awakenings, morning headaches, restless sleep, daytime somnolence.
  - Stress.
  - Medications.

Considerations for Laboratory Evaluation and Other Testing

Two different considerations determine laboratory evaluation for patients with weight gain. The first is evaluation aimed at determining the etiology of the weight gain, and the second is evaluation of any possible comorbidities of obesity, if present.

Evaluation of Etiology Depending on Associated Presenting Factors

- Poor linear growth with persistent weight gain: Consider Cushing syndrome and obtain 24-hour urinary cortisol levels and or midnight salivary cortisol levels [10].
- Symptoms of cold intolerance, poor linear growth, hair loss, constipation: Consider hypothyroidism and obtain thyroid-stimulating hormone (TSH) and free thyroxine (FT4).
- History of menstrual irregularity (oligomenorrhea, amenorrhea, menorrhagia, menometrorrhagia), along with acne and hirsutism: Consider polycystic ovary syndrome (PCOS, see Chap. 45) and obtain total testosterone, sex hormone–binding globulin (SHBG), and dehydroepiandrosterone-sulfate (DHEA-S) [16].
- Tall stature, increased lean mass, hyperphagia with early onset weight gain: Consider MC4R mutation testing [2].
- History of snoring with frequent awakenings, morning headaches, restless sleep, daytime somnolence: Consider obstructive sleep apnea and obtain polysomnography.
- Poor feeding with failure to thrive in infancy, hypotonia, developmental delays, short stature, dysmorphic features, global cognitive impairment, behavioral abnormalities: Consider Prader-Willi syndrome (PWS) and obtain methylation studies for PWS [1].
- Short stature, round facies, short fourth and fifth metacarpals and metatarsals: Consider pseudohypoparathyroidism and obtain calcium, phosphorus and PTH.

Evaluation for Comorbidities of Obesity

- If the cause of weight gain is unclear, a fasting lipid profile is recommended for all children with BMI >95th percentile.
- Transaminases and fasting blood glucose or hemoglobin A1c are recommended for all children with BMI >95th percentile starting at 10 years of age even in the absence of risk factors [8].

Additional Evaluation

- If concern for Cushing syndrome persists or results of preliminary studies are equivocal, consider dexamethasone suppression test (DST) [11].
- If history of elevated transaminases, abdominal pain, concern for gall stones, obtain abdominal ultrasonography.

Next Steps in Diagnosis and Management

- If there is an underlying cause recognized such as an endocrinologic issue, monogenic/syndromic cause of obesity or hypothalamic obesity, management is directed to the fundamental disease (discussed in separate chapters, respectively). If no underlying endocrinologic/genetic/intracranial/psychological cause is identified, then a staged approach is used as per the American Academy of Pediatrics (AAP) [14].
- After a comprehensive evaluation is complete (as elucidated above), the management is guided by the parameters below. Management is discussed in more detail in Chap. 58.

The following parameters are the primary determinants for the intensity of intervention needed.

1. The BMI and severity of obesity at presentation
2. The associated comorbidities
3. Age of the child
4. Previous lifestyle therapies or failed attempts of weight loss or weight stabilization

The stages of intervention are directed to address intervention and resources based on the severity of the disease. All children start with Stage 1. If weight maintenance and/or BMI improvement cannot be achieved at each level, a higher stage is recommended.

- Stage 1: Prevention plus
- Stage 2: Structured weight management
- Stage 3: Comprehensive multidisciplinary evaluation
- Stage 4: Tertiary care intervention

Stage 1 and 2 can be provided by a primary care physician with some additional help from a registered dietician.

Stage 3 and 4 are therapies delivered in the setting of a multidisciplinary team comprising a pediatric obesity medicine specialist, mental health specialist, a registered dietician, exercise physiologist, or physical therapist and potential collaboration with the metabolic and bariatric surgeon [15].

Bibliography

1. Elena G, Bruna C, Benedetta M, Stefania DC, Giuseppe C. Prader-Willi syndrome: clinical aspects. J Obes. 2012;2012:13.
2. Farooqi IS, Yeo GS, Keogh JM, Aminian S, Jebb SA, Butler G, Cheetham T, O'Rahilly S. Dominant and recessive inheritance of morbid obesity associated with melanocortin 4 receptor deficiency. J Clin Invest. 2000;106(2):271–9.
3. Fernandez JR, Redden DT, Pietrobelli A, Allison DB. Waist circumference percentiles in nationally representative samples of

African-American, European-American, and Mexican-American children and adolescents. J Pediatr. 2004;145:439.
4. Flegal KM, Wei R, Ogden CL, Freedman DS, Johnson CL, Curtin LR. Characterizing extreme values of body mass index-for-age by using the 2000 Centers for Disease Control and Prevention growth charts. Am J Clin Nutr. 2009;90:1314–20.
5. Freedman DS, Sherry B. The validity of BMI as an indicator of body fatness and risk among children. Pediatrics. 2009;124(suppl 1):S23–34.
6. Han JC, Lawlor DA, Kimm SY. Childhood obesity. Lancet. 2010;375(9727):1737–48.
7. Juonala M, Magnussen CG, Berenson GS, Venn A, Burns TL, Sabin MA, Srinivasan SR, Daniels SR, Davis PH, Chen W, Sun C. Childhood adiposity, adult adiposity, and cardiovascular risk factors. N Engl J Med. 2011;365(20):1876–85.
8. Krebs NF, Himes JH, Jacobson D, Nicklas TA, Guilday P, Styne D. Assessment of child and adolescent overweight and obesity. Pediatrics. 2007;120(suppl 4):S193–228.
9. Kuczmarski RJ, Ogden CL, Grummer-Strawn LM, Flegal KM, Guo SS, Wei R, Mei Z, Curtin LR, Roche AF, Johnson CL. CDC growth charts: United States. Adv Data. 2000;(314):1–27.
10. Magiakou MA, Mastorakos G, Oldfield EH, Gomez MT, Doppman JL, Cutler GB Jr, Nieman LK, Chrousos GP. Cushing's syndrome in children and adolescents. Presentation, diagnosis, and therapy. N Engl J Med. 1994;331:629.
11. Nieman LK, Biller BM, Findling JW, Newell-Price J, Savage MO, Stewart PM, Montori VM. The diagnosis of Cushing's syndrome: an Endocrine Society clinical practice guideline. J Clin Endocrinol Metab. 2008;93:1526.
12. Barlow SE. Expert committee. Expert committee recommendations regarding the prevention, assessment, and treatment of child and adolescent overweight and obesity: summary report. Pediatrics. 2007;120(suppl 4):S164–92.
13. Skinner AC, Perrin EM, Skelton JA. Prevalence of obesity and severe obesity in US children, 1999-2014. Obesity (Silver Spring). 2016;24:1116–23.
14. Spear BA, Barlow SE, Ervin C, Ludwig DS, Saelens BE, Schetzina KE, Taveras EM. Recommendations for treatment of child and adolescent overweight and obesity. Pediatrics. 2007;120(Suppl 4):S254.
15. Srivastava G, Fox CK, Kelly AS, Jastreboff AM, Browne AF, Browne NT, Pratt JS, Bolling C, Michalsky MP, Cook S, Lenders CM. Clinical considerations regarding the use of obesity pharmacotherapy in adolescents with obesity. Obesity. 2019;27:1.
16. Witchel SF, Oberfield S, Rosenfield RL, Codner E, Bonny A, Ibáñez L, Pena A, Horikawa R, Gomez-Lobo V, Joel D, Tfayli H. The diagnosis of polycystic ovary syndrome during adolescence. Horm Res Paediatr. 2015;83(6):376–89.

Weight Loss

20

Juanita K. Hodax

Introduction

Weight loss is defined as any decrease in weight over time. In growing children a lack of weight gain, as evidenced by a decrease in weight percentile, can have a similar differential diagnosis as weight loss. Failure to thrive is a term used in infants and toddlers with poor weight gain, and also has a similar differential. The definition of failure to thrive can be variable but is typically described as weight or body mass index below the 5th percentile for age and sex, or a decrease in 2 major percentile lines in weight on the standard growth chart [1–3]. Any weight loss or inappropriate decrease in weight gain, even without meeting the definition of failure to thrive, should lead to additional history and physical examination to elucidate any concern for organic causes.

The majority of patients with weight loss or failure to thrive have non-organic causes of inadequate caloric intake [2]. In infants, this can be due to incorrect mixing of formula, inadequate amounts of formula offered, or insufficient breast milk production. In older children and adolescents, this can be due to an eating disorder, inadequate food sources, or neglect [1]. While non-organic causes may be more common, organic causes of weight loss should be evaluated through additional history, physical exam, and laboratory or imaging evaluation when indicated.

Differential Diagnosis

As unintentional weight loss is uncommon in healthy individuals, any weight loss or poor weight gain in children should be a signal for concern. Weight loss occurs if nutrient intake is insufficient compared to metabolic demands. This can be intentional, e.g., purposeful weight loss in a patient who is overweight, or potentially due to an eating disorder in someone who has body dysphoria and/or is limiting food intake. Decreased intake of nutrients can also occur if someone has decreased appetite, which may be due to psychiatric disease such as depression, neurologic disease affecting appetite, or diseases causing increased thirst, leading to increased water intake and decreased food intake (such as diabetes insipidus). In addition, inadequate food sources can lead to insufficient nutrient intake. Weight loss also occurs if there is decreased absorption of nutrients. This can occur in diabetes mellitus, where there is significant glucosuria and inability to utilize glucose. This can also occur in a variety of gastroenteric diseases, such as celiac disease, causing inflammation in the small intestine and poor absorption of nutrients, or other illnesses causing diarrhea and poor absorption. Lastly, diseases such as hyperthyroidism, congenital cardiac disease, chronic inflammatory disease, or chronic infections can cause increased metabolism and higher nutrient requirements, resulting in weight loss if nutrient intake is not increased.

Weight loss is a very nonspecific finding with an extensive differential diagnosis spanning multiple organ systems. This broad differential diagnosis is listed in Table 20.1.

Endocrine causes of weight loss include hyperthyroidism, adrenal insufficiency, diabetes mellitus, and diabetes insipidus.

Hyperthyroidism, discussed further in Chaps. 25 and 42, often presents with weight loss or failure to gain weight. Hyperthyroidism is most often caused by Graves' disease, which is an autoimmune stimulation of the thyroid gland [4, 5]. Less commonly, hyperthyroidism can be caused by an autonomously functioning thyroid nodule or subacute thyroiditis. Symptoms associated with hyperthyroidism include tremor, palpitations, heat intolerance, frequent stools, and difficulty sleeping. Weight loss is a common finding, found in 64% of patients at presentation in one study [5]. Physical examination reveals a goiter or thyroid nodule, and, in Graves' disease, proptosis is common as well. Linear growth acceleration and advanced bone age can occur in children with hyperthyroidism, and these are uncommon findings in other causes of weight loss [4]. Laboratory evaluation shows

J. K. Hodax (✉)
Pediatric Endocrinology, Seattle Children's Hospital and University of Washington, Seattle, WA, USA
e-mail: Juanita.Hodax@seattlechildrens.org

T. Stanley, M. Misra (eds.), *Endocrine Conditions in Pediatrics*, https://doi.org/10.1007/978-3-030-52215-5_20

Table 20.1 Differential diagnosis for the causes of weight loss

Organ system	Diagnosis	Associated symptoms/signs
Endocrine	Hyperthyroidism Adrenal insufficiency Diabetes mellitus Diabetes insipidus	Tachycardia, heat intolerance, diarrhea, jitteriness, insomnia Hyperpigmentation, fatigue, salt craving, hypotension, morning nausea Polydipsia, polyuria, polyphagia Polydipsia, polyuria
Gastroenteric	Celiac disease Milk protein allergy Inflammatory bowel disease Liver disease Chronic infectious diarrhea	Diarrhea, bloating, decreased growth Blood in stools Blood in stools Jaundice, diarrhea Prolonged diarrhea, fever, blood in stools
Cardiac	Congenital cardiac disease	Tachycardia, tachypnea, murmur, cyanosis
Oncologic	Malignancy	Various symptoms depending on type (mass, easy bruising, pallor, fatigue)
Renal	Chronic kidney disease	Polyuria, edema, elevated blood pressure
Pulmonary	Cystic fibrosis	Respiratory illnesses, steatorrhea
Infectious	HIV Tuberculosis	Immune deficiency, secondary infections Chronic cough, night sweats, fever
Rheumatologic	Chronic inflammatory diseases	Various symptoms depending on type (rash, joint pain)
Neurologic	Increased intracranial pressure due to various causes	Vomiting, decreased appetite, headaches, visual disturbances
Genetic	Various genetic syndromes associated with poor growth	Dysmorphic features, developmental delays
Psychiatric	Eating disorder Depression	Body dysphoria, restricting intake, desire to lose additional weight Depressed mood, flat affect, low motivation, sleep disturbance

suppressed TSH levels and elevated T4 and T3 levels. Additional details on presentation, evaluation, and management of hyperthyroidism are discussed in Chap. 42.

Adrenal insufficiency is also most often autoimmune in nature, with Addison's disease being the most common cause of primary adrenal insufficiency. Weight loss is a classic symptom, reported in 100% of patients [6]. Additional symptoms include fatigue, nausea, and vomiting. Salt craving can also occur due to mineralocorticoid deficiency. Physical exam findings include hyperpigmentation, often most prominent in the palmar creases and gums, caused by extremely elevated levels of ACTH and melanocyte stimulating hormone, which is a component of the prohormone for ACTH. Laboratory evaluation may show hyponatremia, hyperkalemia, hypercalcemia, hypoglycemia, low morning cortisol, and elevated ACTH levels in primary adrenal insufficiency [6]. An ACTH stimulation test can confirm the diagnosis [7]. The causes, diagnosis, and treatment of adrenal insufficiency are further discussed in Chap. 49.

Type 1 diabetes mellitus is the most common type of diabetes in pediatrics, but the incidence of type 2 diabetes in youth is increasing [8]. Both type 1 and type 2 diabetes can present with weight loss. Additional symptoms include polydipsia, polyuria, and polyphagia. A random blood glucose >200 mg/dl in the presence of these symptoms is diagnostic of diabetes mellitus. Hemoglobin A1c and oral glucose tolerance testing can be used for further evaluation if needed. Diagnosis and treatment of type 1 and type 2 diabetes are discussed in Chaps. 52 and 53.

Diabetes insipidus is caused by the inadequate production or action of antidiuretic hormone. Central diabetes insipidus is caused by decreased secretion of antidiuretic hormone by the posterior pituitary gland, and nephrogenic diabetes insipidus is caused by a defect in the vasopressin receptor or downstream actions in the collecting duct of the kidney. Patients with diabetes insipidus are unable to concentrate urine, leading to polyuria, hyperosmolarity, and subsequent polydipsia. Patients with diabetes insipidus typically have a thirst for water, and this may lead to a decreased intake of higher calorie liquids or foods causing weight loss [9]. Weight loss may be exacerbated by acute dehydration. The causes, diagnosis, and initial management of diabetes insipidus are further discussed in Chap. 5.

Important Clarifying Questions in the Medical History

Because the differential diagnosis is broad, a thorough history and physical examination are crucial to narrow the differential. Table 20.2 lists important clarifying questions that can be used for further evaluation of the severity and cause of weight loss. Assessing for the severity of the weight loss is an important step in determining the cause. This may be difficult to assess in pediatric patients who are continuing to grow and may have had weight gain and then weight loss since the last visit. If weight loss is severe and chronic, linear growth may be affected as well, as appropriate weight gain is necessary for continued linear growth. In addition, a thorough

Table 20.2 Important clarifying questions for the patient or caregiver

Purpose	Question
Assess the severity of weight loss	How long has weight loss been occurring? How much weight has been lost? Is linear growth affected?
Nutritional intake evaluation	How many meals and snacks are eaten each day? Is there a routine for meals and snacks? How much liquid is typically consumed in a day? Are there any food restrictions or allergies? Has there been a change in the amount of food or liquid consumed? Has the family struggled to afford food?
Assess for signs of malabsorption or increased metabolic state	Any symptoms of diarrhea, frequent stools, or fat in stools? Any symptoms of polydipsia or polyuria? Any change in activity levels?

review of systems focusing on evaluating for symptoms listed in Table 20.1 can help to narrow the differential diagnosis to the organ system involved.

Important Aspects of the Physical Examination

Because of the broad differential diagnosis associated with weight loss, a complete physical examination is important to evaluate for an organic cause. Various exam findings that may be associated with different causes of weight loss are listed in Table 20.3.

Considerations for Laboratory Evaluation

There is no consensus for a standard laboratory evaluation for all patients with weight loss or failure to thrive. In patients who are substantially underweight, a basic metabolic panel is advisable to assess for electrolyte abnormalities that may accompany undernutrition and may require urgent intervention. The remainder of the laboratory evaluation should be tailored to the additional symptoms and physical exam findings that may indicate a specific diagnosis or organ system involvement (see Table 20.4). If there are no additional findings and nutritional intake is reportedly appropriate by history, or if weight loss does not improve after an increase in nutrition intake, a general laboratory evaluation including complete blood count, electrolytes, liver function tests, thyroid function tests, and celiac screening should be considered [2, 3]. Further evaluation with additional laboratory tests, imaging evaluation, or specialist referral should be considered if abnormalities are found on the initial laboratory evaluation.

While laboratory evaluation is often necessary to evaluate the organic causes of weight loss, many laboratory abnormalities may be present as a result of an eating disorder or other non-organic cause of weight loss. Induced vomiting or laxative use can lead to electrolyte abnormalities including hypokalemia, hypophosphatemia, metabolic alkalosis, or metabolic acidosis [10]. Severe malnutrition can lead to

Table 20.3 Important physical examination findings of various causes of weight loss

Exam location	Exam finding	Potential cause
HEENT	Dysmorphic features Papilledema Proptosis	Genetic syndromes Intracranial mass Graves' disease
Neck	Thyromegaly, thyroid nodule Lymphadenopathy	Hyperthyroidism Malignancy, HIV, tuberculosis
Lungs	Respiratory distress, crackles	Cystic fibrosis, tuberculosis
Cardiovascular	Murmur Tachycardia	Congenital heart disease Hyperthyroidism
Abdomen	Hepatomegaly	Liver disease
Skin	Hyperpigmentation Bruising Pallor Rash	Adrenal insufficiency Malignancy Malignancy Rheumatologic diseases
Extremities	Joint swelling Tremor Edema	Rheumatologic diseases Hyperthyroidism Chronic kidney disease

Table 20.4 Possible elements of laboratory evaluation for weight loss, tailored based on clinical suspicion

Differential diagnosis	Recommended labs
Endocrine	
Hyperthyroidism	TSH and free T4, ± total T3, please see Chap. 25
Adrenal insufficiency	8 am cortisol and ACTH, electrolytes
Diabetes mellitus	Fingerstick or plasma glucose, urine glucose and ketones, HbA1c
Diabetes insipidus	Serum and urine electrolytes and osmolality, please see Chap. 17
Other systemic illness	
Celiac disease	Tissue transglutaminase IgA and total IgA
Liver disease	Comprehensive metabolic panel
Kidney disease	Creatinine, urinalysis
Leukemia	CBC with differential
Infectious	Consider HIV testing, Tuberculosis testing, CBC
Cystic fibrosis	Sweat test
Other systemic	c-reactive protein, ESR, comprehensive metabolic panel

leukopenia, anemia, and renal insufficiency. Endocrine abnormalities, including low thyroxine, low insulin growth factor-1, low gonadotropin and sex hormones, and elevated cortisol, may also occur [10, 11]. Therefore, any laboratory abnormalities must be interpreted in the context of the clinical setting.

Additional Evaluation

The need for further evaluation with imaging should be determined based on the findings of the initial history, physical examination, and laboratory evaluation. Because of the broad differential diagnosis, there is no standard imaging evaluation recommended for the evaluation of weight loss.

Next Steps

Referral to a specialist is not indicated unless initial evaluation suggests an organic cause of weight loss that requires further evaluation by a specialist [2, 3]. Referral to a nutritionist may be beneficial in some patients with non-organic causes of decreased oral intake. In patients with suspected eating disorders, a multidisciplinary approach including therapists and nutritionists is often beneficial, and many specialty centers provide these services in a single setting [10]. Hospitalization is rarely required for weight loss alone but can be considered if the child is severely malnourished or if an observation in a structured feeding environment is needed [2].

References

1. Weiss R, Lustig RH. Obesity, metabolic syndrome, and disorders of energy balance. In: Sperling MA, editor. Pediatric endocrinology. 4th ed. Philadelphia: Elsevier; 2014. p. 956–1014.
2. Homan GJ. Failure to thrive: a practical guide. Am Fam Physician. 2016;94(4):295–9.
3. Larson-Nath C, Biank VF. Clinical review of failure to thrive in pediatric patients. Pediatr Ann. 2016;45(2):e46–9. https://doi.org/10.3928/00904481-20160114-01.
4. Hanley P, Lord K, Bauer AJ. Thyroid disorders in children and adolescents: a review. JAMA Pediatr. 2016;170(10):1008–19. https://doi.org/10.1001/jamapediatrics.2016.0486.
5. Williamson S, Greene SA. Incidence of thyrotoxicosis in childhood: a national population based study in the UK and Ireland. Clin Endocrinol. 2010;72(3):358–63. https://doi.org/10.1111/j.1365-2265.2009.03717.x.
6. Charmandari E, Nicolaides NC, Chrousos GP. Adrenal insufficiency. Lancet. 2014;383(9935):2152–67. https://doi.org/10.1016/S0140-6736(13)61684-0.
7. Bornstein SR, Allolio B, Arlt W, et al. Diagnosis and treatment of primary adrenal insufficiency: an Endocrine Society clinical practice guideline. J Clin Endocrinol Metab. 2016;101(2):364–89. https://doi.org/10.1210/jc.2015-1710.
8. Katsarou A, Gudbjörnsdottir S, Rawshani A, et al. Type 1 diabetes mellitus. Nat Rev Dis Primers. 2017;3:17016. Published 2017 Mar 30. https://doi.org/10.1038/nrdp.2017.16.
9. Jain V, Ravindranath A. Diabetes insipidus in children. J Pediatr Endocrinol Metab. 2016;29(1):39–45. https://doi.org/10.1515/jpem-2014-0518.
10. Campbell K, Peebles R. Eating disorders in children and adolescents: state of the art review. Pediatrics. 2014;134(3):582–92. https://doi.org/10.1542/peds.2014-0194.
11. Schorr M, Miller KK. The endocrine manifestations of anorexia nervosa: mechanisms and management. Nat Rev Endocrinol. 2017;13(3):174–86. https://doi.org/10.1038/nrendo.2016.175.

21 Fatigue or Weakness

Takara Stanley

General Approach to Fatigue or Weakness

Fatigue is one of the most common symptomatic complaints in the pediatric age group, particularly among adolescents. Thirty percent of adolescent girls report morning fatigue more than once per week [1], and 20.5% of girls and 6.5% of boys meet the criteria for severe fatigue [2]. Most complaints of fatigue are related to inadequate sleep and/or excessive stress, and roughly 50% of children and adolescents will have improvement within 6 months [3]. Fatigue may also signal underlying systemic illness or endocrine disease, however, such that a careful history, physical examination, and, in some cases, additional evaluation are warranted. Table 21.1 shows the broad differential diagnosis of fatigue. Complaints of weakness often accompany complaints of fatigue [4], and the differential diagnosis is similar. Objective findings of significant muscle weakness on physical exam, however, should broaden the differential to include neurological and neuromuscular diseases that are beyond the scope of this chapter.

Table 21.1 Differential diagnosis of fatigue and/or weakness

Endocrine
Hypothyroidism
Hyperthyroidism
Adrenal insufficiency
Chronic hyperglycemia (undiagnosed diabetes mellitus)
Hypercalcemia
Gastrointestinal
Celiac disease
Inflammatory bowel disease
Hepatitis
Parasitic infection
Infectious
Endocarditis
Tuberculosis
Human immunodeficiency virus infection
Mononucleosis
Cytomegalovirus
Other systemic causes
Pregnancy
Rheumatologic disease
Autoimmune disease (systemic lupus erythematosus, multiple sclerosis)
Obstructive sleep apnea or central sleep apnea
Cardiac or pulmonary disease
Chronic kidney disease
Anemia and/or iron deficiency
Post-concussive syndrome/traumatic brain injury
History of CNS surgery and/or radiotherapy
Ehlers-Danlos syndrome
Familial Mediterranean fever or periodic fever, aphthous stomatitis, pharyngitis, and adenitis (PFAPA)
Psychiatric
Disordered eating and/or anorexia nervosa
Depression or bipolar disorder
Anxiety
Trauma and/or post-traumatic stress disorder
Medications/substances
Antihistamines
Antidepressants
Sedatives, opioids, muscle relaxants
Antihypertensives
Chronic alcohol use
Substance abuse

Abbreviations: *CNS* central nervous system

The first step in the evaluation of fatigue and/or weakness is careful history and physical examination. Although most complaints of fatigue are due to "physiologic fatigue," resulting from inadequate sleep, stress, and physical and/or mental overexertion, any red flags on history and physical examination, as well as persistence of fatigue that limits participation

T. Stanley (✉)
Division of Pediatric Endocrinology, Massachusetts General Hospital and Harvard Medical School, Boston, MA, USA
e-mail: tstanley@mgh.harvard.edu

T. Stanley, M. Misra (eds.), *Endocrine Conditions in Pediatrics*, https://doi.org/10.1007/978-3-030-52215-5_21

in daily activities and/or results in repeated school absences should prompt further evaluation.

There are limited data in the pediatric population regarding the outcomes of children presenting with fatigue and/or weakness. In a systematic review of outcomes of evaluations for "tiredness" in primary care, presumably based on adult patients, depression was found in a high percentage of patients, whereas a significant underlying medical condition was found in 4.3% of cases [5]. The most commonly diagnosed medical diseases were diabetes, hypothyroidism, and anemia [5]. Chronic fatigue syndrome (CFS), also known as myalgic encephalitis (ME), is defined as disabling fatigue that persists for 6 months or longer [6]. CFS/ME has an estimated prevalence of 0.1–2% in secondary school children and is a diagnosis of exclusion [6]. Pediatric CFS/ME is beyond the scope of this chapter; readers are referred to recent reviews on the topic [6, 7].

Important Clarifying Questions in the Medical History

Careful review of sleeping habits, nutrition, and exercise are critical to identify lifestyle factors that may be contributing to fatigue. Children and adolescents generally need more sleep than adults: the American Academy of Sleep Medicine statement, endorsed by the American Academy of Pediatrics, recommends that children 3–5 yo should sleep 10–13 hours per 24-hour period, children 6–12 yo should sleep 9–12 hours, and children 13–18 yo should sleep 8–10 hours [8]. In addition to sleep duration, quality of sleep should be assessed, with questions about difficulty getting to sleep, frequent awakening, and parental observations of snoring, as well as questions addressing sleep hygiene, including screen time before bed.

Depression and anxiety are strongly associated with fatigue in the pediatric population [2]. Depression screening and careful interviewing regarding anxiety symptoms, life stressors, and adverse experiences are warranted. Relationships with friends and family, as well as romantic or sexual relationships when applicable, should also be explored.

Severity of fatigue is assessed by asking if the patient has missed school and/or abstained from any activities they used to enjoy because of the symptom. Changes in school performance should also be queried. Since many non-specific physical symptoms may accompany fatigue, it is helpful to ask patients to list other symptoms in the order of severity. Symptoms that may be associated with endocrine causes of fatigue are listed in Table 21.2.

Table 21.2 Signs, symptoms, and laboratory findings of endocrine causes of fatigue

Hypothyroidism	*Symptoms:* cold intolerance, constipation, hair loss, decreased appetite, exercise intolerance, oligo/amenorrhea *Signs:* decreased growth in height; dry, coarse skin; delayed relaxation phase of deep tendon reflexes; loss of outer part of eyebrows; "puffiness"; and/or delayed puberty, myxedema and bradycardia in severe cases; absence of goiter does not exclude diagnosis *Labs:* Primary hypothyroidism: Elevated TSH >10 μU/mL ± frankly low free T4, positive thyroid peroxidase antibodies; central hypothyroidism: normal, slightly high, or low TSH with low free T4 *See also:* Chaps. 25 and 41
Hyperthyroidism	*Symptoms:* heat intolerance, frequent bowel movements, increased appetite, exercise intolerance, dizziness, palpitations, anxiety, inability to concentrate, oligo/amenorrhea *Signs:* increased growth velocity; weight loss; tachycardia; hypertension; "thyroid stare"; lid lag; ± proptosis; moist, velvety skin; extremity tremor; tongue fasciculations; bounding pulse and/or hyperdynamic precordium; brisk reflexes; goiter typically present ± audible bruit; absence of goiter does not exclude diagnosis *Labs:* Suppressed TSH < 0.1 μU/mL, elevated free T4 and total T3; positive thyroid-stimulating immunoglobulins and/or TSH receptor-binding antibodies; ± positive thyroid peroxidase antibodies *See also:* Chaps. 25 and 42
Adrenal insufficiency	*Symptoms:* decreased appetite, lethargy, dizziness, weakness, nausea and/or vomiting, "fogginess"/inability to concentrate, salt craving (if primary) *Signs:* hyperpigmentation and/or axillary freckling (if primary); hypotension; weight loss; ± decreased growth velocity; dry mucous membranes; reduced skin turgor *Labs:* hyponatremia and hyperkalemia (if primary), hypoglycemia, morning (8 AM) cortisol usually <5 mcg/dL (morning cortisol 5–10 mcg/dL does not exclude diagnosis), elevated ACTH (if primary), usually need ACTH stimulation test to confirm diagnosis *See also:* Chaps. 29 and 49
Chronic hyperglycemia (undiagnosed diabetes mellitus)	*Symptoms:* polyuria, polydipsia, polyphagia, weakness *Signs:* weight loss, acanthosis nigricans (suggests type 2 diabetes) *Labs:* glucosuria ± ketonuria; random glucose ≥200 mg/dL and/or fasting glucose ≥126 mg/dL; HbA1c ≥ 6.5% *See also:* Chaps. 9, 30, 52, and 53

Table 21.2 (continued)

Hypercalcemia	*Symptoms:* bone pain, depression and/or malaise, abdominal pain, constipation, excessive thirst, muscle weakness, lethargy and "fogginess," anxiety *Signs:* often asymptomatic, but may present with dehydration and/or altered mental status *Labs:* Serum calcium above the upper limit of normal for the lab (usually >10–11 mg/dL); subsequent studies should include PTH, 25-hydroxyvitamin D, phosphate and magnesium *See also:* Chap. 6
Cushing syndrome	*Symptoms:* weakness, especially in proximal muscle groups; easy bruising; menstrual irregularities *Signs:* hypertension; decreased growth in height; refractory weight gain; hirsutism; acne; thick purplish striae; "moon facies"; dorsocervical fat pad; increased supraclavicular fat; central adiposity with relatively thinner extremities; difficulty standing from squatting position *Labs:* two of the following: (i) late night salivary cortisol (ii) 24-hour urine free cortisol >2 times upper limit of normal on ≥2 collections, or (iii) non-suppressed 8 AM cortisol (>1.8 mcg/dl) following a 1 mg dexamethasone dose at 11 PM the previous night; hyperglycemia; possible hypernatremia and/or hypokalemia from cortisol acting on mineralocorticoid receptors *See also:* Chaps. 29 and 50

Abbreviations: *ACTH* adrenocortocotropic hormone, *HbA1c* hemoglobin A1c, *PTH* parathyroid hormone, *T3* triiodothyronine, *T4* thyroxine, *TSH* thyroid-stimulating hormone

Several prescribed and over-the-counter medications can cause fatigue (Table 21.1), as can alcohol and substance abuse, necessitating thorough medication and substance use histories. Given the breadth of the differential diagnosis, a thorough family history and review of systems are also warranted to guide further evaluation.

Important Aspects of the Physical Examination

Complete physical examination (with vital signs) should be performed with particular attention to the relevant aspects discussed below. Orthostatic vital signs are also helpful if there are accompanying complaints of dizziness. Signs that may be associated with elements in the endocrine differential diagnosis of fatigue and/or weakness are listed in Table 21.2.

Review of growth charts: Decreased growth velocity in height and/or weight loss or failure to gain weight should increase suspicion for an underlying disease. Significant weight gain, particularly in the context of slowed growth in height that is not attributable to the completion of puberty, raises the possibility of Cushing syndrome, although this condition is rare.

Skin examination should include assessment of possible hyperpigmentation and/or axillary freckling, pallor, bruising, texture (coarse or soft), whether the skin is dry or moist, and whether skin turgor is normal. Hyperpigmentation may be most visible in palmar creases and/or on the gums. Thick purplish striae should raise suspicion of Cushing syndrome, whereas thin, pale striae are normal findings in adolescents. Any rashes that may indicate a rheumatological process should also be noted.

Visual field and fundoscopic examination should be performed to assess for possible visual field deficits and/or papilledema that may occur with CNS pathology.

Musculoskeletal examination should include particular focus on any joint findings that may indicate rheumatologic disease. Additionally, strength should be carefully assessed. Optimal technique for assessing extremity strength is shown in the *Reference Box*. Muscle tenderness should also be assessed.

Deep tendon reflexes should be elicited at the biceps, triceps, brachioradialis, patellar, and Achilles tendons.

Lymphatic examination should assess for lymph node enlargement that may suggest an oncologic or infectious process.

Reference Box: Assessing Strength on Physical Examination

- Muscle strength is rated as follows
  - 0: paralysis
  - 1: muscle contraction but no movement
  - 2: movement with gravity eliminated, but not against gravity
  - 3: movement against gravity, but not against resistance
  - 4: partial movement against resistance
  - 5: full movement against resistance
- *Full examination of extremity strength with the examiner providing resistance includes*
  - *Shoulder*: abduction (raise arms to shoulder level and resist downward pressure)
  - *Upper arms*: flexion (bend arms and resist pressure to extend) and extension (bend arms and resist pressure to flex further)
  - *Wrist*: flexion (bend wrist and resist pressure to extend) and extension (keep wrist "straight" and resist pressure to flex)
  - *Fingers*: flexion (squeeze examiner's fingers), extension (hold fingers straight and resist down-

ward pressure), and abduction (spread the fingers and resist pressure pushing them together)
- *Hip:* (supine position required) flexion (hold straight leg up and resist downward pressure) and extension (keep leg on bed/table and resist upward pressure); abduction (abduct at hip and resist inward pressure) and adduction (resist outward pressure to abduct leg at hip)
- *Knee:* flexion (bend at knee and resist upward pressure against calf) and extension (bend slightly at knee and resist downward pressure against shin)
- *Ankle:* plantar flexion (resist downward pressure against dorsum of feet) and dorsiflexion (resist upward pressure against soles of feet); eversion (resist pressure against lateral foot) and inversion (resist pressure against medial foot).

Considerations for Laboratory Evaluation

In the absence of an obvious cause for persistent fatigue or weakness, a general initial laboratory evaluation may be warranted to "cast a wide net" for possible underlying causes. A recommended initial laboratory evaluation is shown in Table 21.3, with further recommended evaluation based on signs, symptoms, or initial laboratory findings shown in Table 21.4.

Table 21.3 Recommended initial evaluation for significant fatigue and/or weakness

Test	Associated conditions
Complete blood count with differential	Hematologic or oncologic disease; IBD (anemia and elevated PLT)
Comprehensive metabolic panel	Liver disease, kidney disease, hypercalcemia
TSH and free T4	Thyroid disease
HbA1c and/or fasting glucose	Diabetes mellitus
Erythrocyte sedimentation rate and c-reactive protein	General systemic disease, rheumatologic disease, chronic infection
Tissue transglutaminase IgA and total IgA	Celiac disease
Urinalysis	Diabetes mellitus, renal disease
Iron studies	Iron deficiency

Abbreviations: *HbA1c* hemoglobin A1c, *IBD* inflammatory bowel disease, *PLT* platelets, *T4* thyroxine, *TSH* thyroid-stimulating hormone

Table 21.4 Additional evaluation based on symptoms and signs

Signs/symptoms	Recommended additional testing
Weight loss or lack of weight gain, hyperpigmentation, family history of autoimmune disease	Early morning (8 AM) cortisol; endocrine referral for ACTH stimulation testing if (i) morning cortisol <10 mcg/dL and high suspicion of adrenal insufficiency, or (ii) morning cortisol <5 mcg/dL even with low/moderate suspicion of adrenal insufficiency
Weight gain, decreased growth (before the end of puberty), hirsutism, acne, reduced strength, wide purple striae	Late-night salivary cortisol sampling × 2–3 samples on separate nights, or 24-hour urine free cortisol collection × 2–3 samples on separate occasions, or overnight low-dose dexamethasone suppression test
Snoring and/or obesity or tonsillar hypertrophy	Polysomnography
Fever, weight loss, night sweats	Consider TB screening, HIV test, ECHO for endocarditis, testing for other chronic infections
Sore throat, pharyngitis, lymphadenopathy	Consider testing for mononucleosis or cytomegalovirus
Amenorrhea/irregular menses	Pregnancy testing; assess for functional hypothalamic amenorrhea, and other causes of menstrual irregularity
Myalgia, muscle weakness, or muscle tenderness	Creatine Kinase
Objectively decreased strength or abnormal reflexes	Neurology referral

Next Steps in Diagnosis and Management

Any laboratory abnormalities should guide further referral. Children with normal laboratory evaluation for whom no underlying cause of fatigue or weakness is found should be followed relatively frequently in the primary care setting to assess the evolution of signs and symptoms. Children with severe or chronic fatigue with normal laboratory evaluation may warrant referral to counseling, psychiatry, and/or sleep medicine. Children with weight loss and normal laboratory findings should be referred to gastroenterology or, if disordered eating is suspected, psychiatry or adolescent medicine.

References

1. Ghandour RM, Overpeck MD, Huang ZJ, Kogan MD, Scheidt PC. Headache, stomachache, backache, and morning fatigue among adolescent girls in the United States: associations with behavioral, sociodemographic, and environmental factors. Arch Pediatr Adolesc Med. 2004;158(8):797–803.

2. ter Wolbeek M, van Doornen LJ, Kavelaars A, Heijnen CJ. Severe fatigue in adolescents: a common phenomenon? Pediatrics. 2006;117(6):e1078–86.
3. Bakker RJ, van de Putte EM, Kuis W, Sinnema G. Risk factors for persistent fatigue with significant school absence in children and adolescents. Pediatrics. 2009;124(1):e89–95.
4. van de Putte EM, Engelbert RH, Kuis W, Kimpen JL, Uiterwaal CS. How fatigue is related to other somatic symptoms. Arch Dis Child. 2006;91(10):824–7.
5. Stadje R, Dornieden K, Baum E, Becker A, Biroga T, Bosner S, et al. The differential diagnosis of tiredness: a systematic review. BMC Fam Pract. 2016;17(1):147.
6. Brigden A, Loades M, Abbott A, Bond-Kendall J, Crawley E. Practical management of chronic fatigue syndrome or myalgic encephalomyelitis in childhood. Arch Dis Child. 2017;102(10):981–6.
7. Rowe PC, Underhill RA, Friedman KJ, Gurwitt A, Medow MS, Schwartz MS, et al. Myalgic encephalomyelitis/chronic fatigue syndrome diagnosis and management in young people: a primer. Front Pediatr. 2017;5:121.
8. Paruthi S, Brooks LJ, D'Ambrosio C, Hall WA, Kotagal S, Lloyd RM, et al. Recommended amount of sleep for pediatric populations: a consensus statement of the American Academy of Sleep Medicine. J Clin Sleep Med. 2016;12(6):785–6.

Dizziness or "Spells": An Endocrine Approach

22

Takara Stanley

Dizzinesss

What Is Dizziness?

The first priority in addressing complaints of dizziness is to establish what the patient is actually experiencing. The term "dizziness" is often used synonymously with lightheadedness, or the sensation of being about to faint, with or without visual changes. However, patients may also be using "dizziness" to refer to any of the following: *oscillopsia*, the sensation that stationary objects are moving; *vertigo*, a sense of spinning of either the surroundings or the individual, while the other remains stationary; *disequilibrium*, a loss of balance or coordination; *confusion* or *disorientation*; or *generalized weakness* [1, 2].

In patients who refer to vertigo or oscillopsia, issues with the peripheral or central vestibular systems should be investigated – these issues are beyond the scope of this chapter, and the reader is referred to other reviews on the topic [1]. Neurologic causes should also be sought for patients complaining of disequilibrium, although disequilibrium may also be a symptom of some of the entities discussed further below. This chapter primarily deals with lightheadedness, or the sensation of fainting, that is, pre-syncope or near-syncope.

Navigating the Differential Diagnosis

Dizziness and balance problems are present in roughly 5% of children aged 3–17 years, with a higher prevalence among adolescents than younger children [3]. The differential diagnosis of dizziness is shown in Table 22.1. A cross-sectional study of several thousand emergency department visits by those 16 years or older for dizziness found the following prevalence of varying etiologies: otologic/vestibular (32.9%), cardiovascular (11.5%), neurologic (11.2%), metabolic (11%), injury/poisoning (10.6%), psychiatric (7.2%), digestive (7.0%), genitourinary (5.1%), and infectious (2.9%) [4].

A thorough history, including the use of medications, substance use, and trauma or fall history, and a thorough physical examination including orthostatic testing and full neurological examination are warranted for patients presenting with dizziness. Highly pertinent aspects of the history include the following [5]:

- Whether dizziness is persistent or episodic
- If episodic, triggers and duration of episodes
- Whether onset was sudden or gradual
- Associated otologic symptoms such as aural fullness, hearing loss, or tinnitus
- Associated systemic symptoms such as fatigue, nausea, vomiting, diaphoresis
- History of falls, head injury, traumatic brain injury
- History of medication use, substance use, any potential poison exposure

Causes of dizziness are often separated into "central" and "peripheral" causes [5]. Dizziness from CNS pathology (i.e., central) is more likely to be gradual in onset, and persistent rather than episodic. It is likely to present with other neurological symptoms, but rarely other systemic symptoms such as nausea, vomiting, or diaphoresis. Nystagmus may be present, is not fatigable, and does not decrease with visual fixation [5]. Peripheral causes of dizziness (e.g., peripheral vestibular etiology or other etiology) are more likely to have sudden onset and be episodic in nature, with associated systemic symptoms such as nausea, vomiting, and diaphoresis, and also associated auditory symptoms such as hearing loss, tinnitus, and aural fullness [5]. Nystagmus may be present with peripheral vestibular causes but is generally fatigable and decreases with visual fixation [5].

T. Stanley (✉)
Division of Pediatric Endocrinology, Massachusetts General Hospital and Harvard Medical School, Boston, MA, USA
e-mail: tstanley@mgh.harvard.edu

T. Stanley, M. Misra (eds.), *Endocrine Conditions in Pediatrics*, https://doi.org/10.1007/978-3-030-52215-5_22

Clinical Key
Dizziness that is insidious in onset and persistent is more likely to be associated with a CNS etiology, whereas episodic dizziness with systemic symptoms such as nausea, vomiting, and diaphoresis is more likely to be associated with a peripheral etiology.

Patients with apparent central causes of persistent dizziness or vertigo should be referred to neurology. In those with peripheral causes, directed history, otoscopic examination, and positional testing should be performed to evaluate for possible vestibular or otologic causes. Dizziness on lying down suggests benign paroxysmal positional vertigo [2]. In patients who do not appear to have vestibular or otologic etiology, cardiovascular, endocrine, and other causes should be considered as shown in Table 22.1. Postural dizziness, particularly in the morning, should raise concern for adrenal insufficiency, especially if weight loss is also present.

Table 22.1 Differential diagnosis of dizziness

Neurological
Vasovagal
Migraine
Concussion or traumatic brain injury
Postural tachycardia syndrome (POTS)
Multiple sclerosis
CNS lesion or cerebellar disease
Cerebral ischemia and/or cerebrovascular accident
Cervical disorders
Meningitis or encephalitis
Otologic/vestibular
Benign paroxysmal vertigo
Motion sickness
Otitis media or middle ear effusion
Vestibular neuritis
Cardiovascular
Arrhythmia
Orthostatic hypotension
Cardiomyopathy
Endocrine/metabolic
Hyperthyroidism
Hypothyroidism
Hypercalcemia
Hypocalcemia
Hypoglycemia
Adrenal insufficiency
Other
Anemia
Dehydration
Heat stroke
Intoxication or poisoning
Hyperventilation
Medications (beta-blockers, quinolones, neuroleptics, sedatives, anticonvulsants, aminoglycosides, alkylating agents, cyclophosphamide, aspirin, NSAIDS, loop diuretics [5])
Psychogenic, including anxiety, depression
Pregnancy

Table 22.2 Elements of the initial evaluation of dizziness

Test	Comments
TSH and free T4	See Chap. 25 for comprehensive thyroid testing
Calcium	Ensure albumin is normal for interpretation
Glucose	Consider giving patient glucose meter
8 AM cortisol	See Chap. 29 for interpretation and further testing
CBC	Assess for anemia
ECG	Assess for arrhythmia
Pregnancy test	Post-menarchal females
Toxicology screening	Suspected drug abuse or poisoning

Abbreviations: *CBC* complete blood count, *ECG* electrocardiogram, *T4* thyroxine, *TSH* thyroid-stimulating hormone

Laboratory Testing and Additional Evaluation

In patients with a possible endocrine etiology for dizziness, an initial laboratory evaluation should include morning (8 AM) cortisol along with the measurement of serum calcium, thyroid-stimulating hormone (TSH), and free thyroxine (free T4). Glucose may also be measured, but, if hypoglycemia is suspected, it is advisable to provide the patient with a glucose meter to carry with them and use at the time of symptoms (please see Chap. 8). A comprehensive initial approach, including the evaluation of endocrine and non-endocrine causes, is shown in Table 22.2.

Spells

What Constitutes a Spell?

Patients may use the terms "spell" or "episode" to connote a cluster of any of the following symptoms: dizziness, syncope, chest pain, palpitations, headache, nausea, abdominal pain, diarrhea, diaphoresis, flushing, pallor, tremulousness, or shortness of breath. The differential diagnosis of "spells" is broad and includes psychogenic causes as well as underlying endocrine disorders such as pheochromocytoma. Very careful attention to the specific nature and timing of symptoms, as well as precipitating factors and temporal relationship to food intake, hydration, exercise, and emotional or physical stressors will guide further evaluation.

Table 22.3 Characteristic signs and symptoms of different etiologies of spells

	Panic attack	Hypoglycemic episode	Pheochromocytoma	Carcinoid syndrome	Mastocytosis
Anxiety	++	++	++		
Altered mental status		++			
Dizziness	++	++			
Hypotension				+	++
Hypertension	+	+	++		
Chest pain	++				
Palpitations and/or tachycardia	++	+	++	+	
Shortness of breath	++			++	
Headache	+	+	++		
Nausea	++	++	+		++
Abdominal pain	++		++	++	++
Diarrhea				++	++
Diaphoresis	++	++	++		
Flushing			+	++	++
Pallor		++	++		
Pruritus					++
Paresthesias	++	++			
Tremulousness	++	++			

Although psychogenic causes of spells, including panic attacks, are likely the most common etiology, care should be taken to consider possible underlying medical conditions as shown in Table 22.3. Hypoglycemia is relatively common and may cause spell-like episodes, and rare but serious conditions including pheochromocytoma, carcinoid syndrome, and mastocytosis should also be considered. Seizures should be considered, particularly in the presence of post-ictal symptoms after the episode.

Key Clarifying Questions on History and Physical Examination

Critical phenotypic descriptors of spells include the following:

- Sequence of symptoms
- Precipitating and alleviating factors
- Timing, frequency, and duration
- Status after the spell
- Any atypical features

Careful attention to whether the spells are associated with pallor or flushing is highly relevant. Pheochromocytoma usually presents with pallor, although it can also present with flushing, whereas carcinoid syndrome and mastocytosis usually present with flushing. Additionally, "wet" flushing should be differentiated from "dry" flushing (see Clinical Key).

Clinical Key: Wet Flushing Versus Dry Flushing [6]

Wet flushing	Dry flushing
Definition: flushing accompanied by sweating Mechanism: neurogenic (sympathetic cholinergic neurons) Causes: pheochromocytoma, blushing, hot flashes	Definition: flushing with dry skin/no sweating Mechanism: vasoactive compounds (histamine, kinins, prostaglandins) Causes: mast cell activation, carcinoid syndrome

Outside the context of an active episode, physical examination may be relatively unrevealing. Hypertension is likely to be present in patients with pheochromocytoma. Careful palpation for abdominal masses should be performed, as well as careful skin examination to look for lesions associated with mastocytosis.

Hypoglycemia

A diagnosis of hypoglycemia requires fulfillment of Whipple's Triad: (1) symptoms of hypoglycemia along with (2) a low measured blood glucose level, (3) with the resolution of symptoms after glucose ingestion. Hypoglycemic events in children and adolescents often occur in the morning after an overnight fast, or after a period of several hours without eating. "Reactive hypoglycemia" is a controversial entity outside the context of dumping syndrome following GI surgery, but children may present with symptoms several hours after a high-carbohydrate meal. The etiology and management of hypoglycemia are discussed in Chaps. 8, 31, and 51. In the adolescent age group, less common causes of hypoglycemia should also be considered, including early Type 1 diabetes, in which beta cell dysregulation can lead to excessive insulin release; antibodies to insulin or insulin receptor; and factitious hypoglycemia from surreptitious use of insulin or oral anti-diabetic medications. Liver failure, adrenal insufficiency, and alcohol intoxication are important causes of hypoglycemia. Insulinoma may occur but is very rare in the pediatric age group.

Careful history is a critical element of the diagnosis of hypoglycemia, whereas no findings are expected on physical examination unless the patient is acutely hypoglycemic at the time of exam. Provision of a glucose meter for testing during episodes is helpful if confirmation of Whipple's triad is required. For patients with confirmed hypoglycemia, referral to endocrinology is appropriate for further diagnostic evaluation (see Chap. 31).

Pheochromocytoma/Paraganglioma

Pheochromocytoma and paraganglioma are neuroendocrine tumors arising from chromaffin cells in the adrenal gland (pheochromocytoma) or elsewhere (paraganglioma) that secrete catecholamines. Although quite rare in the pediatric age group, pheochromocytoma/paraganglioma should be considered in patients with hypertension who also complain of spells. The classic "5 P's" of pheochromocytoma are pallor, perspiration, pressure (hypertension), palpitations, and pain (abdominal and/or headache). In children, hypertension is more commonly chronic than paroxysmal in pheochromocytoma [7]; episodes with a triad of headache, sweating, and tachycardia in the context of underlying hypertension should also prompt suspicion of pheochromocytoma/paraganglioma [8].

Again, a thorough understanding of the episodic symptoms is critical to achieving the diagnosis. Most episodes are <1 hour in duration [8], with signs and symptoms as shown in Table 22.3. Examination is likely to show hypertension, and careful palpation of the abdomen should be performed to assess for possible mass. Other examination findings are not likely outside the context of an episode.

Testing for pheochromocytoma/paraganglioma begins with sending plasma-free metanephrines or 24-hour urine fractionated metanephrines (see Chap. 34). These first-line screening tests are highly sensitive. Positive testing should prompt urgent endocrine referral.

Carcinoid Syndrome

Carcinoid tumors are malignant neuroendocrine tumors, some of which overproduce serotonin, histamine, dopamine, and prostaglandins, leading to carcinoid syndrome. Carcinoid syndrome is characterized by episodes of flushing, diarrhea, abdominal pain, edema, and bronchospasm. In the pediatric age group, carcinoid tumors are rare, and most carcinoid tumors do not present with carcinoid syndrome [9, 10]. Carcinoid tumors typically arise from the bronchial tree or the gastrointestinal tract. In children, appendiceal carcinoid tumors are by far the most common, followed by bronchial tumors [10]. Carcinoid tumors are the most common bronchial tumor in children and are often initially mistaken for asthma [9, 11].

Children with bronchial carcinoid may have wheezing, shortness of breath, or hemoptysis. Otherwise, examination is likely to be benign, and detailed history of the episodes is required to raise suspicion. Testing for carcinoid is through measurement of 24-hour urine 5-hydroxyindoleacetic acid (5-HIAA). Elevated 5-HIAA in the context of symptoms suggestive of carcinoid syndrome should prompt referral to oncology.

Mastocytosis

Mastocytosis is characterized by pathologic clonal proliferation of mast cells. Cutaneous mastocytosis is the most common form, particularly in the pediatric age group, and is characterized by a variety of possible skin lesions including urticaria pigmentosa; large, elevated, yellowish, or skin-colored lesions; purpuric flat macules or patches; brown macules or patches; or nodular lesions [12]. Systemic mastocytosis is a more diffuse form of the disease, in which mast cell release of histamine and prostaglandins can cause the systemic symptoms listed in Table 22.3. Although systematic mastocytosis appears uncommon in the pediatric age group, its prevalence may be underestimated [13]. Additionally, cutaneous mastocytosis in children may be associated with the same symptoms found in systemic mastocytosis.

Lesions on skin examination along with the episodic symptoms characteristic of mastocytosis should raise suspicion for the disease. Dermatographism may also be present. Mastocytosis is a clinical diagnosis, and standard laboratory testing is generally unhelpful, although serum tryptase may be used to estimate mast cell burden [13]. Suspicion of mastocytosis should prompt referral to an allergist or dermatologist.

References

1. Sorathia S, Agrawal Y, Schubert MC. Dizziness and the otolaryngology point of view. Med Clin North Am. 2018;102(6):1001–12.
2. Whitman GT. Dizziness. Am J Med. 2018;131(12):1431–7.
3. Li CM, Hoffman HJ, Ward BK, Cohen HS, Rine RM. Epidemiology of dizziness and balance problems in children in the United States: a population-based study. J Pediatr. 2016;171:240–7 e1-3.
4. Newman-Toker DE, Hsieh YH, Camargo CA Jr, Pelletier AJ, Butchy GT, Edlow JA. Spectrum of dizziness visits to US emergency departments: cross-sectional analysis from a nationally representative sample. Mayo Clin Proc. 2008;83(7):765–75.
5. Kutz JW Jr. The dizzy patient. Med Clin North Am. 2010;94(5):989–1002.
6. Young WF Jr, Maddox DE. Spells: in search of a cause. Mayo Clin Proc. 1995;70(8):757–65.
7. Lenders JW, Eisenhofer G, Mannelli M, Pacak K. Phaeochromocytoma. Lancet. 2005;366(9486):665–75.
8. Reisch N, Peczkowska M, Januszewicz A, Neumann HP. Pheochromocytoma: presentation, diagnosis and treatment. J Hypertens. 2006;24(12):2331–9.
9. Cogen JD, Swanson J, Ong T. Endobronchial carcinoid and concurrent carcinoid syndrome in an adolescent female. Case Rep Pediatr. 2016;2016:2074970.
10. Degnan AJ, Tocchio S, Kurtom W, Tadros SS. Pediatric neuroendocrine carcinoid tumors: management, pathology, and imaging findings in a pediatric referral center. Pediatr Blood Cancer. 2017;64(9):e26477.
11. Rizzardi G, Marulli G, Calabrese F, Rugge M, Rebusso A, Sartori F, et al. Bronchial carcinoid tumours in children: surgical treatment and outcome in a single institution. Eur J Pediatr Surg. 2009;19(4):228–31.
12. Matito A, Carter M. Cutaneous and systemic mastocytosis in children: a risk factor for anaphylaxis? Curr Allergy Asthma Rep. 2015;15(5):22.
13. Torrelo A, Alvarez-Twose I, Escribano L. Childhood mastocytosis. Curr Opin Pediatr. 2012;24(4):480–6.

Excessive Sweating and Heat Intolerance

23

Madhusmita Misra

Definition

Excessive Sweating The medical term for excessive sweating is hyperhidrosis. This refers to sweating that is more than what one would expect for the ambient temperature, and more than is required for thermoregulation. It is seen in 1–3% of the population. Hyperhidrosis may impact the entire body (generalized, 10%), or only certain areas (localized or focal, 90%), such as the axillae (underarms), soles, palms, forehead, or groin, in that order of prevalence [1, 2]. If hyperhidrosis exceeds an area of 100 cm^2, it is considered generalized [1]. Focal hyperhidrosis is also called primary or idiopathic hyperhidrosis and is usually symmetrical. In general, hyperhidrosis occurs as a consequence of increased activation of the sympathetic nervous system. It may be precipitated by the intake of coffee, tea, cola drinks, chocolate, and spices. Medications such as antidepressants, acetaminophen, aspirin, and insulin, alcohol (and alcohol withdrawal), and drugs such as opiates and cocaine may also precipitate hyperhidrosis. The differential diagnosis of excessive sweating is shown in Table 23.1 [3].

Heat Intolerance This condition refers to a greater perception of and inability to tolerate (higher) temperatures that are well tolerated by others in the same environment. Hyperthyroidism is a well-known endocrine cause of heat intolerance. Other causes include anxiety, the use of medications for allergies and hypertension, amphetamines, caffeine, and multiple sclerosis. While heat intolerance may cause increased sweating, not all patients with hyperhidrosis have heat intolerance.

Confirmation and Quantification of Hyperhidrosis Usually, the diagnosis is evident on history and examination and additional testing is not necessary to confirm increased sweating. However, when this is not clear, the following measures have been described to quantify hyperhidrosis [2]:

1. *Physical examination and visualization*
   (a) Axillary: Sweat stain with a diameter of <5 cm is considered normal; between 5 and 10 cm is considered mild hyperhidrosis, 10–20 cm moderate hyperhidrosis and stains >20 cm reaching the waistline may occur with severe hyperhidrosis.
   (b) Palmar: Moist palmar surface without visible droplets of sweat is considered mild, sweating extending to the fingertips is considered moderate, and sweat dripping off the palm and reaching all fingertips is described as severe hyperhidrosis.
2. *Starch iodine test*: An iodine solution is applied to the area of hyperhidrosis and starch is then sprinkled over this area. Areas of excessive sweat are characterized by the color turning dark blue/purple. This does not allow for quantification of hyperhidrosis, but does allow definition of areas that may need treatment.
3. *Pre-weighed filter paper test*: Weighing the blotting paper after placing this over the area of hyperhidrosis for a defined period of time (to soak up the sweat) allows for quantification of hyperhidrosis (rate of sweat production in mg/minute).

Treatment

- Avoid precipitating factors.
- Treat the underlying condition.
- Antiperspirants, particularly those that contain aluminum chloride.
- Topical anticholinergic agents that prevent nerve stimulation of the sweat glands [1]: These have variable efficacy because of variable absorption.
- Oral anticholinergic drugs such as glycopyrrolate or oxybutynin hydrochloride [1]: These medications have associated side effects, such as blurred vision, dryness of the

M. Misra (✉)
Division of Pediatric Endocrinology, Massachusetts General Hospital and Harvard Medical School, Boston, MA, USA
e-mail: MMISRA@mgh.harvard.edu

T. Stanley, M. Misra (eds.), *Endocrine Conditions in Pediatrics*, https://doi.org/10.1007/978-3-030-52215-5_23

mouth with loss of taste, constipation, urinary retention, tachycardia, drowsiness, increased risk of heat exhaustion and heat stroke.

- Botulinum toxin A injections can be useful for focal hyperhidrosis (e.g., of the axilla) as the toxin blocks the neuronal signal to the sweat gland [1–4]. Side effects include local injection site pain, pruritus and also headache.
- Iontophoresis: This entails passing an electric current through water in which each hand or foot is placed. While the mechanism of action is not clear, this strategy can be effective in reducing sweat production [2, 4]. It can also lead to dry or peeling skin.
- Endoscopic thoracic sympathectomy: This reduces or eliminates sympathetic stimulation of the sweat glands [2, 4].
- For focal hyperhidrosis, it may be possible to excise the local sweat glands [2, 4].

Table 23.1 Differential diagnosis and evaluation of excessive sweating (with a focus on endocrine conditions associated with this symptom)

Differential diagnosis of excessive sweating	Work-up and next steps
Occurs at the time of the precipitating event	
Higher ambient temperature	History (including the use of medications such as hypoglycemic drugs), other associated symptoms Physical examination (including vitals) If hypoglycemia is suspected, finger-stick glucose testing at the time of symptoms (see Chap. 8); consult pediatric endocrinology
Excessive physical activity	
Emotional stress; anxiety	
Fever, particularly when it remits	
Hypoglycemia	
May occur at all times but is exacerbated by higher ambient temperature, excessive physical or emotional stress, and sometimes at night	
Hyperthyroidism (see Chap. 42)	History for symptoms of (i) hyperthyroidism: heat intolerance, mood changes, palpitations, increased appetite, weight loss, difficulty falling asleep, frequent stools, prominence of the eyes; (ii) growth hormone excess: tall stature, increases in ring and hat size, coarsening of features over time, mass effects (headaches, nausea, vomiting, vision changes), polyuria and polydipsia (associated hyperglycemia or diabetes insipidus), galactorrhea (co-secreting adenomas), gynecomastia; family history of genetic conditions causing endocrine tumors, (iii) autonomic neuropathy: postural dizziness and syncopal episodes, gastrointestinal and urinary symptoms Review of the growth chart for patterns of weight and height changes over time: this provides clues to GH excess vs. exogenous obesity. Crossing of height percentiles over time indicative of increased growth velocity is characteristic of GH excess before epiphyseal fusion Physical examination for signs of (i) hyperthyroidism: fine tremor of outstretched hands, tongue fasciculations, warm, velvety skin, tachycardia and hypertension with wide pulse pressure, proptosis or exophthalmos; (ii) GH excess: coarse facial features and coarse skin, prominence of the forehead, jaw and nose, thick lips, skin tags, large hands and feet, acanthosis nigricans, (iii) obesity, (iv) autonomic neuropathy: postural hypotension using the tilt test *Laboratory work-up, and imaging studies* If hyperthyroidism is suspected: TSH, free T4, total T3, consider getting thyroid-stimulating immunoglobulins or TSH receptor-binding antibodies (diagnostic for autoimmune hyperthyroidism or Graves' disease), may consider a Technetium 99 or Iodine 123 scan and/or a thyroid ultrasound depending on presentation (to diagnose a hyperfunctioning nodule or subacute thyroiditis as causes of hyperthyroidism); consult pediatric endocrinology If GH excess is suspected: IGF-1 ± IGFBP-3 levels, followed by a GH suppression test if levels are elevated (using an oral glucose load); pituitary MRI to rule out a GH-secreting pituitary tumor if GH levels do not suppress to <1 ng/ml on this suppression test; may consider testing for prolactin as some GH-secreting tumors also secrete prolactin; may consider testing for deficiency of other pituitary hormones from mass effect; consult pediatric endocrinology In patients with GH excess, genetic studies may be necessary when there are concerns of multiple endocrine neoplasia type 1 (MEN1), *AIR* or XLAG mutations, McCune Albright syndrome, or Carney complex In patients with suspected autonomic neuropathy, additional testing may require a specialist, e.g., gastric emptying tests, quantitative sudomotor axon reflex test, thermoregulatory sweat test, urodynamic tests, and bladder ultrasound
Growth hormone (GH) excess, which may be associated with hyperprolactinemia (see Chap. 56)	
Obesity (see Chap. 58)	
Disorders of the autonomic system (a cause of focal hyperhidrosis)	

Table 23.1 (continued)

Differential diagnosis of excessive sweating	Work-up and next steps
Random and intermittent, but may be triggered by certain situations such as physical activity, anxiety and stress, certain kinds of foods and medications	
Pheochromocytoma and paraganglioma (symptoms may be triggered by physical exertion, anxiety, stress, changes in body position, anesthesia, surgery, food rich in tyramine such as certain cheeses, certain types of alcohol, chocolate, dried and smoked meat, medications such as MAO inhibitors, stimulants such as amphetamines)	History: inquire into associated symptoms such as headaches, pallor or flushing, tremors, palpitations, shortness of breath, wheezing, anxiety, bowel disturbances, weight loss or weight gain; family history of pheochromocytoma, paraganglioma or neurofibromatosis 1 (NF1) Physical examination including vitals: tachycardia and hypertension are clues to a pheochromocytoma or paraganglioma; Cushingoid features may suggest a bronchial carcinoid *Laboratory work-up and imaging studies* If pheochromocytoma or paraganglioma are suspected: plasma free metanephrines, 24-hour urine catecholamines, metanephrines, vanillylmandelic acid, and homovanillic acid; imaging studies for tumor location if labs are positive; consult pediatric endocrinology Depending on presentation, consider genetic studies and work-up for MEN2, von Hippel Lindau disease, familial paraganglioma syndrome and NF1 in patients with a diagnosed pheochromocytoma or paraganglioma If a carcinoid tumor is suspected: 24-hour urine for 5-hydroxy indole acetic acid (5HIAA), serum chromogranin A, whole blood serotonin; followed by imaging studies for tumor location if labs are positive; consult pediatric endocrinology
Carcinoid tumors (may occur in the lungs or digestive tract, and symptoms depend on the location of the tumor)	
Predominantly night sweats	
Lymphoma, leukemia, others	History including the use of medications for acute and chronic infections, antidepressants, history of chemotherapy or radiotherapy (may cause POI) Physical examination including vitals If hematological conditions are suspected: CBC with differential, bone marrow studies, imaging studies, biopsies and additional testing may be necessary; consult pediatric hematology-oncology If TB or other infectious conditions are suspected, consult a pediatric infectious disease specialist If endocarditis is suspected, a CBC with differential, basic metabolic panel, urinalysis, blood culture, ECHO, cardiac Doppler may be necessary, consult pediatric cardiology If POI is suspected, it is necessary to get gonadotropins (FSH and LH) and gonadal steroid levels; gonadotropins are elevated and gonadal steroid levels are low in POI. If POI is diagnosed, genetic studies may be necessary to determine the etiology (such as Turner syndrome, other conditions of gonadal dysgenesis, FMR premutation). Testing for other autoimmune conditions such as Addison's disease should be considered if POI appears to be autoimmune in nature (see Chap. 49); consult pediatric endocrinology
Tuberculosis (TB)	
HIV infection/AIDS	
Endocarditis	
Other infections	
Sleep disorders	
Antidepressant medications	
Premature ovarian insufficiency (POI) (see Chaps. 47 and 49): hot flashes with sweating may occur, particularly at night	
Idiopathic hyperhidrosis	*Diagnosis of exclusion*

References

1. http://www.hyperhidrosis.ca/prevalence.htm.
2. https://www.aboutkidshealth.ca/Article?contentid=799&language=English.
3. https://emedicine.medscape.com/article/1073359-overview.
4. https://www.aad.org/public/diseases/dry-sweaty-skin/hyperhidrosis.

Part II

Interpretation of Endocrine Laboratory Values and Imaging

24 Growth Factors

Eray Savgan-Gurol

Growth Factors (IGF-1 and IGFBP-3)

Growth hormone is secreted from the pituitary gland, mostly at night and in a pulsatile manner. Serum growth hormone levels are very low between secretory pulses. Due to pulsatile secretion and short half-life of growth hormone, random growth hormone measurement cannot be utilized in the work-up of short stature. Instead, insulin-like growth factor 1 (IGF-1) and Insulin-like growth factor binding protein 3 (IGFBP-3), which are produced in response to growth hormone stimulation and which remain stable throughout the day, are used as initial screening labs.

Clinical Key
Circulating levels of GH are very low in between secretory pulses. Measuring random GH levels is not useful in the evaluation of short stature and/or decreased growth velocity.

Insulin-Like Growth Factors (IGFs)

Anabolic and growth-promoting effects of growth hormone such as cell proliferation, protein synthesis, and skeletal growth are mostly mediated by insulin-like growth factors (IGFs) acting in an endocrine, autocrine, and paracrine fashion [1]. Insulin-like growth factors belong to a family of closely related growth factors with high homology to insulin and insulin-like activity. Most organs synthesize IGFs, but the majority of *circulating* IGFs are produced in the liver in response to growth hormone signaling. Insulin-like growth factors in circulation are bound to IGF binding proteins (IGFBPs), which prolong their serum half-life and transport them to target cells.

Insulin-Like Growth Factor-1

Insulin-like growth factor-1 (IGF-1) is a 70 amino acid peptide that plays an important role in both fetal and postnatal growth. In serum, 75% of the circulating IGF-1 is bound to IGFBP-3 and the acid labile subunit (ALS), forming a ternary complex which further prolongs its half-life to close to 16 hours. Levels of IGF-1 vary significantly throughout life, with levels being low at birth, then showing a slow, steady rise in prepubertal children and followed by a steep rise at the time of puberty [2, 3]. The normal range for IGF-1 in healthy young children overlaps with those who are growth hormone deficient, especially in children who are younger than 5 years of age. Therefore, IGF-1 levels should be interpreted with caution in this age group. Rising gonadal steroids with puberty stimulate GH secretion and IGF-1 production, and pubertal IGF-1 levels reach peaks that are 2–3 times higher than the adult levels. Serum IGF-1 levels are influenced by age, degree of pubertal maturation, and nutritional status. Studies have shown that maximal IGF-1 levels are seen at Tanner Stage 3–4 in girls and Tanner stage 4 in boys [4]. After puberty, IGF-1 levels start to show a slow decline that continues through adulthood.

Assay Considerations Commercial IGF-1 assays use various methods – IRMA, ELISA, ICMA (Immunochemiluminometric assay), and liquid chromatography/mass spectrometry (LC/MS) – and have varying validity and reliability. There may be interference by IGFBP's in radioimmunoassay, radioreceptor assays, and bioassays. Serum IGF-1 levels are typically measured after dissociation from binding sites, and the efficiency of this process may affect results. *The ideal IGF-1 assay will be performed by LC/MS and will provide a raw value along with a z-score that is adjusted for age and sex.*

E. Savgan-Gurol (✉)
Pediatric Endocrine Division, Massachusetts General Hospital, Harvard Medical School, Boston, MA, USA
e-mail: esgurol@mgh.harvard.edu

T. Stanley, M. Misra (eds.), *Endocrine Conditions in Pediatrics*, https://doi.org/10.1007/978-3-030-52215-5_24

IGF-1 assays show significant variability between manufacturers and platforms, and assay-specific normal ranges should be used. Comparison or serial assessment of IGF-1 levels between different platforms could be misleading. IGF-1 and IGFBP-3 levels are usually well correlated, and discrepant results should prompt evaluation of pre-analytical or analytical error.

Interpretation IGF-1 levels are low in children younger than 5 years of age and show significant overlap between healthy children and those with growth hormone deficiency. Nutritional status is a major determinant of IGF-1 gene expression both in liver and in other tissues, and fasting reduces serum IGF-1 levels. Conditions associated with low IGF-1 levels are shown in Table 24.1, and conditions associated with high levels are shown in Table 24.2. Children who have poor nutrition, hypothyroidism, chronic disease, renal disease and diabetes have low IGF-1 levels, and IGF-1 cannot be a reliable screening test for short stature in such conditions. Children with delayed puberty typically may appear to have lower IGF-1 levels, but bone age or puberty adjusted levels are usually normal.

The role of IGF-1 by itself in diagnosis of growth hormone deficiency is controversial, and there is no gold-standard cutoff for establishing the diagnosis of growth hormone deficiency. In general, very low IGF-1 levels (z-score below −2, that is, level less than 2 standard deviations below the mean) are highly suggestive of disorders of growth hormone axis if other causes of low IGF-1 are excluded. When the IGF-1 level is above z-score of −1, the diagnosis of growth hormone deficiency is less likely [5].

High IGF-1 levels are associated with growth hormone excess from conditions such as gigantism or growth hormone overtreatment. During pregnancy, serum IGF-1 levels increase up to fourfold of baseline levels.

Table 24.1 Conditions associated with Low IGF-1 levels

Disorders of growth hormone axis
Delayed puberty
Hypothyroidism
Poor nutrition
Chronic disease
Renal disease
Hypothyroidism
Diabetes

Table 24.2 Conditions associated with high IGF-1 levels

Growth hormone excess
Gigantism
Acromegaly
Growth hormone overtreatment
Pregnancy

Insulin-Like Growth Factor Binding Proteins (IGFBPs)

Insulin-like growth factors (IGFs) circulate in plasma bound to a family of binding proteins which are called insulin-like binding proteins (IGFBPs). IGFBPs are a family of peptides which extend serum half-life of IGFs and transport them to target cells. There are six IGFBPs that have been identified and, among those, IGFBP-3 is the major binding protein, transporting more than 90% of IGF-1. IGFBP-3 is mostly produced in the liver in a growth hormone–dependent manner and plays a significant role in functional regulation of IGF-1. The major factors that play a role in IGFBP3 production are growth hormone, nutrition, and age. Reference levels for IGFBP-3 in children, adolescents, and adults have been established by several cohort studies, and despite variations in raw values, studies show a similar pattern across the lifespan [2, 6] . The lowest levels of IGFBP3 are seen at birth, followed by a rapid increase in the first weeks of life and a gradual increase thereafter until puberty. The highest levels are seen in puberty, with levels being higher in females than males, and levels start to decline slowly after late adolescence [4].

Assay Considerations Commercial assays that are commonly used are IRMA, ELISA, and ICMA (Immunochemiluminometric assay). Heterophile antibodies in human serum can interfere with immunoassays and cause falsely high levels. This type of erroneous result can be seen in autoimmune disorders or from individuals who are exposed to animals or animal serum products.

Interpretation Serum levels of IGF-1 and IGFBP-3 levels are GH dependent, and they are both low in conditions that are associated with impaired GH secretion. Like IGF-1 levels, serum IGFBP-3 levels should be adjusted for age, sex, and pubertal stage before interpretation. Age, sex, and pubertal adjusted IGF-1 and IGFBP-3 levels below −2 SD are highly suggestive of disorders of growth hormone axis after excluding conditions that are associated with low levels such as poor nutrition and poorly controlled diabetes [7]. High IGFBP-3 levels are seen in conditions associated with growth hormone excess such as gigantism, acromegaly, or growth hormone overtreatment. Serum IGFBP-3 levels are also high in chronic renal failure. Please see Table 24.3 for suggested interpretation of IGF-1 and IGFBP-3 values.

In conclusion, the diagnosis of growth hormone deficiency is based on clinical expertise, auxological, radiologic, and laboratory data. Low IGF-1 and IGFBP 3 levels may be helpful in initial screening for growth hormone deficiency

Table 24.3 Interpretation of IGF-1 and IGFBP-3

Lab results (IGF-1 and IGFBP-3)	Interpretation	Action
Low (< −2 SD for age and gender)	Highly suggestive of growth hormone (GH) deficiency if child is normal weight and has no other conditions that can affect IGF-1 level (see Table 24.1)	Consider referral to pediatric endocrine for further evaluation
Higher than – 1SD	Less likely to be GH deficient	Follow height velocity (HV) and consider referral if HV is low for age
>1 SD	Very unlikely to be GH deficient	Follow height velocity (HV) and consider referral if HV is low for age

but cannot be used solely for diagnosis due to lack of specificity and sensitivity. This is partly due to technical issues related with utilized assays and the complexity in the physiological regulation of GH-IGF-IGFBP system. Low IGF-1 and IGFBP3 levels should be confirmed with provocative GH testing.

Growth Hormone Stimulation Testing

A next step in testing for GH deficiency, performed by pediatric endocrinologists, is growth hormone stimulation testing. Although GH stimulation testing is controversial due to flaws in both methodology and interpretation, it is generally considered to be more definitive than IGF-1 and IGFBP-3. The rationale behind GH stimulation testing is to administer pharmacologic stimuli that provoke GH secretion and measure the "peak" of serum GH levels in response to one or more of these stimuli. Whereas random serum GH levels have no utility, serial measurement of serum GH following provocative stimulus is thought to reflect GH secretory capacity. Multiple different pharmacologic stimuli are used in pediatric practice: arginine, clonidine, levodopa, propranolol, glucagon, insulin, or, less commonly, exercise. GH stimulation testing generally takes 2–4 hours and involves administration of one or more of the stimuli above, either sequentially or simultaneously. A peak GH of level 6-10mcg/L is generally considered demonstrative of GH "sufficiency," with cutoff values varying by country and a value of 10 mcg/L most commonly in use in the United States at the time of this writing. Peak serum GH values below the designated "cutoff" are considered diagnostic of GH deficiency.

Summary

For patients with short stature and/or decreased growth velocity, IGF-1 and IGFBP-3 measurement in the primary care setting can inform further steps. Whereas low IGF-1 and IGFBP-3 provide further indication for referral to pediatric endocrinology, robust values make GH deficiency less likely. In the interpretation of these values, it is critical to use age- and sex-appropriate normal ranges and to remember factors that may influence these levels, particularly factors that may independently reduce IGF-1 as shown in Table 24.1.

References

1. Yakar S, Werner H, Rosen CJ. Insulin-like growth factors: actions on the skeleton. J Mol Endocrinol. 2018;61(1):T115–37.
2. Brabant G, et al. Serum insulin-like growth factor I reference values for an automated chemiluminescence immunoassay system: results from a multicenter study. Horm Res Paediatr. 2003;60(2):53–60.
3. Chanson P, et al. Reference values for IGF-I serum concentrations: comparison of six immunoassays. J Clin Endocrinol Metabol. 2016;101(9):3450–8.
4. Juul A, et al. Serum insulin-like growth factor-I in 1030 healthy children, adolescents, and adults: relation to age, sex, stage of puberty, testicular size, and body mass index. J Clin Endocrinol Metab. 1994;78(3):744–52.
5. Ranke MB, et al. Significance of basal IGF-I, IGFBP-3 and IGFBP-2 measurements in the diagnostics of short stature in children. Horm Res. 2000;54(2):60–8.
6. Juul A, et al. Serum levels of insulin-like growth factor (IGF)-binding protein-3 (IGFBP-3) in healthy infants, children, and adolescents: the relation to IGF-I, IGF-II, IGFBP-1, IGFBP-2, age, sex, body mass index, and pubertal maturation. J Clin Endocrinol Metab. 1995;80(8):2534–42.
7. Society GR. Consensus guidelines for the diagnosis and treatment of growth hormone (GH) deficiency in childhood and adolescence: summary statement of the GH Research Society. J Clin Endocrinol Metabol. 2000;85(11):3990–3.

Thyroid Studies

25

Julia R. Donner and Lisa Swartz Topor

Introduction

Thyroid disorders are very common and affect more than 10% of the population in the United States [1]. Given the high prevalence of thyroid disease, thyroid function tests are the most frequently ordered endocrine tests in the outpatient setting [1]. Understanding thyroid physiology allows for selection of appropriate thyroid studies and helps inform interpretation of results. This chapter will discuss relevant thyroid function assays and imaging studies, the interpretation of abnormal results, and the next steps in addressing abnormal values in pediatric patients. Additional information about pediatric thyroid diseases can be found in Part III, Chaps. 41 and 42.

Thyroid Hormone Physiology

Thyroid hormone production and secretion are tightly regulated by the hypothalamic-pituitary-thyroid axis in a classic endocrine feedback loop. With normal hypothalamus, pituitary, and thyroid function, thyroid hormone levels are tightly regulated and remain relatively constant, reflecting an individual's physiologic set-point [2]. Thyrotropin-releasing hormone (TRH) from the hypothalamus stimulates the secretion of thyroid-stimulating hormone (TSH) [also known as thyrotropin] from the anterior pituitary. TSH stimulates production of thyroxine (T4) and triiodothyronine (T3). T3 is bioactive and derived from conversion of T4 by deiodinases. Over 99% of T4 and T3 molecules in circulation are tightly bound to carrier proteins (thyroid-binding globulin (TBG), transthyretin, and albumin), and a small percentage circulate as free hormones (free T4 and free T3). The free thyroid hormones act on target tissues and provide negative feedback to the hypothalamus and pituitary gland [2, 3]. See Fig. 25.1.

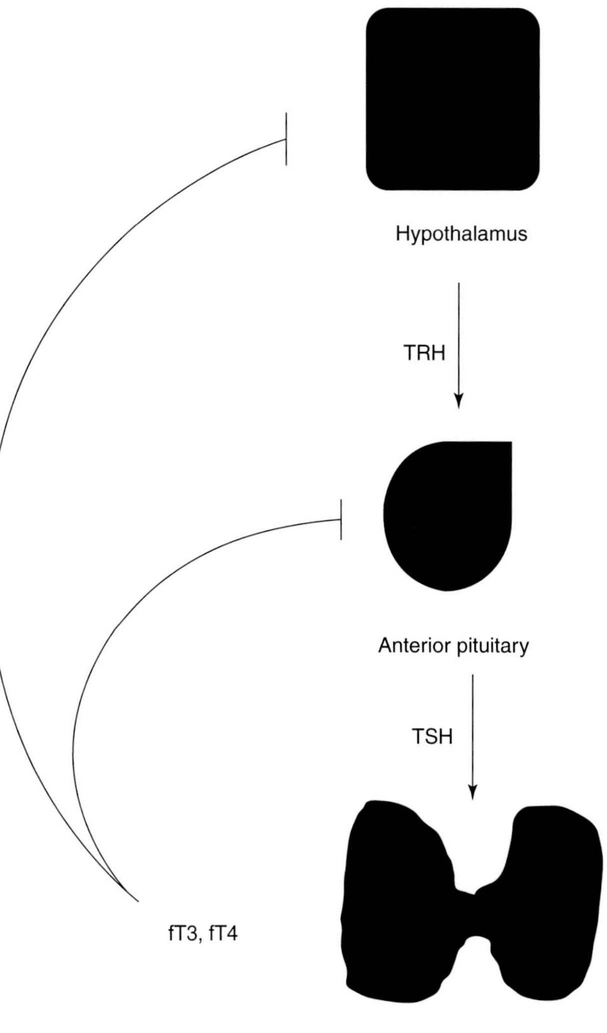

Fig. 25.1 Hypothalamic-pituitary-thyroid axis

J. R. Donner
The Warren Alpert Medical School of Brown University, Providence, RI, USA
e-mail: Julia_donner@brown.edu

L. S. Topor (✉)
Pediatric Endocrinology, The Warren Alpert Medical School of Brown University and Hasbro Children's Hospital, Providence, RI, USA
e-mail: lisa_swartz_topor@brown.edu

T. Stanley, M. Misra (eds.), *Endocrine Conditions in Pediatrics*, https://doi.org/10.1007/978-3-030-52215-5_25

Table 25.1 Laboratory studies of thyroid function

Test	Comments
TSH	First line in nearly all cases, except for known hypopituitary/hypothalamic dysfunction
Free T4	First line in nearly all cases, except for known substantial alterations in TBG; free T4 by equilibrium dialysis is gold-standard and accurate even at extremes of TBG
Free T3	Currently not commonly used; free T4 preferred
Total T4	Useful in conjunction with thyroid-binding assay when free T4 assay is unreliable; useful in infants to determine the severity of congenital hypothyroidism
Total T3	Useful adjunctive test in hyperthyroidism
THBR, T3RU, or T7	Can be used in conjunction with total T4 if free T4 is unreliable
TBG	Rarely useful; could be used to identify hormone binding disorders
Reverse T3	Rarely useful; increased in euthyroid sick syndrome, but not routinely measured in this setting
Thyroglobulin	Useful as a tumor marker following thyroidectomy for thyroid cancer

Abbreviations: *T3* triiodothyronine, *T3RU* T3 resin uptake, *T4* thyroxine, *TBG* thyroid-binding globulin, *THBR* thyroid hormone binding ratio, *TSH* thyroid-stimulating hormone

Thyroid Function Tests Changes in thyroid status lead to fluctuations in thyroid function tests, mainly T4, T3, and TSH levels, which can reflect over- or underactivity of the gland [2]. The most common laboratory tests used to understand thyroid function are shown in Table 25.1 and include TSH, total and free T4, and total and free T3. Additional thyroid laboratory studies that help with understanding thyroid disease include thyroid antibodies: thyroglobulin antibodies (Tg-Ab), thyroid peroxidase antibodies (TPO-Ab), TSH receptor antibodies (TRAb), and thyroid-stimulating immunoglobulins (TSI) [1]. Less commonly used thyroid studies to evaluate and monitor specific aspects of thyroid disease include thyroglobulin (Tg) and thyroid-binding globulin (TBG).

Thyroid-Stimulating Hormone (TSH) The most sensitive test to detect primary dysfunction of the thyroid gland is measurement of TSH [2]. Abnormal TSH levels can be detected and associated with early thyroid dysfunction before changes in thyroid hormone levels develop [1]. In many laboratories, a highly sensitive TSH assay (second or third generation, with usual limits of detection <0.1 μIU/mL or <0.01 μIU/mL, respectively) may be sufficient for screening of primary thyroid dysfunction [4]. The reference range for TSH varies by assay, typically with a lower limit around 0.5 μIU/mL and an upper limit around 5 μIU/mL.

Though TSH is the most sensitive indicator of primary thyroid function, the use of TSH alone (or "TSH with reflex" that measures thyroxine only if TSH is abnormal) may miss other thyroid abnormalities. When central thyroid dysfunction due to pituitary or hypothalamic disease is in the differential diagnosis, it is important to measure thyroid hormone (free T4 or total T4) concentration along with TSH to avoid missing these conditions [1, 2].

TSH levels change slowly after treatment initiation or adjustments. In most cases outside of the newborn period, TSH should be repeated no sooner than 4–6 weeks after a medication adjustment.

Free T4 and Free T3 Measurement of free thyroid hormones, the biologically active thyroid hormones, is now common practice in the United States as the assays have improved in recent years [1]. The two-step assay for free T4 is run by extracting T4 from serum with specific high-affinity antibodies. Antibody-bound thyroid hormones are incubated and labeled with a thyroid hormone probe. Unoccupied antibody binding sites are inversely proportional to free thyroid hormone level [1]. Free T4 is preferred compared to free T3 because free T4 circulates in the bloodstream at levels two to three times higher than free T3, so the precision of the free T4 assay is better than that of the free T3 assay [1]. As the free thyroid hormone measurements are less affected by protein binding variation, free T4 is the optimal thyroid hormone measurement in nearly all conditions if a reliable assay is available [5]. Standard free T4 and free T3 assays may not be reliable in states of altered circulating thyroid-binding globulin (TBG), such as pregnancy (high TBG) or renal failure (low TBG). In these cases, measurement of free T4 by equilibrium dialysis is the gold-standard assay. Alternatively, total thyroxine with the measurement of thyroid hormone binding (see below) could be performed.

Total T3 and Total T4 Total thyroid hormone assays were previously the standard tests used for thyroid assessment, until recent improvements in free thyroid hormone assays. The total T4 or T3 assay measures the bound and free hormone. Total thyroid hormone assays are affected by changes in binding protein concentration or affinity. TBG, discussed below, can vary based on genetic and exogenous factors, and the total thyroid hormone measurements may not reflect thyroid status as accurately.

Measurement of Thyroid Hormone Binding Examples of measurements of thyroid-binding protein include the thyroid hormone binding ratio (THBR), the T3 resin uptake (T3RU) assay, and the T7 assay [4]. *THBR* measures the uptake of T3 or T4 tracer by TBG, estimating available binding sites on TBG in the serum sample. The THBR is calculated by the T3 solid-state (resin) uptake divided by the serum uptake. *T3RU* is an indirect measurement of serum thyroid hormone binding capacity [6]. T3RU is measured by mixing a low affinity solid phase T3 resin binder with patient serum which has a trace amount of ^{125}I-labeled T3. This labeled T3 splits between solid phase and serum-binding sites. The value is calculated by ^{125}I- T3 activity left on the resin binder divided by ^{125}I- T3 added, to get a percent. Normal values are between 25% and 50% [6]. A free T4 index (FTI) is usually provided in conjunction with THBR or T3RU measurements. The free T4 index "adjusts" the total thyroxine level for the amount of thyroid-binding protein. The free T4 index should be normal in euthyroid patients with isolated abnormalities in binding protein, whereas it should be high in patients with hyperthyroidism and low in patients with hypothyroidism. Similarly, the *T7 assay* is a measure that adjusts the total T4 for the T3RU. This adjustment corrects for alterations in thyroid hormone binding, including medication interference or altered binding protein concentrations. Measurements of thyroid hormone binding are only necessary when measuring the total thyroid hormone concentrations.

Thyroid-binding globulin (TBG) is one of the major transport proteins that binds and transports thyroid hormones to tissues throughout the body [7]. The main role of TBG is to maintain a constant level of free thyroid hormone in the serum. TBG levels are affected by medications, hormones, and nonthyroidal illness. Changes in the function and amount of TBG can alter the total amount of T4 in the serum. When there is a decrease in TBG, free T4 transiently increases and provides negative feedback to the hypothalamus and pituitary, leading to a decrease in thyroxine production [7]. Shortly after, the free T4 value returns to its steady state. Measurement of serum TBG levels is done to identify hormone-binding disorders and is rarely indicated.

Reverse T3 is a biologically inactive byproduct of thyroid hormone deiodination that is elevated in euthyroid sick syndrome and is currently not recommended for routine evaluation of thyroid disorders.

Thyroglobulin (Tg) is a glycoprotein produced by thyroid follicular cells. It is measured using immunometric assays [1]. Thyroglobulin is also a tumor marker for differentiated thyroid carcinoma (DTC) following thyroidectomy and radioiodine remnant ablation. As many as 25% of patients with DTC have thyroglobulin antibodies. Elevated thyroglobulin antibodies lead to falsely low serum thyroglobulin measurement, so it is important to always measure the Tg level together with Tg-Ab for optimal interpretation of results.

Table 25.2 Common patterns of thyroid function tests and differential diagnoses

TSH	FT4	Differential diagnosis
High	Low (primary hypothyroidism)	Hashimoto's thyroiditis Iodine deficiency H/o radioactive iodine or surgery
	Normal (subclinical hypothyroidism)	
	High	Thyroid hormone resistance
Low	Low (secondary hypothyroidism)	Pituitary tumor H/o pituitary surgery or radiation Other pituitary hormone deficiencies
	Normal (subclinical hyperthyroidism)	Graves' disease Toxic nodule Thyroiditis
	High (primary hyperthyroidism)	
Normal	Low	Pituitary disease

Patterns of Thyroid Function Tests and Corresponding Diagnoses (Table 25.2)

Elevated TSH with low FT4 is seen in primary hypothyroidism. Due to the negative feedback between serum thyroid hormones and TSH, a decrease in thyroid hormone production will stimulate a rise in TSH. Common causes include autoimmune or Hashimoto's thyroiditis (the most common cause of primary hypothyroidism in iodine replete areas), congenital hypothyroidism, the use of antithyroid drugs, history of radioactive iodine therapy, or thyroidectomy. Worldwide, the most common cause of primary hypothyroidism is iodine deficiency. Treatment of primary hypothyroidism is with thyroid hormone (levothyroxine) replacement.

Elevated TSH with normal FT4 is seen in a milder subtype of primary hypothyroidism known as subclinical hypothyroidism. This condition occurs in 3–8% of the general population and is more common in women [8]. It is of clinical significance because there is an increased likelihood of progression to overt hypothyroidism compared to the general population. Periodic screening is recommended, but treatment with levothyroxine therapy generally should not be initiated until TSH ≥10 μIU/mL. Treatment below this threshold has not been shown to be beneficial for health-related quality of life or symptoms [9]. Exceptions to the treatment threshold of TSH ≥10 μIU/mL include infants and toddlers younger than 3 years old and pregnant women.

Low TSH and elevated FT4 (and/or T3) establish the diagnosis of thyrotoxicosis [10]. Thyrotoxicosis is a disorder of excess thyroid hormone often associated with hyperthyroidism but can also occur in the absence of increased thyroid hormone secretion [11]. TSH is usually undetectable (typically <0.03 μIU/mL) in modern ultrasensitive TSH assays [2]. Etiologies of thyrotoxicosis include Graves' disease, subclinical thyroiditis, and functional (or hot) nodules.

Low TSH and normal FT4 are seen in subclinical hyperthyroidism and occurs in about 0.5% of children [12]. Subclinical hyperthyroidism can be divided into Grade I or mild (TSH 0.1–0.2 μIU/mL) and Grade II or severe (<0.1 μIU/mL). Grade I subclinical hyperthyroidism is much more common than Grade II and is much less likely to progress to overt hyperthyroidism. Careful monitoring is important through continued assessment of thyroid function. Treatment is generally not warranted. As described above, etiologies include mild Graves' disease, subclinical thyroiditis, and functional nodules.

Low FT4 and low or inappropriately normal TSH can reflect secondary hypothyroidism due to pituitary or hypothalamic disease. Patients should be evaluated for a history of brain/pituitary surgery, injury, or disease, or a history of congenital combined pituitary hormone deficiencies. Rare genetic causes of isolated thyrotropin-releasing hormone (TRH) or TSH deficiency can occur. Evaluation for secondary or central hypothyroidism includes a full anterior pituitary evaluation including assessment of growth hormone (GH) production, adrenal function, gonadal function, and prolactin.

Isolated abnormalities of one thyroid test with normal TSH in otherwise asymptomatic children often reflect laboratory/assay issues rather than pathology. Exceptions are cases of secondary hypothyroidism, as above, and thyroid hormone resistance, a rare genetic condition in which TSH may be normal but measures of T4 and T3 are high. Otherwise, TSH is a sensitive indicator of thyroid dysfunction, such that normal TSH in a child with normal physical examination and no "red flags" on history generally indicates normal thyroid function. In cases of asymptomatic children with normal TSH and a mild abnormality of another thyroid test (e.g., slightly low or slightly high free T4), prudent next steps include (1) ensuring the normal range being used is appropriate for age and thyroid status (e.g., normal range for thyroglobulin may be for individuals status-post thyroidectomy) and (2) repeating studies in 1–3 months. These steps can often save unnecessary family anxiety and referral.

Markers of Thyroid Autoimmunity

Autoimmune thyroid diseases are often accompanied by the presence of autoantibodies including thyroid peroxidase (TPO-Ab), thyroglobulin (Tg-Ab), and thyroid-stimulating hormone receptor (TRAbs) [13]. TPO-Ab and Tg-Ab are associated with thyroid dysfunction and damage. In individuals with primary hypothyroidism or subclinical hypothyroidism, the measurement of TPO-Ab titers is a useful adjunct to help guide decision-making. Subclinical hypothyroidism is more likely to progress to overt hypothyroidism in the setting of elevated anti-thyroid antibodies.

Once elevated antibodies are associated with Hashimoto's thyroiditis, there is no need to repeat these laboratory tests again as there is no value in trending these antibodies. Elevated TPO-Ab and Tg-Ab titers indicate the presence of autoimmune thyroid disease but do not correlate with disease activity. In contrast, the TRAbs seen in Graves' disease reflect disease activity and can be used to help inform treatment decisions as detailed below.

Thyroid peroxidase antibodies (TPO-Ab) are found in 5–10% of the general population and are almost always elevated in patients with Hashimoto's thyroiditis [1]. If a patient with subclinical hypothyroidism is found to have positive TPO-Ab, there is a higher risk of progression to overt hypothyroidism [2] compared to those without elevated antibodies. Given the risk of overt hypothyroidism, the American Thyroid Association recommends pregnant euthyroid women with elevated TPO-Ab have TSH monitored monthly to decide on treatment during pregnancy [14]. In asymptomatic children with elevated TPO-Ab, surveillance of TSH and free T4 is advisable every 12 months or with the emergence of new symptoms consistent with hypothyroidism.

Thyroglobulin antibodies (Tg-Ab) are another marker of thyroid autoimmunity. Serum levels are elevated in 10% of the general population, and Tg-Ab is not as sensitive or specific as TPO-Ab is for Hashimoto's thyroiditis [1]. In the absence of TPO-Ab, Tg-Ab alone is not significantly associated with thyroid disease. The main clinical use of this antibody is to ensure accurate clinical measurement in monitoring Tg levels in patients with differentiated thyroid carcinoma (DTC).

TSH receptor antibodies (TRAbs) are used in diagnosis of hyperthyroidism (Graves' disease) and are useful in the prediction of remission after treatment for Graves' disease. TRAbs are also used in the prediction of fetal/neonatal thyrotoxicosis in later stages of gestation in pregnant women with Graves' disease and are helpful in the assessment of Graves' ophthalmopathy [15]. Higher concentration of TRAbs help identify patients who are less likely to sustain remission after therapy with antithyroid medications [16].

Three types of TRAbs bind to TSH receptors: stimulating, blocking, or neutral antibodies. TRAbs can be measured by two types of assays: (1) competitive TSH-binding inhibition using thyroid-binding inhibitory immunoglobulin or (2) thyroid-stimulating immunoglobulin (TSI) assays. The different assay types have different benefits and costs. Thyroid-binding inhibitory immunoglobulin (TBII) measures TRAbs in serum samples based on the ability to inhibit binding of TSH receptors with known TSH receptor ligands. This assay cannot differentiate stimulating antibodies from blocking or neutral antibodies and is not as specific as TSI. The TSI assay is a functional bioassay, typically costs more than the competitive binding assay, and is highly specific for the diagnosis of Graves' disease [1, 17]. The TSI assay is especially useful in cases where a low autoantibody level is anticipated, as it is more sensitive and reproducible than that TBII assay, while still having a similar predictive value [18]. In addition, there is a close correlation of TSI level and severity of Graves' ophthalmopathy [18]. From a clinical standpoint, it is typically unnecessary to differentiate TSI from nonstimulating (TBII) antibodies in the diagnosis of Graves' disease when measuring TRAbs in patients with thyrotoxicosis [17]. Laboratory terminology can be confusing with regard to TRAbs. "TBII" and "TRAb" are often used synonymously in assay naming, whereas TSI specifically indicates the functional assay described above.

Laboratory Assay Interference Thyroid function tests should be interpreted in the context of the clinical status of a patient: hypothyroid, euthyroid, or hyperthyroid. Thyroid function test interpretation also requires consideration of potential assay interference [2] and patient-factor interference (other medications, nonthyroidal illness).

Fluctuation in thyroid-binding globulin (TBG) levels is an essential factor in the interpretation of total thyroid function tests, as alterations in the concentration of TBG will impact serum T4 concentration [10]. Factors that increase TBG include oral contraceptives, pregnancy, estrogens, infectious hepatitis, chronic active hepatitis, neonatal state, and acute intermittent porphyria. Factors that decrease TBG include androgens, corticosteroids, severe illness, cirrhosis, and nephrotic syndrome [1, 10].

An increase in TBG synthesis will lead to increased total T4 levels due to an increase in the total bound T4 in the serum. Similarly, decreased TBG production will lead to low measurement of total T4. Free T4, the active free hormone, is not affected by binding protein status [2]. Therefore, it is advisable to measure free T4 hormone concentration instead of total serum thyroid hormone concentration whenever possible. At extremes of TBG levels, free T4 by equilibrium dialysis may be required for accurate measurement.

Genetic Mutations Impacting Thyroid Hormone Binding Congenital TBG deficiency leads to low concentrations of total T4 with normal TSH and normal fT4. TBG deficiency is inherited in an X-linked pattern. The prevalence of complete TBG deficiency is 1:15000 newborns, while partial TBG deficiency occurs with a prevalence of 1:4000–1:12000 [19]. TBG deficiency is often missed during newborn screening that uses primary TSH detection, as TSH values are normal. However, it will be detected with newborn screening programs that use a primary T4 approach [20]. TBG deficiency does not require treatment, and if there are clinical concerns about thyroid dysfunction, TSH and free T4 should be measured, as total T4 will always be low.

Familial dysalbuminemic hyperthyroxinemia (FDH) is a rare autosomal dominant condition with increased total thyroid binding to albumin, leading to increased measurement of total T4 [1]. In FDH, albumin binds T4 with increased affinity, while T3 binding is much less affected. The typical laboratory pattern in FDH is a normal TSH with an increased total T4, normal or reduced free T4 based upon the characteristics of the free T4 assay, and normal total T3 [5, 21].

High-Dose Biotin Biotin, a water-soluble B vitamin that functions as a coenzyme for carboxylases [22], is commonly used in immunoassay platforms to capture antigens (including TSH and free T4) or antibodies onto the solid phase. In competitive binding assays, such as the free T4 assay, biotinylated T4 in the assay platform competes with serum free T4 for binding sites on a specific antibody. High biotin levels in the serum sample will inhibit the formation of solid phase complex, leading to a low signal and a falsely elevated free T4 measurement [1]. In many TSH assays, the patient serum sample is incubated with biotinylated TSH-Ab and a second ruthenium-labeled TSH-specific antibody is added. This complex is captured in solid phase on an electrode causing a chemiluminescent signal proportionate to sample TSH levels. Elevated serum biotin levels interfere with formation of the solid phase complex, and the low or absent signal will produce a falsely low TSH result [23]. The low TSH coupled with an elevated free T4 gives a false hyperthyroid result, which can lead to additional testing and treatments that are unnecessary. Biotin interference occurs in patients who are taking high doses of biotin such as 10–15 mg/kg daily, most often a dose taken by patients with inborn errors of biotin metabolism. Interference is unlikely to occur with most multivitamins with a biotin dose <1–3 mg per tablet; however, some supplements that are marketed to promote healthy hair and nails provide biotin in doses up to 5 mg (5000 mcg) per tablet. Thus, it is essential to inquire about medical history and use of supplements before proceeding with thyroid function testing. In pediatric populations, biotin interference was found up to 2 days after the last dose of biotin (10 mg/d for 4 days) and disappeared at 1 week in infants and young children receiving between 2 and 15 mg/kg/d [24]. In order to reduce risk of interference and only if medically advisable, patients should discontinue biotin supplementation at least 2 days before thyroid labs are to be drawn [23]. Alternatively, biotin can be neutralized by pre-treating the patient's serum sample with streptavidin.

Clinical Key
Use of high-dose biotin may cause assay interference in thyroid studies as well as other lab testing that utilizes immunoassays, yielding falsely abnormal results. Unless medically unsafe, patients should hold biotin for 1 week prior to testing.

Other Antibody Interactions Anti-animal antibodies, heterophile antibodies, or other antibodies in patient's serum can interfere with TSH assays. If they block TSH binding, negative interference can cause falsely low TSH levels. If they cross-link, positive interference can occur, causing falsely elevated TSH levels. In addition, autoantibodies to T4 can also falsely elevate free T4 levels [2]. The use of an alternate assay platform that uses different antibodies can help differentiate between abnormal thyroid function and assay interference.

Medications A variety of medications interfere with thyroid function. Dopamine agonists, glucocorticoids, and somatostatin analogues cause decreased pituitary TSH secretion. In patients with underlying hypothyroidism or subclinical hypothyroidism, metformin can lead to lower TSH measurements without effect on T3 or T4 [25, 26]. Lithium and tyrosine kinase inhibitors can cause primary hypothyroidism. Amiodarone inhibits type 1 deiodinases and can cause transient mild elevation in free T4, decreased free T3, and elevated TSH. Patients can also develop amiodarone-induced hypothyroidism due to direct cytotoxicity on thyroid follicular cells.

Pregnancy In normal pregnancy, there is a change in thyroid function resulting in increased TBG, T3, and T4 [27]. The increase in estrogen in pregnancy leads to increases in TBG production and subsequent increases in total thyroid hormone levels to around 150% of pre-pregnancy values [2]. In addition, high levels of hCG during early pregnancy stimulate TSH receptors because of homology between the alpha subunits of hCG and TSH [28] and homology of their receptors, resulting in increased thyroid hormone production and decreased TSH levels.

Non-thyroidal Illness Acute illness causes a decrease in free T3 in the first 24 hours, followed by decrease in TSH. In recovery, TSH increases, followed by a rise and normalization of thyroid hormone levels. The impact of non-thyroidal illness on thyroid hormone levels has a variety of causes including reduced deiodinase activity, reduced thyroid hormone-binding protein concentrations, increased circulating pro-inflammatory cytokines, and the use of medicines that impact the hypothalamic-pituitary-thyroidal axis. *Unless there is a very high clinical suspicion of thyroid disease, due to the impact of non-thyroidal disease on thyroid hormone measurement, it is highly recommended to avoid checking TFTs during acute illness and in the immediate recovery period after acute illness.*

Clinical Key
Unless there is a very high suspicion of thyroid disease requiring diagnostic data, avoid checking TFTs during acute illness and in the immediate recovery period.

Thyroid Imaging (See Also Chap. 38)

Imaging has long been a mainstay in the diagnosis of clinically significant thyroid pathology. Thyroid ultrasound and radionucleotide scintigraphy are used for the evaluation of thyroid anatomy and function. Thyroid imaging should be performed in individuals with abnormalities on physical examination of the thyroid (e.g., palpable nodules) and is often useful in differentiating causes of hyperthyroidism, but it is not routine for all individuals with suspected thyroid dysfunction.

Thyroid ultrasound is the first-line imaging study for the identification of thyroid pathology. As the thyroid is a relatively superficial structure, high-frequency sonography allows for the detection of nodules 2–3 mm in size as well as characterization of the lesions. It is also used to measure the thyroid gland and differentiate thyroid masses [29]. A normal thyroid appears homogeneously echogenic with uniform echotexture [30] and is slightly hyper-echogenic with regard to muscle [31]. In Hashimoto's thyroiditis, diffuse enlargement of the gland is often seen. Sonography allows measurement of nodules, can be used to identify figures of suspicious nodules, and can guide fine needle aspiration if indicated [31]. Features often associated with benign nodules in pediatrics include size <1 cm, dimensions that are more wide than tall, smooth margins, and isoechoic echotexture without echogenic foci [31]. In contrast, sonographic findings associated with DTC include nodule size >1 cm, hypoechoic echotexture, dimensions that are taller than wide, irregular margins, and microcalcifications or punctate echogenic foci [31, 32].

Radionucleotide imaging utilizes ^{99m}Technetium pertechnetate or ^{123}Iodine in order to assess physiologic thyroid function as well as characterize thyroid nodules as physiologically active (hot), or inactive (cold), measured by the level of uptake of the radioactive isotope [29, 30]. Radioactive iodine uptake (RAIU) and scan allow for a definitive assessment of thyroid physiology and morphology and are a particularly important diagnostic tool for the assessment of patients with hyperthyroidism for the differentiation of potential causes [17, 33, 34].

RAIU is a measurement of thyroid function that measures metabolism in the thyroid based on incorporation of radioactive iodide. The amount of radioactivity taken up into the gland is reported as a percent of the original dose administered [34]. Increased RAIU may be an indicator of hyperthyroidism or goiter. Decreased RAIU may indicate hypothyroidism, subacute thyroiditis, or iodine overload. The RAIU test does not involve imaging, whereas a thyroid scan provides an image of radioactive tracer uptake using the location and intensity of rays to examine the structure of the thyroid. Normal thyroid tissue displays uniform uptake of radiotracer in both lobes. The ^{99m}Technetium pertechnetate scan is similar to the RAIU but uses a different radioisotope to assess thyroid function. Diagnosis of Graves' disease does not require a scan, as increased uptake of the tracer can confirm the diagnosis. However, if evaluating for a hot nodule, a scan is necessary.

Next Steps in Addressing Abnormal Values and Monitoring TFTs

Primary hypothyroidism: In most cases, TSH is sufficient to monitor thyroid status in primary hypothyroidism [35]. FT4 will improve before TSH in primary hypothyroidism. Repeat measurement of TSH should be done approximately 6 weeks after initiating levothyroxine and after any dose change. For clinically asymptomatic Hashimoto's thyroiditis not requiring treatment, annual TSH monitoring is sufficient. One exception is that thyroid function monitoring should include both TSH and a measure of thyroxine in infants and toddlers <3 years old with primary hypothyroidism.

Secondary hypothyroidism: TSH will remain low/normal, so only FT4 should be monitored to assess response to levothyroxine treatment.

Hyperthyroidism: FT4, total T3, and TSH levels should be regularly monitored during treatment of hyperthyroidism. Free T4 will respond faster than TSH to anti-thyroid therapy by several months. Medication doses should be titrated to free T4 and/or total T3 levels.

Mildly abnormal thyroid function tests in the setting of acute illness: unless clinical signs and symptoms of thyroid dysfunction are present, recommend repeating TFTs 1–2 months after acute illness resolves.

Palpable nodule in thyroid: Obtain thyroid ultrasound and refer to pediatric endocrinology for nodule >1 cm or for any nodule with suspicious features.

Take Home Points

1. TSH is the best indicator of thyroid function or thyroid hormone replacement in the setting of primary thyroid disease.
2. Free T4 is useful to assess the need for and effectiveness of thyroid hormone replacement in the setting of central hypothyroidism due to pituitary or hypothalamic dysfunction.
3. Thyroid function tests are affected by factors outside of thyroid activity, such as severe illness and medications/dietary supplements including biotin. Make sure to take into account the underlying health status and treatments of individual patients when interpreting TFTs.
4. Unless there is a high level of concern for thyroid dysfunction, TFTs should not be checked in the setting of acute illness.
5. If needed, thyroid ultrasound is first-line imaging for thyroid pathology.
6. Once Hashimoto's thyroiditis is diagnosed based upon elevated thyroid antibody levels (TPO-Ab, Tg-Ab), there is no clinical utility in repeating the thyroid antibodies as antibody titers do not correlate with disease activity or progression. In contrast, the antibodies seen with Graves' disease (TSI, TRAbs) correlate with disease activity and are useful to understand clinical course and predict response to treatment.
7. TSH levels change slowly after treatment initiation or adjustments. Accordingly, in most cases TSH should be repeated no sooner than every 4–6 weeks to assess response to levothyroxine or other treatment of primary thyroid disease [36].

References

1. Soh SB, Aw TC. Laboratory testing in thyroid conditions – pitfalls and clinical utility. Ann Lab Med. 2019;39(1):3–14. https://doi.org/10.3343/alm/2019/39.1.3.
2. Koulouri O, Gurnell M. How to interpret thyroid function tests. Clin Med (Lond). 2013;13(3):282–6. https://doi.org/10.7861/clinmedicine.13-3-282.
3. van der Spek AH, Fliers E, Boelen A. The classic pathways of thyroid hormone metabolism. Mol Cell Endocrinol. 2017;458:29–38.
4. Dayan CM. Interpretation of thyroid function tests. Lancet. 2001;357:619–24.
5. Welsh KJ, Soldin SJ. Diagnosis of endocrine disease: how reliable are free thyroid and total T3 hormone assays? Eur J Endocrinol. 2016;175(6):R255–63. https://doi.org/10.1530/EJE-16-0193.
6. Dunlap DB. Chapter 142: Thyroid function tests. In: Walker HK, Hall WD, Hurst JW, editors. Clinical methods: the history, physical, and laboratory examinations. 3rd ed. Boston: Butterworths; 1990.

7. Chakravarthy V, Ejaz S. Thyroxine-binding globulin deficiency. Treasure Island: StatPearls Publishing; 2019.
8. Fatourechi V. Subclinical hypothyroidism: an update for primary care physicians. Mayo Clin Proc. 2009;84(1):65–71. https://doi.org/10.1016/S0025-6196(11)60809-4.
9. Villar HC, Saconato H, Valente O, Atallah AN. Thyroid hormone replacement for subclinical hypothyroidism. Cochrane Database Syst Rev. 2007;(3):CD003419.
10. Surks MI, Chopra IJ, Mariash CN, Nicoloff JT, Solomon DH. American Thyroid Association guidelines for use of laboratory tests in thyroid disorders. JAMA. 1990;263(11):1529–32.
11. Franklyn JA, Boelaert K. Thyrotoxicosis. Lancet. 2012;379(9821):1155–66. https://doi.org/10.1016/S0140-6736(11)60782-4.
12. Santos Palacios S, Pascual-Corrales E, Galofre JC. Management of subclinical hyperthyroidism. Int J Endocrinol Metab. 2012;10(2):490–6. https://doi.org/10.5812/ijem.3447.
13. Fröhlich E, Wahl R. Thyroid autoimmunity: role of anti-thyroid antibodies in thyroid and extra-thyroidal diseases. Front Immunol. 2017;8:521.
14. Alexander EK, Pearce EN, Brent GA, Brown RS, Chen H, Grobman WA, Laurberg P, Lazarus JH, Mandel SJ, Peeters RP, Sullivan S. 2017 Guidelines of the American Thyroid Association for the diagnosis and management of thyroid disease during pregnancy and the postpartum. Thyroid. 2017;27(3):315–89. https://doi.org/10.1089/thy.2016.0457.
15. Winter WE, Jialal I, Deveraj S. Thyrotropin receptor antibody assays. Am J Clin Pathol. 2013;139(2):140–2. https://doi.org/10.1309/ajcpx5vnauyn8mub.
16. Orgiazzi J, Madec AM. Reduction of the risk of relapse after withdrawal of medical therapy for Graves' disease. Thyroid. 2002;12:849–53.
17. Barbesino G, Tomer Y. Clinical review: clinical utility of TSH receptor antibodies. J Clin Endocrinol Metab. 2013;98(6):2247–55. https://doi.org/10.1210/jc.2012-4309.
18. Leschik JJ, Diana T, Olivo PD, König J, Krahn U, Li Y, Kanitz M, Kahaly GJ. Analytical performance and clinical utility of a bioassay for thyroid-stimulating immunoglobulins. Am J Clin Pathol. 2013;139(2):192–200. https://doi.org/10.1309/AJCPZUT7CNUEU7OP.
19. Jain V, Agarwal R, Deorari AK, Paul VK. Congenital hypothyroidism. Indian J Pediatr. 2008;75:363. https://doi.org/10.1007/s12098-008-0040-7.
20. Büyükgebiz A. Newborn screening for congenital hypothyroidism. J Clin Res Pediatr Endocrinol. 2013;5(Suppl 1):8–12. https://doi.org/10.4274/jcrpe.845.
21. Melmed S, Williams RH. Williams textbook of endocrinology. Philadelphia: Elsevier Saunders; 2011.
22. Zempleni J, Hassan YI, Wikeratne SSK. Biotin and biotinidase deficiency. Expert Rev Endocrinol Metab. 2008;6:715–24. https://doi.org/10.1586/17446651.3.6.715.
23. Burch HB. Drug effects on the thyroid. N Engl J Med. 2019;381:749–61. https://doi.org/10.1056/NEJMra1901214.
24. Li D, Radulescu A, Shrestha RT, et al. Association of biotin ingestion with performance of hormone and nonhormone assays in healthy adults. JAMA. 2017;318(12):1150–60. https://doi.org/10.1001/jama.2017.13705.
25. Cappelli C, Rotondi M, Pirola I, et al. TSH-lowering effect of metformin in type 2 diabetic patients: differences between euthyroid, untreated hypothyroid, and euthyroid on L-T4 therapy patients. Diabetes Care. 2009;32(9):1589–90. https://doi.org/10.2337/dc09-0273.
26. Lupoli R, Di Minno A, Tortora A, Ambrosino P, Lupoli GA. Effects of treatment with metformin on TSH levels: a meta-analysis of literature studies. J Clin Endocrinol Metab. 2014;99(1):143–8. https://doi.org/10.1210/jc.2013-2965.
27. Glinoer D, De Nayer P, Bourdoux P, Lemone M, Robyn C, Van Steirteghem A, Kinthaert J, Lejeune B. Regulation of maternal thyroid during pregnancy. J Clin Endocrinol Metabol. 1990;71(22):276–8. https://doi.org/10.1210/jcem-71-2-276.
28. Nwabuobi C, Arlier S, Schatz F, Guzeloglu-Kayisli O, Lockwood CJ, Kayisli UA. hCG: biological functions and clinical applications. Int J Mol Sci. 2017;18(10):2037. Published 2017 Sept 22. https://doi.org/10.3390/ijms18102037.
29. Chaudhary V, Bano S. Imaging of the thyroid: recent advances. Indian J Endocrinol Metab. 2012;16(3):371–6. https://doi.org/10.4103/2230-8210.95674.
30. Nachiappan AC, Metwalli ZA, Hailey BS, Patel RA, Ostrowski ML, Wynne DM, et al. The thyroid: review of imaging features and biopsy techniques with radiologic-pathologic correlation. Radiographics. 2014;34(2):276–93. https://doi.org/10.1148/rg.342135067.
31. Xie C, Cox P, Taylor N, LaPorte S. Ultrasonography of thyroid nodules: a pictorial review. Insights Imaging. 2016;7(1):77–86. https://doi.org/10.1007/s13244-015-0446-5.
32. Francis GL, Waguespack SG, Bauer AJ, Angelos P, Benvenga S, Cerutti JM, Dinauer CA, Hamilton J, Hay ID, Luster M, Parisi MT, Rachmiel M, Thompson GB, Yamashita S, American Thyroid Association Guidelines Task Force. Management guidelines for children with thyroid nodules and differentiated thyroid cancer. Thyroid. 2015;25(7):716–59. https://doi.org/10.1089/thy.2014.0460.
33. Pelletier-Galarneau M, et al. Reproducibility of radioactive iodine uptake (RAIU) measurements. J Appl Clin Med Phys. 2017;19(1):239–42. https://doi.org/10.1002/acm2.12217.
34. Ke CC, He ZM, Hsieh YJ, et al. Quantitative measurement of the thyroid uptake function of mouse by Cerenkov luminescence imaging. Sci Rep. 2017;7(1):5717. https://doi.org/10.1038/s41598-017-05516-5.
35. Nasr C. Is a serum TSH measurement sufficient to monitor the treatment of primary hypothyroidism? Cleve Clin J Med. 2016;83(8):571–3.
36. Chakera AJ, Pearce SH, Vaidya B. Treatment for primary hypothyroidism: current approaches and future possibilities. Drug Des Devel Ther. 2012;6:1–11. https://doi.org/10.2147/DDDT.S12894.

Calcium, Phosphate, Vitamin D, Parathyroid Hormone, and Alkaline Phosphatase

26

Deborah M. Mitchell

Introduction

Accurate interpretation of laboratory tests of bone and mineral ion metabolism can be challenging, in large part as the reference ranges for many of these tests are quite different in children than in adults. An understanding therefore of what is normal and abnormal for children at different ages is critically important. In addition, calcium and phosphate are regulated by endocrine feedback loops; labs which appear to be "normal" may be inappropriately normal in the face of low or high serum calcium or phosphate.

Calcium

Overview Of the body stores of calcium, 99% are within the skeleton; the remainder is in extracellular fluid with low, though critically important, intracellular concentrations [1].

Measurement Considerations Approximately 50% of circulating calcium is protein-bound, primarily to albumin, while it is the unbound, ionized fraction (iCa) that is under physiologic regulation [2]. Significant deficiency of serum albumin, as in nephrotic syndrome, therefore leads to a lower total serum calcium, while iCa is preserved. Calculations which account for altered serum albumin can generate a "corrected" calcium:

Correcting Total Calcium for Serum Albumin

$$\text{"Corrected"}[\mathrm{Ca}](\mathrm{mg/dL}) = \mathrm{Total}[\mathrm{Ca}](\mathrm{mg/dL}) + (0.8 \times (4.0 - [\mathrm{albumin}(\mathrm{g/dL})]))$$

By altering the affinity of calcium for albumin, acidosis raises the fraction of total calcium which is ionized, while alkalosis lowers the fraction. Direct measurement of ionized calcium is possible but is challenging in the primary care setting, as contact with air, such as in an incompletely filled blood tube or after delayed sample processing, will raise the sample pH and thus lower the iCa concentration. Measurement of iCa may be useful in the critical care setting and in advanced chronic kidney disease, situations in which the "corrected" calcium calculation may be less accurate [3].

Reference Range Serum calcium decreases soon after birth, likely due to immature parathyroid glands, with a nadir at approximately 24 hours of life, a nadir which is more dramatic among premature infants and infants of diabetic mothers [4, 5]. Serum calcium rises over the next several days, and then is slightly higher in the first 1 year of life than in later childhood and adulthood [6] (Fig. 26.1).

Hypocalcemia In the setting of hypocalcemia, the appropriate homeostatic response is a rise in the production and secretion of parathyroid hormone (PTH). Therefore, as detailed in Chap. 5, the finding of a low or inappropriately normal range PTH concentration in the setting of hypocalcemia is evidence of *hypoparathyroidism.* This may be congenital, as in 22q11 deletion syndrome, CHARGE syndrome, or other disorders that affect the development of the parathyroid gland. Congenital hypoparathyroidism is also seen in activating disorders of the calcium-sensing receptor, which effectively decrease the setpoint of circulating calcium. Acquired hypoparathyroidism may be autoimmune, iatrogenic following thyroid or other neck surgery, or infiltrative such as in patients requiring frequent blood transfusions or in Wilson's disease [7].

Hypocalcemia with an appropriately elevated parathyroid hormone is most commonly due to severe dietary calcium deficiency, vitamin D deficiency, or, often, a combination of these two factors [8]. Rare genetic disorders impairing acti-

D. M. Mitchell (✉)
Massachusetts General Hospital, Harvard Medical School, Boston, MA, USA
e-mail: dmmitchell@mgh.harvard.edu

T. Stanley, M. Misra (eds.), *Endocrine Conditions in Pediatrics*, https://doi.org/10.1007/978-3-030-52215-5_26

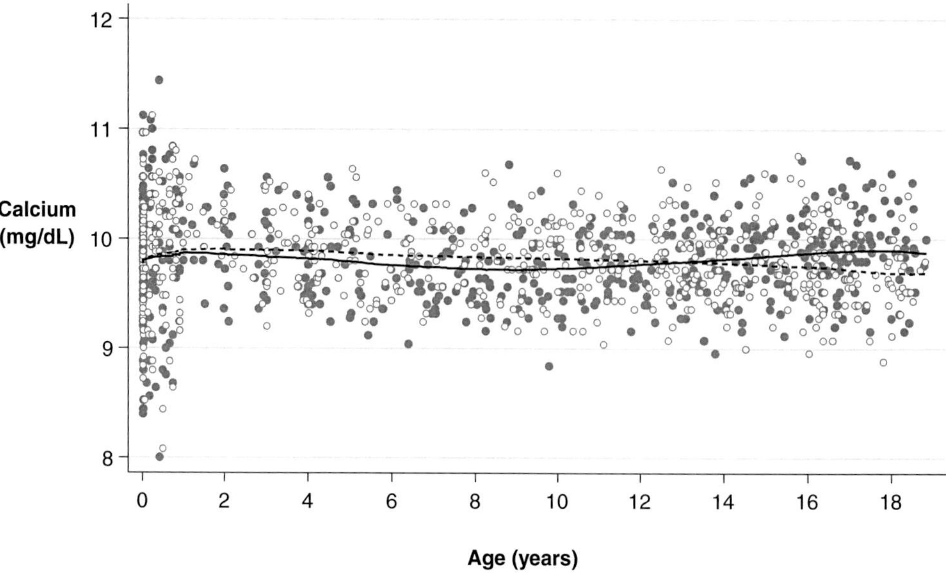

Fig. 26.1 Scatterplot of serum calcium by age. Filled circles, male. Open circles, female. Locally weighted regression lines; solid line, male; dashed line, female. (Adapted from Colantonio et al. [6])

vation of vitamin D or the function of the vitamin D receptor may present similarly [9]. *Pseudohypoparathyroidism* (PHP) is a disorder of impaired signaling downstream of the PTH receptor. In this disorder, circulating PTH is high in the setting of hypocalcemia due to PTH resistance [10]. This disorder can often be distinguished from vitamin D and dietary calcium deficiency by the serum phosphate: phosphate is typically low or low-normal in vitamin D and dietary calcium deficiency due to the effect of elevated PTH to promote renal phosphate excretion, while serum phosphate is elevated in PHP due to resistance to the renal effects of PTH.

Hypercalcemia The appropriate homeostatic response to hypercalcemia is suppression of PTH production and secretion. As detailed in Chap. 6, if PTH is inappropriately normal or frankly elevated in the setting of hypercalcemia, this is consistent with PTH-dependent disease [11]. This may be due to primary hyperparathyroidism from a parathyroid adenoma, either sporadic or associated with a syndrome conferring a predisposition, most commonly multiple endocrine neoplasia syndrome type 1 or 2 [12]. Heterozygous inactivating mutations of the calcium-sensing receptor or mutations in downstream signal transducers lead to *familial hypocalciuric hypercalcemia (FHH)*, which typically presents with a mild and asymptomatic hypercalcemia, low urinary calcium excretion, and high-normal or mildly elevated PTH [13]. Patients taking lithium may also present with hypercalcemia and mildly elevated PTH, thought to be due to inhibition of calcium-sensing receptor activity [14].

If PTH is appropriately suppressed, hypercalcemia can be due to excess vitamin D, either from toxic ingestion or inability to appropriately catabolize vitamin D, as in mutations of the vitamin D 24-hydroxylase [15]. Autonomous production of $1,25(OH)_2$ vitamin D, the activated form of vitamin D, may cause hypercalcemia in granulomatous disease including sarcoidosis, tuberculosis, and subcutaneous fat necrosis of the newborn, and in both Hodgkin and non-Hodgkin lymphoma [16]. Additional causes of hypercalcemia include excess bone turnover as seen in thyrotoxicosis, immobilization, vitamin A toxicity, and malignant bone lesions as well as Williams syndrome.

A summary of typical laboratory findings in various disorders of hypo- and hypercalcemia is shown in Table 26.1. *It is important to note that labs will not always follow the specified pattern, however.*

Phosphate

Overview The human body contains phosphorus in many forms – both as inorganic phosphorus (P_i) and as part of many organic molecules including nucleic acids, phospholipids, and proteins. The majority of extracellular fluid phosphorus is in the form of phosphate (PO_4^{3-}), which is what is measured in standard laboratory assays [17].

Measurement Considerations Redistribution of phosphate from the extracellular fluid into the cytoplasm is stimulated by insulin (either endogenous after carbohydrate ingestion or exogenous), vigorous muscle activity, and respiratory alkalosis. In addition, there is circadian variability of serum phosphate, with a nadir between 8 and 11 am [18]. For these reasons, the measurement of serum phosphate is ideally done early in the morning in the fasting state. If there is clinical concern for hypophosphatemia, serum creatinine, and urine phosphate and creatinine should be measured in tandem with serum phosphate to enable calculation of the tubular reab-

Table 26.1 Usual laboratory findings in various disorders with hypo- or hypercalcemia

	Calcium	Phosphate	PTH	25-OHD	1,25-(OH)$_2$D
Hypocalcemia					
Hypoparathyroidism	↓	↑	↓/↔inapp	Variable	↓/↔
Pseudohypoparathyroidism	↓	↑	↑↑	Variable	↓/↔
Dietary calcium deficiency	↓	↓/↔	↑	Variable	↑
Vitamin D resistance	↓	↓	↑	Variable	↑↑
Vitamin D deficiency	↓/↔	↓/↔	↑	↓	Variable
Hypercalcemia					
Primary hyperparathyroidism	↑	↓	↔inapp/↑	Variable	↔/↑
Vitamin D excess	↑	↔/↑	↓	↑↑	↓/↔
Familial hypocalciuric hypercalcemia	↑	↓/↔	↔inapp/↑	Variable	↔/↑
Granulomatous disease	↑	↔/↑	↓	Variable	↑

[Inapp]indicates that the PTH value is "inappropriate" for the physiology of the condition; for example, a normal PTH during hypercalcemia is considered inappropriately normal

sorption of phosphate (TRP) as shown in the reference box. Urine should be collected in the fasting state and should be from the second void of the day to eliminate variability based on dietary intake.

Reference Box: Calculation of Tubular Reabsorption of Phosphate

$$\left(1-\frac{\dfrac{\text{Urine Phosphate mEq / L}}{\text{Serum Phosphate mEq / L}}}{\dfrac{\text{Urine Creatinine mg / dL}}{\text{Serum Creatinine mg / dL}}}\right)*100$$

Reference range Serum phosphate is physiologically higher in children than in adults; it is therefore vitally important to compare results with age- and sex-specific reference ranges [6]. In particular, serum phosphate is quite high in neonates, likely reflecting renal immaturity, and rapidly declines over the first 2 weeks of life. It then slowly declines over the next few years, remains steady through mid-childhood, and then declines again in late puberty to the adult reference range (Fig. 26.2). Maintaining circulating phosphate in the age-appropriate range is crucial to skeletal health; serum phosphate concentrations in the normal adult range can cause rickets and osteomalacia in children.

Hypophosphatemia In the setting of hypophosphatemia, calculated TRP should be at least 90%, and typically >95%. TRP lower than this threshold implies inappropriate renal phosphate losses. There are several causes of phosphate wasting. Elevations in the two hormones which inhibit renal phosphate reabsorption, parathyroid hormone (PTH) and fibroblast growth factor 23 (FGF23), cause phosphaturia. Elevated PTH is seen in primary hyperparathyroidism and, more commonly, in secondary hyperparathyroidism due to dietary calcium or vitamin D deficiency. Elevated FGF23 is the cause of hypophosphatemia in several rare conditions including *X-linked hypophosphatemic rickets, autosomal dominant hypophosphatemic rickets, fibrous dysplasia*, and *tumor-induced osteomalacia* [19]. Nonendocrine causes of phosphaturia include nonspecific proximal tubule dysfunction (*Fanconi syndrome*) and rare mutations in the sodium-phosphate transporters which mediate renal phosphate reabsorption (*hereditary hypophosphatemic rickets with hypercalciuria*).

If TRP is appropriately elevated, hypophosphatemia may be due to low GI intake, such as in severe malnutrition. Importantly, in very premature infants, rapid skeletal mineralization may outstrip the phosphorus content of total parenteral nutrition, unfortified breast milk, or standard formulas, leading to metabolic bone disease of prematurity [20]. Use of antacids containing calcium, magnesium, or aluminum can cause hypophosphatemia by binding phosphate in the intestines, and chronic diarrhea can interfere with phosphorus absorption. Intracellular redistribution, or transport of phosphate from the extracellular fluid into the cytoplasm, can occur in refeeding syndrome, recovery from diabetic ketoacidosis, respiratory alkalosis, and in conditions leading to rapid cell turnover including hungry bone syndrome and treatment of anemia.

Hyperphosphatemia Elevated serum phosphate can be the result of impaired renal clearance, excess gastrointestinal absorption, or redistribution from the intracellular space to extracellular fluid. Impaired renal clearance can occur in severe renal failure but can also be due to insufficient PTH (*hypoparathyroidism*) [7] or PTH resistance (*pseudohypoparathyroidism*) [10]. Impaired renal clearance is also seen with several rare mutations that lower FGF23 concentration

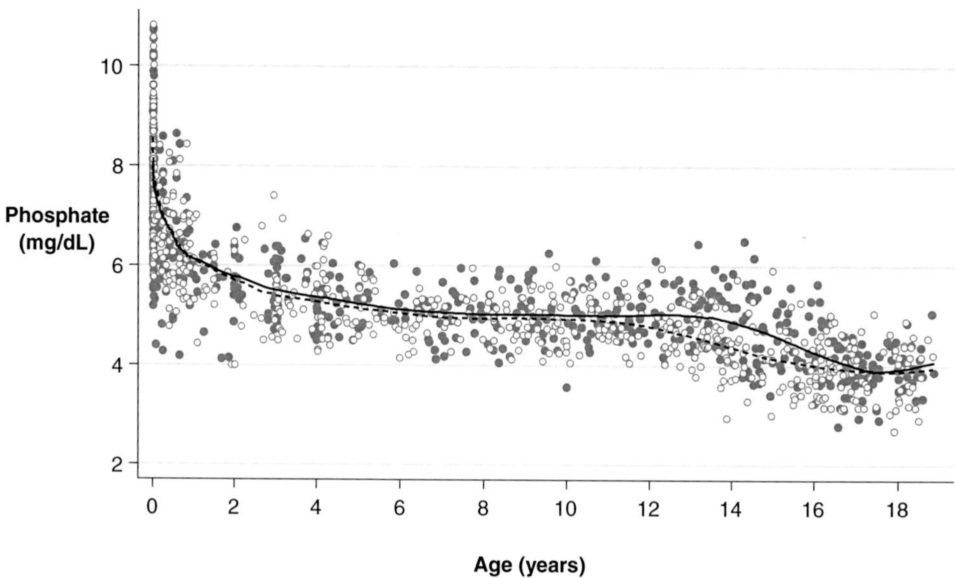

Fig. 26.2 Scatterplot of serum phosphate by age. Filled circles, male. Open circles, female. Locally weighted regression lines; solid line, male; dashed line, female. (Adapted from Colantonio et al. [6])

or activity (*familial tumoral calcinosis*) [21]. Excess gastrointestinal intake is rare but can be seen with the use of phosphate-containing enemas, leading to Food and Drug Administration guidance to avoid use in children under age 2 years and to use with caution in children under age 5 years [22]. Redistribution into the extracellular space is seen in the setting of overwhelming cell breakdown such as in tumor lysis syndrome or rhabdomyolysis, as well as in metabolic acidosis including diabetic ketoacidosis.

Vitamin D

Overview The production of vitamin D in the skin is catalyzed by exposure to ultraviolet light, which generates vitamin D_3 (cholecalciferol). Naturally occurring dietary sources of vitamin D_3 include fish oils, organ meats, and egg yolk, and certain mushrooms contain vitamin D_2 (ergocalciferol). In the United States, many dairy products and cereals are supplemented with vitamin D; supplementation practices vary in other parts of the world. Vitamin D is required to optimize dietary calcium absorption. Data from preclinical and clinical studies suggest that vitamin D may have extraskeletal health benefits as well [23].

Measurement Considerations The best index of vitamin D availability is circulating 25-hydroxyvitamin D (25OHD), a vitamin D metabolite produced in the liver with a half-life of 2–3 weeks. 25OHD may be measured by an immunoassay which reports total 25OHD or by liquid chromatography/mass spectrometry which distinguishes $25OHD_2$ and $25OHD_3$. The total 25OHD is calculated as the sum of the two isoforms. 1,25-dihydroxyvitamin D ($1,25(OH)_2D$) has a half-life of 4–6 hours and is tightly regulated by PTH and by serum phosphate to rapidly respond to changing mineral ion demand [24]. Measurement of this metabolite is rarely required in the primary care setting but may be useful in the evaluation of rare metabolic bone diseases.

Reference Range The threshold which defines vitamin D sufficiency remains controversial. The Institute of Medicine (IOM) advised that a 25OHD concentration of 20 ng/mL is sufficient to support bone health in the general population [25] (IOM report), and a recent consensus guideline of pediatric specialists concurred with this threshold [26]. However, other organizations including the Endocrine Society recommend a higher target of 30 ng/mL, particularly among patients known to be at risk of low bone mineral density and fractures [27]. The safe upper limit of circulating 25OHD also remains poorly defined. The IOM points to concern for adverse events at serum concentrations >50 ng/mL, while the Endocrine Society guidelines suggest a safe upper limit of 100 ng/mL [25, 27].

Low Vitamin D Causes of low vitamin D include low cutaneous synthesis of vitamin D, low vitamin D intake or absorption, and increased vitamin D catabolism. Cutaneous vitamin D synthesis depends on ultraviolet light absorption; thus, people with deeply pigmented skin produce less vitamin D than those with less pigmentation. Less time spent outdoors and clothing styles with less exposed skin are also associated with low circulating vitamin D. Decreased vitamin D intake is seen among infants who are exclusively breastfed without vitamin D supplementation, those with allergies, and those with restricted diets including children with autism [28]. Infants born to mothers with vitamin D deficiency are at a particular risk of low 25OHD due to a high correlation of maternal and cord blood 25OHD [29]. Impaired vitamin D absorption is a result of disorders associated with steatorrhea including inflammatory bowel disease, cystic fibrosis, and celiac disease. Medications that induce cytochrome p450 enzymes increase the catabolism of 25OHD; these include several antiepileptic medications (phenobarbital, phenytoin, carbamazepine, and primidone) as well as rifampin [30, 31].

Elevated Vitamin D Cutaneous synthesis of vitamin D does not lead to vitamin D excess as previtamin D_3 is converted to inactive metabolites after prolonged ultraviolet exposure [32]. Vitamin D toxicity has been reported with high-dose supplementation, including during treatment of rickets as well as due to excessive intake due to dosing errors and manufacturing errors [33].

Parathyroid Hormone

Overview Parathyroid hormone (PTH) is a peptide hormone that regulates serum ionized calcium (iCa). Given this, the interpretation of circulating PTH depends on the ambient iCa [34].

Measurement Considerations The standard laboratory PTH assay, sometimes referred to as the "second-generation" or "intact" assay, is a two-site assay designed to measure full-length PTH, in contrast to older assays which also detected PTH fragments [35]. Because the second-generation assay does detect very large C-terminal fragments which may accumulate in renal failure, a "third-generation" or "biointact" assay has been developed; however, the clinical utility of this assay has not been well established [36].

Elevated PTH The interpretation of elevated PTH in the context of hypo- and hypercalcemia is discussed above. Elevated PTH with *normal* calcium may be secondary to conditions in which there is insufficient calcium intake or excess loss; the PTH in these cases rises as a homeostatic response to protect the serum calcium. Secondary hyperparathyroidism is thus seen with dietary calcium deficiency, vitamin D deficiency, and renal hypercalciuria [37]. Secondary hyperparathyroidism is also seen in chronic kidney disease, as a homeostatic response to rising serum phosphate [38]. Rarely, mild primary hyperparathyroidism may present with normal calcium and elevated PTH in adults [39]; the extent to which this occurs in children remains unknown.

Low PTH The interpretation of low PTH in the context of hypo- and hypercalcemia is discussed above. Low PTH with normal calcium can be seen as an acute response following calcium ingestion [40]. Whether mild hypoparathyroidism can present with this constellation of laboratory values remains unclear [41].

Alkaline Phosphatase

Overview While alkaline phosphatase (ALP) is produced in many tissues, circulating ALP derives primarily from the skeleton (osteoblasts and hypertrophic chondrocytes) and the liver [42]. While these two isoforms can be differentiated based on their post-translational modifications in specialized assays, standard laboratory testing measures the sum of all circulating isoforms of ALP. In the skeleton, ALP functions to cleave pyrophosphate, an inhibitor of calcium and phosphate crystallization, thereby regulating bone formation and mineralization [43].

Reference Range Due to bone growth and thus higher production of bone-specific alkaline phosphatase in childhood, serum ALP activity is physiologically higher in children than in adults. ALP activity is particularly high in early infancy, decreases slightly in childhood, and then rises again during the pubertal growth spurt, before decreasing to adult levels in late adolescence (Fig. 26.3). Due to these dynamic changes in ALP production, age- and sex-specific reference ranges have been constructed, and it is critically important for clinicians caring for children to ensure that they are comparing results to appropriate reference ranges to prevent misinterpretation of results [6, 44].

Low Alkaline Phosphatase Activity Low ALP activity may be seen in several conditions including celiac disease, hypothyroidism, undernutrition, glucocorticoid use, vitamin C deficiency, Wilson's disease, Zn^{2+} deficiency, and Mg^{2+} deficiency. Low ALP is also the hallmark of *hypophosphatasia*, a rare disorder caused by a mutation in the gene encoding tissue nonspecific ALP [45]. In its most severe perinatal and infantile forms, hypophosphatasia presents with rickets-like bony deformities, poor growth, profound muscle weakness, and craniosynostosis, and may be fatal in the perinatal period. Milder childhood forms may present with premature deciduous tooth loss (before age 5 years), bone pain, muscle weakness with delayed attainment of gross motor milestones and a waddling gait, or short stature. Measurement of serum pyridoxal 5′-phosphate (elevated in hypophosphatasia) or genetic testing can help confirm this diagnosis.

Elevated Alkaline Phosphatase Activity Elevated ALP may derive from either excess bone production or cholestatic liver disease [46]. Concomitant measurement of other liver-derived enzymes including gamma-glutamyl transpeptidase (GGTP) can help determine if ALP is of hepatic origin, as GGTP typically rises along with hepatic ALP in cholestasis. Elevated ALP of skeletal origin can be seen in conditions of increased bone turnover including healing fractures, bone tumors, hyperthyroidism, hyperparathyroidism, and osteomalacia (often associated with rickets). Rarely, intestinal

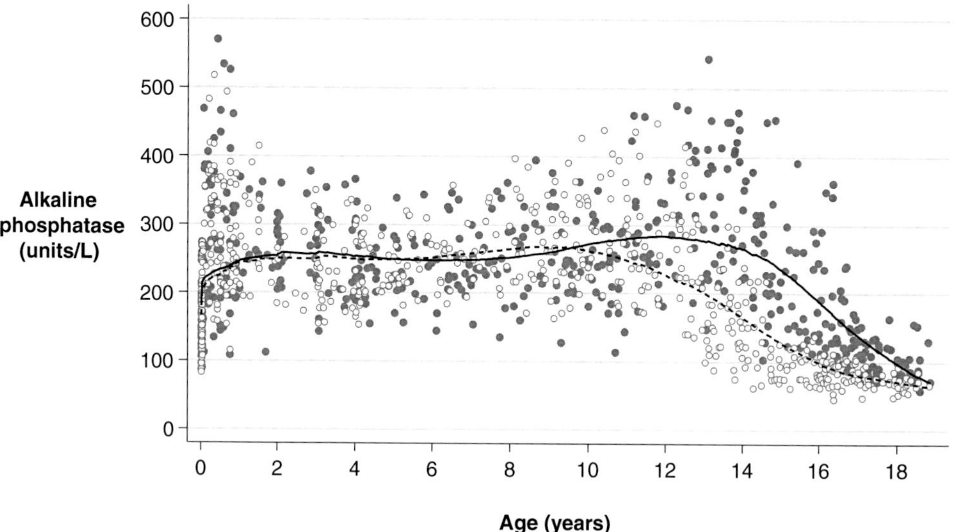

Fig. 26.3 Scatterplot of serum alkaline phosphatase by age. Filled circles, male. Open circles, female. Locally weighted regression lines; solid line, male; dashed line, female. (Adapted from Colantonio et al. [6])

ALP may contribute significantly to circulating ALP concentrations, particularly after a high-fat meal among people with blood types O and B. Placental ALP is also detected in standard assays, leading to slightly elevated concentrations during the third trimester of pregnancy.

Elevated ALP is also observed in *transient hyperphosphatasemia*, a benign condition observed in children under 5 years old, with a prevalence of 3–6% in two recent cross-sectional studies [44, 47]. In most cases, ALP activity is elevated at least five-fold over the upper limit of normal, and may be of skeletal, hepatic, or mixed origin [48]. Affected children have no clinical or laboratory evidence of hepatic or skeletal disease including normal GGT, 25OHD, PTH, calcium, and phosphate concentrations [47]. The pathophysiology of this condition remains unclear but may involve impaired clearance of circulating alkaline phosphatase. While few studies have systematically evaluated the natural history of transient hyperphosphatasemia, a literature review reported a median time to resolution of 10 weeks [49].

References

1. Bringhurst FR, Demay MB, Kronenberg HM. Hormones and disorders of mineral metabolism. In: Melmed S, editor. Williams textbook of endocrinology. 14th ed. Philadelphia: Elsevier, Inc; 2019. p. 1196–255.
2. Walser M. Ion association. VI. Interactions between calcium, magnesium, inorganic phosphate, citrate and protein in normal human plasma. J Clin Invest. 1961;40:723–30.
3. Calvi LM, Bushinsky DA. When is it appropriate to order an ionized calcium? J Am Soc Nephrol. 2008;19(7):1257–60.
4. David L, Anast CS. Calcium metabolism in newborn infants. The interrelationship of parathyroid function and calcium, magnesium, and phosphorus metabolism in normal, "sick," and hypocalcemic newborns. J Clin Invest. 1974;54(2):287–96.
5. Mitchell DM, Juppner H. Regulation of calcium homeostasis and bone metabolism in the fetus and neonate. Curr Opin Endocrinol Diabetes Obes. 2010;17(1):25–30.
6. Colantonio DA, Kyriakopoulou L, Chan MK, Daly CH, Brinc D, Venner AA, Pasic MD, Armbruster D, Adeli K. Closing the gaps in pediatric laboratory reference intervals: a CALIPER database of 40 biochemical markers in a healthy and multiethnic population of children. Clin Chem. 2012;58(5):854–68.
7. Mannstadt M, Bilezikian JP, Thakker RV, Hannan FM, Clarke BL, Rejnmark L, Mitchell DM, Vokes TJ, Winer KK, Shoback DM. Hypoparathyroidism. Nat Rev Dis Primers. 2017;3:17080.
8. Carpenter TO, Shaw NJ, Portale AA, Ward LM, Abrams SA, Pettifor JM. Rickets. Nat Rev Dis Primers. 2017;3:17101.
9. Malloy PJ, Feldman D. Genetic disorders and defects in vitamin d action. Endocrinol Metab Clin North Am. 2010;39(2):333–46, table of contents.
10. Mantovani G, Bastepe M, Monk D, de Sanctis L, Thiele S, Usardi A, Ahmed SF, Bufo R, Choplin T, De Filippo G, Devernois G, Eggermann T, Elli FM, Freson K, Garcia Ramirez A, Germain-Lee EL, Groussin L, Hamdy N, Hanna P, Hiort O, Juppner H, Kamenicky P, Knight N, Kottler ML, Le Norcy E, Lecumberri B, Levine MA, Makitie O, Martin R, Martos-Moreno GA, Minagawa M, Murray P, Pereda A, Pignolo R, Rejnmark L, Rodado R, Rothenbuhler A, Saraff V, Shoemaker AH, Shore EM, Silve C, Turan S, Woods P, Zillikens MC, Perez de Nanclares G, Linglart A. Diagnosis and management of pseudohypoparathyroidism and related disorders: first international Consensus Statement. Nat Rev Endocrinol. 2018;14(8):476–500.
11. Stokes VJ, Nielsen MF, Hannan FM, Thakker RV. Hypercalcemic disorders in children. J Bone Miner Res. 2017;32(11):2157–70.
12. Kollars J, Zarroug AE, van Heerden J, Lteif A, Stavlo P, Suarez L, Moir C, Ishitani M, Rodeberg D. Primary hyperparathyroidism in pediatric patients. Pediatrics. 2005;115(4):974–80.
13. Pollak MR, Brown EM, Chou YH, Hebert SC, Marx SJ, Steinmann B, Levi T, Seidman CE, Seidman JG. Mutations in the human Ca(2+)-sensing receptor gene cause familial hypocalciuric hypercalcemia and neonatal severe hyperparathyroidism. Cell. 1993;75(7):1297–303.
14. McKnight RF, Adida M, Budge K, Stockton S, Goodwin GM, Geddes JR. Lithium toxicity profile: a systematic review and meta-analysis. Lancet. 2012;379(9817):721–8.

15. Schlingmann KP, Kaufmann M, Weber S, Irwin A, Goos C, John U, Misselwitz J, Klaus G, Kuwertz-Broking E, Fehrenbach H, Wingen AM, Guran T, Hoenderop JG, Bindels RJ, Prosser DE, Jones G, Konrad M. Mutations in CYP24A1 and idiopathic infantile hypercalcemia. N Engl J Med. 2011;365(5):410–21.
16. Tebben PJ, Singh RJ, Kumar R. Vitamin D-mediated hypercalcemia: mechanisms, diagnosis, and treatment. Endocr Rev. 2016;37(5):521–47.
17. Imel EA, Carpenter TO. A practical clinical approach to paediatric phosphate disorders. Endocr Dev. 2015;28:134–61.
18. Kemp GJ, Blumsohn A, Morris BW. Circadian changes in plasma phosphate concentration, urinary phosphate excretion, and cellular phosphate shifts. Clin Chem. 1992;38(3):400–2.
19. Bergwitz C, Juppner H. FGF23 and syndromes of abnormal renal phosphate handling. Adv Exp Med Biol. 2012;728:41–64.
20. Backstrom MC, Kuusela AL, Maki R. Metabolic bone disease of prematurity. Ann Med. 1996;28(4):275–82.
21. Topaz O, Shurman DL, Bergman R, Indelman M, Ratajczak P, Mizrachi M, Khamaysi Z, Behar D, Petronius D, Friedman V, Zelikovic I, Raimer S, Metzker A, Richard G, Sprecher E. Mutations in GALNT3, encoding a protein involved in O-linked glycosylation, cause familial tumoral calcinosis. Nat Genet. 2004;36(6):579–81.
22. Mendoza J, Legido J, Rubio S, Gisbert JP. Systematic review: the adverse effects of sodium phosphate enema. Aliment Pharmacol Ther. 2007;26(1):9–20.
23. Rosen CJ, Adams JS, Bikle DD, Black DM, Demay MB, Manson JE, Murad MH, Kovacs CS. The nonskeletal effects of vitamin D: an Endocrine Society scientific statement. Endocr Rev. 2012;33(3):456–92.
24. Fraser DR, Kodicek E. Regulation of 25-hydroxycholecalciferol-1-hydroxylase activity in kidney by parathyroid hormone. Nat New Biol. 1973;241(110):163–6.
25. Institute of Medicine. Dietary reference intakes for calcium and vitamin D. Washington, DC: National Academies Press; 2011.
26. Munns CF, Shaw N, Kiely M, Specker BL, Thacher TD, Ozono K, Michigami T, Tiosano D, Mughal MZ, Makitie O, Ramos-Abad L, Ward L, DiMeglio LA, Atapattu N, Cassinelli H, Braegger C, Pettifor JM, Seth A, Idris HW, Bhatia V, Fu J, Goldberg G, Savendahl L, Khadgawat R, Pludowski P, Maddock J, Hypponen E, Oduwole A, Frew E, Aguiar M, Tulchinsky T, Butler G, Hogler W. Global consensus recommendations on prevention and management of nutritional rickets. J Clin Endocrinol Metab. 2016;101(2):394–415.
27. Holick MF, Binkley NC, Bischoff-Ferrari HA, Gordon CM, Hanley DA, Heaney RP, Murad MH, Weaver CM. Evaluation, treatment, and prevention of vitamin D deficiency: an Endocrine Society clinical practice guideline. J Clin Endocrinol Metab. 2011;96(7):1911–30.
28. Ward LM, Gaboury I, Ladhani M, Zlotkin S. Vitamin D-deficiency rickets among children in Canada. CMAJ. 2007;177(2):161–6.
29. Bouillon R, Van Baelen H, De Moor P. 25-hydroxyvitamin D and its binding protein in maternal and cord serum. J Clin Endocrinol Metab. 1977;45(4):679–84.
30. Gough H, Bissesar A, Goggin T, Higgins D, Baker M, Crowley M, Callaghan N. Factors associated with the biochemical changes in vitamin D and calcium metabolism in institutionalized patients with epilepsy. Ir J Med Sci. 1986;155(6):181–9.
31. Wang Z, Lin YS, Zheng XE, Senn T, Hashizume T, Scian M, Dickmann LJ, Nelson SD, Baillie TA, Hebert MF, Blough D, Davis CL, Thummel KE. An inducible cytochrome P450 3A4-dependent vitamin D catabolic pathway. Mol Pharmacol. 2012;81(4):498–509.
32. Holick MF, MacLaughlin JA, Doppelt SH. Regulation of cutaneous previtamin D3 photosynthesis in man: skin pigment is not an essential regulator. Science. 1981;211(4482):590–3.
33. Vogiatzi MG, Jacobson-Dickman E, DeBoer MD, Drugs, Therapeutics Committee of the Pediatric Endocrine Society. Vitamin D supplementation and risk of toxicity in pediatrics: a review of current literature. J Clin Endocrinol Metab. 2014;99(4):1132–41.
34. Brown EM. Extracellular Ca2+ sensing, regulation of parathyroid cell function, and role of Ca2+ and other ions as extracellular (first) messengers. Physiol Rev. 1991;71(2):371–411.
35. Segre GV. Advances in techniques for measurement of parathyroid hormone: current applications in clinical medicine and directions for future research. Trends Endocrinol Metab. 1990;1(5):243–7.
36. Boudou P, Ibrahim F, Cormier C, Chabas A, Sarfati E, Souberbielle JC. Third- or second-generation parathyroid hormone assays: a remaining debate in the diagnosis of primary hyperparathyroidism. J Clin Endocrinol Metab. 2005;90(12):6370–2.
37. Eastell R, Arnold A, Brandi ML, Brown EM, D'Amour P, Hanley DA, Rao DS, Rubin MR, Goltzman D, Silverberg SJ, Marx SJ, Peacock M, Mosekilde L, Bouillon R, Lewiecki EM. Diagnosis of asymptomatic primary hyperparathyroidism: proceedings of the third international workshop. J Clin Endocrinol Metab. 2009;94(2):340–50.
38. Wesseling-Perry K, Salusky IB. Chronic kidney disease: mineral and bone disorder in children. Semin Nephrol. 2013;33(2):169–79.
39. Schini M, Jacques RM, Oakes E, Peel NFA, Walsh JS, Eastell R. Normocalcemic hyperparathyroidism: study of its prevalence and natural history. J Clin Endocrinol Metab. 2020;105(4):dgaa084.
40. Deroisy R, Zartarian M, Meurmans L, Nelissenne N, Micheletti MC, Albert A, Reginster JY. Acute changes in serum calcium and parathyroid hormone circulating levels induced by the oral intake of five currently available calcium salts in healthy male volunteers. Clin Rheumatol. 1997;16(3):249–53.
41. Cusano NE, Maalouf NM, Wang PY, Zhang C, Cremers SC, Haney EM, Bauer DC, Orwoll ES, Bilezikian JP. Normocalcemic hyperparathyroidism and hypoparathyroidism in two community-based nonreferral populations. J Clin Endocrinol Metab. 2013;98(7):2734–41.
42. Millan JL, Whyte MP. Alkaline phosphatase and hypophosphatasia. Calcif Tissue Int. 2016;98(4):398–416.
43. Millan JL. The role of phosphatases in the initiation of skeletal mineralization. Calcif Tissue Int. 2013;93(4):299–306.
44. Ridefelt P, Gustafsson J, Aldrimer M, Hellberg D. Alkaline phosphatase in healthy children: reference intervals and prevalence of elevated levels. Horm Res Paediatr. 2014;82(6):399–404.
45. Whyte MP. Hypophosphatasia – aetiology, nosology, pathogenesis, diagnosis and treatment. Nat Rev Endocrinol. 2016;12(4):233–46.
46. Shipman KE, Holt AD, Gama R. Interpreting an isolated raised serum alkaline phosphatase level in an asymptomatic patient. BMJ. 2013;346:f976.
47. Huh SY, Feldman HA, Cox JE, Gordon CM. Prevalence of transient hyperphosphatasemia among healthy infants and toddlers. Pediatrics. 2009;124(2):703–9.
48. Kraut JR, Metrick M, Maxwell NR, Kaplan MM. Isoenzyme studies in transient hyperphosphatasemia of infancy. Ten new cases and a review of the literature. Am J Dis Child. 1985;139(7):736–40.
49. Gualco G, Lava SA, Garzoni L, Simonetti GD, Bettinelli A, Milani GP, Provero MC, Bianchetti MG. Transient benign hyperphophatasemia. J Pediatr Gastroenterol Nutr. 2013;57(2):167–71.

27 Gonadotropins, Gonadal Steroids, SHBG, and Related Labs

Seth Tobolsky and Takara Stanley

General Principles for Measuring Gonadotropins, Sex Steroids, and Related Hormones

The physiology of the mini-puberty of infancy and adolescent puberty is directly relevant to the measurement of gonadotropins and sex steroids.

- In infancy:
  - Males: Testosterone is high at day 1 of life but drops substantially by day 2 and begins to rise again around 1–2 weeks, reflecting the "mini-puberty" of infancy, which ends around 6 months of life in males. *The optimal time to measure gonadotropins and testosterone in a male infant is thus between 2 weeks and about 4 months of life*. Outside of that window, low or undetectable values do not necessarily indicate pathology.
  - Females: Mini-puberty lasts longer in girls, approximately 9–12 months, with measurable FSH for 2 years or more. The timing of laboratory evaluation is not as restrictive as in males but should *ideally be done within the first 9 months of life*, as low or undetectable values outside that window do not necessarily indicate pathology.
- In adolescent puberty:
  - *Labs should be sent in the morning whenever possible for both males and females*. This is because the hypothalamic–pituitary–gonadal axis is primarily active overnight during the early stages of puberty.
  - *Undetectable gonadotropins do not exclude early puberty*. LH is pulsatile, and an undetectable level at any given time does not exclude the possibility that a child is in puberty. On the other hand, an LH $\geq$ 0.3 mIU/mL along with clinical signs of puberty is generally a reliable indicator of pubertal onset [1].

S. Tobolsky (✉)
Massachusetts General Hospital for Children, Boston, MA, USA
e-mail: seth.tobolsky@mgh.harvard.edu

T. Stanley
Division of Pediatric Endocrinology, Massachusetts General Hospital and Harvard Medical School, Boston, MA, USA
e-mail: tstanley@mgh.harvard.edu

Hormones of the HPG Axis

Gonadotropin-Releasing Hormone: Not Clinically Measurable

Pulsatile release of GnRH from GnRH-secreting neurons in the hypothalamus drives the pulsatile release of gonadotropic hormones (LH and FSH) from the anterior pituitary. Serum quantities are extremely low, and the measurement of GnRH is not used clinically. Continuous release of GnRH inhibits the release of gonadotropins from the pituitary.

Luteinizing Hormone (LH)

This is one of two gonadotropins released from pituitary gonadotrophs in response to pulsatile GnRH. *In males,* the pulsatile release of LH directly stimulates Leydig cells of the testis, leading to the synthesis and secretion of testosterone. *In females,* pulsatile LH stimulates the theca cells, stimulating the production of ovarian androgens (which are aromatized to estrogen in granulosa cells). The mid-cycle LH surge during the menstrual cycle is followed by ovulation and subsequently "luteinization" of the dominant follicle into the corpus luteum, which in turn secretes progesterone, necessary to sustain a pregnancy.

Assay Considerations for LH

- An ideal assay for pediatric use will be sensitive/ultrasensitive with a lower limit of detection $\leq$0.1 mIU/mL.
- The reference range is dependent on biological sex, days of life/age, and timepoint during the menstrual cycle.

T. Stanley, M. Misra (eds.), *Endocrine Conditions in Pediatrics*, https://doi.org/10.1007/978-3-030-52215-5_27

- Blood samples for LH should be sent in the morning whenever feasible.
- During early puberty, undetectable levels do not exclude pubertal activity, whereas LH ≥ 0.3 mIU/mL is generally a reliable indicator of pubertal onset [1].

Follicle-Stimulating Hormone (FSH)

This is the other gonadotropin released from pituitary gonadotrophs in response to pulsatile GnRH. *In males,* release of FSH directly stimulates Sertoli cells of the testis, leading to expression of various protein products and activation of cell signaling pathways that promote spermatogenesis and other male reproductive functions. *In females*, FSH binds to receptors on granulosa cells in ovarian follicles and promotes growth and development of these follicles. Ultimately, one follicle will develop into the dominant follicle, which will then release its oocyte in response to the LH surge.

Assay Considerations for FSH

- An ideal assay for pediatric use will be sensitive/ultrasensitive with a lower limit of detection ≤0.1 mIU/mL.
- The reference range is dependent on biological sex, days of life/age, and timepoint during the menstrual cycle.
- The half-life of FSH in serum is longer than that of LH, such that the timing of sampling is less critical.

Gonadal/Sex Steroid Hormones

Testosterone

Testosterone is secreted by the Leydig cells of the testes and theca cells of the ovaries in response to LH. Much of the circulating testosterone is bound tightly to sex-hormone-binding globulin (SHBG). The remaining testosterone in the serum (~35%) is either free testosterone (unbound) or weakly bound to albumin.

Assay Considerations for Testosterone

- Reference ranges differ by age and sex. For newborns, gestational age and postnatal age determine the reference range. After 1 year of life, reference ranges change every 1–2 years of life until age 18.
- The gold standard for the measurement of *total testosterone* is via *isotope dilution mass spectroscopy.*
- The gold standard for the measurement of *free testosterone* is via *equilibrium dialysis or ultrafiltration.*
- At the time of this writing, *most labs use immunoassays for measurement of total and free testosterone unless gold-standard methods are available and specifically requested.* For this reason, standard measures of total testosterone can be inaccurate in females and adolescents, since assay performance is often calibrated for adult male levels. Further, *immunoassay-based measures of free testosterone can be inaccurate in both males and females.*
- Because of the above, we recommend the measurement of *total testosterone and sex hormone-binding globulin.* Unless gold standard free testosterone assays are available, this provides a better approximation of bioavailable testosterone [2, 3]. Bioavailable testosterone calculators, or "free androgen index" calculators, are available online and are sometimes provided by labs, with the Vermeulen equation [3] being one of the most widely used and well-validated [2].

Dihydrotestosterone (5′-DHT)

DHT is formed from testosterone by 5-alpha-reductase in peripheral tissues. Its synthesis is impaired in 5-alpha-reductase deficiency syndrome, one of a class of syndromes leading to presentation with ambiguous genitalia. *Circulating levels of DHT do not necessarily correspond to local tissue levels, and measurement of DHT is generally confined to circumstances in which 5-alpha-reductase deficiency is suspected.* With suspicion of 5-alpha reductase deficiency, the testosterone-to-DHT ratio is investigated, both basally and after human chorionic gonadotropin (HCG) stimulation testing. There is not a single agreed-upon diagnostic cutoff for this ratio, with ratios of higher than 10-to-1 generally being considered diagnostic.

Estrogens: Estrone (E1), Estradiol (E2), Estriol (E3)

Estrone, primarily produced in peripheral tissues through aromatization of androstenedione from the adrenal, is the predominant form of estrogen in men and post-menopausal women. Estradiol, primarily produced in the ovary from aromatization of testosterone, is the predominant circulating estrogen in premenopausal women. Estriol is most prominent during pregnancy, as it is synthesized by the placenta.

Assay Considerations for Estrogens

- Estradiol is generally the most clinically useful measurement.
- Estrone may be clinically helpful in certain clinical circumstances but is not routinely used.
- Estriol is generally not measured outside of pregnancy.

- *High-sensitivity estradiol* assays are needed for evaluation of early puberty and may need to be specifically requested.
- The reference range for estrogens depends on biological sex, age, and timing in the menstrual cycle. Ranges for pre-menopausal and post-menopausal women are also different.

Progesterone

Progesterone is primarily released by the corpus luteum in the luteal phase of the menstrual cycle. Except for individuals in the luteal phase or those who are pregnant, circulating levels are generally low and are not clinically helpful. Reference ranges are dependent on biological sex, menstrual phase, menopausal status, and trimester of pregnancy. The day 19–21 progesterone can provide information regarding ovulatory vs. non-ovulatory cycles.

Sex Hormone-Binding Globulin (SHBG)

Most circulating testosterone is bound to SHBG. Measurement of SHBG along with total testosterone allows for the estimation of bioavailable testosterone, which is more accurate than immunoassays for free testosterone. Norms for SHBG are age- and sex-specific. For interpretation, it is also important to understand conditions that elevate or diminish circulating SHBG levels, as shown in Table 27.1.

Alpha-Subunit and hCG Beta-Subunit

Alpha-Subunit

The same alpha-subunit is common to FSH, LH, TSH, beta-hCG, and MSH (melanocyte-stimulating hormone). The alpha-subunit is not commonly sent, but it can be useful in the workup of a child suspected to have a non-functioning or TSH-secreting pituitary tumor, both of which may result in an elevated circulating alpha-subunit. The reference range depends on months/years of life, biological sex, and menopausal status.

Table 27.1 Conditions that alter SHBG [4]

Increase SHBG	Decrease SHBG
Estrogen use (greatest from oral administration, particularly with ethinyl estradiol)	Hyperinsulinism/insulin resistance (insulin suppresses SHBG)
Pregnancy	Androgen excess/testosterone use
Hyperthyroidism	Hypothyroidism
Cirrhosis/chronic significant liver disease	Hyperprolactinemia
Phenobarbital, phenytoin, carbamazepine	Growth hormone excess (gigantism/acromegaly)

Beta-hCG (Human Chorionic Gonadotropin)

Beta-hCG is primarily produced by the placenta and has a diverse range of functions in maintaining pregnancy. Serum beta-hCG may also be elevated in multiple pregnancies, hyperemesis during pregnancy, molar pregnancy, and certain malignancies, including choriocarcinoma of the placenta, ovary, or testis, and germ cell tumors. A normal serum beta-hCG does not rule out a germ cell tumor in children, but an elevated value outside of pregnancy in an adolescent is suggestive of possible germ cell tumor.

Anti-Müllerian Hormone (AMH) and Inhibin B

Anti-Müllerian Hormone

AMH is secreted by the Sertoli cells of the developing testis as well as the granulosa cells of the ovaries. In utero, it promotes regression of the Müllerian ducts (structures that would ultimately develop into a uterus/cervix/vagina) and stabilization of the Wolffian ducts (structures that would develop into the male analogs). Normal levels are age- and sex-specific. AMH has the following clinical utility in pediatrics:

- In the evaluation of atypical genitalia in infants (see Chap. 12), an AMH level in the normal male range is an indicator of functioning testicular tissue.
- AMH levels may also be used as a marker of functioning gonadal tissue in younger males for whom there may be a question of testicular failure or anorchia.
- AMH levels are lower in females than males and serve as a marker of ovarian reserve. In girls with suspected ovarian failure due to alkylating agents or other causes, a low AMH supports this diagnosis.
- AMH is elevated in polycystic ovary syndrome, but, at the time of this writing, AMH is not in routine use for the diagnosis of PCOS.

Inhibin B

Inhibin B is also synthesized by Sertoli cells of the testes and the granulosa cells of the ovary. In addition to age- and sex-dependent norms, the inhibin B reference range depends on the menstrual phase, as Inhibin B is primarily synthesized in early developing follicles. In pediatrics, Inhibin B is used most commonly in the evaluation of boys with delayed puberty, in whom Inhibin B can be used in combination with gonadotropins to help differentiate constitutional delay of growth and development versus idiopathic hypogonadotropic hypogonadism [5].

Interpretation of Lab Results

Table 27.2 provides a guide to the interpretation of lab results. The first step in thinking about the results is generally to determine whether LH and FSH are elevated or suppressed, as discussed in the Clinical Key.

Table 27.2 Usual lab findings in common diagnostic scenarios

Diagnosis	Gonadotropins	Gonadal steroid	Other findings
Atypical genitalia			
Androgen insensitivity	High/normal	Testosterone very high	Female phenotype in complete androgen insensitivity syndrome, intermediate phenotype in partial androgen insensitivity syndrome
Aromatase deficiency (46,XX)	High	Testosterone high, estrogen low/ undetectable	AMH in female range, ultrasound may show polycystic ovaries due to elevated FSH
Hypopituitarism	Low/ low-normal	Low/low-normal	Other pituitary hormone deficiencies, mid-line abnormalities, hypoglycemia
Early puberty			
Central precocious puberty	Pubertal range	Pubertal range	Early signs of puberty; in males, pubertal testicular size concordant with pubertal exam.
Peripheral precocious puberty	Suppressed	Pubertal range	Early signs of puberty. In males, small testes discordant with remainder of pubertal exam. Differential diagnosis includes congenital adrenal hyperplasia, exposure to exogenous androgens, and McCune Albright syndrome, in which there could also be hyperthyroidism, café au lait macules, fibrous dysplasia.
Familial male limited precocious puberty (LH-receptor activating mutation)	Suppressed	Pubertal range	Smaller than expected, firm testes discordant with remainder of pubertal exam
Delayed or stalled puberty, or secondary amenorrhea			
Turner syndrome	Elevated	Low/low-normal	Usually low AMH. Wide-spaced nipples, shield chest, wide carrying angle, webbed neck, short stature
Klinefelter syndrome	Elevated	Low/low-normal	Tall stature; small, firm testes; gynecomastia. Delayed puberty is *not* characteristic but pubertal stalling may occur.
Premature ovarian failure	Elevated	Low	AMH low. 21-hydroxylase antibodies often but not always positive in autoimmune causes. Fragile X premutation may be present.
Functional hypothalamic hypogonadism (includes hypothalamic amenorrhea)	Low/ low-normal	Low/low-normal	Underlying systemic disease, low weight, and/or several hours of strenuous physical activity per week. Clinical diagnosis and diagnosis of exclusion.
Idiopathic hypogonadotropic hypogonadism	Low/ low-normal	Low	In males, low LH response to gonadotropin-releasing hormone (GnRH) or GnRH agonist and low Inhibin B support diagnosis
Polycystic ovary syndrome	LH:FSH usually >2:1	Normal estrogen, high-normal or elevated testosterone	Suppressed or low-normal SHBG; prolactin may be very mildly elevated; adrenal androgens may be elevated

Patients will not uniformly fit these descriptions, however, and clinical judgment should always be primary

Clinical Key: Hypogonadism

In hypogonadism, assessment of LH, FSH, and the sex-appropriate gonadal steroid (estrogen and testosterone) level is critical to determine if the issue is primary/gonadal, in which case FSH and LH will be elevated and the gonadal steroid low or low-normal, versus a secondary/hypothalamic-pituitary issue, in which FSH and LH will be low or normal in the setting of reduced gonadal steroid levels.

References

1. Harrington J, Palmert MR, Hamilton J. Use of local data to enhance uptake of published recommendations: an example from the diagnostic evaluation of precocious puberty. Arch Dis Child. 2014;99(1):15–20.
2. Fiers T, Wu F, Moghetti P, Vanderschueren D, Lapauw B, Kaufman JM. Reassessing free-testosterone calculation by liquid chromatography-tandem mass spectrometry direct equilibrium dialysis. J Clin Endocrinol Metab. 2018;103(6):2167–74.
3. Vermeulen A, Verdonck L, Kaufman JM. A critical evaluation of simple methods for the estimation of free testosterone in serum. J Clin Endocrinol Metab. 1999;84(10):3666–72.
4. Selby C. Sex hormone binding globulin: origin, function and clinical significance. Ann Clin Biochem. 1990;27(Pt 6):532–41.
5. Coutant R, Biette-Demeneix E, Bouvattier C, Bouhours-Nouet N, Gatelais F, Dufresne S, et al. Baseline inhibin B and anti-Mullerian hormone measurements for diagnosis of hypogonadotropic hypogonadism (HH) in boys with delayed puberty. J Clin Endocrinol Metab. 2010;95(12):5225–32.

Sodium, Osmolality, and Antidiuretic Hormone

28

Luz E. Castellanos

Introduction

Endocrinopathies that disrupt water homeostasis are complex and differential diagnosis can be challenging, as an abnormal water balance can result from a variety of disorders. Appropriate diagnosis relies on clinical observation and proper laboratory evaluation. This section reviews relevant labs and their interpretations as well as the next steps in addressing abnormal values.

Polyuria and Polydipsia

When concerned for an endocrinopathy like diabetes insipidus, it is necessary to initially confirm that the patient truly has polyuria. Polyuria is defined as one of the following: urine output greater than 2 L/m^2/day, 150 ml/kg/ day in neonates, 100–110 ml/kg/day in children up to age 2, and 40–50 ml/kg/day in older children. It is also important to quantify liquid intake and assess for polydipsia resulting from thirst. Children with excessive thirst often exhibit a preference for water, whereas children with excessive consumption of juice or other sugary beverages may be driven by taste or other behavioral issues rather than thirst. One must ask how polyuria and polydipsia interfere with normal activities, including if behaviors are nocturnal, and whether there is a possibility of a psychosocial component (see also Chap. 55).

Once polyuria or polydipsia is established, the next step is to obtain first-morning labs ideally after the child has discontinued drinking including serum osmolality, urinary osmolality, serum sodium, potassium, calcium, glucose, blood urea nitrogen (BUN), and urinalysis [1, 2]. *Appropriate interpretation of these labs requires simultaneous measurement of both urine and serum samples.*

L. E. Castellanos (✉)
Pediatric Endocrine Division, Massachusetts General Hospital and Harvard Medical School, Boston, MA, USA
e-mail: Lcastellanos2@mgh.harvard.edu

Serum and Urine Osmolality

Sodium, glucose, and blood urea nitrogen (BUN) are the primary contributors to serum osmolality under normal physiologic conditions. With known concentrations of these three compounds, *calculated serum osmolality* can be estimated by (2 * Serum Na + Serum glucose + BUN), with all concentrations in mmol/L or by ([2 * Serum Na in mmol/L] + [Serum glucose in mg/dL/18] + [BUN in mg/dL/18]). When calculated serum osmolality differs from the measured serum osmolality by more than 10 mOsm/kg, this "gap" indicates the presence of another osmotically active compound in circulation, such as ketones, ethanol, or toxins like ethylene glycol.

In the urine, sodium, urea, potassium, and chloride are the primary contributors to osmolality under normal physiologic conditions, with glucose also contributing significantly if glucosuria is present. Urine osmolality is considered a more precise measurement than urine specific gravity, discussed below, although the two are highly correlated when urine has a neutral pH and is "clean" from other substances such as protein, ketones, and bilirubin [3].

Diabetes insipidus is generally characterized by high or high-normal serum sodium and serum osmolality in the presence of hypotonic urine osmolality (see Table 28.1). A serum osmolality greater than 300 mOsm/kg at the same time of urine osmolality less than 300 mOsm/kg is reflective of diabetes insipidus due to inappropriately dilute urine. In contrast, a urine osmolality of greater than 600 mOsm/kg in the setting of normal serum osmolality (<300 mOsm/kg) confirms adequate water reabsorption in the kidneys and strongly suggests against diabetes insipidus. If serum osmolality is greater than 300 mOsm/kg and urine osmolality is less than 600 mOsm/kg, the result is indeterminate and a water deprivation test should be the next step in confirmation of diabetes insipidus diagnosis as discussed in Chap. 55 [1, 2].

In cases of syndrome of inappropriate antidiuretic hormone secretion (SIADH), urine osmolality is usually inappropriately concentrated (greater than 100 mOsm/kg) in the presence of hypotonic serum osmolality (less than

T. Stanley, M. Misra (eds.), *Endocrine Conditions in Pediatrics*, https://doi.org/10.1007/978-3-030-52215-5_28

Table 28.1 Key facts reference box

Diabetes insipidus
May be hypovolemic due to polyuria >2 L/m^2/day Serum osmolality >300 mOsm/kg in the presence of urine osmolality <300 mOsm/kg Hypernatremia in the presence of dilute urine *Next steps: water deprivation test (see Part III)*
SIADH
Clinical euvolemia Serum osmolality <275 mOsm/kg in the presence of urine osmolality >100 mOsm/kg Urinary sodium >40 mmol/L Hyponatremia in the presence of inappropriately concentrated urine *Next steps: fluid restriction (consult with endocrinology)*

275 mOsm/kg, see Table 28.1) [4, 5]. Treatment with fluid restriction is typically preferred and should be performed in consultation with a pediatric endocrinologist or nephrologist.

Sodium

A sodium level assessment and a volume status assessment can also be helpful in obtaining a diagnosis. In patients with hypovolemia and hypernatremia (>145 mmol/L), diabetes insipidus should be suspected [1]. Conversely, hyponatremia (<135 mmol/L) with clinical euvolemia should raise concerns for SIADH [4]. Urinary sodium >40 mmol/L with normal dietary salt intake further suggests SIADH [5].

In the interpretation of serum sodium, it is important to remember that both severe hypertriglyceridemia and severe hypercholesterolemia can cause "pseudohyponatremia" in some types of sodium assays, in which the reported serum sodium concentration is falsely low due to incorrect quantification of the water content of the sample. Additionally, hyperglycemia causes osmotic shifts of water extracellularly, temporarily lowering serum sodium concentrations without lowering total body sodium. A "corrected" sodium concentration can be calculated using the formula: [measured Na] + [1.6 * (serum glucose in mg/dL – [6])].

Urine Specific Gravity

Urine specific gravity can also be helpful in endocrine evaluation although one must keep in mind that the result can be affected by the size of particles in the urine and variations in urine pH. Urine specific gravity is normally between 1.001 and 1.035. A low urine specific gravity helps support the diagnosis of diabetes insipidus or primary polydipsia [7, 8].

Serum Antidiuretic Hormone and Copeptin

Serum concentrations of antidiuretic hormone (ADH, also called vasopressin, arginine vasopressin, or AVP) will not generally be useful in the primary care setting. Measurement of serum ADH is challenging due to several factors, including a very short half-life, small molecular size, instability in plasma or serum, and a high level of binding to platelets [9]. ADH assays are thus difficult and time-consuming and are generally used only in the setting of a water deprivation test (see Chap. 55), in which measurement of ADH may help differentiate central versus nephrogenic DI, with the former having low ADH levels and the latter having very high levels due to resistance at the level of the kidney.

Copeptin, which is part of the precursor peptide of ADH, is secreted along with ADH in equimolar amounts and shows promise as an emerging diagnostic marker for DI. Copeptin has a larger size, greater stability, and longer half-life in serum [9], facilitating easier and more accurate measurement in serum compared to ADH. Although there is limited commercial availability of the copeptin assay at the time of this writing, and pediatric protocols are not well-validated, copeptin is likely to emerge in the next few years as an important diagnostic tool, with very high baseline levels suggestive of nephrogenic DI and levels following diagnostic infusion of hypertonic saline able to distinguish between DI and primary polydipsia.

Excluding Other Causes

Primary polydipsia is a common cause of polyuria, as discussed in Chap. 55. Polyuria can also be caused by osmotic diuresis as most commonly seen in diabetes mellitus, which results in glycosuria [10]. A normal blood glucose value and urinalysis can help rule this out. Other causes of osmotic diuresis include urea and sodium. A urea diuresis can occur in patients recovering from acute kidney injury, whereas sodium diuresis is typically secondary to saline fluid administration or recovery from urinary tract obstruction [11–13]. In these cases, it is necessary to determine specific testing from the history. One should also evaluate for renal abnormalities (e.g. intrinsic renal disease) by measuring BUN and serum creatinine. Hypokalemia and hypercalcemia can also cause polyuria and induce nephrogenic diabetes insipidus [14, 15]. These electrolyte abnormalities should be corrected prior to proceeding with central diabetes insipidus evaluation.

References

1. Sperling M, editor. Pediatric endocrinology. 4th ed. Philadelphia: Elsevier/Saunders; 2014. 1061 p.
2. Di Iorgi N, Morana G, Napoli F, Allegri AEM, Rossi A, Maghnie M. Management of diabetes insipidus and adipsia in the child. Best Pract Res Clin Endocrinol Metab. 2015;29(3):415–36.
3. Imran S, Eva G, Christopher S, Flynn E, Henner D. Is specific gravity a good estimate of urine osmolality? J Clin Lab Anal. 2010;24(6):426–30.
4. Jones DP. Syndrome of inappropriate secretion of antidiuretic hormone and hyponatremia. Pediatr Rev. 2018;39(1):27–35.
5. Ellison DH, Berl T. The syndrome of inappropriate antidiuresis. N Engl J Med. 2007;356(20):2064–72.
6. Penne EL, Thijssen S, Raimann JG, Levin NW, Kotanko P. Correction of serum sodium for glucose concentration in hemodialysis patients with poor glucose control. Diabetes Care. 2010;33(7):e91.
7. Andropoulos DB. Appendix B: pediatric normal laboratory values. In: Gregory GA, Andropoulos DB, editors. Gregory's pediatric anesthesia [Internet]. Oxford: Wiley-Blackwell; 2011. [cited 2019 Nov 6]. p. 1300–14. Available from: http://doi.wiley.com/10.1002/9781444345186.app2.
8. Simerville JA, Maxted WC, Pahira JJ. Urinalysis: a comprehensive review. Am Fam Physician. 2005;71(6):1153–62.
9. Fenske WK, Schnyder I, Koch G, Walti C, Pfister M, Kopp P, et al. Release and decay kinetics of copeptin vs AVP in response to osmotic alterations in healthy volunteers. J Clin Endocrinol Metabol. 2018;103(2):505–13.
10. Ferrannini E. Learning from glycosuria: FIG. 1. Diabetes. 2011;60(3):695–6.
11. Drummer C, Heer M, Baisch F, Blomqvist CG, Lang RE, Maass H, et al. Diuresis and natriuresis following isotonic saline infusion in healthy young volunteers before, during, and after HDT. Acta Physiol Scand Suppl. 1992;604:101–11.
12. Ghazali S, Barratt TM. Sodium excretion after relief of urinary tract obstruction in children. Br J Urol. 1974;46(2):163–7.
13. Lindner G, Schwarz C, Funk G-C. Osmotic diuresis due to urea as the cause of hypernatraemia in critically ill patients. Nephrol Dial Transplant. 2012;27(3):962–7.
14. Berl T, Linas SL, Aisenbrey GA, Anderson RJ. On the mechanism of polyuria in potassium depletion. J Clin Investig. 1977;60(3):620–5.
15. Goldfarb S, Agus ZS. Mechanism of the polyuria of hypercalcemia. Am J Nephrol. 1984;4(2):69–76.

Adrenal Steroids, Adrenocorticotropic Hormone, and Plasma Renin Activity

29

Marwa Tuffaha

Glucocorticoids

Cortisol, the primary active glucocorticoid, is synthesized and secreted from the adrenal cortex in response to adrenocorticotropic hormone (ACTH) produced by the pituitary gland. ACTH is secreted in response to corticotropin-releasing hormone (CRH) from the neurons in the paraventricular nucleus of the hypothalamus. The same neurons also produce antidiuretic hormone (ADH, also known as arginine vasopressin or AVP). In response to stress, both CRH and ADH travel down the axons of the median eminence into the pituitary and stimulate the production and release of ACTH, which stimulates the uptake of cholesterol and its conversion to steroidal products. The principal pathway of adrenal steroid hormone synthesis is shown in Fig. 29.1.

Considerations for Measurement of Cortisol

Types of Measurement

Cortisol is most commonly measured in serum (*serum cortisol*). It is important to recognize that this is a *total* cortisol measurement, which quantifies both the small fraction of circulating "free" cortisol, unbound to protein carriers, and the much larger fraction of circulating cortisol that is bound to cortisol-binding globulin (CBG, also known as transcortin) or to a lesser extent, albumin.

Other measures of cortisol are *salivary cortisol*, in which free cortisol is quantified from a saliva sample extracted from a "salivette" provided by the patient, usually late at night, and *24-hour urine-free cortisol*. Both of these assays measure free cortisol and both are used in the evaluation for Cushing's syndrome (see Chap. 50).

M. Tuffaha (✉)
Pediatric Endocrine Division, Massachusetts General Hospital and Harvard Medical School, Boston, MA, USA
e-mail: mtuffaha@mgh.harvard.edu

Timing of Measurement

Cortisol is secreted in pulses throughout the day; however, pulse amplitude is much greater in the morning than at other times of the day. ACTH levels usually peak between 4 and 6 AM, resulting in peak cortisol levels at about 8 AM; cortisol levels reach nadir around 11 PM to midnight. This diurnal rhythm does not begin to be established until 3–12 months of age. Physical stress can increase section of ACTH and thus cortisol, such that ACTH and cortisol secretion in an emergent setting, such as severe illness should already be maximal.

The diurnal rhythm of cortisol has important implications with respect to the timing of testing. To assess for adrenal insufficiency, cortisol should be drawn in the morning, ideally at 8 AM, to take advantage of the peak level at that time. A low cortisol during other times of the day is not necessarily indicative of insufficiency. In contrast, patients with Cushing's syndrome lose the diurnal rhythm of cortisol, making late-night cortisol testing diagnostically useful in that setting. Both late-night serum and salivary cortisol levels, which should be low in healthy individuals, can be useful in the diagnosis of Cushing's syndrome, as further described in Chap. 50.

Infants (<12 months of age) may not yet have established a diurnal rhythm of cortisol secretion. In infants <3 months old, random cortisol levels can be used, followed by ACTH stimulation testing if necessary (see below). Infants between 3 and 12 months of age may or may not have established the diurnal rhythm, such that sending a morning cortisol may be helpful if it is robust but will not be definitive if it is low.

Interference by Other Medications or Physiologic States

Administration of exogenous glucocorticoids will decrease cortisol secretion due to a negative feedback loop. Megestrol acetate, used for appetite stimulation, also suppresses cortisol secretion. Depending on the cortisol assay, the different exogenous corticosteroids may or may not be quantified in the assay. For example, exogenous hydrocortisone is typi-

T. Stanley, M. Misra (eds.), *Endocrine Conditions in Pediatrics*, https://doi.org/10.1007/978-3-030-52215-5_29

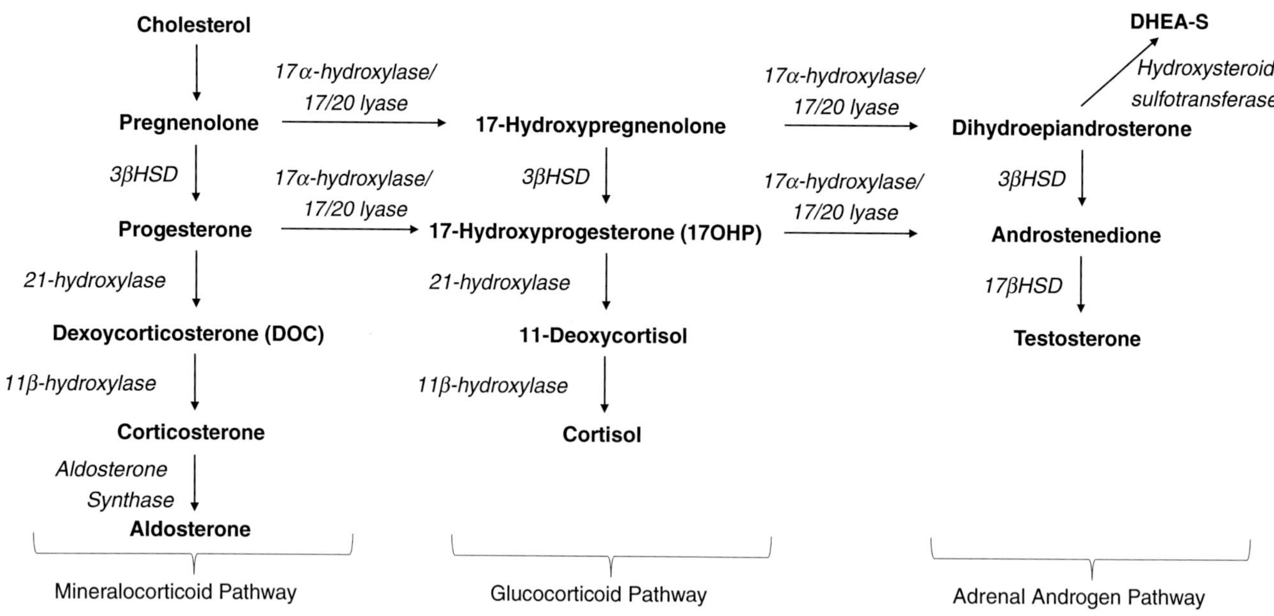

Fig. 29.1 Adrenal steroid synthesis pathways. Abbreviations: 3βHSD, 3-beta hydroxysteroid dehydrogenase type 2; 17βHSD, 17-beta hydroxysteroid dehydrogenase; DHEA-S, dehydroepiandrosterone sulfate

cally reflected in a serum cortisol measurement, whereas exogenous dexamethasone is not. For patients receiving exogenous glucocorticoids, discussing the specific assay with the lab is critical to correctly interpret results.

Patients on ketoconazole, megestrol acetate, mitotane, or metyrapone may have low serum cortisol levels, as all of these medications interfere with cortisol biosynthesis.

Because the serum measurement of cortisol quantifies total cortisol, medications or physiologic states that increase cortisol-binding globulin increase the serum cortisol level, whereas medications or physiologic states that decrease cortisol-binding globulin will decrease the serum cortisol level. *CBG is increased* in pregnancy, hyperthyroidism, and in individuals using oral estrogen (including combined hormonal contraceptives [COC]). *CBG is decreased* in individuals with a critical illness, cirrhosis/liver failure, hypothyroidism, and nephrotic syndrome. In addition, infants generally have relatively low levels of CBG, such that low random serum cortisol levels do not necessarily indicate adrenal insufficiency.

Assay Considerations

Cortisol is measured either by immunoassay or liquid chromatography–tandem mass spectrometry (LC–MS/MS), with LC–MS/MS being a more reliable and valid measure. Serum cortisol has traditionally been measured with immunoassay, and our current thresholds for determining adrenal sufficiency are based on immunoassay. Immunoassay lacks specificity; measuring some cortisol-like compounds in addition to cortisol itself results in serum cortisol values that are likely higher than the true value [1]. Consequently, "normal" cortisol values from LC–MS/MS may be lower than those defined by immunoassay. At the time of this writing, there are not agreed-upon changes to the diagnostic thresholds for cortisol by LC–MS/MS, but this general principle should be kept in mind when interpreting results from LC–MS/MS.

Recommendations for Testing and Interpretation of Serum Cortisol Measurement

Based on the considerations above, recommendations for assessment and interpretation of cortisol *in children ≥1 year old* are as follows:

- A random cortisol measurement is generally not clinically helpful.
- An 8 AM cortisol level is a good first step in assessing adrenal sufficiency:
  - 8 AM cortisol >10 mcg/dL is reassuring for adrenal sufficiency.
  - 8 AM cortisol <5 mcg/dL in the context of symptoms/signs suggestive of adrenal insufficiency is of concern and should prompt an ACTH stimulation test.
  - 8 AM cortisol between 5 and10 mcg/dL is generally considered indeterminant and may require further testing and/or clinical follow-up depending on clinical suspicion.
- Levels must be interpreted with caution in individuals who may have alterations in CBG, including girls on oral estrogen/combined oral contraceptives. When possible, girls should stop COC a few weeks prior to testing.
- In the setting of severe acute illness, for example, acute presentation to the emergency department, "random" cortisol can be sent along with ACTH, as these are expected to be maximally stimulated values. These should be

treated similarly to morning cortisol values, with equivocal values followed up by stimulation testing.

Considerations for *infants*, as discussed above, are the use of random cortisol in infants <3 months of age and use of morning cortisol in older infants. In both cases, values must be interpreted with caution because the infant's diurnal rhythm may not yet be established and CBG levels may be relatively low. ACTH stimulation testing may be necessary.

ACTH Stimulation Testing

Because of the pulsatile release of cortisol, morning values or values during critical illness may not be sufficient to definitively establish diagnoses. In these cases, an ACTH stimulation test or corticotropin test is performed to assess the capacity for cortisol secretion. After baseline blood sampling, synthetic ACTH is administered, with follow-up blood sampling at 30–60 minutes. Although a comprehensive review of ACTH stimulation testing is beyond the scope of this discussion, brief guidelines are presented below.

"High-Dose" Stimulation Testing

A conventional or "high-dose" stimulation test is recommended for the diagnosis of primary adrenal insufficiency, congenital adrenal hyperplasia, and in some circumstances, other types of adrenal insufficiency. In this test, baseline ACTH and cortisol are obtained followed by administration of IV corticotropin: 250 mcg for children ≥2 years old, 125 mcg for children ages 1–2 years, and 15 mcg/kg for infants [2].

For the diagnosis of primary adrenal insufficiency, follow-up serum cortisol levels are obtained at 60 minutes, and peak cortisol levels <18 mcg/dL are considered diagnostic of adrenal insufficiency, although norms for LC–MS/MS may be somewhat lower.

For the evaluation of congenital adrenal hyperplasia, various panels of intermediate steroid precursors are also sent depending on the type of CAH suspected. (This should be done by or in consultation with a pediatric endocrinologist.) The goal of the test is to stimulate steroidogenesis, which results in the accumulation of all steroids proximal to the enzymatic block.

In 21-hydroxylase deficiency (21-OHD), responsible for up to 95% of all CAH cases, the conversion of 17α-hydroxyprogesterone (17-OHP), the main substrate of 21-hydroxylase, to 11-deoxycortisol is impaired and precursors are shunted down the pathway of androgen biosynthesis. The diagnosis of classic 21-OHD is based upon a very high serum concentration of 17-OHP. Most affected neonates have random concentrations greater than 3500 ng/dL (105 nmol/L), and nearly all have concentrations greater than 1200 ng/dL (36 nmol/L). If newborn screening raises concern for CAH, this should be followed with a random 17-OHP sent to the laboratory and electrolytes. If the 17-OHP level remains high, immediate referral to a pediatric endocrinologist is warranted for further management. If the random 17-OHP level is not diagnostic, an ACTH stimulation test can help make the diagnosis by the detection of extremely high concentrations of stimulated 17-OHP.

"Low-Dose" Stimulation Testing

For the diagnosis of secondary adrenal insufficiency, that is, dysfunction of CRH or ACTH secretion, a "low-dose" ACTH test is thought to be more sensitive than conventional/high-dose testing. This test is quite similar to the standard/high-dose test, except that the dose of corticotropin is typically 1 mcg, and the cortisol value is obtained at 30 minutes (although data now suggest that adding sampling at 15 and 60 minutes may increase the sensitivity of the test). For situations in which the origin of suspected adrenal insufficiency is uncertain, some centers perform low-dose testing followed by high-dose testing as follows: (1) baseline cortisol and ACTH samples; (2) 1 mcg IV corticotropin at 0 minutes; (3) cortisol sample at 30 minutes; (4) high-dose IV corticotropin at 30 minutes; and (5) repeat serum cortisol sampling at 60 and/or 90 minutes.

The diagnostic threshold of 18mcg/dL is currently the same for both low-dose and high-dose testing, although clinical judgment is important based on the pretest probability of adrenal insufficiency, the method of testing, and the assay used for cortisol.

It should also be noted that patients with new-onset secondary adrenal insufficiency may respond normally to ACTH stimulation testing. A "failed" response to testing in secondary adrenal insufficiency depends on adrenal atrophy due to lack of ACTH stimulation, which takes time to develop.

Mineralocorticoids: The Renin–Angiotensin–Aldosterone System (RAAS)

Mineralocorticoid (aldosterone) release is determined by the renin–angiotensin system and, to a lesser extent, by ACTH. Decreases in vascular volume result in increased secretion of renin by the renal juxtaglomerular apparatus. Renin cleaves angiotensin into angiotensin I, which is then converted into angiotensin II by angiotensin-converting enzyme. Angiotensin II both increases sodium reabsorption in the proximal convoluted tubule and stimulates the release of aldosterone. Aldosterone causes renal sodium retention, potassium excretion, and a resulting increase in intravascular volume and blood pressure.

Measurement of electrolytes (discussed in Chap. 28) is the first step in evaluating an appropriately functioning RAAS. If mineralocorticoid deficiency or excess is suspected based on electrolytes, measurement of plasma renin

Table 29.1 Laboratory findings of congenital adrenal hyperplasia

Enzyme deficiency	Presentation	Laboratory finding
21-Hydroxylase deficiency	Classic form: Includes salt wasting and simple virilizing subtypes: Females present with ambiguous genitalia Non-classic form: Premature adrenarche, polycystic ovary syndrome	↑ 17OH before and after stimulation testing ↑ serum androgens ↓ mineralocorticoids ↑ ACTH and PRA
11β-Hydroxylase deficiency	Female ambiguous genitalia; hypertension	↑ DOC, 11-deoxycortisol ↑ serum androgens ↑ACTH and ↓PRA
17-Alpha-hydroxylase deficiency	Ambiguous genitalia in males; suboptimal feminization during puberty in females; hypertension	↑ DOC, corticosterone ↓ serum androgens ↑ mineralocorticoids ↑ ACTH and ↓PRA
3-Beta-hydroxysteroid dehydrogenase deficiency	Ambiguous genitalia in males and females	↑ DHEA, 17-hydroxypregnenolone ↓ serum androgens (in males) ↓ mineralocorticoids ↑ ACTH and PRA

17OHP 17-hydroxyprogesterone, *DOC* deoxycorticosterone, *DHEA* dehydroepiandrosterone

activity and aldosterone are useful next steps in diagnosis. Assessment of the mineralocorticoid axis is also critical in cases of suspected CAH; typical lab findings in various types of CAH are shown in Table 29.1.

Plasma Renin Activity

Rather than measuring renin directly in circulation, the more common assay is plasma renin activity (PRA), in which the renin in the patient's plasma is allowed to act on the plasma's endogenous angiotensinogen to generate Angiotensin I, which is subsequently measured by either immunoassay or liquid chromatography–tandem mass spectrometry (LC–MS/MS). Elevated PRA in the setting of hyponatremia and/or hyperkalemia is consistent with aldosterone deficiency. PRA is elevated in 21-OHD CAH, whereas it is low in some less common forms of CAH that are accompanied by excessive production of aldosterone precursors that have mineralocorticoid activity. PRA may also be used to monitor the sufficiency of mineralocorticoid dosing in CAH. In that setting, elevated PRA may indicate insufficient dosing, whereas suppressed PRA may indicate excessive dosing. Patient posture during testing, concomitant medication use, and sodium consumption are the primary considerations in the interpretation of PRA. Norms for age, sex, and body position should be used, and patients may need to discontinue medications that affect the RAAS.

Aldosterone

Aldosterone may be measured in serum or with 24-hour urine collections. Like PRA, aldosterone concentrations vary substantially depending on patient posture, sodium intake, and concomitant medications. In pediatric endocrinology, serum aldosterone levels are sent primarily to confirm aldosterone deficiency in cases of adrenal insufficiency and congenital adrenal hyperplasia. Norms for age, sex, and body position should be used, and patients may need to discontinue medications that affect the RAAS.

Adrenal Androgens

The zona reticularis secretes androgen precursors [e.g., dehydroepiandrosterone (DHEA), dehydroepiandrosterone sulfate (DHEA-S), and androstenedione] that can be peripherally converted to testosterone. After the newborn period, the concentration of the androgen precursors falls until the onset of adrenarche.

In the clinical setting, adrenal androgens are measured for evaluation of possible congenital adrenal hyperplasia, polycystic ovary syndrome, or androgen-secreting tumors. DHEA has a very short half-life and is sulfated into the much more stable DHEA-S, which is the predominant form in circulation. For this reason, *serum measurement of DHEA-S is generally performed in lieu of DHEA*. Pediatric endocrinologists generally send both DHEA-S and androstenedione to assess adrenal androgens, although the two are well correlated and measurement of DHEA-S may be sufficient in some contexts.

Plasma ACTH

In conjunction with serum cortisol measurements, plasma ACTH may be useful in differentiating between primary and secondary adrenal insufficiency or in a separate clinical context between pituitary versus ectopic Cushing's syndrome (see Chap. 50). ACTH is generally measured by immunoassay, and normal ranges are assay-specific. The assay is subject to interference by heterophile antibodies, and values that do not fit the clinical context should prompt a conversation with the lab and/or measurement in another laboratory.

In cortisol deficiency, the appropriate pituitary response is increased secretion of ACTH due to the absence of negative feedback by cortisol. Thus, low cortisol with markedly elevated ACTH is consistent with primary adrenal insufficiency, whereas low cortisol with low or low-normal ACTH values is suggestive of secondary adrenal insufficiency.

In cortisol excess, the appropriate pituitary response is decreased secretion of ACTH due to excessive negative feedback by cortisol. Thus, cortisol excess, simultaneous with elevated or normal plasma ACTH, is consistent with pituitary Cushing disease or an ectopic source of ACTH or CRH production, while cortisol excess with a suppressed plasma ACTH is consistent with an adrenal cause of hypercortisolemia (further testing is described in Chap. 50).

References

1. El-Farhan N, Aled Rees D, Evans C. Measuring cortisol in serum, urine, and saliva – are our assays good enough? Ann Clin Biochem. 2017;54(3):308–22.
2. Bornstein SR, Allolio B, Arlt W, et al. Diagnosis and treatment of primary adrenal insufficiency: an endocrine society clinical practice guideline. J Clin Endocrinol Metab. 2016;101:364–89.

30 Labs Related to Glucose Metabolism and Diabetes

Rachel Whooten

This chapter addresses laboratory studies used in (1) diagnosis of diabetes, (2) initial evaluation of diabetes, and (3) long-term monitoring of glycemic control and risk of ketosis in diabetes.

Initial Laboratory Evaluation for Diabetes

Diabetes and prediabetes diagnosis and screening may be performed through either plasma glucose levels [fasting plasma glucose or 2-hour plasma glucose following an oral glucose tolerance test (OGTT)] or hemoglobin A1c. The diagnostic criteria for each test are shown in Table 30.1. While these tests are equally appropriate, each test has different advantages and disadvantages as outlined below (Table 30.2). Diabetes is diagnosed when two tests are abnormal in an asymptomatic individual or when hyperglycemia is noted in an individual with classic signs of diabetes (e.g., polyuria, polydipsia, and weight loss). It is important to note that there is not perfect concordance between these tests for diagnosing diabetes [1].

Table 30.1 Criteria for the diagnosis of diabetes and prediabetes [1]

		Diabetes	Prediabetes
2 of the following	Fasting plasma glucose	≥126 mg/dL (7.0 mmol/L)	100 mg/dL (5.6 mmol/L) to 125 mg/dL (6.9 mmol/L) *(Impaired Fasting Glucose)*
	or		
	2-hour plasma glucose[a]	≥200 mg/dL (11.1 mmol/L)	140 mg/dL (7.8 mmol/L) to 199 mg/dL (11.0 mmol/L) *(Impaired Glucose Tolerance)*
	or		
	A1C	≥6.5% (>47 mmol/mol)	5.7–6.4% (39–47 mmol/mol)
	Random plasma glucose	≥200 mg/dL (11.1 mmol/L) *with* classic symptoms of diabetes	

[a]OGTT should be performed as described by WHO, with 75 g of anhydrous glucose dissolved in water [20]

Hemoglobin A1C

Red blood cells are freely permeable to glucose, which allows for the formation of stable hemoglobin components containing glucose or glycated hemoglobin. Hemoglobin A1c (HgbA1c or HbA1c) measurement reflects this and provides an estimate of glycemic control over the prior 3 months, reflecting the average red blood cell lifespan of 120 days [2]. HgbA1c values are more highly influenced by glycemia during the month right before the test and much less so by circulating glucose levels 2–3 months before the test.

While epidemiologic studies using HgbA1c have only been performed within adult populations [3], the 2019 American Diabetes Association (ADA) guidelines recommend HgbA1c as appropriate for diagnosing prediabetes or type 2 diabetes in children and adolescents [4]. For children with classic symptoms of diabetes and hyperglycemia, a normal HgbA1c may suggest a short-term duration of disease but does not rule out disease [5].

Assay Considerations

For the initial diagnosis of diabetes, HgbA1c should be measured using a standardized lab assay; point-of-care measurement should be avoided unless necessary. Compared to plasma glucose measurement, HgbA1c is convenient, as there is no need to fast, and the sample is stable from the time of drawing to analysis. As a reflection of average glycemia

R. Whooten (✉)
Massachusetts General Hospital for Children, Boston, MA, USA
e-mail: RWHOOTEN@MGH.HARVARD.EDU

T. Stanley, M. Misra (eds.), *Endocrine Conditions in Pediatrics*, https://doi.org/10.1007/978-3-030-52215-5_30

Table 30.2 Relative advantages and disadvantages of HgbA1c, fasting glucose, and 2-hour glucose

	Advantages	Disadvantages
HgbA1c	High convenience – can be performed at any time of day Relatively low assay variability, good reproducibility Good correlation with diabetes complications	Less well validated in children compared to adults Not reliable in cystic fibrosis or states of abnormal red blood cell turnover May not reflect acute changes in glycemia
Fasting plasma glucose	Moderate convenience – requires fasting Relatively low assay variability, good reproducibility	One of the last parameters to become abnormal in the progression of diabetes – may lack sensitivity
2-hour glucose (OGTT)	Generally, the first parameter to become abnormal in the progression of diabetes Recommended for diagnosis in children with cystic fibrosis	Low convenience – requires fasting and a 2-hour test Poor reproducibility for diagnosing diabetes in youth with obesity [21]

over the past 2–3 months, HgbA1c measurement is not affected by acute stress or illness [1]. However, as it reflects the average glycemia over this period, it is less sensitive than plasma glucose-based testing and may not identify all cases of diabetes [3].

As an indirect measure of glycemia, HgbA1c is dependent on red blood cell turnover and is unreliable in conditions that affect this. This includes hemoglobinopathies, glucose 6-phosphate dehydrogenase (G6PD) deficiency, recent history of blood transfusion or erythropoietin use, pregnancy and the postpartum setting, HIV treatment with certain drugs, and iron deficiency anemia. HgbA1c is not recommended for the diagnosis of diabetes in children with cystic fibrosis [1].

Plasma Glucose

Diabetes may also be diagnosed through an abnormal fasting plasma glucose or 2-hour plasma glucose after a 75-g glucose load in an oral glucose tolerance test (OGTT) [1].

Assay Considerations

For both tests, the patient must fast for a minimum of 8 hours before, as any food intake may affect the results. If plasma glucose samples are not spun and separated promptly upon drawing, sitting at room temperature for a prolonged period may lead to falsely low results. Plasma glucose-based strategies are ideal for diagnosis in situations where red blood cell turnover may be affected, as described above [1].

Interpretation of Abnormal Values

Diabetes diagnostic criteria are met with either (1) classic symptoms of diabetes in the setting of hyperglycemia (defined as a random plasma glucose >200) or (2) two abnormal results above the threshold for diabetes (Table 30.1). If one screening or diagnostic test is abnormal in an asymptomatic individual, a second (either using the same or a different strategy) should be repeated. If the results are discordant, the measure that is above the threshold for diagnosis should be repeated to confirm the diagnosis [1].

> **Clinical Key**
> In asymptomatic individuals undergoing screening for diabetes, a single abnormal value for HbA1c, fasting plasma glucose, or 2-hour plasma glucose should prompt a second test to confirm the diagnosis, using either the same or a different testing strategy.

Next Steps in Addressing Abnormal Values

In concern for new-onset diabetes, the patient should be referred emergently to a pediatric endocrinologist/diabetes specialist. A basic metabolic panel or venous blood gas, along with urinalysis for ketones, if feasible, should be obtained to evaluate for diabetic ketoacidosis (DKA). The presence of ketones and/or evidence of acidosis (pH < 7.3, bicarbonate <15 mEq/L) requires emergent evaluation and treatment [5]. Additional laboratory evaluation can assist with distinguishing type 1 vs type 2 diabetes. Overweight and obesity are common among children with type 1 diabetes [6], and ketosis can be present in youth with type 2 diabetes [7]. Consequently, the ADA recommends sending autoantibodies (*discussed below*) at the presentation of new-onset diabetes in all overweight youth [8]. C-peptide and insulin levels (*discussed below*) may also be helpful in distinguishing between diabetes subtypes. Borderline values near or at the prediabetic range should be closely followed; increasing values of HgbA1c reflect a higher risk of progression to diabetes [4].

Labs Used in Distinguishing Type 1 vs Type 2 Diabetes

Autoantibodies

Diabetes-associated autoantibodies are serological markers of beta-cell autoimmunity diagnostic of type 1 diabetes.

Assay Considerations
Commercially available panels can detect autoantibodies against glutamic acid decarboxylase (GAD), insulinoma antigen 2 (IA2), islet cell antibody 512 (ICA512), insulin (IAA; insulin autoantibody), and zinc transporter 8 (ZnT8). Levels of autoantibodies may decrease with disease progression [9].

Interpretation of Abnormal Values
Laboratory evaluation including four autoantibodies (e.g., IAA, IA2, GAD, and ZnT8) detects 98% of individuals with type 1 diabetes at onset. The prevalence of autoantibodies is age- and sex-dependent, with IAA and ZnT8 more common in patients <10 years of age and GAD more common among females [9]. The presence of one positive autoantibody in the setting of diabetes diagnosis confirms type 1 diabetes [5]. Of note, in children who have a first-degree relative with type 1 diabetes, the presence of ≥2 autoantibodies is associated with ≈70% risk of progression to type 1 diabetes over 10 years [10]. There is currently limited clinical utility for screening outside of the research setting. Individuals with a family history of Type 1 Diabetes and positive autoantibodies may be referred to Trialnet, a coordinated research effort to both understand and modify the natural history of diabetes progression [11].

C-peptide

C-peptide is co-secreted with insulin from pancreatic beta-cells in an equimolar fashion and provides a measure of endogenous insulin secretion and beta-cell function.

Assay Considerations
C-peptide levels should be drawn fasting. C-peptide is degraded more slowly than insulin and provides a more stable measurement. Measurements may be inaccurate in kidney disease, as C-peptide is metabolized via the kidneys and excreted in the urine. C-peptide levels do not reflect exogenous insulin administration or the presence of anti-insulin antibodies [12].

Interpretation of Abnormal Values
Increased endogenous insulin production results in increased C-peptide levels. C-peptide levels are usually elevated at diagnosis in individuals with type 2 diabetes and low in those with type 1 diabetes. Cohort studies of children presenting with diabetes suggest thresholds for distinguishing subtypes, with C-peptide levels of <0.6 ng/mL excluding type 2 diabetes and >3.0 ng/mL making type 1 diabetes unlikely [13], and a C-peptide level of 0.85 ng/mL providing 83% sensitivity and 89% specificity for distinguishing between Type 1 (<0.85 ng/mL) and type 2 (≥0.85 ng/mL) diabetes [14].

Insulin

An elevated insulin level can provide early evidence of insulin resistance while the beta cells can secrete enough insulin to maintain normoglycemia [4]. Existing evidence suggests a strong association between elevated fasting insulin and metabolic syndrome [15]. Despite this, there is limited clinical understanding of how elevated insulin levels are related to the progression of insulin resistance toward diabetes [16]. If fasting insulin concentration is elevated, one of the recommended screening tests for prediabetes should be performed for further evaluation.

Assay Considerations
Insulin levels should be drawn fasting. To better interpret the value, a fasting serum glucose should be drawn as well. Serum concentrations may be variable, as up to 50–60% of insulin produced is metabolized by the liver before reaching the circulation [17]. The insulin immunoassay cannot distinguish between exogenous and endogenous insulin, so it cannot be used in a patient treated with insulin. Given few trials for examining the predictive power of insulin levels and the lack of a standardized assay, the clinical utility of insulin levels is limited [16].

Interpretation of Abnormal Values
Similar to C-peptide levels, fasting insulin levels will be low in type 1 diabetes. In type 2 diabetes, they may be high initially and then decrease with continued loss of beta-cell mass.

Labs Used in Long-Term Management of Diabetes

HgbA1c

In addition to use in diagnosis, HgbA1c levels are monitored quarterly in most pediatric diabetes patients to (1) assess glycemic control, (2) guide insulin therapy decisions, and (3) provide a prediction of future risk of diabetes complications. The goal for children and adolescents with type 1 diabetes is a HgbA1c <7.5%. Among patients with type 2 diabetes, the ADA supports a goal of HgbA1c <6.5–7.0% if it can be achieved without hypoglycemia [8].

Fructosamine

Fructosamine refers to any glycated protein and provides an alternative strategy for measuring average glycemia if HgbA1c cannot be used due to alterations in red blood cell turnover. As serum proteins have a shorter half-life

(≈14–20 days) than red blood cells, glycated serum proteins provide information on glycemia over a shorter period [2]. Measurement may be affected by conditions affecting protein synthesis or clearance, such as systemic illness or liver disease. Fructosamine measurements do not translate easily into average glucose levels, are not equivalent to HgbA1c, and there are no data on related levels and associated diabetes-related complications [18]. Thus, they are not routinely used but may have clinical utility in patients for whom HbA1c is not reliable.

Ketones

Ketones are a marker of insulin deficiency, resulting from a shift in energy production to the breakdown of free fatty acids and the production of ketone bodies for energy in the absence of insulin-stimulated glucose transport. Beta-hydroxybutyrate and acetoacetate are the primary ketone bodies [17]. Ketone measurement is important in the setting of hyperglycemia, illness, or insulin omission to prevent diabetic ketoacidosis (DKA).

Assay Considerations

Ketones may be measured in either urine or serum. Urine ketone measurement is painless, inexpensive, and requires no technical skills or quality assurance. However, the results are inexact and depend on voiding, which may be difficult if the patient is dehydrated. Additionally, urine measurement reflects the average ketone concentration since the last void, which may overestimate current ketone level, and only measures acetoacetate. Serum ketones reflect beta-hydroxybutyrate and may be measured as point-of-care testing or via a laboratory. Point-of-care testing provides accurate and timely information that may guide treatment but requires a meter and test strips that must be tested for quality assurance and may be expensive. Delays in processing laboratory samples may limit clinical utility as well [19].

Interpretation of Values

Negative ketone measurement – either serum or urine – suggests a low likelihood of DKA. Elevated ketones raise concern for diabetic ketoacidosis, although certainly patients can be ketotic without having acidosis. A serum ketone level of >0.6 mmol/L is considered elevated, while a level >3.0 mmol/L is associated with an increased risk of diabetic ketoacidosis. A ketone level up to 0.25 mmol/L may be found following an overnight fast, so it is considered normal [19].

Next Steps in Addressing Abnormal Values

Elevated ketones require urgent attention to prevent progression to DKA. Patients should follow the recommendations of their endocrinologists, which should include frequent insulin administration and continued monitoring of ketone/blood glucose levels. If a patient has a pump, insulin should be administered via injections until evidence of ketone resolution.

References

1. American Diabetes A. 2. Classification and diagnosis of diabetes: standards of medical care in diabetes-2019. Diabetes Care. 2019;42(Suppl 1):S13–28.
2. Goldstein DE, et al. Tests of glycemia in diabetes. Diabetes Care. 2004;27(7):1761–73.
3. Cowie CC, et al. Prevalence of diabetes and high risk for diabetes using A1C criteria in the U.S. population in 1988–2006. Diabetes Care. 2010;33(3):562–8.
4. Arslanian S, et al. Mel evaluation and management of youth-onset Type 2 diabetes: a position statement by the American Diabetes Association. Diabetes Care. 2018;41(12):2648–68.
5. Mayer-Davis EJ, et al. ISPAD clinical practice consensus guidelines 2018: definition, epidemiology, and classification of diabetes in children and adolescents. Pediatr Diabetes. 2018;19(Suppl 27):7–19.
6. DuBose SN, et al. Obesity in youth with type 1 Diabetes in Germany, Austria, and the United States. J Pediatr. 2015;167(3):627–32 e1-4.
7. Dabelea D, et al. Trends in the prevalence of ketoacidosis at diabetes diagnosis: the SEARCH for diabetes in youth study. Pediatrics. 2014;133(4):e938–45.
8. American Diabetes A. 13. Children and adolescents: standards of medical Care in Diabetes-2019. Diabetes Care. 2019;42(Suppl 1):S148–64.
9. Watkins RA, et al. Established and emerging biomarkers for the prediction of type 1 diabetes: a systematic review. Transl Res. 2014;164(2):110–21.
10. Ziegler AG, et al. Seroconversion to multiple islet autoantibodies and risk of progression to diabetes in children. JAMA. 2013;309(23):2473–9.
11. Bingley PJ, et al. Type 1 diabetes TrialNet: a multifaceted approach to bringing disease-modifying therapy to clinical use in type 1 diabetes. Diabetes Care. 2018;41(4):653–61.
12. Besser RE. Determination of C-peptide in children: when is it useful? Pediatr Endocrinol Rev. 2013;10(4):494–502.
13. Cho MJ, et al. Fasting serum C-peptide is useful for initial classification of diabetes mellitus in children and adolescents. Ann Pediatr Endocrinol Metab. 2014;19(2):80–5.
14. Katz LE, et al. Fasting c-peptide and insulin-like growth factor-binding protein-1 levels help to distinguish childhood type 1 and type 2 diabetes at diagnosis. Pediatr Diabetes. 2007;8(2):53–9.
15. Pataky Z, et al. Fasting insulin at baseline influences the number of cardiometabolic risk factors and R-R interval at 3years in a healthy population: the RISC study. Diabetes Metab. 2013;39(4):330–6.
16. Staten MA, et al. Insulin assay standardization: leading to measures of insulin sensitivity and secretion for practical clinical care. Diabetes Care. 2010;33(1):205–6.
17. Williams Textbook of Endocrinology. 2015: Elsevier.
18. Welsh KJ, Kirkman MS, Sacks DB. Role of glycated proteins in the diagnosis and management of diabetes: research gaps and future directions. Diabetes Care. 2016;39(8):1299–306.
19. Dhatariya K. Blood ketones: measurement, interpretation, limitations, and utility in the management of diabetic ketoacidosis. Rev Diabet Stud. 2016;13(4):217–25.
20. WHO/IDF, Definitions and diagnosis of diabetes and intermediate hyperglycemia. 2006. Geneva, Switzerland.
21. Libman IM, et al. Reproducibility of the oral glucose tolerance test in overweight children. J Clin Endocrinol Metab. 2008;93(11):4231–7.

Laboratory Evaluation of Hypoglycemia

31

Liya Kerem

Who Should Be Evaluated and What Is the Threshold to Obtain the Laboratory Evaluation?

In adults, the Endocrine Society recommends an evaluation of hypoglycemia in patients who fulfill Whipple's triad: (1) Symptoms and/or signs consistent with hypoglycemia (please see Chap. 8 for common presenting signs and symptoms of hypoglycemia); (2) documented low plasma glucose concentration; and (3) resolution of signs/symptoms with treatment and a documented increase in plasma glucose levels [1]. While the Pediatric Endocrine Society's recommendations also emphasize the importance of Whipple's triad, they specifically establish a plasma glucose level threshold of 60 mg/dL (3.3 mmol/L) to perform an evaluation in patients who cannot reliably communicate their symptoms, such as infants and toddlers [2].

In children and adults, there is no single value of plasma glucose that determines hypoglycemia, and rather it is a clinical diagnosis defined as a plasma glucose concentration low enough to alter and impair brain function and evoke defensive counter-regulatory hormonal response [1]. An average plasma glucose level of 68 mg/dL would usually initiate an autonomic hormonal response, while an average level of 55 mg/dL would present with noticeable signs and/or symptoms of hypoglycemia [3]. Importantly, these thresholds can shift in the setting of recurrent hypoglycemic events causing an adaptive response.

For the purpose of diagnostic blood tests, a plasma glucose level of 50–55 mg/dL is considered sufficient to delineate the underlying etiology of the hypoglycemic event, using the more stringent threshold of 50 mg/dL in controlled diagnostic fasts [2, 3]. Importantly, a plasma glucose level of 70 mg/dL (3.9 mmol/L) is considered the therapeutic goal in the management of pediatric hypoglycemia. The management of hypoglycemia in neonates in the nursery/inpatient setting is beyond the scope of this chapter. It is important to emphasize that after the first 48 hours of age, glucose homeostasis is similar to that of older children and adults [2, 3]. Also, certain neonates at increased risk for hypoglycemia can be identified by pertinent findings in their perinatal history and physical examination (see Chap. 8), and consultation with a pediatric endocrinologist may help in planning the appropriate diagnostic investigation.

Clinical Key
In older children/adolescents, it is preferable to confirm Whipple's triad (hypoglycemia on testing, symptoms or signs of hypoglycemia, and resolution of symptoms or signs with treatment) prior to proceeding with further diagnostic testing or endocrine referral. Prescription of a glucose meter to be used at the time of symptoms to document hypoglycemia can be helpful, along with a physician's letter listing the critical sample labs (the diagnostic blood tests) that the patient can provide to an emergency department at the time of hypoglycemia.

Laboratory Evaluation of Hypoglycemia

As mentioned earlier, a careful history and a detailed physical exam are critical in the initial evaluation of a child presenting with hypoglycemia (please see Chap. 8). When the clinical presentation is suspicious for hypoglycemia, the first step is a prompt evaluation of the glucose levels with a point-of-care (POC) glucometer, which provides a convenient and rapid screening method.

L. Kerem (✉)
Pediatric Endocrinology Unit, Massachusetts General Hospital for Children, Boston, MA, USA

T. Stanley, M. Misra (eds.), *Endocrine Conditions in Pediatrics*, https://doi.org/10.1007/978-3-030-52215-5_31

Clinical Key

Point-of-care glucose meters can be used for initial evaluation, but a plasma glucose level is needed to confirm hypoglycemia. Point-of-care meters have 10–20% variability.

A POC glucose level <60 mg/dL should be repeated and, if confirmed, an attempt should be made to collect the critical sample prior to providing appropriate treatment. The critical sample should always include a plasma glucose level since the accuracy of POC meters is limited in the hypoglycemic range and can vary by more than 10–20% [4]. The elements of the critical sample that should be obtained appear in Box 31.1.

Box 31.1: Elements of the "Critical Sample," in Order of Priority

Blood tests:

- Plasma glucose
- Beta-hydroxybutyrate (BOHB)
- Comprehensive metabolic panel (CMP) with bicarbonate levels
- Insulin
- Free fatty acids (FFAs)
- Lactate (should be sent on ice)
- Cortisol
- C-peptide
- Ammonia (should be sent on ice)
- Growth hormone
- Acyl-carnitine profile
- Plasma free and total carnitine profiles
- Blood tests that should be taken with specific clinical suspicion—lipid panel, serum amino acids, and proinsulin

Urine tests:

Organic acids

If a blood test for BOHB is not available, a urine dip for ketones should be obtained instead.

In children with known hypoglycemia for whom a critical sample cannot be obtained as an outpatient, referral to pediatric endocrinology is appropriate for performance of a "diagnostic fast," which is a supervised fast in the hospital so that the critical sample can be obtained.

Interpretation of the Critical Sample

Clues for the initial differential diagnosis of the hypoglycemic disorder are provided by the critical sample. A general categorization of the different main etiologies of hypoglycemia is provided according to the results of the laboratory evaluation. Figure 31.1 shows an algorithm for the workup of hypoglycemia according to these categories.

Clinical Key

Possible reasons for falsely low glucose readings

- Falsely low capillary ("finger stick"/point-of-care) readings
  - Poor extremity perfusion (e.g., acrocyanosis, Raynaud phenomenon)
  - Expired testing strips and equipment malfunction
  - Certain drugs at high doses (e.g., ascorbic acid or acetaminophen, depending on the technology used by the meter)
  - Acidosis
- Falsely low plasma glucose readings
  - Delay in sample processing (red blood cells and white blood cells metabolize glucose)
  - Polycythemia (red blood cells metabolize glucose)
  - Significant leukocytosis/leukemia (white blood cells metabolize glucose)

1. *Confirm hypoglycemia*: In order for the critical sample to accurately reflect the etiology of hypoglycemia, the plasma glucose level should be below 50–55 mg/dL. Notably, delays in processing and separation of the blood samples can falsely result in lower glucose levels due to red blood cells' glycolysis, estimated to reduce the plasma glucose concentration by up to 6 mg/dL/h (0.3 mmol/L/h, see Clinical Key).
2. *Establish the state of acidosis*: This is done by studying the levels of Beta-hydroxybutyrate (BOHB), bicarbonate, FFAs, and lactate. Bicarbonate, sent as part of a comprehensive metabolic panel, and lactate, which should be sent on ice, are both readily available in most medical centers. If BOHB testing is not available, urine ketones are an excellent alternative, and they remain informative even if obtained following treatment to correct the hypoglycemia. Importantly, the presence of acidosis and spe-

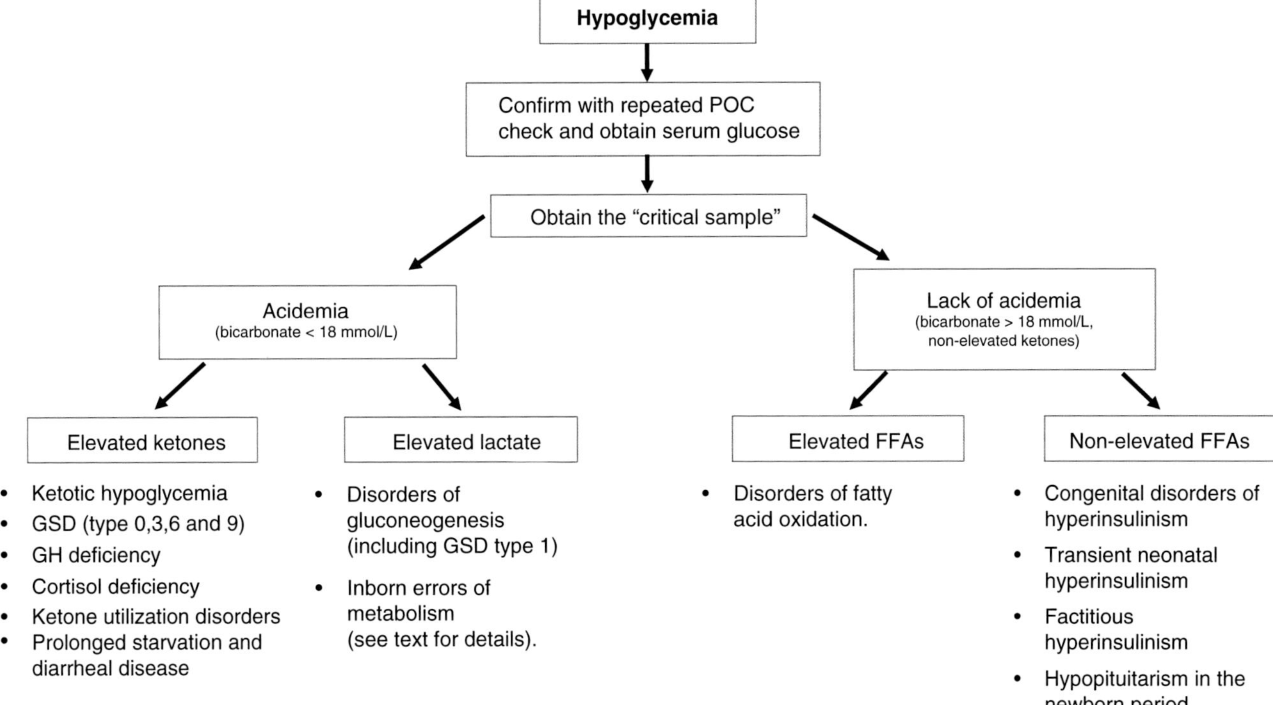

Fig. 31.1 Workup of hypoglycemia depending on the results of the critical samples

cifically elevated blood or urine ketones (BOHB >2.5 mmol/L, positive urine ketones) would usually exclude disorders of hyperinsulinism and fatty acid oxidation (FAO) defects. If acidosis has been established (bicarbonate <18 mmol/L), the differential diagnosis can be advanced by recognizing the cause of acidosis—elevated ketones versus elevated lactate. In the absence of acidosis, disorders of hypoglycemia can be differentiated by studying the levels of the FFA as detailed below and presented in Fig. 31.1.

(a) *Acidosis and elevated ketones*:
    (i) *Idiopathic ketotic hypoglycemia*: This is a diagnosis of exclusion (see Chap. 51) and a relatively common cause of childhood hypoglycemia for which the pathophysiology is still not well understood [5]. It can occur in the setting of a skipped evening meal in children aged 2–8 years. Of note, elevated ketones in a child with a classical presentation support this diagnosis; however, establishing it as the underlying cause of recurrent hypoglycemia requires exclusion of other etiologies by examining the rest of the critical samples or as part of a supervised diagnostic fast. An acyl-carnitine profile should always be obtained and studied prior to performing a controlled fast since prolonged fasting can be life threatening in children with fatty acid oxidation defects.
    (ii) *Glycogen-storage diseases* (GSD; specifically types 0, 3, 6, and 9): GSD can be associated with elevated liver enzymes and hyperlipidemia. Type 3 is also specifically associated with elevated creatine kinase due to disordered glycogen metabolism in the muscle.
    (iii) *Growth hormone (GH) and/or cortisol deficiencies*: Both cortisol and GH play a secondary role in the counter-regulatory response to acute hypoglycemia, and GH is specifically important for prolonged fasting. Hypoglycemia should act as a "stimulation test" for both cortisol and GH, but definitive diagnosis of glucocorticoid or GH deficiencies cannot be based on a single low level of cortisol or GH during hypoglycemia. Rather, low levels should prompt endocrinology referral for additional formal stimulation tests [6]. When primary adrenal insufficiency is suspected in a child presenting with hypoglycemia, plasma adrenocorticotropic hormone (ACTH) could be added to the critical sample and is expected to be significantly elevated.
    (iv) *Disorders of ketone utilization*: Deficiencies of succinyl-CoA:3-ketoacid CoA transferase (SCOT), monocarboxylate transporter 1 (MCT1), and alpha-methylacetoacetic aciduria present with mild hypoglycemia and significantly elevated ketone levels that resolve rela-

tively slowly with feeding. These disorders can be diagnosed by an abnormal urine organic acid and acylcarnitine profiles with further confirmation by enzyme assays or genetic testing.

(v) *Prolonged starvation and diarrheal disease*: Hypoglycemia in the setting of infectious acute gastroenteritis associated with severe diarrhea would present with elevated ketones. While it is uncommon in healthy children, it can occur if associated with prolonged starvation without repletion of appropriate fluids containing glucose [7].

(b) *Acidosis and elevated lactate*:

(i) *Disorders of gluconeogenesis*: With prolonged fasting (12 to 16 hours) and after liver glycogen stores have been depleted, gluconeogenesis is required to maintain stable glucose levels. Genetic defects of the four major enzymes of gluconeogenesis (pyruvate carboxylase, phosphoenolpyruvate carboxykinase, fructose 1,6-diphosphatase, and glucose 6-phosphatase) can lead to hypoglycemia, resulting in elevated levels of lactic acid. Deficiency of glucose 6-phosphatase is the pathophysiology underlying GSD type 1, which is associated with significantly elevated lipids, hypophosphatemia, and hyperuricemia. Deficiency of pyruvate carboxylase is associated with elevated levels of alpha-ketoglutarate when examining the urine organic acids. Phosphoenolpyruvate carboxykinase deficiency presents with early liver failure. Genetic testing for gluconeogenesis disorders is now commercially available.

(ii) *Late-onset maple syrup urine disease and glycerol kinase deficiency*: These are two rare inborn errors of metabolism that present with hypoglycemia accompanied by elevated ketones and lactic acidosis.

(c) *Lack of acidosis (bicarbonate > 18 mmol/L) and elevated FFA*: During fasting, fatty acid oxidation (FAO) has an important role in maintaining stable glucose levels. Genetic disorders causing defects in transport and oxidation of fatty acids are associated with *hypoketotic* hypoglycemia due to impaired ketone body generation. Many of these disorders are tested as part of the newborn screening, results of which should be reviewed if a FAO disorder is suspected [8]. Abnormal plasma acylcarnitine profile and/or urine organic acid levels (especially dicarboxylic aciduria) are suggestive of a fatty acid oxidation disorder and should prompt metabolic and genetic evaluation. Depending on the type of FAO defect, patients can present with liver dysfunction (associated with elevated aspartate aminotransferase (AST) and alanine aminotransferase (ALT) levels) and myopathy or rhabdomyolysis, which can occur in long-chain FAO defects (associated with elevated creatine kinase levels). A patient with FAO defect presenting in acute crisis can have hyperammonemia on laboratory evaluation.

(d) *Lack of acidosis and low FFA*: Hypoglycemia associated with suppressed blood ketones (BOHB <1.5 mmol/L; <15 mg/dL), together with low levels of FFA (<1–1.5 mmol/L; <28–42 mg/dL), suggests *disorders of hyperinsulinism* (insulin inhibits the mobilization of FFA from adipose tissue and further beta-oxidation to ketones). From a practical diagnostic standpoint, in most cases, the insulin levels will be available prior to the results of FFAs, and therefore a laboratory profile showing low plasma glucose level together with inappropriately suppressed blood ketones and a measurable insulin level would suggest hyperinsulinism. Traditionally, an insulin level >2.5 uU/mL (18 pmol/L) concurrent with hypoglycemia was considered indicative of hyperinsulinism [3]. However, more sensitive insulin assays are now available, and therefore any detectable insulin level during hypoglycemia (plasma glucose <50 mg/dL) suggests hyperinsulinism [9]. Importantly, undetectable insulin levels do not exclude hyperinsulinism. When hyperinsulinism is suspected and insulin is undetectable, a glucagon stimulation test (0.5–1 mg given intravenously, intramuscularly, or subcutaneously) is required and would show an increase in glucose levels by more than 30 mg/dL (1.7 mmol/L), indicating that liver glycogen release was inhibited by insulin. This test is usually performed at the end of a controlled supervised diagnostic fast when the plasma glucose level is <50 mg/dL when hyperinsulinism is suspected.

(i) *Congenital disorders of hyperinsulinism*: The clinical presentation of these disorders is discussed in detail in Chap. 51. Congenital hyperinsulinism usually presents early on in life, characterized by severe hypoglycemia (glucose levels <30 mg/dL) and a high glucose infusion rate (GIR) > ~8 mg/kg/min.

(ii) *Transient neonatal hyperinsulinism*: Hyperinsulinism in the setting of perinatal stress, gestational diabetes, birth asphyxia, and intrauterine growth restriction would also present with a similar profile, including hypoglycemia associated with detectable insulin levels, suppressed ketones and FFA. In these cases, the hypoglycemia is not as severe as in congenital hyperinsulinism, and the GIR required to maintain normoglycemia is lower.

(iii) *Factitious hyperinsulinism*: If exogenous administration of insulin is suspected as the underlying cause of hypoglycemia, C-peptide should be added to the critical samples and is expected to be undetectable, reflecting suppression of endogenous insulin production. A C-peptide level ≥0.5 ng/dL indicates that inappropriate endogenous insulin production occurred [9]. Of note, not all commercially available insulin assays detect insulin analogues (e.g., lispro, aspart, glargine, glulisine, detemir, and degludec), and therefore low insulin levels are not sufficient to exclude superstitious insulin administration. When exogenous insulin administration is suspected, it is important to consult with the local lab to consider use of an appropriate assay [10]. Hyperinsulinism can also be the result of sulfonylureas, which induce insulin secretion. In this case, both insulin levels and C-peptide would be elevated, and a specific toxicology screen study for sulfonylurea can be performed.

(iv) *Insulinomas*: Insulin-producing adenomas of the pancreas are exceedingly rare in the pediatric population and present in older children and adolescents. The laboratory evaluation would reveal significantly elevated insulin, proinsulin, and C-peptide levels concurrent with suppressed ketones.

(v) *Hypopituitarism in the newborn period*: It is important to emphasize that in newborns, hypoglycemia concurrent with suppressed ketones and FFA can occur due to hypopituitarism, which is not associated with hyperinsulinism. Careful history and specific findings on physical exam (micropenis, midline defects, jaundice, findings on brain magnetic resonance imaging scan) could suggest hypopituitarism.

Additional Laboratory Evaluation for Specific Etiologies

1. When hypoglycemia is suspected to result from drug exposure, specific drug screens should be done (e.g., for alcohol, beta-blockers, and salicylates).
2. An oral glucose or mixed-meal tolerance test can be performed when hypoglycemia occurs postprandially and is suspected to result from a complication of fundoplication or gastric bypass bariatric surgery [11].
3. Many of the organic or amino acid metabolism defects are included in the newborn screening and will be associated with an abnormal urine organic acid profile.

In summary, the laboratory evaluation of clinical hypoglycemia is crucial to decipher underlying etiology and to recognize life-threatening conditions in a timely manner. The initial evaluation done by the pediatrician when a child presents with hypoglycemia can fundamentally advance the investigation of the underlying cause and to promote implementation of appropriate treatment.

References

1. Cryer PE, Axelrod L, Grossman AB, Heller SR, Montori VM, Seaquist ER, et al. Evaluation and management of adult hypoglycemic disorders: an Endocrine Society clinical practice guideline. J Clin Endocrinol Metab. 2009;94(3):709–28.
2. Thornton PS, Stanley CA, De Leon DD, Harris D, Haymond MW, Hussain K, et al. Recommendations from the Pediatric Endocrine Society for evaluation and management of persistent hypoglycemia in neonates, infants, and children. J Pediatr. 2015;167(2): 238–45.
3. Sperling M. Pediatric endocrinology. 4th ed. Philadelphia: Elsevier/Saunders; 2014. xv, 1061 pages
4. Rebel A, Rice MA, Fahy BG. Accuracy of point-of-care glucose measurements. J Diabetes Sci Technol. 2012;6(2):396–411.
5. Huidekoper HH, Duran M, Turkenburg M, Ackermans MT, Sauerwein HP, Wijburg FA. Fasting adaptation in idiopathic ketotic hypoglycemia: a mismatch between glucose production and demand. Eur J Pediatr. 2008;167(8):859–65.
6. Kelly A, Tang R, Becker S, Stanley CA. Poor specificity of low growth hormone and cortisol levels during fasting hypoglycemia for the diagnoses of growth hormone deficiency and adrenal insufficiency. Pediatrics. 2008;122(3):e522–8.
7. Reid SR, Losek JD. Hypoglycemia complicating dehydration in children with acute gastroenteritis. J Emerg Med. 2005;29(2):141–5.
8. Ziadeh R, Hoffman EP, Finegold DN, Hoop RC, Brackett JC, Strauss AW, et al. Medium chain acyl-CoA dehydrogenase deficiency in Pennsylvania: neonatal screening shows high incidence and unexpected mutation frequencies. Pediatr Res. 1995;37(5): 675–8.
9. Ferrara C, Patel P, Becker S, Stanley CA, Kelly A. Biomarkers of insulin for the diagnosis of Hyperinsulinemic hypoglycemia in infants and children. J Pediatr. 2016;168:212–9.
10. Moriyama M, Hayashi N, Ohyabu C, Mukai M, Kawano S, Kumagai S. Performance evaluation and cross-reactivity from insulin analogs with the ARCHITECT insulin assay. Clin Chem. 2006;52(7):1423–6.
11. Palladino AA, Sayed S, Levitt Katz LE, Gallagher PR, De Leon DD. Increased glucagon-like peptide-1 secretion and postprandial hypoglycemia in children after Nissen fundoplication. J Clin Endocrinol Metab. 2009;94(1):39–44.

Lipid Profiles

32

Bhuvana Sunil and Ambika P. Ashraf

Abbreviations

(apo B)	Apolipoprotein B
HDL-C	High-density lipoprotein cholesterol
IDL-C	Intermediate-density lipoprotein cholesterol
LDL-C	Low-density lipoprotein cholesterol
Lp (a)	Lipoprotein (a)
NCEP	The National Cholesterol Education Program
NHLBI	National Heart, Lung, and Blood Institute
TC	Total cholesterol
TG	triglycerides
VLDL-C	Very-low-density lipoprotein cholesterol

Introduction

The Pathobiological Determinants of Atherosclerosis in Youth and Bogalusa Heart study have shown that atherosclerosis begins in early childhood [1, 2]. According to the World Health Organization, ischemic heart disease and stroke are the world's leading causes of death [3]. Most primary, and some secondary causes of dyslipidemia have no physical stigmata, but have serious clinical consequences, including myocardial infarction and strokes in the third and fourth decade of life if left unrecognized. Initiation of statin therapy during childhood in patients with familial hypercholesterolemia can reduce the risk of cardiovascular disease in adulthood [4]. This underlines the importance of pediatricians understanding lipid screening guidelines and interpretation of lipid profiles.

Definition of Dyslipidemia

Dyslipidemia is defined as an abnormality in any of the following: increased levels of total cholesterol (TC), low-density lipoprotein cholesterol (LDL-C), and/or triglycerides (TG), and/or decreased levels of high-density lipoprotein cholesterol (HDL-C). Another consideration is elevated non-HDL cholesterol (calculated as TC minus HDL-C); this measure is a single marker of all of the atherogenic apolipoprotein B (apoB)-containing lipoproteins in the circulation, including very-low-density lipoprotein (VLDL-C) and intermediate-density lipoprotein cholesterol (IDL-C). Dyslipidemia could be primary (monogenic or polygenic) or secondary to other disorders, conditions, or exposures.

Considerations of Secondary Causes of Dyslipidemia with Potential Mechanisms

The National Cholesterol Education Program (NCEP) guidelines recommend evaluation of underlying conditions that could be causing or exacerbating dyslipidemias before initiating or intensifying treatment in patients with dyslipidemias [5]. Some conditions to consider include diabetes mellitus (Type 1 or 2), hypothyroidism, Cushing's syndrome, obesity-induced metabolic syndrome, growth hormone deficiency, pregnancy, use of certain medications/recreational drugs, acute and chronic hepatitis, nephrotic syndrome, chronic kidney disease, metabolic and storage disorders, etc. [8–14]. It is important for the pediatrician to consider these conditions, as some conditions such as hypothyroidism may have subtle clinical manifestations that may only be recognized on laboratory testing, whereas some such as nephrotic syndrome may be clinically obvious.

B. Sunil · A. P. Ashraf (✉)
Department of Pediatrics, Division of Endocrinology and Diabetes, University of Alabama at Birmingham, Birmingham, AL, USA
e-mail: bsunil@uabmc.edu; aashraf@peds.uab.edu

T. Stanley, M. Misra (eds.), *Endocrine Conditions in Pediatrics*, https://doi.org/10.1007/978-3-030-52215-5_32

Obtaining a Lipid Profile

In 1992, the NCEP made initial recommendations for "targeted screening" for pediatric lipid disorders [5]. Recommendations since then have now changed from targeted screening alone, as family history alone is an insensitive predictor of familial hyperlipidemia [6]. In 2011, the National Heart, Lung, and Blood Institute (NHLBI), endorsed by the American Academy of Pediatrics, recommended "universal screening" for all children to be screened for dyslipidemia once between the ages of 9 years and 11 years and again between 17 years and 21 years [7]. On the contrary, the US Preventive Services Task Force stated insufficient evidence for or against screening for pediatric dyslipidemia [8]. Figure 32.1 illustrates the current screening and approach recommendations adopted from the 2011 Expert Panel on Integrated Guidelines for Cardiovascular Health and Risk Reduction in Children and Adolescents [6].

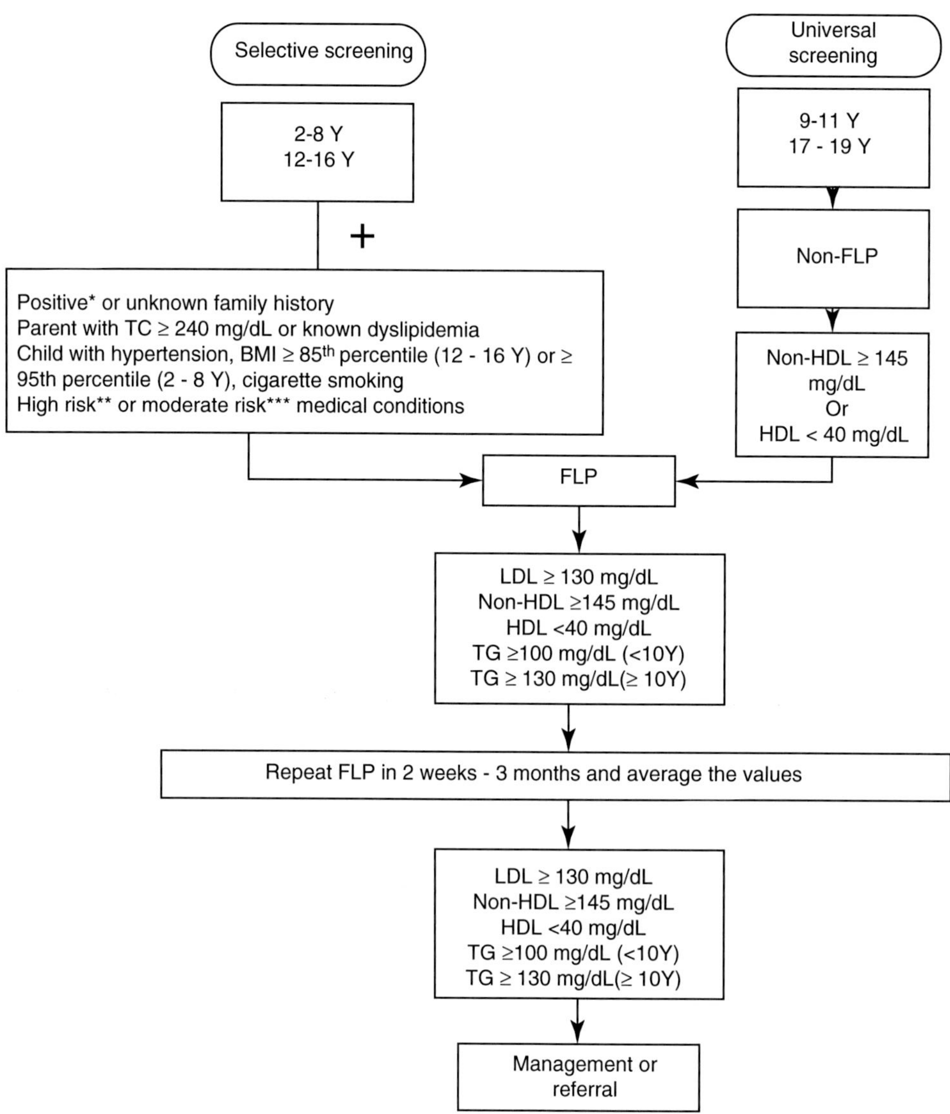

Fig. 32.1 Guidelines for dyslipidemia screening in the pediatric population. Based on recommendations from the Expert Panel on Integrated Guidelines for Cardiovascular Health and Risk Reduction in Children and Adolescents in 2011. Abbreviations: Y – years, FLP – fasting lipid profile, TC – total cholesterol, LDL – low-density lipoprotein cholesterol, HDL – high-density lipoprotein cholesterol, TG – triglyceride, BMI – body mass index. *Positive family history: Parent, grandparent, aunt, uncle, or sibling with any of these before the age 55 Y in a male or 65 Y in a female – myocardial infarction, stroke, angina, coronary artery bypass, stent, angioplasty, sudden cardiac death, parent with total cholesterol >240 mg/dL . **High-risk medical condition: Type 1 or 2 diabetes, chronic renal disease/end-stage renal disease/postrenal transplant, post-orthotopic heart transplant, and Kawasaki disease with current aneurysms. ***Moderate-risk medical condition: Kawasaki disease with regressed coronary aneurysms, systemic lupus erythematosus, juvenile rheumatoid arthritis, human immunodeficiency virus (HIV) infection, and nephrotic syndrome

Components of a Standard Lipid Profile

A standard lipid profile includes measurements of TC, TG, LDL-C, and HDL-C. The LDL-C may be directly measured or calculated. Some labs also report VLDL-C and calculate the non-HDL-C. The importance of these components is elaborated in section "Considerations of Secondary Causes of Dyslipidemia with Potential Mechanisms".

Assay Considerations

In general, the standard lipid profile is performed by enzymatic/spectrophotometric methods. Total cholesterol is measured by standard enzymatic methods, the HDL-C by modified enzymatic assay, and direct LDL-C by an elimination-detergent and selective assay.

Depending on the lab, the reported LDL-C may be directly measured using enzymatic/spectrophotometric assays or calculated using the Friedewald equation: LDL-C = TC − HDL-C − TG/5 [9]. Since the TG values are utilized in the LDL-C calculation, the formula is not applicable at higher TG levels, especially when the TG is >400 mg/dL. When directly measured, there is no significant interference in direct LDL-C value from hemolysis up to 10.0 g/L hemoglobin, from bilirubin up to 30 mg/dL, and from triglycerides up to 1200 mg/dL.

Newer Assays and Utility

The vertical autoprofile test directly measures and routinely reports all five lipoprotein classes and subclasses, including LDL-C, HDL-C, IDL, VLDL-C, and lipoprotein (a) and is unaffected by TG levels. The nuclear magnetic resonance spectroscopy lipoprotein profile assay can quantify specific lipoprotein particle concentrations and sizes. Other measurements are apolipoprotein B and lipoprotein (a). Measurement of particle sizes, concentration or number, and apoB are not routinely recommended in pediatrics at this time. Moreover, pediatric reference intervals for these newer measures are not available.

Considerations in the Interpretation of the Lipid Profile

Age The lipid profile values are age and gender dependent. Table 32.1 indicates age-appropriate normal values for a lipid panel in children and adolescents based on NCEP report [5].

Typically, TC and LDL-C increase until 2 years and then stay relatively stable until adolescence. Although the exact mechanisms are not known, a 10–20% reduction of TC and LDL-C occurs during puberty both in normal children and in children with genetic dyslipidemias such as familial hypercholesterolemia, such that testing for hyperlipidemia during puberty could result in false-negative testing [8]. It is important to repeat lipid levels between ages 17 years and 19 years.

Race There are racial variations in circulating lipid concentrations, with African-American children having higher TC and HDL-C, and lower TG levels compared to other ethnic groups despite higher incidence of obesity, insulin resistance, and prediabetes/diabetes [10, 11].

Fasting versus non-fasting sample TG is the component of the lipid profile most affected by non-fasting status, with TG increasing after food ingestion. The LDL-C and non-HDL-C are mostly unaffected or minimally affected, [12–15], so a non-fasting lipid profile (FLP) is reliable for screening.

Table 32.1 Standard lipid profile: expected values by age

	TC	LDL-C	Non-HDL-C	TG (0–9 years)	TG (10–19 years)	HDL-C
Acceptable	<170	<110	<120	<75	<90	>45
Borderline All values > 75th percentile HDL-C < 25th percentile	171–199	110–129	120–144	75–99	90–129	40–45
Abnormal All values > 95th percentile HDL-C < 10th percentile	>200	≥130	≥145	≥100	≥130	<40

Values from the National Cholesterol Education Program [5]. All fasting values in mg/dL. To convert to SI units, divide total cholesterol, LDL-C, HDL-C, and non-HDL-C by 38.6; for TG, divide by 88.6

Abbreviations: *TC* total cholesterol, *LDL-C* low-density lipoprotein cholesterol, *HDL-C* high-density lipoprotein cholesterol, *TG* triglyceride

Other variations The lipid profile is postulated to have slight postural and seasonal variations [16] and can be affected by stress and intercurrent illnesses. Inter-laboratory value differences of up to 14% have been reported in TC levels [8]. Although rarer in pediatrics, presence of monoclonal proteins in circulation may produce assay interference, especially with causing falsely low HDL-C values [17].

Initial Workup

Children with borderline lipid levels (Table 32.1) need recommendations for diet and lifestyle modifications as outlined in section "Considerations of Secondary Causes of Dyslipidemia with Potential Mechanisms". Confirmed average high or low values on a repeat level merit evaluation for secondary dyslipidemia. Some considerations include liver function testing, serum albumin, blood glucose level or hemoglobin A1C, renal function tests, serum thyroid–stimulating hormone, and a pregnancy screen.

Immediate Referral to a Lipid Specialist

- Children with average LDL-C ≥ 250 mg/dL.
- Fasting TG level of ≥500 mg/dL, which may indicate postprandial elevations to >1000 mg/dL and risk of pancreatitis.
- When considering therapeutic initiation of niacin, fibrates, and cholesterol-absorption inhibitors or combination therapy of lipid-lowering agents with statins.

Knowledge of what constitutes a positive family history, high risk and moderate risk factors, and medical conditions is necessary before determining if the pediatrician will initiate therapy with an HMG Co-A reductase inhibitor (statin) or make a referral to the lipid specialist for further pharmacotherapy.

*Positive family history: Parent, grandparent, aunt, uncle, or sibling with any of these before the age 55 years in a male or 65 years in a female – myocardial infarction, stroke, angina, coronary artery bypass, stent, angioplasty, sudden cardiac death, and parent with total cholesterol > 240 mg/dL.

**High risk condition: Type 1 or 2 diabetes, chronic renal disease/end-stage renal disease/post-renal transplant, post-orthotopic heart transplant, and Kawasaki disease with current aneurysms.

**High risk factor: Hypertension requiring drug therapy (BP ≥ 99th percentile + 5 mmHg), current smoking, and BMI ≥ 97th percentile.

***Moderate risk condition: Kawasaki disease with regressed coronary aneurysms, systemic lupus erythematosus, juvenile rheumatoid arthritis, human immunodeficiency virus (HIV) infection, and nephrotic syndrome.

***Moderate risk factor: Hypertension not requiring drug therapy, BMI ≥ 95th percentile but < 97th percentile, HDL-C < 40 mg/dL.

Considerations for Either Initiation of Statin Therapy by the Pediatrician or Referral to a Lipid Specialist

- Children between 8years and 9 years with LDL-C ≥ 190 mg/dL + positive family history* or at least one high-level risk factor or risk condition** or at least two moderate-level risk factors or risk conditions***.

After a 6-month trial of diet/lifestyle management in children ≥10 years:

- LDL–C ≥ 190 mg/dL.
- LDL–C ≥ 160 to 189 mg/dL + positive family history* or at least one high-level risk factor or risk condition**, or at least two moderate-level risk factors or risk conditions***.
- LDL–C ≥ 130 to 159 mg/dL + two high-level risk factors or risk conditions** or one high-level risk factor or condition, together with at least two moderate-level risk factors or conditions***.

Considerations Based on Abnormal Lipid Profiles

Once secondary causes of dyslipidemias have been ruled out, if it is determined that the abovementioned abnormal criteria are met, considering the following diagnoses based on the predominant lipid measure encountered is necessary. Details of the conditions are listed in Table 32.2, as well as principles of management are found in section "Etiology and Key Pathophysiology", Chap. 57, of this book.

Table 32.2 Common diagnostic considerations based on abnormal lipid profiles

Disorders of LDL-C metabolism	Disorders of TG metabolism	Disorders of HDL-C metabolism
Familial hypercholesterolemia LDL-C receptor mutation Gain of function PCSK9 mutation Familial defective apo B-100. Polygenic hypercholesterolemia LDL-C receptor adaptor protein defects Autosomal-recessive hypercholesterolemia Sitosterolemia Lysosomal acid lipase deficiency Cholesterol 7α-hydroxylase deficiency *Overproduction of VLDL-C/LDL-C/IDL-C* Familial combined hyperlipidemia *Decreased VLDL-C/IDL/HDL-C levels*: Abetalipoproteinemia Hypobetalipoproteinemia Chylomicron retention disease	Defective or absent lipoprotein lipase or its cofactors Exogenous autoimmune hypertriglyceridemia Familial hypertriglyceridemia Dysbetalipoproteinemia	Familial hypoalphalipoproteinemia Tangier disease Lecithin cholesterol acyl transferase deficiency Cholesterol ester transfer protein deficiency Endothelial lipase deficiency

Abbreviations: *LDL-C* low-density lipoprotein cholesterol, *HDL-C* high-density lipoprotein cholesterol, *TG* triglyceride

Conclusion

Dyslipidemias may be primary (monogenic or polygenic) or secondary. Dyslipidemia is often clinically silent, begins in childhood, and tracks into adulthood. Screening for lipid disorders in childhood allows early identification and control of pediatric dyslipidemia with the goal to reduce cardiovascular morbidity and mortality in adulthood.

References

1. Strong JP, Malcom GT, McMahan CA, Tracy RE, Newman WP III, Herderick EE, et al. Prevalence and extent of atherosclerosis in adolescents and young adults implications for prevention from the pathobiological determinants of atherosclerosis in youth study. JAMA. 1999;281(8):727–35.
2. Urbina EM, Srinivasan S, Kieltyka R, Tang R, Bond M, Chen W, et al. Correlates of carotid artery stiffness in young adults: the Bogalusa Heart Study. Atherosclerosis. 2004;176(1):157–64.
3. Organization WH. World health statistics 2016: monitoring health for the SDGs sustainable development goals: World Health Organization; 2016.
4. Luirink IK, Wiegman A, Kusters DM, Hof MH, Groothoff JW, de Groot E, et al. 20-year follow-up of statins in children with familial hypercholesterolemia. N Engl J Med. 2019;381(16):1547–56.
5. National Cholesterol Education Program (NCEP): highlights of the report of the expert panel on blood cholesterol levels in children and adolescents. Pediatrics. 1992;89(3):495–501.
6. Starc TJ, Belamarich PF, Shea S, Dobrin-Seckler BE, Dell RB, Gersony WM, et al. Family history fails to identify many children with severe hypercholesterolemia. Am J Dis Child (1960). 1991;145(1):61–4.
7. Expert panel on integrated guidelines for cardiovascular health and risk reduction in children and adolescents: summary report. Pediatrics. 2011;128(Supplement 5):S213–S56.
8. Bibbins-Domingo K, Grossman DC, Curry SJ, Davidson KW, Epling JW, García FA, et al. Screening for lipid disorders in children and adolescents: US Preventive Services Task Force recommendation statement. JAMA. 2016;316(6):625–33.
9. Friedewald WT, Levy RI, Fredrickson DS. Estimation of the concentration of low-density lipoprotein cholesterol in plasma, without use of the preparative ultracentrifuge. Clin Chem. 1972;18(6):499–502.
10. Chang MH, Ned RM, Hong Y, Yesupriya A, Yang Q, Liu T, et al. Racial/ethnic variation in the association of lipid-related genetic variants with blood lipids in the US adult population. Circ Cardiovasc Genet. 2011;4(5):523–33.
11. Bentley AR, Rotimi CN. Interethnic variation in lipid profiles: implications for Underidentification of African-Americans at risk for metabolic disorders. Expert Rev Endocrinol Metab. 2012;7(6):659–67.
12. Doran B, Guo Y, Xu J, Weintraub H, Mora S, Maron DJ, et al. Prognostic value of fasting versus nonfasting low-density lipoprotein cholesterol levels on long-term mortality: insight from the National Health and Nutrition Examination Survey III (NHANES-III). Circulation. 2014;130(7):546–53.
13. Eckel RH. LDL-C cholesterol as a predictor of mortality, and beyond: to fast or not to fast, that is the question? Am Heart Assoc. 2014;130(7):528–9.
14. Nordestgaard BG, Langsted A, Mora S, Kolovou G, Baum H, Bruckert E, et al. Fasting is not routinely required for determination of a lipid profile: clinical and laboratory implications including flagging at desirable concentration cut-points—a joint consensus statement from the European Atherosclerosis Society and European Federation of Clinical Chemistry and Laboratory Medicine. Eur Heart J. 2016;37(25):1944–58.
15. Craig SR, Amin RV, Russell DW, Paradise NF. Blood cholesterol screening. J Gen Intern Med. 2000;15(6):395–9.
16. Orchard TJ, Rodgers M, Hedley A, Mitchell J. Serum lipids in a teenage population: geographic, seasonal and familial factor. Int J Epidemiol. 1981;10(2):161–70.
17. Tsai LY, Tsai SM, Lee SC, Liu SF. Falsely low LDL-C-cholesterol concentrations and artifactual undetectable HDL-C-cholesterol measured by direct methods in a patient with monoclonal paraprotein. Clin Chim Acta. 2005;358(1–2):192–5.

Prolactin

33

Madhusmita Misra

Important Considerations in Prolactin Measurements

Prolactin is a hormone secreted by the lactotropes of the anterior pituitary gland with levels that are higher in women than in men (assay-specific normative ranges should thus be used to interpret levels). Prolactin levels increase markedly (10–20 times) during pregnancy because of increasing levels of gonadal steroids, particularly estradiol, and levels remain high for a period following pregnancy, when prolactin is necessary for the milk "let-down" necessary for lactation. In addition to pregnancy, prolactin increases during suckling (which facilitates lactation), other instances of nipple stimulation, and from lesions of the chest wall. Physiological conditions such as sleep [1–3], exercise, and high protein meals [4] may cause prolactin levels to rise, as may physical and emotional stress. Significant prolactin elevations have been noted following stressful venipuncture in children [2].

Prolactin is primarily regulated through tonic inhibition by dopamine, when dopamine binds to D2 receptors on lactotropes. Dopamine reaches the anterior pituitary from the hypothalamus via the portal circulation that traverses the pituitary stalk. Thus, any lesion that compresses or infiltrates the pituitary stalk can cause hyperprolactinemia by interrupting dopamine signaling (see Table 33.1 and Chap. 56, Sellar and Extrasellar Lesions). Further, many medications that antagonize dopamine signaling may cause an increase in prolactin secretion, with some of the greatest elevations observed with risperidone and paliperidone (see Table 33.1). Olanzapine and ziprasidone cause lesser increases in prolactin, quetiapine is typically neutral, and aripiprazole may decrease prolactin [5, 6]. In addition, thyrotropin-releasing hormone (TRH) can stimulate prolactin secretion, and therefore, severe primary hypothyroidism (associated with low free T4 and high TRH and thyrotropin levels) is associated with increased prolactin secretion [7] (see Chap. 41, Hypothyroidism). Renal failure is associated with high prolactin because of increased secretion, decreased clearance, and use of medications that may cause prolactin elevation [7–9].

Because prolactin is secreted by the pituitary lactotropes, pituitary adenomas resulting from lactotrope hyperplasia (prolactinomas) are associated with increased prolactin levels, with the extent of prolactin elevation related to the size of the adenoma. However, large prolactinomas that are cystic or poorly differentiated may not demonstrate the extent of prolactin elevation expected for the size of the tumor. Careful consideration of the differential diagnosis of elevated prolactin is a critical first step in patients with prolactin elevations (Table 33.1).

Low prolactin levels are rare, but may occur (Table 33.1). Although there is no medical consequence of low prolactin in an individual who does not desire lactation, low prolactin may indicate certain underlying conditions. The transcription factor POU1F1 (or Pit1) is necessary for lactotrope differentiation, and mutations in the *POU1F1* gene or the *PROP1* gene (prophet of Pit1) are associated with low prolactin levels. Mutations in *POU1F1* also cause deficiencies of growth hormone (GH) and thyroid-stimulating hormone (TSH), while mutations of *PROP1* can cause deficiencies of prolactin, GH, TSH, the gonadotropins, and, in later life, of adrenocorticotropic hormone (ACTH). Further, severe postpartum hemorrhage may result in hypoxic damage to the anterior pituitary with resultant deficiency of the anterior pituitary hormones, including prolactin (manifests as insufficient or failed lactation).

Falsely Low Prolactin Due to Hook Effect

Prolactin is usually measured by an immunometric assay with prolactin bound to both a solid-phase capture antibody and a detection antibody ("sandwich" complex), with the signal from the detection antibody quantified in the assay.

M. Misra (✉)
Division of Pediatric Endocrinology, Massachusetts General Hospital and Harvard Medical School, Boston, MA, USA
e-mail: MMISRA@mgh.harvard.edu

T. Stanley, M. Misra (eds.), *Endocrine Conditions in Pediatrics*, https://doi.org/10.1007/978-3-030-52215-5_33

Table 33.1 Conditions resulting in high or low prolactin levels

High prolactin levels	Expected prolactin levels
Physiological causes	
Pregnancy and breastfeeding	10–20-fold elevations, typically <400 ng/mL [10, 11]
Anxiety and stress (phlebotomy, critical illness, surgery)	≤100 ng/mL [2, 12], typically <50 ng/mL [13]
Nipple stimulation, chest trauma, and chest wall lesions	≤100 ng/mL for chest wall issues [14, 15], usually lower with nipple stimulation
Exercise	Within normal physiologic range [16, 17]
Sleep	Up to fourfold waking levels [3]
Medical conditions	
Hypothyroidism	≤50–100 ng/mL [18–20]
Renal failure	≤200 ng/mL [8]
Medications	
Estrogen	Minimal increases with lower doses (e.g., hormone replacement or ≤35mcg daily ethinyl estradiol [21–23])
Antipsychotics (typical and atypical)	Risperidone and paliperidone ≤250 ng/mL [24] Others to a lesser degree [5, 6, 23]
Antidepressants (including serotonin selective reuptake inhibitors [SSRIs], monoamine oxidase inhibitors, and tricyclics)	≤50 ng/mL [23, 25]
Metoclopramide	≤300 ng/mL [26]
Domperidone	≤150 ng/mL [27]
Cocaine	≤50 ng/mL [28]
Opiates	≤50 ng/mL [29, 30]
Verapamil	≤50 ng/mL [31, 32]
Stalk compression	Usually ≤ 250 ng/ml
Craniopharyngioma	
Rathke cleft cyst	
Non-functioning adenoma or other functioning adenoma	
Less common: Gliomas, lymphomas, meningiomas, or hamartomas	
Autoimmune hypophysitis	
Germinoma	
Histiocytosis X	
Other granulomatous or infiltrative diseases (sarcoidosis, tuberculosis, IgG4 hypophysitis)	
Prolactinomas	
Microprolactinomas	Variable depending on the size
Macroprolactinomas	Usually ≥250 ng/ml May be lower if cystic or poorly differentiated
Low prolactin levels	
Congenital	
Transcription factor defects (POUF1, PROP1)	Variable, may be low
Acquired	
Pituitary apoplexy	Variable, may be low
Sheehan's syndrome	Variable, may be low

Adapted with permission from: Stanley and Misra [34]

When prolactin levels are very high, excess prolactin saturates the detection antibody in the liquid phase. Much of this detection antibody then gets washed away, with reduced sandwich binding [33], leading to a falsely low assay reading (Hook effect) [34]. The hook shape of the graph demonstrating assay results at varying concentrations gives this effect its name. This is particularly an issue with macroprolactinomas, when a falsely low prolactin level can mislead the clinician into considering other etiologies for hyperprolactinemia, or impact dose adjustments of medications being used to treat the tumor. Hook effect can be prevented by requesting prolactin levels in dilution [33] or by a washout (after prolactin has bound to the capture antibody) to eliminate excess unbound prolactin before adding the detection antibody [34].

Hyperprolactinemia from Macroprolactinemia

An increase in circulating "big big prolactin," or macroprolactin (a high molecular weight, bio-inactive form of prolactin) [35], may cause hyperprolactinemia that is not otherwise clinically relevant. This is usually discovered incidentally, and has been reported in 7.5% of cases of hyperprolactinemia [20, 34]. Polyethylene glycol–mediated precipitation allows removal of macroprolactin but not monomeric prolactin, and precipitation of >50% total prolactin confirms macroprolactinemia [35]. Testing for macroprolactin may be considered in asymptomatic patients with hyperprolactinemia, particularly those with a normal pituitary MRI [7].

Clinical Key: Dealing with Mildly Elevated Prolactin
Patients with a mild elevation in prolactin should have a repeat level drawn in the morning in the fasting state, ideally with any prolactin-raising medications discontinued. If stress may be a contributor, it is ideal to place an IV and wait 60 min after placement to draw the sample. In asymptomatic patients, macroprolactin testing can be requested from the laboratory. After these steps, persistent elevations in prolactin that are not explained by other causes, even when mild, usually warrant a brain MRI.

Interpretation of an Abnormal Level and Next Steps

Sufficiently high prolactin levels can cause galactorrhea, as well as suppression of gonadotropin and gonadal steroid secretion, although the extent of prolactin elevation necessary to cause these symptoms may vary among individuals. Hypogonadism manifests as amenorrhea in females, gynecomastia in males, and decreased libido and infertility in both. An elevated prolactin level should be repeated in the fasting state, preferably earlier in the day, with instructions to the patient to refrain from any nipple stimulation or exercise preceding the test. Pregnancy should be ruled out in girls of childbearing age and pubertal stage, and hypothyroidism and chronic renal failure should be ruled out in all. If stress of venipuncture is a consideration, placing an intravenous catheter and drawing blood at the time of venipuncture and an hour later (when the patient has presumably calmed down) is sufficient to demonstrate the normalization of prolactin levels, following reduction of stress.

Ideally, a normal prolactin level should be documented before beginning a medication known to cause prolactin elevations. Mild prolactin elevations subsequent to starting the medication are then less concerning, but should be monitored. Rising levels may indicate a coincident additional etiology for hyperprolactinemia and may mandate an MRI. In general, when a medication is the suspected cause of hyperprolactinemia, this should be confirmed by documenting normal prolactin after stopping the medication [36]. However, stopping the medication may not be feasible, particularly when it is an antipsychotic. Because the degree of prolactin elevation with certain antipsychotics overlaps that seen with sellar and extrasellar lesion, an MRI should be performed in patients who cannot be safely withdrawn from treatment [7], and in those whose prolactin level is >100 ng/mL.

If a sellar or extrasellar lesion is causing hyperprolactinemia, other manifestations may include headache, nausea, vomiting, vision changes, polyuria, polydipsia, and features of hypopituitarism from deficiency of other pituitary hormones (from mass effects). After making sure that all abovementioned considerations have been ruled out, a pituitary MRI is indicated to diagnose such lesions (see Chap. 56, Sellar and Extrasellar Lesions). When a sizeable (≥10 mm) lesion is found on MRI without the expected degree of elevation in prolactin (i.e., prolactin < 250 ng/mL), sellar masses other than prolactinomas causing prolactin elevation due to stalk compression should be considered. A consultation with radiology and/or neurosurgery may help determine the need for a biopsy.

References

1. Roelfsema F, Pijl H, Keenan DM, Veldhuis JD. Prolactin secretion in healthy adults is determined by gender, age and body mass index. PLoS One. 2012;7(2):e31305.
2. Whyte MB, Pramodh S, Srikugan L, Gilbert JA, Miell JP, Sherwood RA, et al. Importance of cannulated prolactin test in the definition of hyperprolactinaemia. Pituitary. 2015;18(3):319–25.
3. Stawerska R, Smyczynska J, Hilczer M, Lewinski A. Does elevated morning prolactin concentration in children always mean the diagnosis of hyperprolactinemia? Exp Clin Endocrinol Diabetes. 2015;123(7):405–10.
4. Quigley ME, Ropert JF, Yen SS. Acute prolactin release triggered by feeding. J Clin Endocrinol Metab. 1981;52(5):1043–5.
5. Cohen D, Bonnot O, Bodeau N, Consoli A, Laurent C. Adverse effects of second-generation antipsychotics in children and adolescents: a Bayesian meta-analysis. J Clin Psychopharmacol. 2012;32(3):309–16.
6. Fraguas D, Correll CU, Merchan-Naranjo J, Rapado-Castro M, Parellada M, Moreno C, et al. Efficacy and safety of second-generation antipsychotics in children and adolescents with psychotic and bipolar spectrum disorders: comprehensive review of prospective head-to-head and placebo-controlled comparisons. Eur Neuropsychopharmacol. 2011;21(8):621–45.
7. Melmed S, Casanueva FF, Hoffman AR, Kleinberg DL, Montori VM, Schlechte JA, et al. Diagnosis and treatment of hyperprolactinemia: an Endocrine Society clinical practice guideline. J Clin Endocrinol Metab. 2011;96(2):273–88.
8. Yavuz D, Topcu G, Ozener C, Akalin S, Sirikci O. Macroprolactin does not contribute to elevated levels of prolactin in patients on renal replacement therapy. Clin Endocrinol. 2005;63(5):520–4.

9. Sievertsen GD, Lim VS, Nakawatase C, Frohman LA. Metabolic clearance and secretion rates of human prolactin in normal subjects and in patients with chronic renal failure. J Clin Endocrinol Metab. 1980;50(5):846–52.
10. Tay CC, Glasier AF, McNeilly AS. Twenty-four hour patterns of prolactin secretion during lactation and the relationship to suckling and the resumption of fertility in breast-feeding women. Hum Reprod. 1996;11(5):950–5.
11. Abbassi-Ghanavati M, Greer LG, Cunningham FG. Pregnancy and laboratory studies: a reference table for clinicians. Obstet Gynecol. 2009;114(6):1326–31.
12. Heidemann SM, Holubkov R, Meert KL, Dean JM, Berger J, Bell M, et al. Baseline serum concentrations of zinc, selenium, and prolactin in critically ill children. Pediatr Crit Care Med. 2013;14(4):e202–6.
13. Mancini T, Casanueva FF, Giustina A. Hyperprolactinemia and prolactinomas. Endocrinol Metab Clin N Am. 2008;37(1):67–99. viii
14. Katsuren E, Ishikawa S, Honda K, Saito T. Galactorrhoea and amenorrhoea due to an intradural neurinoma originating from a thoracic intercostal nerve radicle. Clin Endocrinol. 1997;46(5):631–6.
15. Saraiya H. Postburn galactorrhea with refractory hypertrophic scars: role of obesity under scrutiny. J Burn Care Rehabil. 2003;24(6):392–4.
16. Chang FE, Richards SR, Kim MH, Malarkey WB. Twenty four-hour prolactin profiles and prolactin responses to dopamine in long distance running women. J Clin Endocrinol Metab. 1984;59(4): 631–5.
17. Cho GJ, Han SW, Shin JH, Kim T. Effects of intensive training on menstrual function and certain serum hormones and peptides related to the female reproductive system. Medicine (Baltimore). 2017;96(21):e6876.
18. Kleinberg DL, Noel GL, Frantz AG. Galactorrhea: a study of 235 cases, including 48 with pituitary tumors. N Engl J Med. 1977;296(11):589–600.
19. Honbo KS, van Herle AJ, Kellett KA. Serum prolactin levels in untreated primary hypothyroidism. Am J Med. 1978;64(5):782–7.
20. Soto-Pedre E, Newey PJ, Bevan JS, Greig N, Leese GP. The epidemiology of hyperprolactinaemia over 20 years in the Tayside region of Scotland: the Prolactin Epidemiology, Audit and Research Study (PROLEARS). Clin Endocrinol. 2017;86(1):60–7.
21. Hwang PL, Ng CS, Cheong ST. Effect of oral contraceptives on serum prolactin: a longitudinal study in 126 normal premenopausal women. Clin Endocrinol. 1986;24(2):127–33.
22. Josimovich JB, Lavenhar MA, Devanesan MM, Sesta HJ, Wilchins SA, Smith AC. Heterogeneous distribution of serum prolactin values in apparently healthy young women, and the effects of oral contraceptive medication. Fertil Steril. 1987;47(5):785–91.
23. Molitch ME. Drugs and prolactin. Pituitary. 2008;11(2):209–18.
24. Kearns AE, Goff DC, Hayden DL, Daniels GH. Risperidone-associated hyperprolactinemia. Endocr Pract. 2000;6(6):425–9.
25. Kim S, Park YM. Serum prolactin and macroprolactin levels among outpatients with major depressive disorder following the administration of selective serotonin-reuptake inhibitors: a cross-sectional pilot study. PLoS One. 2013;8(12):e82749.
26. Cunha-Filho JS, Gross JL, Vettori D, Dias EC, Passos EP. Growth hormone and prolactin secretion after metoclopramide administration (DA2 receptor blockade) in fertile women. Horm Metab Res. 2001;33(9):536–9.
27. Cho E, Ho S, Gerber P, Davidson AG. Monitoring of serum prolactin in pediatric patients with cystic fibrosis who are receiving domperidone. Can J Hosp Pharm. 2009;62(2):119–26.
28. Mendelson JH, Mello NK, Teoh SK, Ellingboe J, Cochin J. Cocaine effects on pulsatile secretion of anterior pituitary, gonadal, and adrenal hormones. J Clin Endocrinol Metab. 1989;69(6):1256–60.
29. Zis AP, Haskett RF, Albala AA, Carroll BJ. Morphine inhibits cortisol and stimulates prolactin secretion in man. Psychoneuroendocrinology. 1984;9(4):423–7.
30. Afrasiabi MA, Flomm M, Friedlander H, Valenta LJ. Endocrine studies in heroin addicts. Psychoneuroendocrinology. 1979;4(2):145–53.
31. Gluskin LE, Strasberg B, Shah JH. Verapamil-induced hyperprolactinemia and galactorrhea. Ann Intern Med. 1981;95(1):66–7.
32. Kelley SR, Kamal TJ, Molitch ME. Mechanism of verapamil calcium channel blockade-induced hyperprolactinemia. Am J Phys. 1996;270(1 Pt 1):E96–100.
33. do Carmo Dias Gontijo M, de Souza Vasconcellos L, Ribeiro-Oliveira A Jr. Hook effect and linear range in prolactin assays: distinct confounding entities. Pituitary. 2016;19(4):458–9.
34. Stanley TK, Misra M. Prolactinomas. In: Kohn B, editor. Pituitary disorders of childhood: diagnosis and clinical management. Gewerbestrasse, Switzerland: Humana Press; 2019. p. 71–88.
35. Overgaard M, Pedersen SM. Serum prolactin revisited: parametric reference intervals and cross platform evaluation of polyethylene glycol precipitation-based methods for discrimination between hyperprolactinemia and macroprolactinemia. Clin Chem Lab Med. 2017;55(11):1744–53.
36. Cazabat L, Bouligand J, Salenave S, Bernier M, Gaillard S, Parker F, et al. Germline AIP mutations in apparently sporadic pituitary adenomas: prevalence in a prospective single-center cohort of 443 patients. J Clin Endocrinol Metab. 2012;97(4):E663–70.

Catecholamines and Catecholamine Metabolites

34

Takara Stanley

Introduction

Catecholamines are a group of three neurotransmitters derived from the amino acid tyrosine: dopamine, norepinephrine, and epinephrine. Norepinephrine is synthesized and secreted from both sympathetic nerves and the adrenal medulla, whereas epinephrine is synthesized and secreted solely in the adrenal medulla [1]. Figure 34.1 illustrates pathways of norepinephrine and epinephrine metabolism that are particularly relevant to diagnostic testing. Norepinephrine is primarily metabolized via monoamine oxidase, with secondary metabolism through catechol-O-methyltransferase (COMT) to normetanephrine and, to a lesser degree, metanephrine. Epinephrine is metabolized via COMT to metanephrine and, to a lesser extent, normetanephrine. Metanephrine and normetanephrine are produced in the adrenal medulla as well as other extraneuronal tissues, with the adrenal medulla being the primary source of circulating metanephrine and normetanephrine [1]. The primary end metabolic product of all these compounds is vanillylmandelic acid (VMA), which is produced in the liver and excreted in urine [1]. Homovanillic acid (HVA) is the primary metabolite of dopamine, also excreted in urine [1].

Measurement of catecholamines and their metabolites assesses the diagnostic possibility of pheochromocytoma or paraganglioma, which are neuroendocrine tumors comprised of an abnormal proliferation of chromaffin cells. The difference between a pheochromocytoma, arising from the adrenal medulla, and a paraganglioma, arising from a non-adrenal source, is solely based on location. Sympathetic paragangliomas arise from the sympathetic chain and secrete catecholamines. Parasympathetic paragangliomas, arising from parasympathetic neurons, usually do not secrete catecholamines and thus would not be detected by the testing discussed in this chapter.

T. Stanley (✉)
Division of Pediatric Endocrinology, Massachusetts General Hospital and Harvard Medical School, Boston, MA, USA
e-mail: tstanley@mgh.harvard.edu

Initial Laboratory Evaluation

For a patient with suspected pheochromocytoma or paraganglioma, the recommended first step in screening is either plasma free metanephrines (also called plasma fractionated metanephrines) or 24-hour urine fractionated metanephrines [2]. Although catecholamine release from tumors may be sporadic, metanephrines provide a relatively stable measurement [2]. Both plasma and urine metanephrines have very high sensitivity and good specificity. Twenty-four-hour urine catecholamine or VMA measurements have lower sensitivity but better specificity.

The diagnostic characteristics and notes regarding each test are shown in Table 34.1. One of the most important considerations in diagnostic testing is a careful medication history, as multiple medications affecting catecholamine metabolism can cause false "positive" screening, as listed in Table 34.2. Other conditions that cause physiological increases in catecholamines, such as acute illness, can also cause false positives (Table 34.2).

Other important principles of testing are as follows:

- The ideal conditions for blood sampling for metanephrines are after the patient has been resting, ideally supine, for 30 minutes. Drawing samples in the seated position and/or without a sufficient resting period increases the likelihood of false-positive results [2].
- Liquid chromatography with mass spectrometry or electrochemical detection should be used for diagnosis. Immunoassays should not be used due to poorer diagnostic performance [2].
- Twenty-four-hour urine collection should be in an acid container (i.e., with acid added to the collection container as a preservative). Urine creatinine should also be measured to ensure sample validity.

Another critical thing to remember in testing for pheochromocytoma and paraganglioma is that these diseases are

T. Stanley, M. Misra (eds.), *Endocrine Conditions in Pediatrics*, https://doi.org/10.1007/978-3-030-52215-5_34

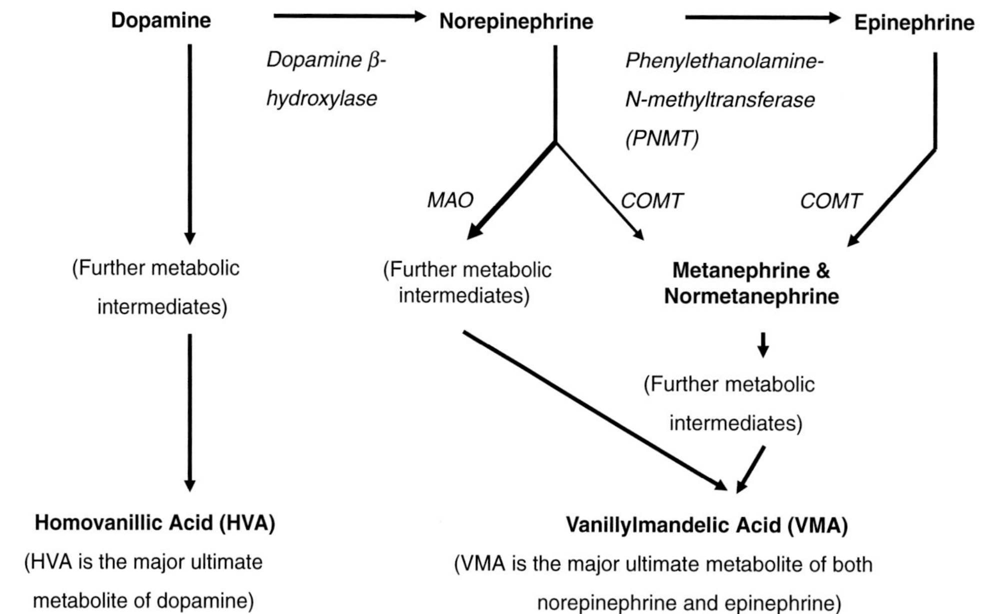

Fig. 34.1 Pathways of catecholamine metabolism relevant to diagnostic testing. Legend: Norepinephrine is primarily metabolized through deamination via monoamine oxidase (MAO) followed by further metabolism to vanillylmandelic acid (VMA). A secondary pathway of metabolism is to normetanephrine and, to a lesser degree, metanephrine via catechol-O-methyltransferase (COMT). Epinephrine is metabolized by COMT to metanephrine and, to a lesser extent, normetanephrine. Subsequent metabolism of metanephrine and normetanephrine also results in the production of VMA [1]. Abbreviations: COMT, catechol-O-methyltransferase; MAO: monoamine oxidase

Table 34.1 Initial laboratory testing for pheochromocytoma and paraganglioma

Test	Diagnostic characteristics	Notes
First-line screening tests		
Plasma free metanephrines	Very high sensitivity (~99%); moderate specificity (~89%) [3]	Ideal sampling is after 30 min rest in supine position. Positive screen should be confirmed with additional testing due to possibility of false-positive result
24-hour urinary fractionated metanephrines	Very high sensitivity (~97%); poor specificity (~69%) [3]	Positive screen should be confirmed with additional testing due to possibility of false-positive result
Other testing		
24-hour urine total metanephrines	Very high specificity (~93%); poor sensitivity (~77%) [3]	Excellent confirmatory test due to high specificity
24-hour urinary VMA	Very high specificity (~95%); poor sensitivity (~64%) [3]	Excellent confirmatory test due to high specificity
24-hour urinary catecholamines	Moderate sensitivity (~86%) and specificity (~88%) [3]	
Plasma catecholamines	Moderate sensitivity (~84%) and specificity (~81%) [3]	
24-hour urinary HVA	(n/a)	Used in testing for neuroblastoma; not part of the diagnostic process for pheochromocytoma or paraganglioma but may be elevated
Sporadic HVA and VMA	(n/a)	"Spot" urine testing for HVA and VMA used for neuroblastoma; not part of the diagnostic process for pheochromocytoma or paraganglioma but may be elevated

quite rare, such that even tests with high specificity will yield a relatively high percentage of false-positive testing.

Urine VMA and HVA are commonly used to test for neuroblastoma. It is important to note that plasma and urine metanephrines and catecholamines are often elevated in patients with neuroblastoma, which is a more common tumor in the pediatric age group than pheochromocytoma or paraganglioma.

Table 34.2 Conditions contributing to false positives in measurement of catecholamines and catecholamine metabolites in plasma and/or urine

Conditions that alter circulating levels
Acute illness
Exercise or significant exertion or stress
Hypoglycemia
Substantial pre-test consumption of fruits (particularly if overripe or dried), nuts, potatoes, tomatoes, beans, aged cheese, aged/smoked/pickled/cured meat/fish/poultry, soy products (which contain high amounts of tyramine)
Medications that alter circulating levels
Tricyclic antidepressants
Monoamine oxidase inhibitors
Selective serotonin reuptake inhibitors
Serotonin norepinephrine reuptake inhibitors
Dopamine antagonists (some antipsychotics and some anti-emetics)
Levodopa
Epinephrine (i.e., "epi-pen")
Cocaine
Sympathomimetics, amphetamines
Phenoxybenzamine
Caffeine and ethanol
Medications that interfere with certain assays [2]
Acetaminophen
Sotalol and labetolol
α-Methyldopa
Buspirone

Clinical Keys

- Plasma free (fractionated) metanephrines are easily obtained and highly sensitive, such that normal plasma free metanephrines makes a diagnosis of pheochromocytoma unlikely.
- Pheochromocytoma and paraganglioma are rare, and specificity of plasma free metanephrines or 24-hour urine metanephrines is imperfect, so positive testing should be confirmed with a second type of test.
- Elevations in metanephrines and catecholamines are typically not subtle in pheochromocytoma and paraganglioma. Rather, they are usually more than twofold the upper limit of the normal of the assay.
- For mild elevations, <2x upper limit of the normal, strongly consider the possibility of a false positive and consider repeat-testing in the supine position after 30 minutes of rest.

Initial Management of Results

Normal plasma free metanephrines or 24-hour urine metanephrines significantly decrease the likelihood of pheochromocytoma and paraganglioma and should prompt a search for other diagnoses related to the patient's symptoms. If pretest probability is moderate to high, however, negative testing could prompt retesting during an episode or spell.

If plasma free metanephrines or 24-hour urine metanephrines are elevated >2 times the upper limit of the normal of the lab, urgent referral to pediatric endocrinology is warranted. In children with pheochromocytoma or paraganglioma, the likelihood of an underlying genetic mutation and/or syndromic cause is high. Consideration should be given to the possibility of commonly associated syndromes (neurofibromatosis, multiple endocrine neoplasia 2, von Hippel-Lindau), and genetic testing should be performed for other associated mutations [2].

For milder elevations in plasma or urine metanephrines, particularly in patients with possible reasons for false-positive results, consider repeating the test with any possible interfering medications temporarily discontinued, and, for plasma free metanephrines, after the patient has rested for 30 minutes in the supine position.

References

1. Eisenhofer G, Kopin IJ, Goldstein DS. Catecholamine metabolism: a contemporary view with implications for physiology and medicine. Pharmacol Rev. 2004;56(3):331–49.
2. Lenders JW, Duh QY, Eisenhofer G, Gimenez-Roqueplo AP, Grebe SK, Murad MH, et al. Pheochromocytoma and paraganglioma: an endocrine society clinical practice guideline. J Clin Endocrinol Metab. 2014;99(6):1915–42.
3. Lenders JW, Pacak K, Walther MM, Linehan WM, Mannelli M, Friberg P, et al. Biochemical diagnosis of pheochromocytoma: which test is best? JAMA. 2002;287(11):1427–34.

Clinical Genetic Testing Options

35

Danielle Renzi and Barbara Pober

Introduction

Genetic disorders diagnosed during childhood can present with complex endocrine abnormalities. As genetic testing assumes an increasingly important role in clinical practice and becomes more widely available, pediatricians need to be aware of the range of clinical genetic testing options. Some tests can be ordered by the pediatrician (chromosome analysis, Fragile X testing), while others are more likely to be ordered by a specialist. Even so, families may want to discuss implications of genetic testing results with their pediatrician. In this chapter, we provide an overview of the most common genetic tests used to diagnose disorders that can present in childhood along with the salient strengths, limitations, and indications for each test.

Organization of Human Genetic Material

The genetic material constituting the human genome is carried on 46 chromosomes, comprising 23 pairs of chromosomes. Deoxyribonucleic Acid (DNA) exists as loosely packed genetic material called chromatin until cell division or replication, when the chromatin condenses into the structures called chromosomes. A normal female and a normal male chromosome complement are designated as 46,XX and 46,XY, respectively.

One member of each chromosome pair is maternally inherited, while the other is paternally inherited. Chromosomes vary in size and, accordingly, in the number of genes and base pairs. The smallest human chromosomes (such as chromosomes #21 and #22) contain approximately 50 million base pairs and 200 genes, while the largest chromosomes (such as #1 and #2) contain approximately 240 million base pairs and just over 2000 genes.

Genetic changes can vary in size and significance. Some changes are not necessarily meaningful for health, while others have great impact. Genetic variation is common between individuals; these differences are known as polymorphisms. A single base pair change is referred to as a *single nucleotide polymorphisms (SNP)*, in which two or more versions of the base pair occur in greater than 1% of the human population. Millions of SNPs have been identified throughout the human genome, and many are not related to disease. In contrast, a single base pair change occurring with less than 1% frequency in the population is more likely to be associated with disease and be classified as a point mutation. Testing, such as DNA sequencing, may be used clinically to identify relationships between point mutations and disease.

Other common larger sources of genetic variation, such as gain or loss of a few hundred to several million base pairs, are called *copy number variants (CNVs)***.** CNVs may or may not have a clear association with negative health impact, depending on the size and specific genes contained within the change.

While it is necessary to acknowledge normal variation in the human genome, the aim of this chapter is to provide an overview of genetic changes that cause medical complications, and to introduce a few common genetic syndromes that are of particular relevance to the clinical scope of pedi-

D. Renzi · B. Pober (✉)
Department of Pediatrics, Genetics Unit, Massachusetts General Hospital, Boston, MA, USA
e-mail: Drenzi3@mgh.harvard.edu;
Pober.barbara@mgh.harvard.edu

T. Stanley, M. Misra (eds.), *Endocrine Conditions in Pediatrics*, https://doi.org/10.1007/978-3-030-52215-5_35

atric endocrinology. The size and type of genetic abnormality that is being considered influences the choice of testing options. Expanded descriptions of abnormalities covered in the following sections are provided in the glossary at the end of this chapter (Table 35.1).

Options for Genetic Testing

Testing options are presented in the following section, beginning with lower resolution tests, which typically detect relatively large genetic changes, and concluding with higher resolution tests, such as DNA sequencing that can detect changes as small as a single DNA base pair. As a general rule, lower resolution tests are ordered first in the clinic setting. If an abnormality is not detected, then increasingly higher resolution tests may subsequently be ordered. Table 35.2 presents a condensed overview of cytogenetic (lower resolution) and clinical molecular cytogenetic (higher resolution) testing options discussed in sections "Cytogenetic Testing" and "Clinical Molecular Cytogenetic Techniques". Table 35.3 follows with an overview of DNA sequencing techniques discussed in section "Gene Sequencing".

Cytogenetic Testing

Clinical use of cytogenetic testing aims to identify structural abnormalities affecting whole chromosomes, or one or more chromosome bands, and is considered a relatively low resolution option.

Chromosome Analysis (Karyotype)

Chromosome analysis results in an image (called a *karyotype*) that displays 46 chromosomes (Fig. 35.1). During mitotic metaphase, the genetic material is maximally condensed, which makes viewing individual chromosomes possible with a microscope. The genetic material is stained with a Giemsa dye that produces a characteristic visible banding pattern.

This test detects various large alterations such as gain or loss of whole chromosomes or chromosome arms, duplications, deletions, and large (greater than ~3 million base pair) chromosome segment abnormalities [1]. While a missing chromosome would be clearly apparent on a karyotype, the banding pattern of each of the chromosomes can also be studied to detect not only large deletions or insertions but also some cases of inversion or translocation.

Common indications for karyotyping include suspicion of aneuploidy, such as Down syndrome. Chromosome analysis is also an option for diagnosing disorders of sexual development related to aneuploidy of the sex chromosomes, such as Klinefelter syndrome or Turner syndrome. Mosaicism commonly occurs in Turner syndrome. Note that mosaicism refers to the presence of at least two cell types with differing chromosomal (or genetic) make-ups in an individual, such as 45,X/46,XX in Turner syndrome.

Understanding Karyotype Notation

- The general notation of a karyotype is "[number of chromosomes],[sex chromosomes], [description of any chromosomal abnormalities]." For example, "47,XY,+21" indicates a male (XY) with an extra copy of the 21st chromosome, i.e., Down Syndrome.
- In the presence of mosaicism, different cell lines are separated by an "/". For example, "46,XX/46,XY" indicates the presence of both XX and XY cell lines and is consistent with a diagnosis of mixed gonadal dysgenesis (see Chap. 46).
- Cytogenetic location on the chromosome is noted using "q" for the long arm and "p" for the short arm of the chromosome, moving outward from the centromere to denote regions, bands, sub-bands. For example, 22q11.2 indicates a position in region 1 (22q**1**1), band 1 (22q1**1**), sub-band 2 (22q11.**2**) on the long arm (q) of chromosome 22.

Clinical Molecular Cytogenetic Techniques

Common clinical molecular cytogenetic testing techniques include chromosomal microarray analysis (CMA) and fluorescence in situ hybridization (FISH). The resolution of CMA has evolved impressively over time. When first discovered, only larger changes of 1–3 million base pairs in size could be detected, whereas now, changes as small as a few hundred base pairs can be appreciated [2].

Table 35.1 Glossary of Chap. 35 relevant terms

Aneuploidy
The gain or loss of one or more entire chromosome(s).
Deletions/duplications/insertions
Gain or loss of some genetic material, ranging in size from a single base pair up to chromosome segments. This change can result in a phenotype by altering the gene dose or, depending on its location, the gene function. Types of gain or loss: *Deletion* is a genetic loss, ranging in size from one or more chromosome segments down to one or a few base pairs. *Insertion* adds genetic material to the genetic sequence, ranging in size from one or more bases to one or more chromosome segments. *Duplication* is a base pair, or chromosome segment, that is copied one or more times.
Copy number variants (CNVs)
CNVs are gains or losses of a segment or section of DNA. CNVs can range in size from 50–100 kb up to millions of base pairs which may involve many genes. Many CNVs have no demonstrable health effects, while others have known associations to genetic disorders. Factors influencing the likely impact of a CNV include its size, the specific genetic content that is either gained or lost, and whether the CNV is familial or de novo.
Single nucleotide polymorphism (SNP)
SNPs are variant versions of a single base pair in the DNA sequence; the alternate versions of the base are typically observed in at least 1% of the population. SNPs are often benign (e.g., have no impact on phenotype) or of uncertain clinical significance. Single base pair changes that are pathogenic occur less commonly than 1%, are more likely to be in the coding or regulatory portions of the gene, and tend to be classified as "mutations" rather than SNPs.
Other chromosome rearrangements
Translocations occur when there is an exchange of chromosome segments between two or more different chromosomes. The exchange can be balanced (i.e., without gain or loss of genetic material) or unbalanced (i.e., with gain or loss of genetic material). The latter is far more likely to be associated with adverse health effects. Inversions occur when a middle segment, bordered by a double break, rotates 180° before rejoining the chromosome.
DNA methylation
DNA methylation is an epigenetic change that can alter gene transcription through binding of a methyl group to a specific DNA base (cytosine). The binding of the methyl group does not change the actual sequence of the DNA but rather can act to repress or silence gene expression. This, in turn, can result in a phenotype.
Mosaicism
Mosaicism describes the existence of two or more genetically different cell types in a person's body. Mosaicism occurs when a mutation, or aneuploidy, arises early during development but in only a subset of cells. The resulting individual harbors both cell types (i.e., "normal," and those with a mutation or aneuploidy) in their body. Mosaicism can exist in the germline (making it possible that the mutation could be passed to offspring), or be restricted to the "soma" (e.g., somatic mosaicism). The latter involves cells in a certain part or parts of the body other than the germline. When there is a relatively low percentage of abnormal cells in the body, this is considered *low-level mosaicism.*
Loss of heterozygosity (LOH)
In LOH, one parental copy of a gene or genes is absent, so that all expression comes from the remaining parental allele. LOH has particular relevance to the inactivation of tumor suppressor genes. In offspring of consanguineous unions, LOH often signifies a different phenomenon. In these circumstances, LOH indicates the presence of identical stretches of DNA that were inherited from a common ancestor through related parents, such as first-cousin unions.

Fluorescent In Situ Hybridization (FISH)

Fluorescent in situ hybridization uses fluorescent probes to detect genetic alterations, such as microdeletions. FISH can also detect other abnormalities (translocations or DNA amplifications), but these are less likely to be associated with disorders that come to the attention of a pediatric endocrinologist. This technique works by applying a single stranded DNA probe with a high degree of sequence homology to the gene or DNA segment (e.g., the "target") being interrogated. If the probe hybridizes to the target in the patient sample, its presence and location can be detected using fluorescence microscopy. Prior to testing, the clinician *must* specify the region to be interrogated in the patient genome. In other words, the FISH technique is only informative when the laboratory utilizes the probe that correctly corresponds to the patient's diagnosis.

Table 35.2 Common clinical molecular cytogenetic and cytogenetic tests

Test Name	Size of DNA change detectable	Types of DNA changes detectable	Test limitations	Common indications	Examples of frequently diagnosed pediatric disorders	Examples of nomenclature
Chromosome analysis (karyotype)	Sensitivity range: change in entire chromosome, chromosome arm, or chromosome sub-band down to approximately 3 mb	Whole chromosome or arm gain or loss Large segment abnormalities including inversion and rearrangement (such as translocation) Deletions, duplications, or insertions >3–5 million base pairs	Changes must be "large" (affecting several million base pairs) to be seen Karyotype is technically labor intensive Low-level mosaicism may not be detected	Patient characteristics, including physical, developmental, or family history that strongly suggest aneuploidy Recurrent miscarriages	Down syndrome (trisomy 21) Klinefelter syndrome Turner syndrome Turner syndrome mosaicism	F: 47, XX, +21 M: 47, XY +21 M: 47, XXY F: 45, X F: 45, X / 46, XX
Fluorescent in situ Hybridization (FISH)	Sensitivity range for metaphase FISH: several hundred kb–1 mb	Clinically used to detect loss of chromosomal regions smaller than what is visible through a microscope (microdeletions)	Detects known abnormalities only; does not lead to discovery of new changes Specific disorder or location in genome must be identified prior to testing, so laboratory knows which probe to use Does not identify full extent of deleted interval in microdeletion disorders Does not detect microduplication disorders Being replaced by CMA (though FISH is cheaper and may be more readily available in certain parts of the world)	Suspected microdeletion disorders	Williams syndrome Deletion 22q11 Prader Willi syndrome (note that ~70% of PWS caused by a chr 15 microdeletion; however, as discussed in the text, other genetic mechanisms also cause PWS, so the single best diagnostic test for PWS is methylation analysis)	ish del(7)(q11.23q11.23)(ELN-) ish del(15)(q11.2q11.2)(SNRPN-)
Chromosomal Microarray Analysis (CMA)	Sensitivity range: Detects gains or losses of stretches of DNA as small as 50–100 kb in length	DNA segment gains or losses smaller than what is visible through a microscope, including: chromosomal imbalances (unbalanced translocations), loss/absence of heterozygosity, microdeletions, and microduplications Gains or losses are typically referred to as CNVs Detects changes throughout the genome (without clinician having to specify, in advance, a disorder or chromosome location) More accurately identifies extent of deletion in microdeletion disorders (compared to FISH)	Detects CNVs of unknown or uncertain clinical significance Does not detect small changes in a single gene Does not sequence DNA (e.g., is not providing base pair information) Does not detect balanced translocations or other balanced rearrangements May not detect low-level mosaicism Does not detect gains or losses below the limits of resolution of the probes More expensive than FISH	Presence of developmental delay, intellectual disability, or physical or congenital abnormalities with no specific suspected condition to explain phenotype CMA can serve as a more detailed and comprehensive alternative to FISH	Williams syndrome Deletion 22q11 Prader Willi syndrome (see note above on PWS testing)	arr 7q11.23 (72718252_7413332) ×1 arr 22q11.21 (18894339_21440514) ×1

Table 35.3 Current clinical applications of DNA sequencing technologies and comparative options

Name of test	Types of DNA changes detectable	Test limitations	Common indications
Single gene sequencing	Can detect single base pair changes (including small substitutions, insertions, deletions) in target gene or area of interest sequenced	If mutations in several genes lead to the same phenotype, then individually sequencing each of these genes, but in a multi-gene panel, is better suited While this method is less expensive and may be technically less difficult to run, larger deletions and duplications of several adjacent genes may not be detected (e.g., CNVs)	Change is suspected in a specific gene or region of a gene; specific mutation is unknown Specific mutation is unknown, but based on clinical presentation, a change in one gene is suspected An advantage of single gene (or multi-gene panel) sequencing is a smaller chance of detecting an incidental finding
Whole exome sequencing	Sequences only the protein coding section of the genome (exome) which makes up about ~2% of the genome May detect CNVs and chromosomal rearrangements	Benefits from a control comparison, or a sequence of other close family members to interpret May be more technically difficult and expensive than single gene sequencing WES does not sequence mtDNA May reveal incidental genetic findings and/or findings of unclear significance	Indicated when there is a genetic mutation suspected and other genetic tests were not revealing
Whole genome sequencing	Sequences both protein coding and non-coding regions of the genome, including regulatory regions May detect CNVs and chromosomal rearrangements	May be more expensive than targeted gene sequencing or other genetic tests May reveal incidental genetic findings and/or findings of unclear significance	Indicated when genetic change suspected and other, more specific tests were not revealing

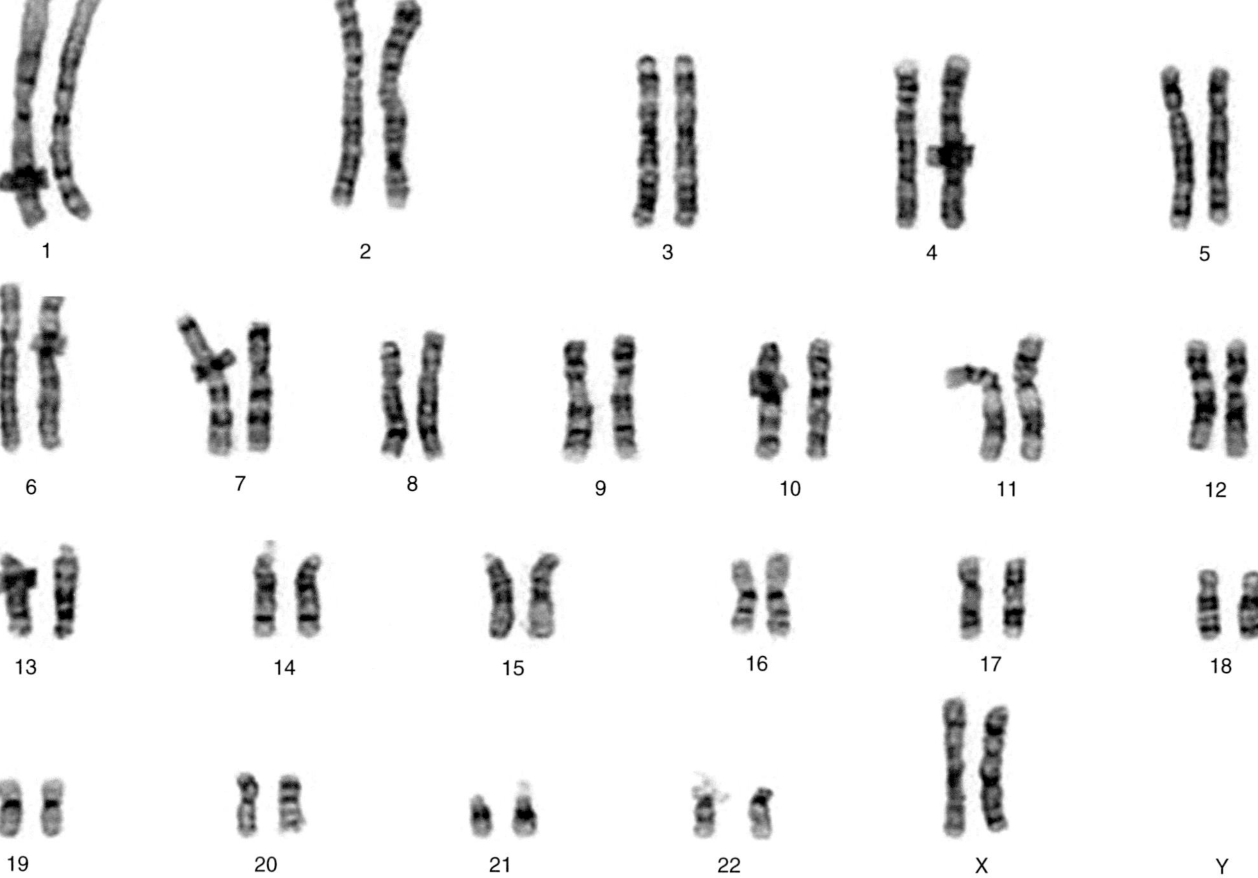

Fig. 35.1 46, XX. A normal female karyotype displays 22 pairs of autosomes and one pair of sex chromosomes. The metaphase chromosomes are arranged according to size and banding pattern. The characteristic dark-and-light banding pattern is the result of staining with Giemsa dye. Changes in the banding pattern may indicate abnormalities not apparent from just examining chromosome size, such as balanced translocations. The small pieces apparently perpendicular to the main chromosome (e.g., on chromosomes 1, 4, and 7) represent other chromosomes, the so-called chromosome "cross-over" in the image

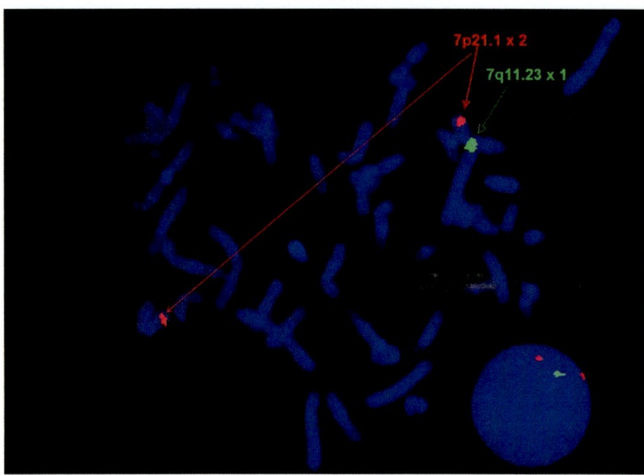

Fig. 35.2 Fluorescent in situ hybridization (FISH) can confirm the clinical diagnosis of Williams syndrome. (**a**) Control probe is a magenta or red probe which identifies chromosome #7; it hybridizes to chromosome 7p21.1. The appearance of two probes, one on either chromosome #7, indicates this region is present on either chromosome #7. (**b**) Elastin probe is a green probe which hybridizes to chromosome 7q11.23, the location of the WS critical interval. The appearance of the probe on only a single chromosome #7 indicates the presence of the Elastin (ELN) gene on one chromosome #7 but deletion of the Elastin gene on the other (and by inference the rest of the WS critical interval)

FISH is often the initial line of testing when a specific microdeletion disorder is clinically suspected. Presenting physical facial characteristics or endocrine abnormalities (such as hypercalcemia in Williams syndrome) may prompt consideration of a specific disorder. In pediatric endocrinology, examples of common microdeletion disorders include Williams syndrome (Fig. 35.2), Prader–Willi syndrome, Angelman syndrome, or 22q11.2 deletion syndrome (aka DiGeorge or Velo-Cardio-Facial syndrome). The probe used in FISH must be selected to target the area of suspected microdeletion. In other words, the diagnosis of Williams syndrome *cannot* be established by using a probe that hybridizes, for example, to a gene in the chromosome 22q11.2 interval. Rather, the laboratory must apply a probe that hybridizes to a gene mapping to the Williams syndrome interval on chromosome 7q11.23. FISH is not used to make discoveries about new areas of microdeletion, nor to detect genetic changes outside the probed region. In contrast to CMA, the FISH technique is also unable to define the limits or actual size of a microdeletion disorder. In certain circumstances it is used in combination with CMA for a more targeted follow-up analysis [3, 4].

Chromosomal Microarray Analysis

Chromosomal microarray analysis (CMA) is a widely available technology that can detect relatively small (smaller than would be visible on a karyotype) gains or losses of genetic material. Over the past decade, CMA has become increasingly higher resolution [2]. Depending on the specific platform used, gains or losses in the 50–100 kilobase (kb) range can be appreciated; however, current practice guidelines (American College of Medical Genetics) recommend that clinically used platforms be able to detect genetic changes of at least 400 kb [5].

To perform CMA, patient and reference DNA are fragmented, differentially labelled, and competitively hybridized to a microarray. The microarray is spotted with reference DNA consisting of millions of small fragments of DNA (aka probes) on a solid support. By utilizing DNA's preference to bind and resume a double-stranded structure with its complimentary probe sequences, CMA compares the ratio of patient to control DNA across the genome. Results from CMA indicate whether the amount of patient DNA for each probe is normal diploid (two copies) or if it deviates from the normal by being in excess (duplication or gain, three copies), or in deficiency (deletion or loss, one copy). If you may, for a minute, visualize the human genome as two sets of encyclopedias, CMA would reveal areas where a person has three copies of a chapter (or part of a chapter) instead of the expected two, or even smaller deletions where several pages were torn out of a book. Genetic gains or losses detected by CMA are generally referred to as CNVs (copy number variants). See Fig. 35.3 for CMA detection of loss of one copy of <2 million base pairs of genetic material on chromosome 7q11.23, which is responsible for Williams syndrome (Fig. 35.3).

As a clinical molecular cytogenetic technique, CMA is becoming the first line option for patients presenting with developmental delay or intellectual disability without a clear suspected genetic cause [6]. The coverage of CMA is comprehensive compared to targeted gene analysis. CMA is useful in detecting deviations from normal diploid genetic content, including: microdeletions, microduplications, unbalanced chromosomal rearrangements, such as translocations, and the loss or absence of heterozygosity (see glossary).

Arrays used in clinical practice contain many, generally millions of, probes that cover the genome; this allows for exploration of all 46 chromosomes in one array and can reveal more precise alterations than a karyotype. CMA has limitations in that it generally does not detect very small intragenic changes or balanced rearrangements, such as balanced translocations, as these rearrangements are not associated with a gain or loss in the actual amount of genetic material. Also, CMA is unable to detect changes in regions not probed. CMA will also fail to detect mosaicism not present in the cells from which DNA was extracted and may still miss low-level mosaicism even when present in tested cells. Much remains to be learned about the frequency and clinical impact of mosaicism and which technology is best suited for detecting it [7]. Finally, CMA is not the same as DNA sequencing (discussed below); CMA identifies gains or losses of small stretches of DNA, whereas sequencing specifies which nucleotide (A, T, G, or C) is present at each base.

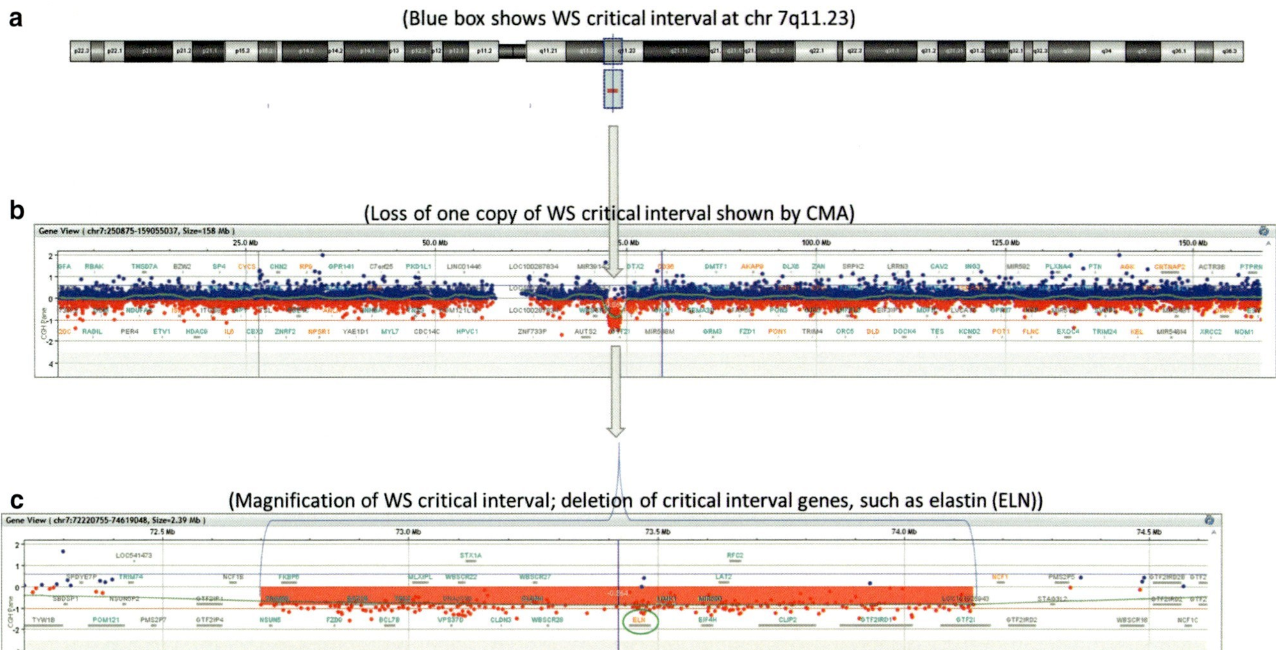

Fig. 35.3 Chromosomal microarray (CMA) is now a widely used genetic test to establish the diagnosis of conditions associated with gain or loss of genetic material. This image shows a CMA diagnostic of Williams syndrome. Array platform is Agilent Human Genome CGH 400 K kit with 292,097 CGH probes and 119,091 SNP probes covering the whole genome. (**a**) Ideogram of chromosome #7 (lying on its side). The WS critical interval is located at chromosome 7q11.23, outlined by the blue box. (**b**) CMA demonstrates genetic imbalance, with deletion of one copy of the WS critical interval, measuring ~1.5 million base pairs, at chromosome 7q11.23 (gray arrow). [Note that the absence of red and blue "dots" (hybridization signals) to the left of the WS critical interval indicates the location of the chromosome #7 centromere.] (**b**) Magnification of the WS critical interval depicting genes, including the Elastin (ELN) gene, that are deleted in persons with WS

Current CMA technology can detect CNVs which vary in size, ranging from millions of base pairs to as small as 50–100 kilobases (kb) [8]. In terms of disease impact, CNVs are classified as being: benign (e.g., gain or loss of the DNA segment does not appear to be associated with disease); pathogenic (e.g., gain or loss confers risk for disease); or of uncertain significance. Factors influencing classification include the size of the CNV, number and nature of genes contained within the gained or lost DNA segment, and whether the CNV is familial or de novo. It is important to note that many CNVs are not associated with disease and commonly exist in varying lengths in healthy individuals in the general population.

Gene Sequencing

DNA sequencing can be performed to determine the sequence of the approximately 3 billion DNA base pairs that exist in the human genome. Historically, the Sanger method was used to sequence DNA, but this has been replaced by next-generation sequencing (NGS) due to its greater speed, labor efficiency, and much lower cost.

NGS, also known as high-throughput or massively parallel sequencing, can be completed on several types of platforms. Each platform utilizes slightly different technology but generally refers to determining the genetic sequence down to the single nucleotide level by sequencing millions of small fragments of the patient's DNA. These millions of fragments are sequenced simultaneously (e.g., in parallel) on a solid surface, such as a glass slide or a bead. Bioinformatic analysis is employed to reassemble the newly sequenced segments of DNA and to compare them to a reference DNA sequence; this allows the presence of DNA sequence changes to be identified. Sequencing technology is continuously evolving, and the literature is replete with new or developing platforms applicable to research and clinical settings [9].

For clinical diagnostic testing, the extent of DNA sequenced can vary from part of or all of a single gene to a panel of genes, to all exons (so-called whole exome sequencing), and finally to every base pair in the whole genome (so-called whole genome sequencing). Further details, with a few examples, are provided below.

Single Gene Sequencing

Single gene sequencing involves sequencing all of one gene or a region of a gene. Focusing on sequencing a single gene is useful when the clinical presentation leads to suspicion of a specific disorder, or likely causative gene, and no familial mutation has been identified to date.

By way of example, single gene sequencing can be used to interrogate the endocrine-related genes MEN1 or MEN2 [10]. Testing is generally indicated due to family history, or patient history or presentation of multiple tumors. Mutations in these genes may be familial and lead to a characteristic constellation of findings, including associations with a variety of endocrine tumor multiplicities.

Also available is the option of sequencing a "panel" of several different genes. Genes selected for the panel are those that, when harboring a mutation, produce a similar or overlapping phenotype. For instance, monogenetic forms of diabetes, such as Maturity-Onset Diabetes of the Young (e.g., MODY), have been associated with mutations in 14 different genes, including HNF1A (MODY 3) and GCK (MODY 2) [11]. Thus, ordering a gene panel containing these 14 genes would be appropriate in the clinical setting of familial early-onset diabetes.

Whole Exome Sequencing

Whole exome sequencing (WES) is targeted sequencing of the protein coding regions (e.g., exons) of the human genes. This technique works by "capturing" the DNA sequences that constitute all the exons (collectively, all the exons are referred to as the exome) and then applying an NGS method to look for genetic mutations and variations. Though the exons constitute only about 2% of the entire human genome, they are the best understood part of the genome. Furthermore, mutations in exons, as opposed to mutations or variations in introns, are more likely to alter the function of the protein the gene encodes. WES has a narrower scope than WGS; in other words, WES sequences <2% of the genome and does not sequence mitochondrial DNA, while NGS sequences virtually the entire genome. Accordingly, WES should be performed prior to WGS, as it is cheaper and less likely to detect incidental findings or variants of unknown significance. Given the complexity surrounding testing, in terms of ethical issues, insurance coverage, and interpretation of results, WES should be ordered by a genetics professional.

Whole Genome Sequencing

Whole genome sequencing (WGS) typically employs the next-generation sequencing (NGS) technique discussed previously, in which parallel fragmented sequencing is applied to the entire genome. WGS may be clinically indicated when a genetic mutation is highly suspected but all other genetic testing methodologies, such as WES and CMA, were not revealing. WGS is becoming a clinical option for undiagnosed rare diseases to replace what may be a tedious and cumulatively expensive process of ordering a series of separate tests in pursuit of a diagnosis.

WGS offers the most coverage of the single nucleotide sequencing options. Similar to WES, it should be ordered by a geneticist. Not only must consideration be given to ethical implications, but sequencing the whole genome comes with a risk of discovering other abnormalities not specifically suspected in testing [12]. WGS may reveal variants that are known to be associated with varying extents of health risks, or even variants of unknown significance (VUS) which may raise questions for the patient and their family. Ethical considerations are vital to the clinical testing process across all resolutions and breadth of coverage, but especially to the aforementioned high-throughput sequencing applications.

Other Considerations for Types of Testing

DNA Methylation

DNA methylation testing aims to detect epigenetic changes. Epigenetic changes do not alter the DNA sequence itself but still have the potential to affect gene function by altering the level of gene expression. Specifically, methylation refers to the binding of a methyl group to a specific DNA base, cytosine. For certain genes, hyper-methylation can result in decreased transcription and ultimately a diminished gene product, whereas hypo-methylation can result in the opposite, namely excess gene product. Various genetic testing techniques have been adapted to identify areas of abnormal methylation throughout the genome, but from a practical clinical perspective, methylation is most relevant to the pediatric endocrinologist for the consideration of imprinting disorders, such as Prader Willi syndrome (PWS) and Beckwith-Wiedemann syndrome. In terms of PWS, several different genetic mechanisms are responsible for the disorder (including deletion of chromosome 15q11.2-q13.1 region on the paternally inherited chromosome 15, maternal disomy of chromosome 15, and imprinting center mutations); however, virtually all result in an abnormal (maternal chromosome specific) pattern of methylation. Thus, methylation analysis is the first line of testing when considering this diagnosis [13].

Fragile X Screening

Fragile X syndrome occurs due to a specific change in the FMR1 gene, which codes for a protein called FMRP. The 5′ untranslated portion of the FMR1 gene harbors a short stretch of three-repeating bases, "CGG," referred to as a trinucleotide repeat; normally the "CGG" stretch repeats 6–44 times. If the stretch of CGGs becomes too long, abnormal methylation ensues, resulting in decreased production of the FMRP protein product. Various phenotypes arise depending on the gender of the patient and the length of trinucleotide repeat expansion. Two phenotypes are of particular relevance to the endocrinologist. Males with Fragile X syndrome, due to a CGG repeat length of >200, display significant cognitive and behavioral deficits, and on physical examination, postpubertal males demonstrate macro-orchidism (with enlarged testicular volume not being appreciated before age 8 years). In females who carry a modest expansion of "CGG"s (e.g., 50/55–200 repeats), on one of their X chromosomes, an increased frequency of premature ovarian failure ensues [14].

Polymerase chain reaction (PCR) is the most commonly used clinical diagnostic test to determine the number of trinucleotide repeats within the FMR1 gene [15].

Ethical and Financial Considerations of Testing

Genetic testing can be associated with several emotional and financial outcomes. It is important to consider that if the results of testing reveal variants of unknown significance, the patient and their family may feel anxious about the unknown. If results lead to a genetic diagnosis, there is not only concern for emotional impact on the patient and their immediate family but also concerns about other family members' health and future planning, if the genetic change can be passed to offspring. Patients and their families might worry about what a genetic diagnosis can mean in the future regarding potential discrimination by employers or insurance companies.

Additionally, an assessment of financial consequences is an essential pre-testing step. Although the cost of genetic testing is decreasing as technology advances, the risk of a financial burden is an important consideration when performing these tests clinically. Finally, guidelines for obtaining genetic testing in minors exist [16]. Clinical testing to establish a diagnosis that impacts care and treatment during childhood is justified, beginning with the most focused genetic testing available (e.g., mutation analysis on a single gene or gene panel as opposed to whole genome sequencing). However, pre-symptomatic screening for adult onset disorders is generally not endorsed.

Acknowledgments Pictures kindly shared by:

Peining Li, PhD, FACMG.
Director of the Cytogenetics Laboratory,
Department of Genetics, Yale School of Medicine
333 Cedar Street, New Haven, CT.
(Tel: 203-785-6317).

References

1. Wallace SE, Bean LJ. Educational materials; Genetic Testing: Current Approaches. GeneReviews. 2018. https://www.ncbi.nlm.nih.gov/books/NBK279899/. Accessed 11 November 2019.
2. Dugoff L, Norton ME, Kuller JA. The use of chromosomal microarray for prenatal diagnosis. Am J Obstet Gynecol. 2016;215(4):B2:B9. https://doi.org/10.1016/j.ajog.2016.07.016.
3. Neill NJ, Ballif BC, Lamb AN, Parikh S, Ravnan JB, Schultz RA, et al. Recurrence, submicroscopic complexity, and potential clinical relevance of copy gains detected by array CGH that are shown to be unbalanced insertions by FISH. Genome Res. 2011;21(4):535–44. https://doi.org/10.1101/gr.114579.110.
4. Kang SHL, Shaw C, Ou Z, Eng PA, Cooper ML, Pursley AN, et al. Insertional translocation detected using FISH confirmation of array-comparative genomic hybridization (aCGH) results. Am J Med Genet. 2010;152A(5):1111–26. https://doi.org/10.1002/ajmg.a.33278.
5. Kearney HM, South ST, Wolff DJ, Lamb A, Hamosh A, Rao KW. American College of Medical Genetics recommendations for the design and performance expectations for clinical genomic copy number microarrays intended for use in the postnatal setting for detection of constitutional abnormalities. Genet Med. 2011;13(7):676–9. https://doi.org/10.1097/GIM.0b013e31822272ac.
6. Miller DT, Adam MP, Aradhya S, Biesecker LG, Brothman AR, Carter NP, et al. Consensus statement: chromosomal microarray is a first-tier clinical diagnostic test for individuals with developmental disabilities or congenital anomalies. Am J Hum Genet. 2010;86(5):749–64. https://doi.org/10.1016/j.ajhg.2010.04.006.
7. Pham J, Shaw C, Pursley A, Hixson P, Sampath S, Roney E, et al. Somatic mosaicism detected by exon-targeted, high-resolution aCGH in 10 362 consecutive cases. Eur J Hum Genet. 2014;22:969–78. https://doi.org/10.1038/ejhg.2013.285.
8. Zhang F, Gu W, Hurles ME, Lupski JR. Copy number variation in human health, disease, and evolution. Annu Rev Genomics Hum Genet. 2009;10:451–81. https://doi.org/10.1146/annurev.genom.9.081307.164217.
9. Kumar KR, Cowley MJ, Davis RL. Next-generation sequencing and emerging technologies. Semin Thromb Hemost. 2019;45(7):661–73. https://doi.org/10.1055/s-0039-1688446.
10. Vannucci L, Marini F, Giusti F, Ciuffi S, Tonelli F, Brandi ML. MEN1 in children and adolescents: data from patients of a regional referral center for hereditary endocrine tumors. Endocrine. 2018;59(2):438–48. https://doi.org/10.1007/s12020-017-1322-5.
11. Hattersley AT, Greeley SAW, Polak M, Rubio-Cabezas O, Njølstad PR, Mlynarski W, et al. ISPAD clinical practice consensus guidelines 2018: the diagnosis and management of monogenic diabetes in children and adolescents. Pediatr Diabetes. 2018;27:46–63. https://doi.org/10.1111/pedi.12772.
12. Biesecker LG, Biesecker BB. An approach to pediatric exome and genome sequencing. Curr Opin Pediatr. 2014;28(6):700–4. https://doi.org/10.1097/MOP.0000000000000418.
13. Beygo J, Buiting K, Ramsden SC, Ellis R, Clayton-Smith J, Kanber D. Update of the EMQN/ACGS best practice guidelines for molecular analysis of Prader-Willi and Angelman syndromes. Eur J Hum Genet. 2019;11:70. https://doi.org/10.1186/1471-2350-11-70.
14. Rajaratnam A, Shergill J, Salcedo-Arellano M, Saldarriaga W, Duan X, Hagerman R. Fragile X syndrome and fragile X-associated disorders. F1000Res. 2017;6:2112. https://doi.org/10.12688/f1000research.
15. Sofocleous C, Kolialexi A, Mavrou A. Molecular diagnosis of fragile X syndrome. Expert Rev Mol Diagn. 2009;9(1):23–30. https://doi.org/10.1586/14737159.9.1.23.
16. Botkin JR, Belmont JW, Berg JS, Berkman BE, Bombard Y, Holm IA, et al. Points to consider: ethical, legal, and psychosocial implications of genetic testing in children and adolescents. Am J Hum Genet. 2015;97(1):6–21. https://doi.org/10.1016/j.ajhg.2015.05.022.

Bone Age

36

Dayna McGill

Anatomical and Physiologic Principles Underlying Bone Age

For each child, clinicians can consider three different "ages." The chronological age (CA) is the child's actual age, based on birth date. The height age (HA) refers to the CA at which a child's height would be at the 50th percentile for age and sex. Finally, the bone age (BA) is an assessment of the degree of skeletal maturation. The child's hand/ wrist X-ray is interpreted based on the appearance and shapes of the bones and growth plates compared against standards for age and sex. The BA represents the CA for which the degree of bone maturation would be average for the child's sex.

Throughout childhood, skeletal maturation follows a highly coordinated progression of changes in the skeleton, including changes in bone contours, the appearance of ossification centers, and the eventual closure of growth plates. Although the pattern is strikingly predictable, the timing and pace of bone age advancement vary greatly. Some factors that contribute to the progression of skeletal maturation include genetics, sex, race/ethnicity, nutritional status, metabolic influences, social and emotional circumstances, illness, stress, environment, and hormones [1]. Sex steroids are required for epiphyseal closure; as such, there is an important relationship between pubertal timing and the progression of skeletal maturation.

Factors that generally lead to delayed bone age are shown in Table 36.1 and include endocrine causes such as constitutional delay, hypothyroidism, and growth hormone deficiency; nonendocrine chronic disease such as celiac disease, chronic kidney disease, inflammatory bowel disease, and congenital heart disease; nutritional deficiency; glucocorticoid use; and genetic syndromes including trisomy 21 and Turner syndrome [2]. Factors that generally lead to advanced bone age include premature adrenarche, precocious puberty, obesity, and hyperthyroidism. Children who are obese frequently have advanced bone age, along with early adrenarche and/or puberty; linear growth may be accelerated earlier in childhood and, subsequently, the pubertal growth spurt may

Table 36.1 Etiologies of delayed and advanced bone age

Delayed bone age	Advanced bone age
Endocrine	
Constitutional delay of growth and development	Premature adrenarche
Hypothyroidism	Precocious puberty
Growth hormone deficiency	Hyperthyroidism
Panhypopituitarism	Congenital adrenal hyperplasia (undertreated)
Hypogonadism (including female athlete triad)	
Corticosteroid excess (Cushing syndrome)	
Nutritional/chronic disease	
Rickets	Obesity
GI: Celiac disease and inflammatory bowel disease	
Chronic kidney disease	
Congenital heart disease	
Liver disease	
Juvenile idiopathic arthritis	
Psychosocial (neglect or abuse)	
Medications	
Glucocorticoids (including inhaled)	Estrogens, testosterone, and oral contraceptives
Amphetamine and dextroamphetamine	Supplements with estrogen-like effects (lavender, tea tree oil)
GnRH analogues and aromatase inhibitors	
Genetic syndromes	
Trisomy 21, trisomy 18, and trisomy 13	Familial male-limited precocious puberty
Turner syndrome	McCune-Albright syndrome
Russell-Silver syndrome	Sotos syndrome
Klinefelter syndrome	Beckwith-Wiedemann syndrome

D. McGill (✉)
Division of Pediatric Endocrinology, Massachusetts General Hospital for Children, Boston, MA, USA
e-mail: dmcgill@mgh.harvard.edu

T. Stanley, M. Misra (eds.), *Endocrine Conditions in Pediatrics*, https://doi.org/10.1007/978-3-030-52215-5_36

be attenuated [3–6]. The mechanisms behind bone age advancement in obese children are not entirely clear, but appear to relate to relative elevations in DHEAS, androgens, estrogens, and insulin [3, 7, 8].

One important caveat to bone age interpretation is that the bone age may "lag behind" clinical status. Clinicians should bear in mind that if a child's clinical exam and laboratory evaluation are consistent with precocious puberty, but the bone age is *not* advanced, this may be an indication of recent exposure to high levels of gonadal or adrenal androgens (i.e., gonadotropin-independent precocious puberty, as in the case of a gonadal or adrenal tumor for instance). Similarly, in cases of recent-onset hypothyroidism or growth hormone deficiency, the bone age may not yet be delayed.

Bone Age Determination

The left hand/wrist is used for bone age determination; this area may be used as a representation of the skeletal maturity of the body as a whole since there are many bones and epiphyses in the hand and wrist, and the area is easy and safe to X-ray on a single small radiograph [9].

The two predominant methods used for bone age determination are the Greulich and Pyle (GP) atlas method and the Tanner-Whitehouse (TW) bone-scoring method [10, 11].

- *Greulich and Pyle method*: The GP atlas method is the fastest and easiest to use, and the most commonly used method for pediatric endocrinologists and radiologists in the United States [1, 9]. It is based on data for bone age norms determined based on the Brush Foundation study conducted in the 1930s–1940s in well-nourished Caucasian children born in the United States [10]. The atlas consists of a series of X-rays in order of increasing age by sex; for male standards, there are 31 radiograph images covering the time period from 0 to 19 years of age, and for female standards, there are 27 radiograph images covering the time period from 0 to 18 years of age [10]. To determine a child's bone age, the child's hand/ wrist bones are matched with the atlas images that are the most similar; all bones are regarded and compared, but the interpreter generally arrives at one bone age, which best represents the overall picture. One drawback to this method is that, commonly, some bones are more mature than others. Many bone age readers de-emphasize the carpals in comparison to other bones, but there is no standardization for weighting of different bones in the GP method [12].
- *Tanner-Whitehouse method*: The TW bone-scoring method is based on a large sample of urban and rural children studied in the 1950s, and it is the preferred method of bone age interpretation in Europe [1, 9]. Each of the 20 bones in the hand/wrist is compared with a set of 8 standard ages and assigned a stage; each stage of each bone has a score, and the sum of the scores for all of the bones is the bone age [11].

The GP method has been shown to be significantly faster than TW; reading one bone age by the GP method takes an average of 1.4 minutes, compared with TW which takes 7.9 minutes [1]. Importantly, bone age interpretation may be slightly different between the two methods, so any time bone ages are being compared (within an individual for clinical or research purposes, or between individuals for research purposes), the same method should be used for all X-rays being interpreted [9].

Bone age determinations for both of the common methods (TW and GP) were based on studies of predominantly white European children and are less generalizable to other populations. Specifically, African American children are more likely to have "advanced" bone ages compared to GP standards, and Southeast Asian boys' bone ages are more likely to be "delayed" compared to GP standards [2, 13, 14].

Due to the inherent subjective nature of bone age interpretation, combined with the heavy weight that is often placed on bone ages in clinical decision-making, most pediatric endocrinologists read and interpret their own bone ages rather than relying solely on the radiologist's interpretation. Indeed, a recent retrospective chart review of bone ages done in 103 children presenting for initial evaluation of short stature of precocious puberty found a discrepancy between radiologist and pediatric endocrinologist interpretations in 68% of bone ages; however, most of the discrepancies were small (56% less than 1 year discrepant, 38% between 1 and 2 years discrepant, and 6% more than 2 years discrepant) [15].

Given the imprecise and time-consuming nature of manual bone age reading, there has been interest in automation of bone age reading. BoneXpert (Visiana, Horsholm, Denmark) was the first fully automated software platform developed to calculate bone age, and it is approved for use in Europe [1, 12, 16]. This software calculates both TW and GP scores with impressive precision (0.18 years, compared to 0.45–0.83 years for manual readings), and interestingly does not consider carpal bones in its algorithm [1, 12]. Height predictions that perform well compared to other methods can also be done by BoneXpert [16, 17]. There has not yet been full uptake of this automated technology for clinical use, likely due to the cost of the software and the ability for providers to assess bone age manually with relatively little training and effort [1].

Criteria for bone age advancement or delay Bone age is delayed or advanced if it is ≥2 standard deviations below or above the mean. Standard deviation scores can be found in bone age atlases, and are usually noted on radiology reports. In older children and adolescents (approximately 12 years of age or older), 1 standard deviation score is about 1 year, so a 2-year difference between the bone and chronological age would be considered delayed or advanced. In younger children, the standard deviation is smaller, such that a smaller difference between bone age and chronological age (~18 months in children between the ages of 4 and 12 years) is typically considered delayed or advanced [10].

Common Clinical Scenarios in Which Bone Age Assessment May Be Useful

The most common clinical scenarios in which a bone age is obtained include the diagnostic workup and monitoring of short stature, tall stature, delayed puberty, precocious puberty, or premature adrenarche. Bone age assessment is also used in the monitoring of treatment effects in children treated for growth disorders (e.g., with growth hormone therapy) or disorders of puberty (e.g., children with precocious puberty treated with a gonadotropin-releasing hormone agonist). There are also uses for bone age assessment related to orthopedic procedures (for scoliosis or leg-length discrepancy), determination of chronological age for adopted children and in immigration and forensics, and issues related to youth sports participation [1, 2].

Although not the primary purpose of bone age assessment, hand X-rays provide other information and useful diagnostic clues related to Turner syndrome (squared off carpals, shortening of the fourth metacarpal, and Madelung deformity with bowing of the radius with irregularities at the distal radial epiphysis), pseudohypoparathyroidism (shortening of the fourth and fifth metacarpals), hypochondroplasia (wider and shorter bones), rickets (metaphyseal cupping and fraying), and history of temporary arrest of long bone growth (Harris lines) [1, 12].

It may be useful to obtain a bone age X-ray in the initial assessment of:

- *Short stature*: length or height that is more than 2 standard deviations below the mean for age and sex, which corresponds to height below the 2.3rd percentile for age and sex.
- *Decreased growth velocity*: crossing of major percentiles of the Centers for Disease Control and Prevention growth charts, and/or annualized growth velocity <4 cm/year in prepubertal children or <8 cm/year in pubertal children.
- *Delayed puberty*: lack of breast enlargement in girls by age 13 or lack of testicular enlargement by age 14 in boys.
- *Early puberty*: development of secondary sexual characteristics before age 8 in girls and before age 9 in boys.

Short stature/decreased growth velocity In children with short stature or decreased growth velocity, a bone age X-ray may provide valuable information. Taken in the context of parental heights, an "average" bone age (not delayed or advanced) may help confirm a diagnosis of familial/genetic short stature. On the other hand, a delayed bone age, together with family history of delayed puberty (typically in at least one parent), may help confirm the diagnosis of constitutional delay of growth and development in a child who has an otherwise reassuring clinical picture. Although delayed bone age with a family history of constitutional growth delay and benign presentation is highly reassuring with regard to final height, multiple underlying diagnoses can also cause delayed bone age (Table 36.1), such that delayed bone age does not rule out underlying pathology.

Delayed puberty In children with delayed puberty, bone age will typically be delayed. Part of the workup for delayed puberty might include a gonadotropin-releasing hormone (GnRH) stimulation test to distinguish delayed puberty (in which case one would expect a rise in gonadotropin level after administration of a GnRH analog) from hypogonadism (where there would be an absent or subnormal rise in gonadotropins). A bone age is essential in the interpretation of a GnRH stimulation test because, regardless of chronological age, a pubertal gonadotropin response would typically only be expected in children with a *bone age* of 13 years or greater [9].

When a child has the combination of reduced growth rate and delayed puberty, several endocrine and non-endocrine causes must be considered, including growth hormone deficiency, hypothyroidism, celiac disease, and other nutritional deficiencies and systemic disorders. It is important to recognize that the bone age may not yet be delayed when these disorders present acutely.

Early puberty In patients with premature adrenarche and/or precocious puberty, bone age assessment can help confirm sexual precocity, give a sense of the time course of puberty, and allow for estimation of potential impact on final height. Advancement in the bone age is more consistent with precocious puberty (central or peripheral), whereas bone age that is within approximately 2 SDs of chronological age is less consistent with precocious puberty and more consistent with benign entities such as isolated premature thelarche.

When the clinical exam reveals signs of puberty (thelarche, enlargement of testes, etc.), gonadotropin levels are elevated, and the bone age is advanced, this is most consistent with central (true) precocious puberty with activation of the hypothalamic-pituitary-gonadotropin axis. When the clinical exam reveals signs of adrenarche, androgens levels are elevated, and the bone age is advanced, this may represent premature adrenarche, or it may be a sign of hyperandrogenism (e.g., congenital adrenal hyperplasia). Depending on the age of the child and the clinical scenario, further evaluation may be warranted to elucidate the cause of precocious puberty/premature adrenarche. Notably, up to 30% of children with premature adrenarche have significantly advanced bone ages (more than 2 years ahead of chronologic age); while this group may be taller and have higher BMI than children with premature adrenarche and less advanced bone ages, hormone levels were similar in the two groups, and there did not appear to be a significant impact on adult height [18].

Using Bone Age for Height Prediction

A bone age provides information about a child's skeletal maturation, which in turn informs potential for future growth, and preliminary prediction of final adult height. The calculation of a predicted adult height uses the bone age, the current height of the child, and considers whether the bone age is advanced, delayed, or average (based on the relationship between a child's chronological age and bone age).

Height predictions are calculated using the methodology of Bayley and Pinneau [19] if the bone age was determined by the GP atlas method, and using the TW height prediction method if the bone age was determined by the TW bone-scoring method. In both cases, the child's bone age is determined, and then—depending on whether the bone age is delayed, average, or advanced—that bone age is translated into a percentage of final adult height, and the current height is divided by that decimal number in order to derive a predicted adult height. This method is valid for children aged 6 years and older, and is most accurate as the child gets older [19].

Height predictions must be made with caution, and families must understand that they are imprecise. An overestimation of predicted adult height may occur in early puberty (when bone age may lag behind true maturation), when a child has an accelerated progression through puberty, and in children with bone age that is delayed more than 2 years [2, 19]. An underestimation of predicted adult height may occur in children with bone age that is accelerated more than 2 years [19].

References

1. De Sanctis V, Di Maio S, Soliman AT, Raiola G, Elalaily R, Millimaggi G. Hand X-ray in pediatric endocrinology: skeletal age assessment and beyond. Indian J Endocrinol Metab. 2014;18(Suppl 1):S63–71.
2. Creo AL, Schwenk WF 2nd. Bone age: a Handy tool for pediatric providers. Pediatrics. 2017;140(6)
3. de Groot CJ, van den Berg A, Ballieux B, Kroon HM, Rings E, Wit JM, et al. Determinants of advanced bone age in childhood obesity. Horm Res Paediatr. 2017;87(4):254–63.
4. De Leonibus C, Marcovecchio ML, Chiavaroli V, de Giorgis T, Chiarelli F, Mohn A. Timing of puberty and physical growth in obese children: a longitudinal study in boys and girls. Pediatr Obes. 2014;9(4):292–9.
5. Denzer C, Weibel A, Muche R, Karges B, Sorgo W, Wabitsch M. Pubertal development in obese children and adolescents. Int J Obes. 2007;31(10):1509–19.
6. He Q, Karlberg J. Bmi in childhood and its association with height gain, timing of puberty, and final height. Pediatr Res. 2001;49(2):244–51.
7. Sopher AB, Jean AM, Zwany SK, Winston DM, Pomeranz CB, Bell JJ, et al. Bone age advancement in prepubertal children with obesity and premature adrenarche: possible potentiating factors. Obesity (Silver Spring). 2011;19(6):1259–64.
8. Lee HS, Shim YS, Jeong HR, Kwon EB, Hwang JS. The association between bone age advancement and insulin resistance in Prepubertal obese children. Exp Clin Endocrinol Diabetes. 2015;123(10):604–7.
9. Spadoni GL, Cianfarani S. Bone age assessment in the workup of children with endocrine disorders. Horm Res Paediatr. 2010;73(1):2–5.
10. Greulich WW, Pyle SI. Radiographic atlas of skeletal development of the hand and wrist. Palo Alto: Stanford University Press; 1959.
11. Tanner JM, Whitehouse RH, Cameron N, Marshall WA, Healy MJR, Goldstein H. Assessment of skeletal maturity and prediction of adult height (TW2 method), Ed 2. London: Academic Press; 1983.
12. van Rijn RR, Thodberg HH. Bone age assessment: automated techniques coming of age? Acta Radiol. 2013;54(9):1024–9.
13. Ontell FK, Ivanovic M, Ablin DS, Barlow TW. Bone age in children of diverse ethnicity. AJR Am J Roentgenol. 1996;167(6):1395–8.
14. Mora S, Boechat MI, Pietka E, Huang HK, Gilsanz V. Skeletal age determinations in children of European and African descent: applicability of the Greulich and Pyle standards. Pediatr Res. 2001;50(5):624–8.
15. Eitel KB, Eugster EA. Differences in bone age readings between pediatric endocrinologists and radiologists. Endocr Pract. 2020;26(3):328–31.
16. Thodberg HH, Kreiborg S, Juul A, Pedersen KD. The BoneXpert method for automated determination of skeletal maturity. IEEE Trans Med Imaging. 2009;28(1):52–66.
17. Thodberg HH, Jenni OG, Caflisch J, Ranke MB, Martin DD. Prediction of adult height based on automated determination of bone age. J Clin Endocrinol Metab. 2009;94(12):4868–74.
18. DeSalvo DJ, Mehra R, Vaidyanathan P, Kaplowitz PB. In children with premature adrenarche, bone age advancement by 2 or more years is common and generally benign. J Pediatr Endocrinol Metab. 2013;26(3–4):215–21.
19. Bayley N, Pinneau SR. Tables for predicting adult height from skeletal age: revised for use with the Greulich-Pyle hand standards. J Pediatr. 1952;40(4):423–41.

Pituitary MRI

37

Takara Stanley

Important Imaging Considerations

Ordering an MRI

In order to assess for pituitary abnormalities, brain magnetic resonance imaging (MRI) should typically be ordered with the "pituitary protocol," meaning that the brain is imaged using "thin cuts" (1-mm cuts) through the sellar and suprasellar region, with imaging performed both pre- and post-administration of gadolinium-containing contrast. Depending on the radiology services available, radiologists may further refine the scanning methodology based on clinical history.

Planning for Sedation or Child Life Services

Younger children will typically require conscious sedation or anesthesia, in order to undergo an MRI of acceptable quality, and older children may benefit from Child Life services to help them tolerate the scanning procedures. The need for anesthesia, conscious sedation, and/or child life support should be planned in advance with the imaging facility.

Other Patient-Related Considerations

Pituitary MRIs should be performed with contrast; thus, children will require intravenous (IV) catheter placement. Gadolinium-containing contrast agents are typically used for MRI and are generally safe, but children with known previous allergic reactions to gadolinium may require pretreatment with diphenhydramine and/or glucocorticoids. In these cases, radiology should be contacted prior to scanning so that a different contrast agent can be used if possible.

Children with metal implants may not be able to safely undergo an MRI, and consultation with a radiologist regarding whether the implant is MRI-safe may be warranted. *Children with braces* may safely undergo MRI, but the images are often quite poor because of artifact from the braces. Whenever possible, it is best to have braces removed before a brain MRI to ensure that the images are usable.

Interpretation of Scans

Interpretation by a radiologist is required for definitive reading of pituitary MRI scans, but we encourage treating physicians to look at the images as well. Helpful pituitary landmarks on coronal and sagittal scans are shown in Fig. 37.1. Table 37.1 lists common imaging terms and anatomical terms that may be helpful when reading pituitary MRI reports. Table 37.2 describes common pathological findings in imaging reports and discusses next steps for managing these findings. Please note that Table 37.2 does not include all possible suprasellar findings, and a finding of suprasellar tumor should generally prompt emergent referral to oncology or an emergency department, as well as urgent endocrine assessment. A pituitary MRI showing a craniopharyngioma is shown in Fig. 37.2. Further management of pituitary and suprasellar lesions is described in Chap. 56.

Tips on discussing results with patients are shown in Table 37.3. Pituitary or suprasellar lesions $\geq$ 10 mm should almost always prompt urgent or emergent referral, but smaller lesions need not necessarily raise substantial alarm. For example, most Rathke's cleft cysts are completely benign and do not require intervention, and most pituitary microadenomas are benign as well, although some will require medical or surgical intervention. Please see Table 37.3 for suggested language around these findings.

T. Stanley (✉)
Division of Pediatric Endocrinology, Massachusetts General Hospital and Harvard Medical School, Boston, MA, USA
e-mail: tstanley@mgh.harvard.edu

T. Stanley, M. Misra (eds.), *Endocrine Conditions in Pediatrics*, https://doi.org/10.1007/978-3-030-52215-5_37

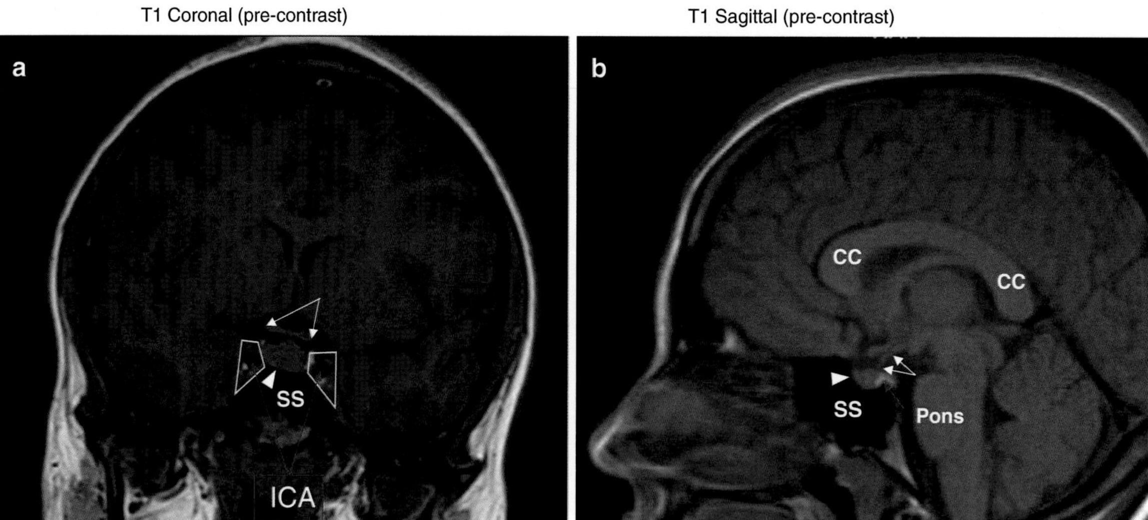

Fig. 37.1 Figure shows T1 coronal (**a**) and sagittal (**b**) pituitary MRIs without visible abnormalities to illustrate landmarks on Pituitary MRI. 1A, Coronal View: The Cavernous Sinuses lie on either side of the pituitary gland and are outlined in yellow. The internal carotid arteries (ICA), indicated with red arrows, run through the cavernous sinuses. The pituitary gland, pointed to by the white arrowhead, lies in the sella turcica, between the cavernous sinuses. The optic chiasm lies above the pituitary gland; its left and right boundaries are demarcated by the white arrows. The stalk is not highly visible on this cut and lies between the pituitary and the optic chiasm. The hypointense (nearly black) area below the pituitary is the sphenoid sinus (SS). 1B, Sagittal View: Again the pituitary is pointed to by the white arrowhead. The pituitary stalk can be seen leading from the hypothalamus to the pituitary, as demarcated by the white arrows. The hyperintense "posterior pituitary bright spot," which results from granules of stored vasopressin, is noted by the red arrow. Again the hypointense (nearly black) area below and anterior to the pituitary is the sphenoid sinus (SS). The pons and corpus callosum (CC) are also noted as important landmarks for the sagittal pituitary view

Table 37.1 Definitions for pituitary imaging and pituitary anatomy

Key imaging terms	
Coronal plane	The anatomical plane parallel to the dorsal and ventral surfaces of the body. Coronal MRIs are viewed as if the person in the image is standing straight in front of the viewer, facing the viewer.
Sagittal	The anatomical plane perpendicular to the dorsal and ventral surfaces of the body, or parallel to the sagittal suture. Sagittal MRIs are viewed as if the person in the image is standing with their left side facing the viewer.
Hypointense	A hypointense structure is darker than the structure it is being compared to. Colloquially often used without a comparator, such that hypointense means "darker" (i.e., blacker) on imaging.
Hyperintense	A hyperintense structure is brighter than the structure it is being compared to. Colloquially often used without a comparator, such that hyperintense means "brighter" (i.e., whiter) on imaging.
T1 versus T2	T1- versus T2-weighted images have different types of timing for acquiring images, resulting in differences in which types of tissues appear bright. On T1-weighted images, the tissues appear bright and fluid appears dark, whereas T2-weighted images are the opposite. Gadolinium-based contrast is also bright on T1-weighted images. T1-weighted images are generally of greater use in interpreting pituitary MRIs, although T2-weighted images are usually obtained as well.
1.5 tesla (1.5 T) vs. 3 tesla (3 T)	Tesla (T) refers to the strength of the magnet used in an MRI machine. 3 T scanners use stronger magnets than 1.5 T scanners and thus generally produce images with better resolution. When possible, pituitary MRIs should be performed on 3 T scanners for best image quality.
Pituitary incidentaloma	A pituitary lesion incidentally found on brain MRI performed for another reason. It is important to know that approximately 10% of adults have pituitary incidentalomas on imaging [1].
Key anatomic terms	
Adenohypophysis	Another name for the anterior pituitary gland
Hypophysis	Another name for the pituitary gland
Infundibulum	Another name for the pituitary stalk
Neurohypophysis	Another name for the posterior pituitary gland
Pars intermedia	Boundary between the anterior and posterior lobes of the pituitary gland; this is where Rathke's cleft cysts and pars intermedia cysts are located
Sella Turcica	The depression in the sphenoid bone that contains the pituitary gland
Sellar	Refers to the Sella turcica itself as well as the area within the Sella turcica; "sellar mass" and "intrasellar mass" have the same meaning, that is, within the Sella
Parasellar	Refers to the region around the Sella, including the cavernous sinuses laterally and the pituitary stalk and hypothalamus superiorly
Suprasellar	Refers to the area immediately superior to the pituitary gland, containing the pituitary stalk and hypothalamus
Macroadenoma	A pituitary adenoma measuring $\geq$ 10 mm in any dimension
Microadenoma	A pituitary adenoma measuring < 10 mm in every direction

Table 37.2 Common pathological findings on pituitary MRI and next steps in evaluation/management

Finding	Definition	Suggested action
Rathke's cleft cyst (RCC), also called Rathke cleft cyst	A benign cyst in the pars intermedia, formed from remnants of Rathke's pouch (though benign, a small subset can grow aggressively and cause problems through mass effect)	An RCC <10 mm in a completely asymptomatic person can generally be followed with serial MRIs to ensure stability, starting with once-annual scanning [2], but non-urgent referral to pediatric endocrinology may be advisable. A non-urgent referral to endocrinology and/or neurosurgery is necessary if the RCC ≥10 mm. Regardless of size, urgent referral is mandated if there are any symptoms suggestive of pituitary dysfunction or symptoms of mass effect such as headaches or visual changes.
Thickened pituitary stalk, also called thickened infundibulum	A pituitary stalk that is wider than published norms	A thickened stalk raises concern for lesions such as germinoma, Langerhans cell histiocytosis, or hypophysitis (inflammation of the pituitary). The patient should be assessed for diabetes insipidus and referred urgently to pediatric endocrinology.
Ectopic posterior pituitary	Posterior pituitary in a location other than posterior to the anterior pituitary gland, typically inferior to the hypothalamus and superior to the pituitary gland	This is caused when the posterior pituitary does not fully complete embryological migration. In an asymptomatic child, this may be a normal finding, but it can be associated with growth hormone deficiency and, less commonly, other pituitary deficiencies. If there are any suggestions of hormonal deficits, decreased growth, or other symptoms, a non-urgent referral to pediatric endocrinology is recommended.
Small pituitary, hypoplastic pituitary, or diminutive pituitary	Pituitary gland that is smaller in volume than published norms	A small pituitary raises concerns for possible hormonal insufficiencies but could also be a normal finding. Non-urgent referral to pediatric endocrinology and/or pituitary hormone assessment[a] for asymptomatic children, with increased urgency of endocrine referral in symptomatic children depending on symptoms.
Pituitary hyperplasia	Pituitary gland that is larger in volume than published norms	This is typically due to increased volume of one or more pituitary cell lines (e.g., somatotrophs, lactotrophs or thyrotrophs) and can be a normal finding during puberty and during pregnancy. In the absence of symptoms, this finding should not raise alarm but may warrant pituitary hormone assessment[a] and/or non-urgent endocrine referral depending on the degree of enlargement and whether other symptoms or signs are present. Severe undiagnosed and untreated primary hypothyroidism can lead to significant thyrotroph hyperplasia from reduced negative feedback, leading to a markedly enlarged pituitary. This normalizes with thyroid hormone replacement. Pituitary hyperplasia may also occur with certain transcription factor defects (such as *PROP-1* mutations).
Microadenoma	A lesion with appearance consistent with an adenoma (benign overgrowth of pituitary cells) that is <10 mm in every measured dimension	A pituitary hormone assessment[a] should be performed. If hormonal deficiencies are suspected, an urgent referral to endocrinology is necessary. If laboratory testing not suggestive of pituitary hormone deficiency, a non-urgent referral to endocrinology should suffice.
Macroadenoma	A lesion with appearance consistent with an adenoma (benign overgrowth of pituitary cells) that is ≥10 mm in every measured dimension	If disturbance/compression/displacement of the optic chiasm is reported, emergent referral to pediatric endocrinology and neurosurgery or an emergency department is mandated. If the optic chiasm is not involved, an urgent referral to endocrinology is usually sufficient. Pituitary hormonal assessment[a] could also be performed in the primary care setting but should not preclude urgent referral.
Craniopharyngioma (see Fig. 37.2)	A technically benign tumor arising from remnants of Rathke's pouch, which can cause significant issues due to mass effect. Symptoms resulting from mass effect typically precede those resulting from hormone deficiency.	This is the most common suprasellar lesion in childhood. Emergent referral to an emergency department is necessary for evaluation by oncology, endocrinology, and neurosurgery.
Hypothalamic hamartoma	Congenital malformation arising from the inferior part of the hypothalamus	Hypothalamic hamartomas are benign and generally do not change in size, but they can cause precocious puberty that is treatable with GnRH agonists. Referral to endocrinology is recommended if there are signs or symptoms of precocious puberty, and referral to neurology is recommended if there are any other signs or symptoms of possible seizure activity or cognitive or behavioral problems. These lesions have been associated with gelastic or 'laughing' seizures.

[a]Pituitary hormone assessment should consist of careful history, including assessment for possible diabetes insipidus, review of the growth chart, and labs, including TSH, thyroxine or free thyroxine, IGF-I and IGFBP-3, morning (8:00 AM) cortisol, prolactin, electrolytes, and, if of pubertal age, FSH, LH, estradiol/testosterone. If there is suspicion of diabetes insipidus, please add serum and urine osmolality and urine sodium

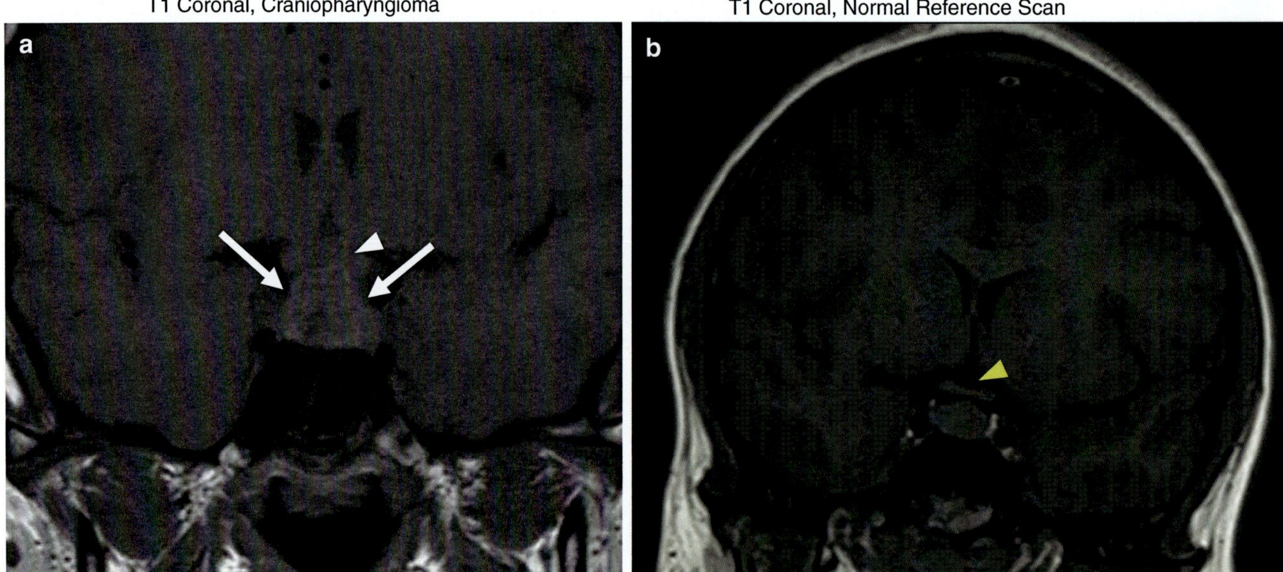

Fig. 37.2 A coronal scan showing a craniopharyngioma (white arrows) in a female child. The optic chiasm is displaced upward, as noted by the white arrowhead, in comparison to the normal horizonal appearance noted by the yellow arrowhead in the coronal reference scan from Fig. 37.1

Table 37.3 Tips on discussing pituitary findings

Ectopic posterior pituitary and *small pituitary gland* can be normal variants—parents should be counseled that there may be hormonal issues, but otherwise these are benign findings.
Rathke's Cleft Cysts are also benign—it can be helpful to reassure parents that "this is not a tumor," but it could potentially cause problems if it grows in size, such that monitoring with MRI is necessary.
Using the term "brain tumor" for pituitary adenomas can cause unnecessary worry and is best avoided. We propose more specific language below.
Pituitary microadenomas can be described as an overgrowth of cells in the pituitary. It is helpful to explicitly note that only a very small percentage of pituitary adenomas are malignant, and a pituitary microadenoma is highly likely to remain stable in size, so this is not considered a "brain tumor."
Prolactinoma is the most common type of pituitary adenoma, and both microprolactinomas and macroprolactinomas can usually be treated with oral medication, such that patients will probably not require surgery.
Non-functioning microadenomas (e.g., microadenomas without any associated abnormal pituitary function) do not require medical or surgical management but do require MRI monitoring.
Adenomas that make growth hormone (causing gigantism/acromegaly) or ACTH (causing Cushing's disease) will often require surgical treatment, but the surgery is usually done transsphenoidally (a nasal approach through the sphenoid sinus) with excellent success.

References

1. Hall WA, Luciano MG, Doppman JL, Patronas NJ, Oldfield EH. Pituitary magnetic resonance imaging in normal human volunteers: occult adenomas in the general population. Ann Intern Med. 1994;120:817–20.
2. Zada G. Rathke cleft cysts: a review of clinical and surgical management. Neurosurg Focus. 2011. 31:1–6. https://doi.org/10.3171/2011.5.FOCUS1183.

38 Thyroid Imaging

Christine E. Cherella

The thyroid gland is butterfly-shaped, composed of right and left lobes joined centrally by the isthmus. Its precursor, the thyroid primordium, first forms at the base of the tongue during the fourth to fifth gestational week, then descends caudally through a small channel (i.e., the thyroglossal duct) down to the lower neck. The final location of the thyroid gland is anterior to the trachea, inferior to the larynx, and sandwiched between neck musculature, with the carotid arteries and internal jugular veins located laterally.

Thyroid imaging is useful in evaluating the size and location of thyroid tissue, suspected focal thyroid disease, thyroid nodules, glandular function, nodular function, and congenital thyroid abnormalities. The primary diagnostic imaging modalities for evaluating thyroid diseases are ultrasound and scintigraphy. Computerized tomography (CT) scans and magnetic resonance imaging (MRI) are less sensitive in detecting and characterizing thyroid lesions because of poor spatial resolution, although occasionally thyroid pathology may be detected incidentally on these scans [1].

Thyroid Ultrasound

Given the superficial location of the thyroid gland in the neck, ultrasonography remains the most sensitive imaging modality for assessing thyroid anatomy and diagnosing intrathyroidal lesions (Table 38.1). An additional advantage of ultrasound is the lack of exposure to ionizing radiation, which is an important consideration in the pediatric population. Ultrasound is the mainstay for detecting and characterizing thyroid nodules and for providing biopsy guidance [2]. Neck ultrasound can also be used to determine the presence of thyroid tissue (i.e., when determining the underlying pathophysiology of congenital hypothyroidism as either secondary to dysgenesis or dyshormonogenesis) and to differentiate adjacent non-thyroid masses from thyroid pathology. Ultrasound is not required to diagnose diffuse thyroid disease (i.e., Graves' disease or Hashimoto's thyroiditis), although affected glands may have a heterogeneous appearance if ultrasound images were to be obtained in these settings.

Table 38.1 Interpreting thyroid imaging

	Ultrasound	Scintigraphy	Diagnoses to consider
Thyroid nodules	Assess for features associated with malignancy	No uptake	Non-functioning
		Uptake localized to nodule (with uptake in the rest of the gland being typically reduced)	Autonomous
Thyrotoxicosis	Less helpful in determining the underlying etiology	Increased uptake	Hyperthyroidism
		No uptake	Thyroiditis
Congenital hypothyroidism	No thyroid tissue seen	No uptake	Dysgenesis: aplasia
	Thyroid visualized along the migration course of thyroid primordium	Uptake in the ectopic gland	Dysgenesis: ectopic
	Normally placed thyroid, possibly enlarged	Absent or high, depending on etiology	Dyshormonogenesis

C. E. Cherella (✉)
Division of Endocrinology, Department of Pediatrics, Boston Children's Hospital, Boston, MA, USA
e-mail: Christine.Cherella@childrens.harvard.edu

T. Stanley, M. Misra (eds.), *Endocrine Conditions in Pediatrics*, https://doi.org/10.1007/978-3-030-52215-5_38

Ultrasound for Detecting Thyroid Nodules and Other Intrathyroidal Lesions

Detecting thyroid nodules on physical examination can be challenging, particularly when the nodules are more posterior than anterior within the gland [3]. If an overt nodule or mass is palpated, or if there is a question of thyroid asymmetry on examination, thyroid ultrasound should be obtained to confirm the presence of a nodule, and characterize additional features that are more likely to be associated with benign versus malignant disease. Approximately 1–2% of pediatric patients have thyroid nodules, and while the majority of pediatric thyroid nodules are benign, the risk of malignancy (approximately 25%) is higher than that in adults [4]. Features associated with malignancy in pediatric thyroid nodules include solid composition, hypoechogenicity, calcifications, irregular borders, and taller than wide orientation [5]. Additionally, a thorough ultrasonographic evaluation of cervical lymph nodes is important in all patients who undergo thyroid ultrasound for known or suspected nodules, as the appearance of abnormal lymph nodes is concerning for thyroid malignancy.

If a thyroid nodule is confirmed by ultrasound, the American Thyroid Association guidelines first recommend obtaining a thyroid-stimulating hormone (TSH) level [2, 6]. If the TSH level is found to be suppressed below the lower limits of normal, thyroid scintigraphy should be pursued to determine if the nodule is autonomous (see the section on "Nuclear Imaging (Thyroid Scintigraphy)" below). Autonomous nodules are considered to have a very low risk of malignancy in adults as well as pediatric patients [7]. Treatment is usually reserved for autonomous nodules causing overt hyperthyroidism, and referral to a pediatric endocrinologist and/or experienced pediatric surgeon for additional management is warranted. A non-suppressed TSH would suggest a non-functioning nodule, and if the nodule is ≥1 cm, the patient should be referred to a pediatric endocrinologist for ultrasound-guided fine-needle aspiration.

Importantly, while ultrasonography is widely available, interpretation of the images by a radiologist who has experience in both thyroid pathology and pediatric physiology is of utmost importance. Occasionally, there may be an incidental discovery of ectopic intrathyroidal thymic tissue, which is unique to the pediatric population [8]. Radiologists who are less comfortable with interpreting pediatric thyroid sonography may confuse the sonographic appearance of this benign lesion with a suspicious thyroid nodule, leading to unnecessary referral and significant family anxiety.

Some neck masses identified on physical examination and ultrasound are not thyroid nodules, but instead are thyroglossal duct cysts. These cysts are the fluid-filled remnants of the thyroglossal duct that served as the tract for thyroid gland descent in the developing embryo. Thyroglossal duct cysts typically present as midline cystic masses, the majority of which are located below the level of the hyoid bone. Acute infection or hemorrhage may occur, leading to sudden pain, tenderness, and difficulty in swallowing. Referral to a pediatric surgeon or orolaryngologist for removal is warranted.

Ultrasound in Primary Congenital Hypothyroidism

Neck ultrasound can also be helpful in clarifying the etiology of primary congenital hypothyroidism. These can be broadly classified as defects of thyroid gland development, that is, thyroid dysgenesis (ranging from complete agenesis to hypoplasia to ectopy) or defects of thyroid hormone production in a structurally normal gland, that is, thyroid dyshormonogenesis (please refer to Chap. 41 for more details on "Congenital Hypothyroidism"). Transient causes of primary congenital hypothyroidism include the transplacental passage of maternal TSH receptor-blocking antibodies or iodine excess/deficiency. Although the presence or lack of thyroid tissue does not change initial management when treating patients with congenital hypothyroidism, imaging results provide insight regarding the need for future therapy. With this information, parents can be counseled on either the certainty of lifelong thyroid hormone supplementation (i.e., complete thyroid aplasia and most ectopic glands) versus the possibility of later discontinuing treatment (i.e., potential transient cause of congenital hypothyroidism).

Nuclear Imaging (Thyroid Scintigraphy)

Thyroid scintigraphy plays an important role in the evaluation of thyroid gland function, particularly in diagnosing the cause of thyrotoxicosis and identifying focal thyroid nodules as autonomously functioning or non-functioning [9]. While beyond the scope of practicing pediatricians, scintigraphy is also used by endocrinologists to determine the presence and location of residual functioning thyroid tissue after treatment of thyroid cancer and for calculating radioactive iodine doses for patients to be treated for hyperthyroidism or thyroid cancer (after surgery).

The most frequently used isotopes for thyroid scintigraphy are Iodine-123 (administered orally by capsule or liquid) or Technetium-99m pertechnetate (administered intravenously). Uptake measurements are obtained at fixed intervals, and capture either the amount of Iodine-123 that has been concentrated into thyroid tissue, or the amount of pertechnetate that is trapped in the gland. Thyroid scans, in which a camera is used to take pictures after the agent has been ingested, can also be obtained with the uptake measurements to generate planar images of the thyroid gland. There are no known adverse effects from the low doses employed, and while the isotopes contain a very small amount of radioactive molecules, the diagnostic benefits (see Table 38.1) oftentimes outweigh the potential radiation risk.

Scintigraphy in Thyrotoxicosis and Thyroid Nodules

Scintigraphy can be helpful in determining the underlying etiology of thyrotoxicosis when the history, physical examination, and laboratory testing are indeterminate. High uptake seen in the setting of a suppressed TSH level is diagnostic of hyperthyroidism, that is, active production of thyroid hormone. This suggests stimulation of the TSH receptor from autoantibodies in the setting of Graves' disease, from constitutive activation or increased activation of the TSH receptor signaling pathway, or increased thyroid hormone production from an autonomous nodule. Lack of uptake is consistent with thyroiditis, that is, passive release of preformed thyroid hormone (as seen in Hashitoxicosis or subacute thyroiditis), or, if a nodule is present, a non-functioning nodule. Please refer to section "Initial Management of Hyperthyroidism" in Chap. 42 for more information about the diagnosis and management of hyperthyroidism.

Scintigraphy in Congenital Hypothyroidism

Thyroid scintigraphy can provide additional insight into the etiology of congenital hypothyroidism [10]. Scintigraphy can identify agenesis (no uptake seen), hypoplasia (less uptake than expected), ectopy (uptake at any point along the pathway of the normal embryological descent), a eutopic thyroid, or large gland in situ with or without abnormally high levels of uptake. Transient etiologies (i.e., iodine excess or maternal TSH receptor-blocking antibodies) or certain forms of dyshormonogenesis can present with no uptake on scintigraphy despite the presence of a eutopic thyroid gland on ultrasound. Together, these imaging studies help to improve the diagnostic accuracy of patients with congenital hypothyroidism.

Conclusion

Thyroid ultrasound and scintigraphy are useful in evaluating the structure and function of the thyroid gland. Pediatricians may consider obtaining these imaging modalities when evaluating patients with thyroid nodules, thyrotoxicosis, or congenital hypothyroidism. Pediatric endocrinologists and/or radiologists with experience in pediatric thyroidology should be consulted if there are questions about result interpretation.

References

1. Hoang JK, Nguyen XV. Understanding the risks and harms of management of incidental thyroid nodules: a review. JAMA Otolaryngol Head Neck Surg. 2017;143(7):718–24.
2. Francis GL, Waguespack SG, Bauer AJ, Angelos P, Benvenga S, Cerutti JM, et al. Management guidelines for children with thyroid nodules and differentiated thyroid cancer. Thyroid. 2015;25(7):716–59.
3. Gupta A, Ly S, Castroneves LA, Frates MC, Benson CB, Feldman HA, et al. How are childhood thyroid nodules discovered: opportunities for improving early detection. J Pediatr. 2014;164(3):658–60.
4. Gupta A, Ly S, Castroneves LA, Frates MC, Benson CB, Feldman HA, et al. A standardized assessment of thyroid nodules in children confirms higher cancer prevalence than in adults. J Clin Endocrinol Metab. 2013;98(8):3238–45.
5. Richman DM, Benson CB, Doubilet PM, Peters HE, Huang SA, Asch E, et al. Thyroid nodules in pediatric patients: sonographic characteristics and likelihood of cancer. Radiology. 2018;288(2):591–9.
6. Haugen BR, Alexander EK, Bible KC, Doherty GM, Mandel SJ, Nikiforov YE, et al. 2015 American Thyroid Association management guidelines for adult patients with thyroid nodules and differentiated thyroid cancer: the American Thyroid Association Guidelines Task Force on thyroid nodules and differentiated thyroid cancer. Thyroid. 2016;26(1):1–133.
7. Ly S, Frates MC, Benson CB, Peters HE, Grant FD, Drubach LA, et al. Features and outcome of autonomous thyroid nodules in children: 31 consecutive patients seen at a single center. J Clin Endocrinol Metab. 2016;101(10):3856–62.
8. Frates MC, Benson CB, Dorfman DM, Cibas ES, Huang SA. Ectopic intrathyroidal thymic tissue mimicking thyroid nodules in children. J Ultrasound Med. 2018;37(3):783–91.
9. Ross DS, Burch HB, Cooper DS, Greenlee MC, Laurberg P, Maia AL, et al. 2016 American Thyroid Association guidelines for diagnosis and management of hyperthyroidism and other causes of thyrotoxicosis. Thyroid. 2016;26(10):1343–421.
10. Leger J, Olivieri A, Donaldson M, Torresani T, Krude H, van Vliet G, et al. European Society for Paediatric Endocrinology consensus guidelines on screening, diagnosis, and management of congenital hypothyroidism. Horm Res Paediatr. 2014;81(2):80–103.

39 Bone Densitometry in Children: What Clinicians Need to Know

Sasigarn A. Bowden

Introduction

Bone health screening and evaluation have become an important aspect of care in children and adolescents with chronic diseases and in those presenting with multiple fractures, due to increased awareness of pediatric osteoporosis. Evaluation of bone health in children often requires measurement of bone mineral density (BMD). In the primary care setting, two common reasons for obtaining BMD testing in children are the following: (1) To identify possible underlying bone fragility in children with recurrent fractures who may benefit from interventions to improve bone health and reduce fracture risk. (2) To determine the magnitude of low bone mass in children with chronic disorders at risk for osteoporotic fractures in order to guide and monitor treatment. Dual-energy X-ray absorptiometry (DXA) is the most widely available and preferred tool to assess BMD in children due to its relatively low radiation, high precision, and well-established pediatric normative data [1, 2]. This chapter summarizes the principles and indications of DXA scans for clinical practice, and the key concepts of interpretation of DXA results according to the International Society of Clinical Densitometry (ISCD) official positions.

Principles of DXA

DXA assesses the transmission of X-rays through the body. It uses high- and low-energy X-rays, allowing for discrimination between soft tissue and bone. Low-energy X-rays are attenuated by soft tissue, whereas high-energy X-rays are attenuated by both soft tissue and bone. Subtraction of the two attenuation values using software algorithms yields bone mineral content (BMC) measurements for the projected area of the bone. BMD is reported as the ratio of BMC and cross-sectional bone area. DXA thus provides a BMD measurement that is based on a two-dimensional projection of a three-dimensional structure and does not account for the depth of the bone being measured. The resultant BMD is called "areal" BMD (aBMD) and is measured in gram/cm^2 (versus true density, which is measured as gram/cm^3). A consequence of this is the underestimation of BMD of smaller bones (as in children with chronic disease and poor growth), and overestimation of BMD of larger bones [3]. Radiation exposure with DXA is very low, approximately 5–8 uSv, similar to the natural background radiation in a day, and is about 10–100 times lower than the radiation dose from lumbar or thoracic spine X-ray.

Which Skeletal Sites Should Be Assessed Using DXA?

The preferred sites of measurements in children are (1) the total body less head (example in Fig. 39.1) and (2) lumbar spine (L1–L4) (example in Fig. 39.2). The rationale for excluding the head in the total body bone density measurement is that the skull constitutes a relatively large percentage of total body bone mass, but does not respond similarly to physical activity or metabolic changes. Inclusion of the skull potentially under or overestimates BMD gains or losses at other skeletal sites. Unlike in adults, DXA measurements of the hip region (total hip or femoral neck) in growing children are unreliable, as the bony landmarks in the hip region that assure accurate positioning are not well developed until mid-adolescence [1]. However, obtaining a DXA measurement of the hip can eventually be helpful in older adolescents for better longitudinal BMD assessment as they transition to adulthood with follow-up DXA at adult healthcare facilities where the hip is the standard site of measurement [4]. It is important to make sure that there are no foreign artifacts overlying the area of scan (e.g., indwelling hardware) as these will invalidate DXA results. In such circumstances, alternate

S. A. Bowden (✉)
Division of Endocrinology, Department of Pediatrics, Nationwide Children's Hospital/The Ohio State University College of Medicine, Columbus, OH, USA
e-mail: Sasigarn.Bowden@nationwidechildrens.org

T. Stanley, M. Misra (eds.), *Endocrine Conditions in Pediatrics*, https://doi.org/10.1007/978-3-030-52215-5_39

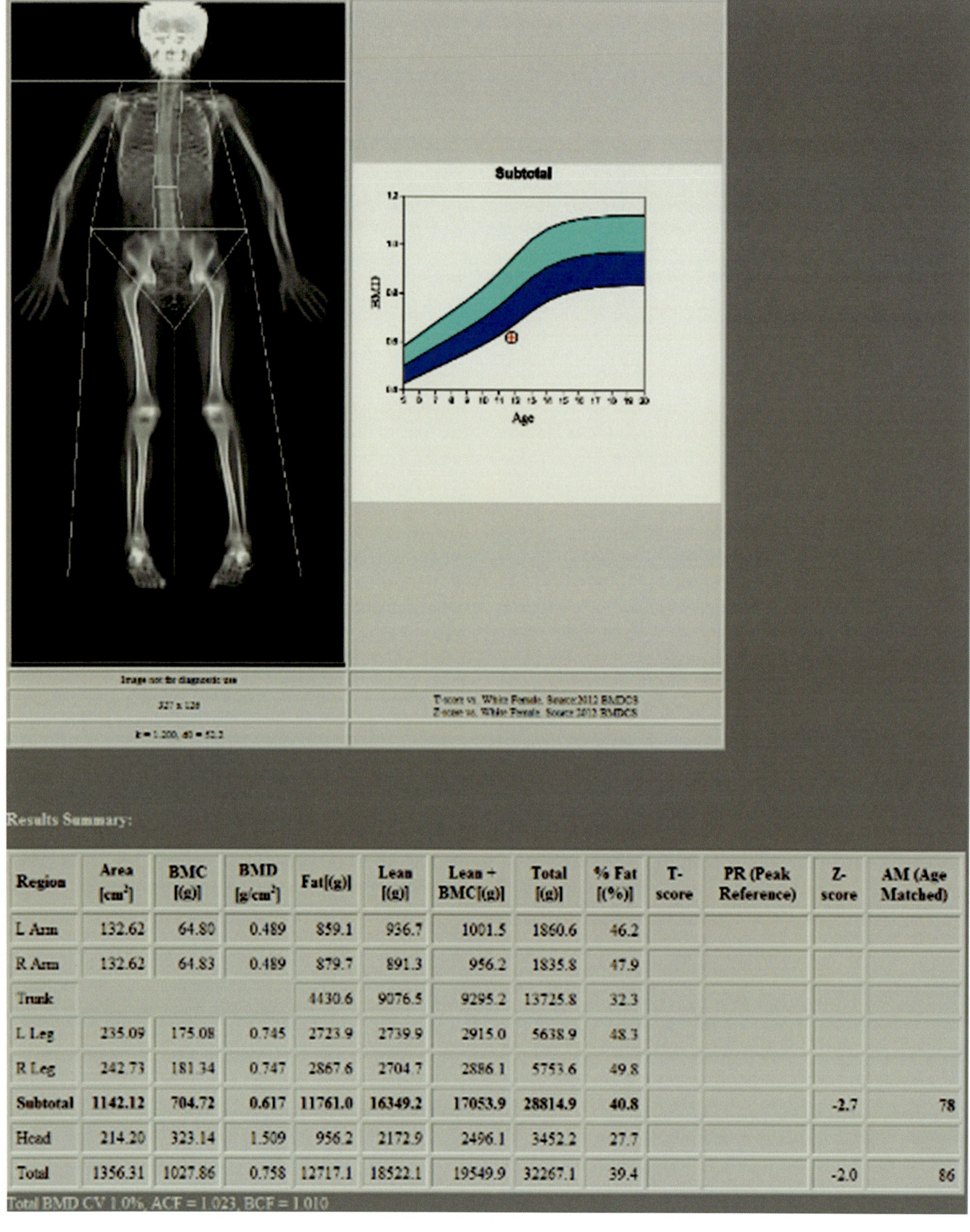

Results Summary:

Region	Area [cm²]	BMC [(g)]	BMD [g/cm²]	Fat[(g)]	Lean [(g)]	Lean + BMC[(g)]	Total [(g)]	% Fat [(%)]	T-score	PR (Peak Reference)	Z-score	AM (Age Matched)
L Arm	132.62	64.80	0.489	859.1	936.7	1001.5	1860.6	46.2				
R Arm	132.62	64.83	0.489	879.7	891.3	956.2	1835.8	47.9				
Trunk				4430.6	9076.5	9295.2	13725.8	32.3				
L Leg	235.09	175.08	0.745	2723.9	2739.9	2915.0	5638.9	48.3				
R Leg	242.73	181.34	0.747	2867.6	2704.7	2886.1	5753.6	49.8				
Subtotal	**1142.12**	**704.72**	**0.617**	**11761.0**	**16349.2**	**17053.9**	**28814.9**	**40.8**			**-2.7**	**78**
Head	214.20	323.14	1.509	956.2	2172.9	2496.1	3452.2	27.7				
Total	1356.31	1027.86	0.758	12717.1	18522.1	19549.9	32267.1	39.4			-2.0	86

Total BMD CV 1.0%, ACF = 1.023, BCF = 1.010

Fig. 39.1 Image of whole-body DXA scan. The total body less head is a preferred skeletal site for bone mineral density (BMD) or bone mineral content (BMC) measurement in pediatric patients (values in bold). This is also referred to as "subtotal BMC/BMD." BMD Z-score is shown in the second column from the right

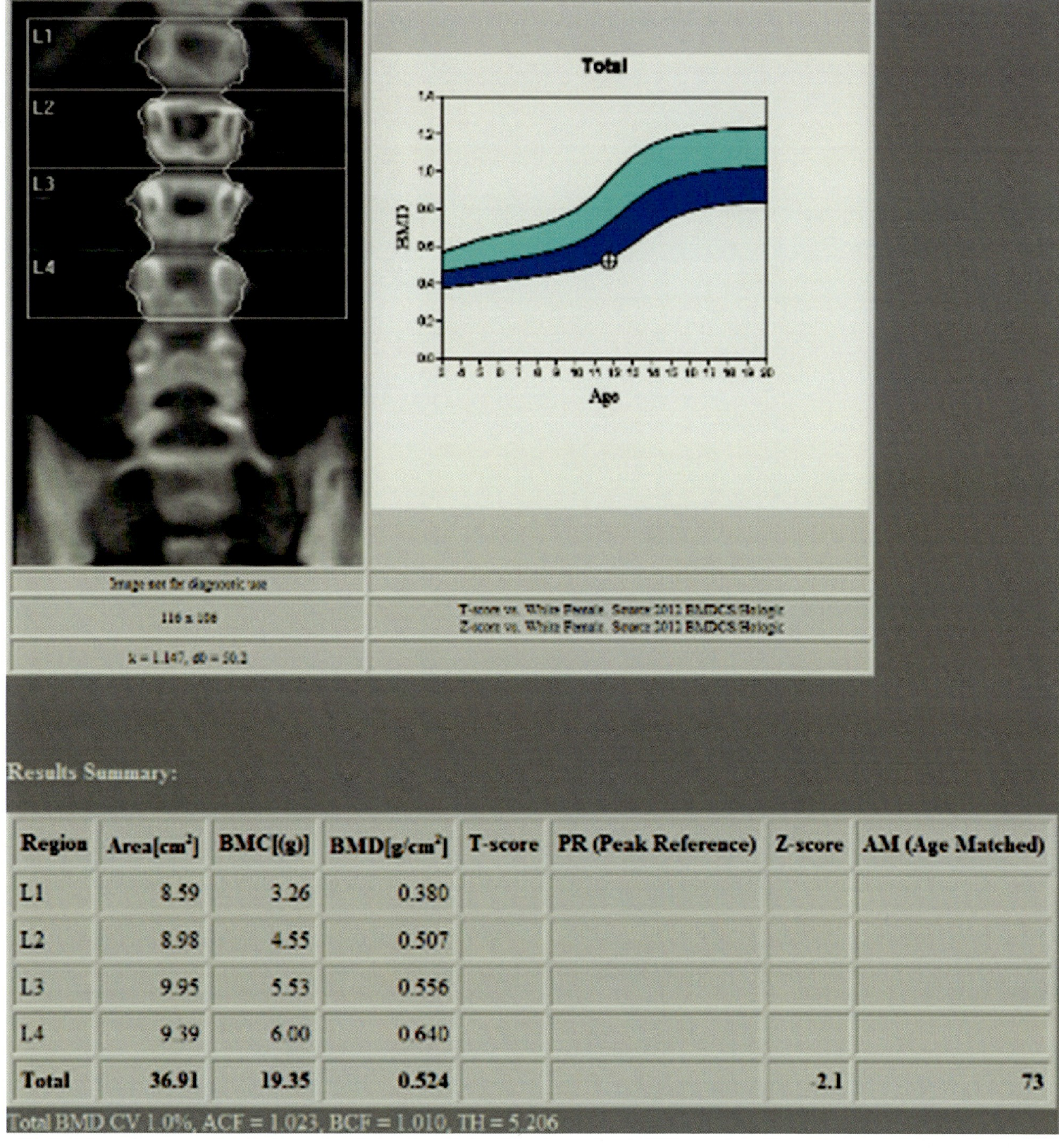

Region	Area[cm²]	BMC[(g)]	BMD[g/cm²]	T-score	PR (Peak Reference)	Z-score	AM (Age Matched)
L1	8.59	3.26	0.380				
L2	8.98	4.55	0.507				
L3	9.95	5.53	0.556				
L4	9.39	6.00	0.640				
Total	36.91	19.35	0.524			-2.1	73

Fig. 39.2 Image of lumbar spine DXA scan. Note that BMC and BMD values incrementally increase from L1 to L4

skeletal sites such as the forearm, proximal, or distal femur can be used [4]. Reference data for these alternate sites are only available for certain DXA machines with special scan software. For the scan, patients should wear a hospital gown or light clothing without metal, plastic, or objects (including casts or splints) that may affect the scan results.

When to Order a DXA Scan?

A DXA scan for BMD assessment should be obtained in children or adolescents with multiple fractures (see Chap. 4) or those with chronic diseases that pose risk factors for compromised bone health. These patients may benefit from

Table 39.1 Indications for DXA testing

1. Children and adolescents (without chronic diseases) with concern for fragility fractures
(a) Clinically significant fracture history
(b) Recurrent fractures
(c) Pathologic fracture(s)
(d) One or more vertebral compression fractures identified by spinal radiograph
2. Children and adolescents with primary bone disease (e.g., osteogenesis imperfecta)
3. Children and adolescents with chronic diseases
(a) Duchenne muscular dystrophy: baseline DXA at the time of glucocorticoid initiation and every 1–2 years [7]. When height-adjusted lumbar spine BMD Z-score is < −2 or if there is a history of back pain, vertebral fracture assessment should be performed
(b) Children and adolescents on long-term (>3 months) corticosteroids [8]
(c) Inflammatory bowel disease: in patients with severe disease, prolonged malnutrition, amenorrhea, delayed puberty, and/or steroid dependency [9]. Repeat DXA every 1–2 years if BMD is suboptimal at baseline (Z-score < −1) [10]
(d) Celiac disease: at presentation if the patient has growth and pubertal delay, fractures, or shows a poor response to a gluten-free diet [11]
(e) Cystic fibrosis: children >8 years if ideal body weight is <90%, FEV_1 (forced expiratory volume in 1 second) < 50% of the predicted value, if the patient has delayed puberty or has received high-dose glucocorticoid treatment for >90 days/year. Follow-up DXA every 5 years if BMD Z score is > −1, every 2 years if BMD Z score is between −2 and −1, or every year if BMD Z score < −2 [12]
(f) Adolescents with functional hypothalamic amenorrhea (from anorexia nervosa, excessive exercise, or emotional stress) when there is a history of ≥6 months of amenorrhea (or earlier when there is a history or suspicion of severe nutritional deficiency, other energy-deficit states, and/or skeletal fragility) [13]
(g) Oncological diseases: childhood cancer survivors previously treated with therapies associated with low bone density and with endocrinopathies should undergo a DXA scan at entry into a long-term follow-up program [14]
4. Children on bone-strengthening therapies (bisphosphonates or denosumab)

This list is not all-inclusive

interventions to decrease their fracture risk, and DXA results may influence management. The primary goals of BMD measurement are to identify patients at risk for fragility fractures and to monitor the effects of ongoing disease and/or therapy. Indications for DXA and published recommendations for the timing of the initial DXA scan for specific chronic childhood disorders (not all-inclusive) are listed in Table 39.1.

Interpretation of Pediatric DXA: Important Facts

- The International Society of Clinical Densitometry (ISCD) official positions state that the diagnosis of osteoporosis in children and adolescents should not be made based on DXA criteria alone [1].
- As children and adolescents grow, their BMD should increase. Therefore, BMD values in children and adolescents are expressed as Z-scores, where values are compared to age-, sex- and race-matched controls.
- Under no circumstance should T scores be used in pediatric BMD assessments because T-scores compare BMD values to those of healthy adults ages 20–30 years (when peak bone mass is achieved).
- The term "osteopenia" or "osteoporosis" should never appear in pediatric DXA reports.
- When aBMD or BMC Z-scores are ≤ −2.0, the term "low bone mineral density for age" is preferred.
- Diagnosis of osteoporosis in children and adolescents can be made when one or more vertebral compression fractures are present (in the absence of local spinal disease or high-energy trauma), regardless of BMD Z-scores.
- Low bone density (BMD Z-scores < −2) does not make a diagnosis of osteoporosis in children, but rather support the diagnosis when a clinically significant fracture history is present (See Chap. 4, Box 4.1 for the definition of pediatric osteoporosis and a clinically significant fracture history).
- A BMC or BMD Z-score greater than −2.0 does not preclude the possibility of skeletal fragility and increased fracture risk.

- BMD Z-scores can be falsely low in short children and falsely elevated in tall children [5, 6]. It is important to use height-adjusted Z scores for these children using a website calculator for BMD measured on Hologic densitometers (https://zscore.research.chop.edu/bmdCalculator.php).
- Lumbar spine BMD values typically increase from L1 to L4 (L1 < L2 < L3 < L4) (Fig. 39.2). Clinicians should review BMD values for each lumbar vertebra on the DXA output. BMD values that do not increase from L1 to L4 in this order may indicate an underlying vertebral fracture or the presence of an artifact. A vertebral fracture can overestimate BMD results (higher values).

When to Refer to a Pediatric Endocrinologist or Bone Specialist?

Patients with low bone density defined by BMD or BMC Z-scores < −2 should be referred to a pediatric bone specialist or pediatric endocrinologist. The presence of one or more vertebral compression fractures, any pathologic fractures, or a clinically significant fracture history (see Chap. 4), regardless of BMD results also warrant a referral to a pediatric bone specialist for a comprehensive evaluation and management.

References

1. Crabtree NJ, Arabi A, Bachrach LK, Fewtrell M, Fuleihan GE-H, Kecskemethy HH, et al. Dual-energy X-ray absorptiometry interpretation and reporting in children and adolescents: the revised 2013 ISCD Pediatric Official Positions. J Clin Densitom. 2014;17(2):225–42.
2. Zemel BS, Kalkwarf HJ, Gilsanz V, Lappe JM, Oberfield S, Shepherd JA, et al. Revised reference curves for bone mineral content and areal bone mineral density according to age and sex for black and non-black children: results of the bone mineral density in childhood study. J Clin Endocrinol Metabol. 2011;96(10):3160–9.
3. Zemel BS, Leonard MB, Kelly A, Lappe JM, Gilsanz V, Oberfield S, et al. Height adjustment in assessing dual energy x-ray absorptiometry measurements of bone mass and density in children. J Clin Endocrinol Metabol. 2010;95(3):1265–73.
4. Weber DR, Boyce A, Gordon C, Hogler W, Keckskemethy H, Misra M, et al. The utility of DXA assessment at the forearm, proximal femur, and lateral distal femur, and vertebral fracture assessment in the pediatric population: the 2019 official pediatric positions of the ISCD. J Clin Densitom. 2019;22(4):567–89.
5. Fewtrell M. Bone densitometry in children assessed by dual x ray absorptiometry: uses and pitfalls. Arch Dis Child. 2003;88(9):795–8.
6. Crabtree NJ, Arabi A, Bachrach LK, Fewtrell M, El-Hajj Fuleihan G, Kecskemethy HH, et al. Dual-energy X-ray absorptiometry interpretation and reporting in children and adolescents: the revised 2013 ISCD Pediatric Official Positions. J Clin Densitom. 2014;17(2):225–42.
7. Birnkrant DJ, Bushby K, Bann CM, Alman BA, Apkon SD, Blackwell A, et al. Diagnosis and management of Duchenne muscular dystrophy, part 2: respiratory, cardiac, bone health, and orthopaedic management. Lancet Neurol. 2018;10:18.
8. Liu D, Ahmet A, Ward L, Krishnamoorthy P, Mandelcorn ED, Leigh R, et al. A practical guide to the monitoring and management of the complications of systemic corticosteroid therapy. Allergy Asthma Clin Immunol. 2013;9(1):30.
9. Turner D, Ruemmele FM, Orlanski-Meyer E, Griffiths AM, De Carpi JM, Bronsky J, et al. Management of paediatric ulcerative colitis, part 1: ambulatory care—an evidence-based guideline from European Crohn's and Colitis Organization and European Society of Paediatric Gastroenterology, Hepatology and Nutrition. J Pediatr Gastroenterol Nutr. 2018;67(2):257–91.
10. Pappa H, Thayu M, Sylvester F, Leonard M, Zemel B, Gordon C. A clinical report on skeletal health of children and adolescents with inflammatory bowel disease. J Pediatr Gastroenterol Nutr. 2011;53(1):11.
11. Duerksen D, Pinto-Sanchez MI, Anca A, Schnetzler J, Case S, Zelin J, et al. Management of bone health in patients with celiac disease: practical guide for clinicians. Can Fam Physician. 2018;64(6):433–8.
12. Aris RM, Merkel PA, Bachrach LK, Borowitz DS, Boyle MP, Elkin SL, et al. Guide to bone health and disease in cystic fibrosis. J Clin Endocrinol Metabol. 2005;90(3):1888–96.
13. Gordon CM, Ackerman KE, Berga SL, Kaplan JR, Mastorakos G, Misra M, et al. Functional hypothalamic amenorrhea: an Endocrine Society clinical practice guideline. J Clin Endocrinol Metab. 2017;102(5):1413–39.
14. Group AAoPSoHOCsO. Long-term follow-up care for pediatric cancer survivors. Pediatrics. 2009;123(3):906–15.

Part III

Common Endocrine Conditions: Overview and Initial Management

40 Short Stature

Monica Serrano-Gonzalez

Abbreviations

AHO Albright hereditary osteodystrophy
ALS Acid labile subunit
BMI Body mass index
CDC Centers for Disease Control
CDGP Constitutional delay of growth and puberty
CF Cystic fibrosis
CNS Central nervous system
CRP C-reactive protein
FDA Food and Drug Administration
FSS Familial short stature
GH Growth hormone
GHD Growth hormone deficiency
GV Growth velocity
IBD Inflammatory bowel disease
IgA Immunoglobulin A
IGF-1 Insulin-like growth factor-1
ISS Idiopathic short stature
MAP Mitogen-activated protein
MRI Magnetic resonance imaging
ONH Optic nerve hypoplasia
PAH Predicted adult height
PSIS Pituitary stalk interruption syndrome
PTH Parathyroid hormone
PWS Prader–Willi syndrome
SDS Standard deviation score
SGA Small for gestational age
SHOX Short stature homeobox-containing gene on the X-chromosome
SRS Silver–Russell syndrome
TS Turner syndrome
TSH Thyroid-stimulating hormone
WHO World Health Organization

M. Serrano-Gonzalez (✉)
Pediatric Endocrinology and Diabetes Center, Hasbro Children's Hospital, The Warren Alpert Medical School of Brown University, Providence, RI, USA
e-mail: monica_serrano@brown.edu

Part I: Overview

Linear growth in childhood is an indicator of overall health [1]. In infants younger than 2 years, the length should be measured at each office visit. After 2 years, standing height should be measured, if possible, at each visit [1], and at least once per year. Please see Chap. 1 for specific considerations on accurately measuring length and height. To monitor length/height, it should be accurately plotted (to the month) on age- and sex-specific growth charts. Length/height can then be expressed as a percentile or a *z*-score (standard deviation score, SDS). Percentiles represent the proportion of the reference population that lies above or below that of the child being measured [2]. The height *z*-score represents the number of standard deviations below or above the mean height for age and sex [3]. It is generally recommended to use the World Health Organization (WHO) growth charts for children <2 years and the Centers for Disease Control (CDC) growth charts for those ≥2 years [4].

A child is considered to have short stature if his or her length/height *z*-score is 2 SDS or more below the mean for age and sex [5]. While individual measurements may reflect the presence of a growth disorder, it is more helpful to assess the trend over time (over at least 6 months) as compared to a single moment in time; crossing two major percentile lines on the growth chart is concerning, even if the height *z*-score is above −2 SDS [1, 6]. The annualized growth velocity (GV) represents the number of centimeters grown in a year, and can be plotted on age- and sex-specific charts (see Chaps. 1 and 2). Between the age of 5 years and puberty, a typical annualized GV is 5–6 cm/year [4]. A persistent annualized GV below the tenth percentile for age and sex is concerning [7].

Weight relative to height should be tracked (weight-to-height or body mass index, BMI), as weight preservation versus a drop in either of these parameters is helpful for diagnostic purposes. Body proportions should also be assessed as described in Chap. 1.

T. Stanley, M. Misra (eds.), *Endocrine Conditions in Pediatrics*, https://doi.org/10.1007/978-3-030-52215-5_40

A child's height should be interpreted in the context of his or her genetics, as short children usually have short parents. This is done by calculating the mid-parental target height, which is obtained by adding maternal height (in inches) plus paternal height (in inches), followed by an adjustment for gender by adding 5 inches in boys and subtracting 5 inches in girls and then dividing by 2.

A bone age (also known as a skeletal age) is a radiograph of the left hand and wrist that is compared to a set of standards (most commonly those found in the Greulich and Pyle atlas) to find the age to which the bone maturation corresponds [5, 8, 9]. The bone age may be delayed or advanced compared to the chronological age in normal variants of growth; however, if it is more than 2 SDS away from the mean, it is more likely due to a pathological condition [4]. Predicted adult height (PAH) is estimated based on the bone age and the concurrent height, most commonly using the Bayley and Pinneau method [5]. This method takes into account the fraction of final height achieved at each level of bone age and estimates adult height by dividing a child's current height by this fraction [8]. A child's predicted adult height is considered discordant from his or her genetic potential if it differs from the mid-parental target height by more than 2 standard deviations, or ~4 inches [4].

Owing to the complex physiology of growth and the pathophysiology of growth disorders, the differential diagnosis of short stature is broad (Table 40.1). It includes normal variants (such as familial short stature and constitutional delay of growth and puberty), as well as pathologic causes spanning intrauterine growth retardation (IUGR), chronic illness, malnutrition, psychosocial deprivation, endocrine disorders (hypothyroidism, growth hormone deficiency, Cushing syndrome or pseudohypoparathyroidism), intrinsic growth plate disorders (i.e., achondroplasia, hypochondroplasia, spondyloepiphyseal dysplasia, short stature homeobox-containing gene-SHOX-haploinsufficiency, and aggrecanopathies), syndromic causes (Turner, Noonan, Silver–Russell, and Prader–Willi syndromes), chronic systemic illnesses (e.g., renal, gastrointestinal, and cardiovascular), iatrogenic, and idiopathic short stature (ISS).

The evaluation of a short child (Table 40.2) should include a thorough medical and family history and physical examination. Targeted laboratory investigation is recommended based on the clues provided by the history and physical examination. Lastly, if the history and physical examination do not provide clues toward a specific diagnosis, nonspecific laboratory and radiographic screening tests can be pursued [3].

Table 40.1 Key pathophysiology

Linear growth is determined by the rate of growth plate chondrogenesis [31].
GH and IGF-1 stimulate growth by acting on the growth plate [1].
Thyroid hormones are essential for linear growth [37].
Sex steroids cause an increase in GH and IGF-1 secretory rates during puberty [38]. In peripheral tissues, androgens are aromatized to estrogen. Estrogen alters growth rate and also accelerates bone maturation, leading to the cessation of growth [31].
During stress and chronic inflammation, concentrations of cortisol and proinflammatory cytokines are higher. They can impede normal growth at the growth plate [31].
Nutritional intake affects longitudinal growth [39].
Supraphysiological concentrations of glucocorticoids cause a slowing of growth through effects on the growth plate [31].
SHOX haploinsufficiency is the main reason for short stature in patients with Turner syndrome [40].

Table 40.2 Items required for diagnosis and items supporting diagnosis

Auxological data
Height z-score < −2 SDS increases the likelihood of a pathological cause for shortness. A normal growth rate points to a normal variant of growth, whereas a slow growth rate may indicate a pathological cause of poor growth. Weight percentiles more affected than height percentiles point to chronic illness or malnutrition as the basis for growth failure.
Physical examination
Midline craniofacial anomalies (cleft lip/palate, single central incisor) increase the likelihood of GH deficiency. Dysmorphic features may suggest the presence of Noonan syndrome, Turner syndrome, Prader–Willi syndrome, AHO, or SHOX deficiency, all of which are associated with a subnormal linear growth velocity. A reduced arm span-to-height ratio or an abnormal upper-to-lower body segment ratio suggests a skeletal dysplasia.
Laboratory evaluation
Determination of a random serum GH concentration is not useful except during the first week of life, during GH stimulation test, or at the time of hypoglycemia (critical sample). Normal GH secretion is pulsatile and greatest during deep sleep; therefore, random values are not likely to be helpful. Low surrogate markers of GH sufficiency (IGF-1 and/or IGFBP-3) suggest GH deficiency. Low free T4 with high TSH is indicative of primary hypothyroidism; low free T4 with low or normal TSH is consistent with central hypothyroidism. Elevated ESR/CRP is consistent with inflammatory conditions that, when chronic, can impair linear growth. A karyotype (chromosome study) is indicated in girls with unexplained short stature (and slow height velocity) so as to identify those with Turner syndrome.
Imaging studies
Delayed bone age will be present in patients with constitutional delay of growth and puberty. An abnormal skeletal survey is expected in those with skeletal dysplasia. A brain/sellar MRI may identify a structural cause of GHD (e.g., congenital causes such as empty sella syndrome, pituitary hypoplasia, ectopic posterior pituitary, interrupted pituitary stalk, optic nerve hypoplasia, or acquired causes such as a brain tumor).

Part II: Etiologies of Short Stature

Familial Short Stature and Constitutional Delay of Growth and Puberty

Children with familial short stature (FSS) are otherwise healthy and nondysmorphic. They have a normal rate of growth (normal annualized GV) and a bone age that is concordant with their chronological age. Their PAH falls within their genetic target range [mid-parental target height +/− 4 inches (~2 SD)] [4]. Given the limited correlation between birth length and adult height, it stands to reason that children with FSS who are long as infants will cross percentile curves in a downward fashion, as they attain their genetically appropriate growth channel. They typically do so during their first 3 years of life [10].

In contrast to children with FSS, children with constitutional delay of growth and puberty (CDGP, often referred to as "late bloomers") typically show a decrease in height percentiles during the peripubertal years, although they also may do so during the first 3 years of life [4]. The age of maternal menarche and age of the paternal adolescent growth spurt are helpful in identifying CDGP, as more than 50% of children with constitutional delay have a positive family history [5]. Children with CDGP will have delayed puberty and/or a slow pubertal tempo, a normal annualized GV, and a skeletal age that is delayed, defined as ≥2 standard deviations below their chronological age [11], which results in a normal or near-normal adult height [4, 7].

Small for Gestational Age (SGA)

SGA may be defined as a weight and/or length more than 2 SDS below the mean for gestational age [12]. It may be due to known causes of impaired in utero growth, such as prenatal infection, or exposure to drugs, smoking, or alcohol during pregnancy. It may also be idiopathic. Infants born SGA typically demonstrate catch-up growth during the first 2 years of life. However, up to 8–12% of children born SGA do not demonstrate this catch-up growth and fail to reach the third percentile for height by 2 years of age [3, 4]. Such a pattern carries a high risk of short stature in later life and is an approved indication by the US Food and Drug Administration (FDA) for growth hormone therapy [12].

Chronic Systemic Illnesses, Malnutrition, and Psychosocial Deprivation

An abnormally low BMI for age/gender (below the second percentile or crossing percentiles downward) may indicate nutritional disorders or chronic systemic illnesses [13, 14], in which case BMI would be disproportionately affected relative to height. Such a situation warrants nonspecific screening. Screening for celiac disease includes an assessment of tissue transglutaminase activity of the immunoglobulin A (IgA) type and total IgA. The latter is indicated because IgA deficiency would hinder the interpretation of the tissue transglutaminase antibody test. It is important to screen for this condition because short stature may be the only or overriding presenting symptom [4]. Inflammatory bowel disease (Crohn's disease and ulcerative colitis) may also impair linear growth; both will typically show an elevated sedimentation rate (ESR) and/or C-reactive protein (CRP). Anemia and/or thrombocytosis may also be present. Other conditions such as chronic renal insufficiency (evaluation includes a basal metabolic panel and urinalysis), chronic anemia (evaluation includes a complete blood count), cardiac disorders (diagnosed by history and physical examination), and cystic fibrosis (evaluation includes a chloride sweat test) should be considered. Severe psychosocial deprivation can also cause poor growth that improves upon changes in the adverse environment [15, 16].

Endocrine Disorders

Growth Hormone Deficiency (GHD)

Normal serum levels of insulin-like growth factor-1 (IGF-1) and insulin-like growth factor-binding protein 3 (IGFBP-3), and a robust GV (>25th percentile) make GH deficiency very unlikely [14], whereas a low IGF-1 and/or IGFBP-3 raise suspicion for GHD and should be followed by a referral to endocrinology for consideration of GH stimulation test. IGF-1 levels should be interpreted in the context of the nutritional status, as undernutrition is associated with lower IGF-1 levels, often frankly low levels [17]. Because of the pulsatile nature and nocturnal predilection of growth hormone secretion, random growth hormone levels should not be sent. Rather, provocative GH testing is the gold standard for diagnosis. Stimulation tests involve the administration of insulin, arginine, glucagon, or clonidine followed by timed sampling for the determination of serum GH concentration [5]. Diagnostic thresholds for stimulated GH levels have varied from <2.5 to <10 ng/mL; <10 ng/mL is the most widely used diagnostic threshold in the United States [5, 14, 18].

GH deficiency may be congenital, associated with syndromes such as the optic nerve hypoplasia (ONH) spectrum, empty sella syndrome, or pituitary stalk interruption syndrome (PSIS). It may also be acquired as a consequence of tumors, such as craniopharyngioma, germinoma or hamartoma (or their treatments) [10]. Midline defects on physical examination (for example, a cleft palate) should suggest the possibility of a growth–hormone axis abnormality [4]. Patients with congenital GH deficiency usually have a normal length at birth and do not show growth deceleration until after 6 months of life [4].

Other Endocrine Disorders

A wide variety of endocrine disorders other than GH deficiency can present as impaired linear growth. Disorders of GH signaling or other components of the GH/IGF-1 axis are rare causes of short stature. Growth hormone insensitivity would present with a pattern of low GH surrogate markers (IGF-1 and IGFBP-3) and a robust GH response during stimulation testing. Causes of acquired GH resistance, such as undernutrition, hepatic disease, or chronic inflammatory disorders, should be excluded [19]. GH insensitivity may be due to abnormalities of the GH receptor (Laron syndrome), the GH signal transduction (i.e. STAT5B), IGF-1 or its receptor, or the acid-labile subunit (ALS), which plays a role in extending the half-life of IGF-1 and IGFBP-3 [8, 20]. Patients with mutations to IGF-1 or the IGF-1 receptor have postnatal linear growth failure, and may have prenatal growth failure, microcephaly, intellectual delay, and deafness [20]. Patients with pathogenic mutations to the GH receptor or STAT5B have a normal birth weight/length [20].

Hypothyroidism, either congenital or acquired, is a common, sometimes profound, and eminently treatable cause of poor linear growth. Congenital hypothyroidism screening is part of the newborn screen panel in the United States. The diagnosis of congenital hypothyroidism is critical given that, in addition to growth retardation, it is a cause of impaired intellectual development if not treated early [4]. Acquired hypothyroidism in childhood and adolescence is most often due to autoimmunity (Hashimoto thyroiditis). This disorder may present with a gradual decrease in height percentiles together with modest weight gain (due to mucinous fluid retention secondary to myxedema, not obesity) and a history of fatigue, dry skin, and constipation. On physical examination, patients may have a goiter, cool/dry skin, delayed relaxation of deep tendon reflexes, and in severe cases, myxedema [21].

Hypercortisolism in the setting of Cushing syndrome is characterized by decreasing height percentiles with concomitantly increasing weight percentiles as well as other features, such as fatigue, easy bruising, thick and reddish purple striae, facial plethora, and proximal muscle weakness [22]. True Cushing syndrome in children is rare.

Albright hereditary osteodystrophy (AHO) is a syndrome characterized by short stature, obesity, rounded face, brachydactyly (short fourth and fifth metacarpals), and subcutaneous ossifications [23]. In the subtype pseudohypoparathyroidism type 1a (PHP-1a), there is also resistance to parathyroid hormone (which presents with hypocalcemia, hyperphosphatemia and an elevated parathyroid hormone) and to other hormones such as thyroid-stimulating hormone. PHP-1a is due to inactivating mutations to the GNAS gene, which encodes the stimulatory alpha subunit of a protein complex called a guanine nucleotide-binding protein (G-protein). Because the gene is imprinted, the presentation of AHO differs depending on whether inheritance is from the mother or father. When the disorder is inherited from the mother, the patient will have resistance to hormones that act through G-protein-coupled receptors. When inherited from the father, the affected individual will typically have the AHO phenotype without hormone resistance [23].

Another endocrine disorder that can be associated with impaired linear growth is diabetes mellitus. Long-standing, poorly controlled type 1 diabetes is a cause of Mauriac syndrome, which is characterized by poor linear growth, pubertal delay, and hepatomegaly [24].

Intrinsic Growth Plate Disorders

This category includes skeletal dysplasias, such as achondroplasia, hypochondroplasia, spondyloepiphyseal dysplasia, SHOX haploinsufficiency, and aggrecanopathies. Abnormal body proportions are strongly suggestive of a skeletal dysplasia. In achondroplasia, patients have short limbs and a large head with a prominent forehead [4]. Patients with SHOX deficiency may have short forearms, reduced arm span-to-height ratio, and an increased upper-to-lower body segment ratio [3, 5, 25]. A skeletal survey of the long bones may be helpful to arrive at a diagnosis [3].

Syndromic Causes

A careful physical examination should assess for dysmorphic features that could indicate a syndromic cause of short stature. Trisomy 21 (Down syndrome) is the most common chromosomal disorder; it has short stature as a prominent feature [26]. Patients with this syndrome usually have an early onset of puberty and reduced pubertal growth spurt, and most have normal stimulated GH levels [1]. Patients with Trisomy 21 should have their height plotted on Trisomy 21-specific growth charts to avoid missing complicating conditions such as hypothyroidism or celiac disease, which have an increased frequency in this population [1, 26].

Turner syndrome (TS) occurs in about 1 in 2000 liveborn girls [14]. The diagnosis is most often based on short stature, hypogonadism, and minor dysmorphic features [14]. However, it may come to clinical attention due to delayed puberty or primary amenorrhea [27] or, in some patients, impaired linear growth with no other prominent phenotypic features. In actuality, 50% of girls with TS may have no associated physical features, except for short stature and delayed or absent puberty. However, some patients may have one or more of the well-characterized physical findings of a webbed neck, cubitus valgus (increased carrying angle), short metacarpals, broad chest with widely spaced nipples, high-arched palate, or low-set ears [1, 4]. A karyotype should be considered in any short girl without an identified cause, even if there are no dysmorphic features on examination [3]. In boys with unexplained short stature and a history of genital abnormalities, it is recommended to obtain a karyotype to rule out a mosaic form of gonadal dysgenesis, 46, XY/45, X [3].

Noonan syndrome is an autosomal dominant condition with a prevalence of 1 in 1000–2500 live births [28]. It is caused by mutations in the *PTPN11* gene in ~50% of the cases and by other genes in the RAS/MAP kinase signaling pathway. Patients with Noonan syndrome have characteristic facial features (webbed neck, low-set, and posteriorly rotated ears, hypertelorism, ptosis, pectus carinatum or excavatum), heart defects (most commonly pulmonary valve stenosis, followed by hypertrophic cardiomyopathy), cryptorchidism in up to 80%, and short stature [28]. GH secretion on provocative testing is usually normal [14]; however, GH is approved by the US FDA for the treatment of patients with Noonan syndrome [28].

Silver–Russell syndrome (SRS, also known as Russell–Silver syndrome) is a condition associated with both prenatal and postnatal growth retardation. Patients with SRS are born SGA, and they have postnatal growth failure with relative macrocephaly at birth, prominent forehead, body asymmetry, and feeding difficulties. The most common cause is the loss of methylation on chromosome 11p15 and maternal uniparental disomy of chromosome 7 [29].

Patients with Prader–Willi syndrome (PWS) often have a history of hypotonia and feeding difficulties during infancy. PWS is due to lack of expression of genes on the paternally inherited chromosome 15q11.2-q13 region. Characteristic facial features include almond-shaped eyes with downslanting palpebral fissures, as well as hypotonia and failure to thrive during infancy followed by hyperphagia, obesity, and developmental delay [30].

Iatrogenic Short Stature

Poor growth can occur in association with chronic exposure to medications that impair growth, such as supraphysiological doses of glucocorticoids for treatment of chronic illness (including inhaled glucocorticoids) or chemotherapy for malignancy, or radiation therapy. Inhaled glucocorticoids at appropriate doses have minimal effect on height, but very high doses of inhaled glucocorticoids are a relatively common reason for reduced growth velocity and/or short stature. Cranial irradiation increases the risk of hypopituitarism, including GH deficiency, in a time- and dose-dependent manner [19]. Radiation also adversely affects growth plates: even a single radiation dose of 10 Gy to the spine can impair linear growth [31].

Idiopathic Short Stature

Idiopathic short stature (ISS) is a diagnosis of exclusion. It is diagnosed when a child has short stature (height *z*-score below −2.25 SDS) and no recognizable cause is found after thorough evaluation [3]. These children have a normal annualized GV and a bone age that is concordant with their chronological age [4]. The importance of this diagnosis is related to GH therapy being approved for the treatment of ISS by the US FDA if the height *z*-score is below −2.25 SDS (<1.2nd percentile) and if PAH is below 63 inches for a boy or 59 inches for a girl [5]. However, this indication for GH treatment has not been without controversy related to the required (most often daily) injections, the frequency with which diagnosed patients are determined to actually have constitutional delay, the modest effect on final height, and the high cost of the treatment [7].

Part III: Urgent or Emergent Considerations and Initial Management

- A comprehensive laboratory evaluation for children with short stature and/or decreased growth velocity is outlined in Chap. 1. This evaluation is advisable for children with decreased growth velocity and/or concerning signs/symptoms on history and physical, but is generally not necessary when growth velocity is normal and presentation is highly consistent with FSS or CDGP.
- It is advised to refer children with decreasing height percentiles who are also showing increased weight percentiles to endocrinology, as they are more likely to have an endocrine cause of impaired linear growth.
- An infant with growth deceleration after 6 months of life and history of hypoglycemia, prolonged jaundice, giant cell hepatitis, micropenis, and/or a midline craniofacial defect may have congenital hypopituitarism, which requires urgent evaluation by an endocrinologist.
- Infants with growth deceleration and nystagmus may have a midline defect such as the optic nerve hypoplasia/septo-optic dysplasia spectrum, which can be associated with hypopituitarism. Such infants, especially if there is a history of hypoglycemia, prolonged jaundice, or micropenis, warrant urgent evaluation by an endocrinologist.
- Children with growth deceleration and signs/symptoms of central nervous system (CNS) pathology (headaches, vision changes, behavior changes, and/or emesis) could have a brain tumor. Children who have not completed pubertal development and have no linear growth in

≥1 year warrant careful evaluation for CNS pathology, potentially including a brain MRI.

- Children with significant growth deceleration who also have prominent fatigue (potentially due to central hypothyroidism or adrenal insufficiency) or polyuria/polydipsia (signs of diabetes insipidus) should be suspected to have CNS disease and concomitant hypopituitarism.
- If hypopituitarism is suspected, brain magnetic resonance imaging (MRI) without and with intravenous contrast dye enhancement, with specific cuts to examine the pituitary/sellar region (and optic pathway), should be obtained to exclude tumors and identify ectopic and hypoplastic pituitary glands, and any findings to suggest the diagnosis of optic nerve hypoplasia/septo-optic dysplasia spectrum.

Part IV: Chronic Management and Considerations for Referral

Recombinant human GH (rhGH) is used for multiple indications in children with short stature or decreased growth (Table 40.3). For children with GHD, rhGH results in an average height gain of 1.5–2 SDS [32]. Factors that affect the response to GH include age and height at the start of GH, continuity, and duration of treatment, and GH dose [33]. GH is approved by the FDA for children born SGA without catch-up growth to the fifth percentile by 2 years of life [12]. It is also approved for ISS if height *z*-score is below −2.25 SDS, and for PAH if <63 inches for males and <59 inches for females; therapy results in an average height gain of 2 inches for children with ISS, though the response to therapy is highly variable [5]. GH therapy is also an approved therapy for individuals with Turner syndrome, Prader–Willi syndrome, Noonan syndrome, and SHOX deficiency. The shorter the child, the more consideration should be given to treatment with GH, especially if the child is concerned about his/her stature [5]. Children who are treated with GH should have monitoring of their height several times per year as well as IGF-1 levels monitored at least annually [18]. IGF-1 levels should be maintained within the normal range for the age/pubertal stage [18].

Table 40.3 Indications for growth hormone in children approved by the US Food and Drug Administration

Growth hormone deficiency
Turner syndrome
Prader–Willi syndrome
Noonan syndrome
Small for gestational age without catch-up growth
Chronic kidney disease
SHOX gene haploinsufficiency or mutation
Idiopathic short stature

Recombinant human IGF-1 is FDA-approved to treat children with GH insensitivity, if their height SDS is below −3.0, their IGF-1 SDS is below −3.0, and they have normal stimulated levels of GH [5, 19].

Hypothyroidism is treated with thyroid hormone replacement (see Chap. 41). It is important to identify acquired hypothyroidism early, as it can lead to a loss of height potential with delay in the onset of treatment. Congenital hypothyroidism is identified by the newborn screen. Treatment with levothyroxine should be started as soon as the diagnosis is made to prevent intellectual disability [34].

The use of gonadotropin-releasing hormone agonists has been proposed and put into limited use to delay pubertal progression in short children, although this practice is not the accepted standard of care. GnRH agonists temporarily return sex steroids to prepubertal levels and thereby allow for a longer period of growth. However, there is a paucity of data addressing the efficacy of this approach. In addition, the potential for adverse psychosocial consequences and risk of long-term bone under-mineralization have prevented their routine use in children with normally timed puberty [35].

Regardless of the likely cause of impaired linear growth, early referral to a pediatric endocrinologist is preferable, as the window for intervention closes with age (once growth plates fuse). Starting GH treatment at an earlier age is associated with a better response [5]. To put the consideration of the timing of treatment into context, boys usually complete 97% of their growth by 15 years and girls by 13–14 years [11].

If a bone age radiograph is obtained prior to the visit to endocrinology, it is helpful to request the image so it can be reviewed by the pediatric endocrinologist.

If weight percentiles are significantly more affected than height, consider initial referral to gastroenterology or parallel referral in addition to endocrinology.

The following more clearly warrant referral to pediatric endocrinology:

- Height below the first percentile (*z*-score below −2.25 SDS) [1, 7].
- Unexplained neonatal hypoglycemia, prolonged jaundice, and/or micropenis [1].
- Having crossed two major percentile lines on the growth chart over a period of 6 months or more [36].
- Persistent growth velocity less than the tenth percentile for age [7] or less than 2 inches per year [4].
- Predicted adult height less than two standard deviations (4 inches) below the mid-parental target height range [7].
- No onset of puberty by 14 years in boys (testicular volume at least 4 mL) or 13 years in girls (onset of thelarche) [4].
- History of SGA at birth without evidence of catch-up growth to the fifth percentile by 2 years of life [4].

- Symptoms and signs consistent with hypopituitarism (e.g., polyuria and polydipsia suggestive of diabetes insipidus, presence of a midline defect, etc.) [1].
- History of cranial irradiation [19].

References

1. Kappy MS, Allen DB, Geffner ME. Pediatric practice endocrinology. 2nd ed. New York: McGraw-Hill Education; 2014.
2. Becker P, Carney LN, Corkins MR, Monczka J, Smith E, Smith SE, et al. Consensus statement of the Academy of Nutrition and Dietetics/American Society for Parenteral and Enteral Nutrition: indicators recommended for the identification and documentation of pediatric malnutrition (undernutrition). Nutr Clin Pract. 2015;30(1):147–61.
3. Oostdijk W, Grote FK, de Muinck Keizer-Schrama SM, Wit JM. Diagnostic approach in children with short stature. Horm Res. 2009;72(4):206–17.
4. Barstow C, Rerucha C. Evaluation of short and tall stature in children. Am Fam Physician. 2015;92(1):43–50.
5. Cohen LE. Idiopathic short stature: a clinical review. JAMA. 2014;311(17):1787–96.
6. Chianese J. In brief-short stature. Pediatr Rev. 2005;26(1):36–7.
7. Allen DB, Cuttler L. Clinical practice. Short stature in childhood – challenges and choices. N Engl J Med. 2013;368(13):1220–8.
8. Rosenfield RL. Essentials of growth diagnosis. Endocrinol Metab Clin N Am. 1996;25(3):743–58.
9. Martin DD, Wit JM, Hochberg Z, Sävendahl L, van Rijn RR, Fricke O, et al. The use of bone age in clinical practice – part 1. Horm Res Paediatr. 2011;76(1):1–9.
10. Rose SR, Vogiatzi MG, Copeland KC. A general pediatric approach to evaluating a short child. Pediatr Rev. 2005;26(11):410–20.
11. Greulich WW, Idell PS. Radiographic atlas of skeletal development of the hand and wrist. 2nd ed. Stanford: Stanford University Press; 1959.
12. Chatelain P, Carrascosa A, Bona G, Ferrandez-Longas A, Sippell W. Growth hormone therapy for short children born small for gestational age. Horm Res. 2007;68(6):300–9.
13. Cole TJ, Flegal KM, Nicholls D, Jackson AA. Body mass index cut offs to define thinness in children and adolescents: international survey. BMJ. 2007;335(7612):194.
14. Maghnie M, Labarta JI, Koledova E, Rohrer TR. Short stature diagnosis and referral. Front Endocrinol (Lausanne). 2017;8:374.
15. Blizzard RM, Bulatovic A. Psychosocial short stature: a syndrome with many variables. Bailliere Clin Endocrinol Metab. 1992;6(3):687–712.
16. Stanhope R, Gohlke B. The aetiology of growth failure in psychosocial short stature. J Pediatr Endocrinol Metab. 2003;16(3):365–6.
17. Hawkes CP, Murray DM, Kenny LC, Kiely M, O'B Hourihane J, Irvine AD, et al. Correlation of insulin-like growth factor-I and -II concentrations at birth measured by mass spectrometry and growth from birth to two months. Horm Res Paediatr. 2018;89(2):122–31.
18. Peters CJ, Dattani MT. How to use insulin-like growth factor 1 (IGF1). Arch Dis Child Educ Pract Ed. 2012;97(3):114–8.
19. Grimberg A, DiVall SA, Polychronakos C, Allen DB, Cohen LE, Quintos JB, et al. Guidelines for growth hormone and insulin-like growth factor-I treatment in children and adolescents: growth hormone deficiency, idiopathic short stature, and primary insulin-like growth factor-I deficiency. Horm Res Paediatr. 2016;86(6):361–97.
20. David A, Hwa V, Metherell LA, Netchine I, Camacho-Hübner C, Clark AJ, et al. Evidence for a continuum of genetic, phenotypic, and biochemical abnormalities in children with growth hormone insensitivity. Endocr Rev. 2011;32(4):472–97.
21. Diaz A, Lipman Diaz EG. Hypothyroidism. Pediatr Rev. 2014;35(8):336–47; quiz 48–9.
22. Nieman LK, Biller BM, Findling JW, Newell-Price J, Savage MO, Stewart PM, et al. The diagnosis of Cushing's syndrome: an Endocrine Society clinical practice guideline. J Clin Endocrinol Metab. 2008;93(5):1526–40.
23. Germain-Lee EL. Short stature, obesity, and growth hormone deficiency in pseudohypoparathyroidism type 1a. Pediatr Endocrinol Rev. 2006;3(Suppl 2):318–27.
24. Myaeng J, Ong B, Pinsker JE. Case 1: hepatomegaly and growth failure in an 11-year-old girl with type 1 diabetes. Pediatr Rev. 2015;36(10):459–61.
25. Binder G. Short stature due to SHOX deficiency: genotype, phenotype, and therapy. Horm Res Paediatr. 2011;75(2):81–9.
26. Myrelid A, Gustafsson J, Ollars B, Annerén G. Growth charts for Down's syndrome from birth to 18 years of age. Arch Dis Child. 2002;87(2):97–103.
27. Practice Committee of American Society for Reproductive Medicine. Current evaluation of amenorrhea. Fertil Steril. 2004;82(Suppl 1):S33–9.
28. Roberts AE, Allanson JE, Tartaglia M, Gelb BD. Noonan syndrome. Lancet. 2013;381(9863):333–42.
29. Wakeling EL, Brioude F, Lokulo-Sodipe O, O'Connell SM, Salem J, Bliek J, et al. Diagnosis and management of Silver-Russell syndrome: first international consensus statement. Nat Rev Endocrinol. 2017;13(2):105–24.
30. Angulo MA, Butler MG, Cataletto ME. Prader-Willi syndrome: a review of clinical, genetic, and endocrine findings. J Endocrinol Investig. 2015;38(12):1249–63.
31. Baron J, Sävendahl L, De Luca F, Dauber A, Phillip M, Wit JM, et al. Short and tall stature: a new paradigm emerges. Nat Rev Endocrinol. 2015;11(12):735–46.
32. Wit JM, Kamp GA, Rikken B. Spontaneous growth and response to growth hormone treatment in children with growth hormone deficiency and idiopathic short stature. Pediatr Res. 1996;39(2):295–302.
33. Frindik JP, Baptista J. Adult height in growth hormone deficiency: historical perspective and examples from the national cooperative growth study. Pediatrics. 1999;104(4 Pt 2):1000–4.
34. Cherella CE, Wassner AJ. Congenital hypothyroidism: insights into pathogenesis and treatment. Int J Pediatr Endocrinol. 2017;2017:11.
35. Dunkel L. Treatment of idiopathic short stature: effects of gonadotropin-releasing hormone analogs, aromatase inhibitors and anabolic steroids. Horm Res Paediatr. 2011;76(Suppl 3):27–9.
36. Canadian Paediatric Society. A health professional's guide to using growth charts. Paediatr Child Health. 2004;9(3):174–88.
37. Kim HY, Mohan S. Role and mechanisms of actions of thyroid hormone on the skeletal development. Bone Res. 2013;1(2):146–61.
38. Mauras N, Attie KM, Reiter EO, Saenger P, Baptista J. High dose recombinant human growth hormone (GH) treatment of GH-deficient patients in puberty increases near-final height: a randomized, multicenter trial. Genentech, Inc., Cooperative Study Group. J Clin Endocrinol Metab. 2000;85(10):3653–60.
39. Lifshitz F. Nutrition and growth. J Clin Res Pediatr Endocrinol. 2009;1(4):157–63.
40. Oliveira CS, Alves C. The role of the SHOX gene in the pathophysiology of Turner syndrome. Endocrinol Nutr. 2011;58(8):433–42.

Hypothyroidism

41

Jennifer M. Barker and Taylor M. Triolo

Hypothyroidism is the most common disorder of the thyroid and may be congenital or acquired (Table 41.1). Thyroid hormone regulates growth, neurocognitive development, and metabolism; and thyroid hormone deficiency negatively impacts well-being. Prompt treatment of hypothyroidism, congenital or acquired, prevents associated neurologic and physiologic sequelae.

In children, the symptoms of hypothyroidism can be nonspecific. Symptoms vary among patients partially due to the degree of biochemical derangement. Symptoms include fatigue, changes in sleep pattern, constipation, cold intolerance, or weight gain. On physical exam, practitioners may appreciate a goiter, bradycardia, delayed reflexes, edema, and dry skin. Longstanding hypothyroidism can result in linear growth retardation, which is disproportionate to weight gain, resulting in an increased BMI. Prolonged acquired hypothyroidism can also cause paradoxical pseudopubertal changes such as testicular enlargement and breast development due to cross-reactivity of elevated TSH with the FSH receptor.

Serum TSH and total or free T4 should be measured when hypothyroidism is suspected. Serum TSH is elevated in primary hypothyroidism. If free or total T4 is low with an inappropriately normal or low TSH, central hypothyroidism should be considered. If serum TSH and serum T4 are both elevated, rare thyroid hormone abnormalities, such as thyroid hormone resistance should be considered. While many laboratories have assays for circulating T3, the evaluation of T4 is sufficient to confirm the diagnosis of hypothyroidism. Serum concentrations of TSH and T4 change through childhood. Therefore, adult reference ranges do not apply to pediatric cohorts.

Thyroid hormone supplementation with levothyroxine treats hypothyroidism. It is typically a well-tolerated medication. If possible, levothyroxine should be taken at the same time each day. Soy formula, iron supplements, calcium carbonate, and sucralfate can bind levothyroxine intraluminally and reduce its absorption. Therefore, these agents should not be taken at the same time as thyroid hormone supplementation. Infants should take levothyroxine as a pill crushed up in a small amount of water or breastmilk. Newly available commercial liquid levothyroxine is an acceptable alternative, but liquid levothyroxine made by compounding pharmacies should not be used. Drugs including phenytoin, rifampin, and carbamazepine can increase the metabolism of levothyroxine.

Congenital Hypothyroidism

Congenital hypothyroidism (CH) is a common and preventable cause of intellectual disability. Since its inclusion in the newborn screen, the prevalence of CH has risen from 1 in 4000 to 1 in 2500 [1] and is thought to be due to the identification of milder forms of hypothyroidism. The most common causes of CH are thyroid dysgenesis or agenesis resulting from abnormalities in thyroid gland development. Additional, rarer causes of CH are due to thyroid dyshormonogenesis, or a pituitary or hypothalamic abnormality causing central hypothyroidism. Dyshormonogenesis results from inherited defects in one of the multiple steps required to synthesize thyroid hormone in the thyroid gland, including defects in iodine trapping, organification of iodine, and thyroglobulin synthesis. Dyshormonogenesis may present with goiter, is thought to result in 10–15% of congenital hypothyroidism, and is generally inherited in an autosomal recessive manner. Patients with dyshormonogenesis as the etiology of their congenital hypothyroidism are treated with levothyroxine, and identification of the underlying genetic defect

J. M. Barker (✉)
Pediatric Endocrinology, University of Colorado School of Medicine, Aurora, CO, USA
e-mail: Jennifer.barker@childrenscolorado.org

T. M. Triolo
Barbara Davis Center for Diabetes, University of Colorado School of Medicine, Aurora, CO, USA
e-mail: Taylor.triolo@cuanschutz.edu

T. Stanley, M. Misra (eds.), *Endocrine Conditions in Pediatrics*, https://doi.org/10.1007/978-3-030-52215-5_41

Table 41.1 Causes of hypothyroidism

Causes of hypothyroidism	Lab findings	Distinguishing physical examination findings	Treatment	Populations to consider screening
Congenital hypothyroidism	T4 ↓ TSH ↑		Levothyroxine 10–15 μg/kg/day	All newborns
Acquired hypothyroidism	T4 ↓ TSH ↑ TPO and Tg antibodies ↑/↔	Declining growth velocity Goiter Delayed reflexes Dry skin	Levothyroxine 2–6 μg/kg/day	Evaluation of inadequate linear growth Children with additional autoimmune disease
Central hypothyroidism	T4 ↓ TSH ↓/↔	Central abnormalities (cleft lip/palate) Jaundice Micropenis	Levothyroxine 1.6 μg/kg/day	Infants with midline abnormalities (cleft lip/palate) Infants with concern for central abnormalities (absent septum pellucidum) Children with acquired central injuries/tumors
Subclinical hypothyroidism	T4 ↔ TSH ↑ TPO and Tg antibodies ↔/↑	Goiter Fatigue Usually normal exam	None	

Cause of hypothyroidism in the pediatric population. Characteristic lab findings, physical exam findings, treatment, if necessary, and populations to consider screening

Abbreviations: *T4* thyroxine, *TSH* thyroid-stimulating hormone, *TPO* thyroid peroxidase, *Tg* thyroglobulin

does not change this management. Congenital hypothyroidism may be transient due to maternal influences, including passage of maternal medications, transplacental passage of maternal blocking antibodies, or maternal iodine deficiency or excess. Thyroid hormone resistance may also be identified on newborn screens with an elevation in both T4 and TSH.

In early gestation, the fetus is dependent on the maternal thyroid hormone. The fetal hypothalamic–pituitary–thyroid axis develops in the first trimester, begins to produce thyroid hormone around mid-gestation, and is mature at term delivery. At delivery, there is a temperature-stimulated surge of TRH and TSH that results in an increase in T4 secretion. TSH levels peak to a mean concentration of 70 μU/mL at 30 minutes after birth. This is typically short-lived, and TSH levels return to normal infant levels by 3–5 days. Infants with CH appear normal at birth, as the fetus appears to be protected by maternal thyroid hormone. Normal neurocognitive outcomes can be achieved if CH is detected early and adequate postnatal therapy is initiated. However, when both maternal and fetal hypothyroidism is present, there is a risk for significant impairment in neuro-intellectual development [2].

CH is screened on state newborn screens and is typically carried out on dried blood samples. Screening programs vary by location and include primary TSH, primary T4, or combined T4, TSH screen. A primary TSH screen tests a TSH on all samples. A primary T4 screen tests T4 on all samples and a TSH on samples with T4 below set cut-offs. A primary screen with TSH will identify infants with primary hypothyroidism but may miss infants with central hypothyroidism because central hypothyroidism presents with low T4 and inappropriately normal TSH. Practitioners should familiarize themselves with their local screening methods.

Typically, CH is clinically silent in neonates, but it is easily treated if detected. Additionally, early treatment is required to prevent intellectual disability associated with CH, prior to the onset of symptoms. Therefore, relying on symptoms to identify infants misses a critical window for the prevention of intellectual disability, and screening for CH is recommended for all newborns. Screening should be obtained after 24 hours of life to avoid identifying infants with an exaggerated or prolonged physiologic TSH surge. Abnormal screening should be confirmed by a formal measurement of serum TSH and T4 in a clinical laboratory. Factors such as prematurity and severe illness can delay the elevation of TSH. If there is clinical concern for hypothyroidism, serum tests should be checked, even if the newborn screen is normal. Radiographic studies such as ultrasound or radionuclide scintigraphy can be performed to characterize the subtype of congenital hypothyroidism (agenesis or dyshormonogenesis), but do not change the management of treatment with levothyroxine.

Levothyroxine is the ideal therapy for CH [3]. The medication is well tolerated, and generic forms are typically equivalent to more expensive brand preparations [4]. Initial dosing is typically 10–15 μg/kg/day in CH. The goal is to normalize thyroid status as soon as possible. Thyroid tests should be measured 2–4 weeks after treatment has started. In CH, thyroid tests should be checked every 1–2 months in the first 6 months of life and then every 3–4 months in the first 3 years. In some cases, at 3 years of age, a trial off levothyroxine can be attempted to assess if the cause of CH was transient. This can be considered if the patient does not need an increased dosage of levothyroxine as they grow. Once a child is over 3 years, thyroid levels should be monitored every 3–6 months to see if a dose adjustment is required as the child grows. Thyroid levels should be measured 4–6 weeks after a dose adjustment.

Autoimmune Hypothyroidism

Autoimmune thyroiditis (Hashimoto's thyroiditis) is the most common cause of childhood thyroid disease. It is associated with antibodies against thyroglobulin and thyroperoxidase (TPO) and results in lymphocytic infiltration of the thyroid parenchyma. In many, but not all, cases there will be resulting thyromegaly. Destruction of the follicular thyroid cells results in hypothyroidism. The degree of hypothyroidism depends on the amount of functional thyroid tissue present and can vary from severe hypothyroidism with no functional thyroid tissue to subclinical hypothyroidism (normal T4 with mildly elevated TSH). Patients are identified based on symptoms of hypothyroidism, decreased linear growth velocity, appreciation of goiter on physical examination, or screening of patients at increased risk for thyroid disease. Laboratory assessment of TSH and T4 levels is adequate to diagnose hypothyroidism.

Anti-TPO antibodies are a more sensitive marker of thyroid autoimmunity than antithyroglobulin antibodies and can be added to the laboratory evaluation if there is suspicion for hypothyroidism, but measurement of anti-TPO antibodies is not necessary for the diagnosis of hypothyroidism. In children, the incidence of anti-TPO antibodies is not well defined. In children with anti-TPO antibodies, about 20% will go on to require treatment for hypothyroidism [5]. Typically, these children will have very elevated antibody titers. If a child is found to have positive thyroid-related antibodies with normal thyroid function testing, it is reasonable to monitor TSH and T4 every 6–12 months or with symptoms of thyroid disease. Measurement of anti-TPO antibodies can be useful in patients with subclinical hypothyroidism, as they may identify patients with a higher likelihood of progressing to overt hypothyroidism.

The prevalence of autoimmune hypothyroidism increases with age and has a female predominance [5]. Presentation in infancy is rare but can occur [6]. There is a strong familial component. Children with Klinefelter, Turner, and Down syndromes are at an increased risk for autoimmune thyroid disease [7]. Children with autoimmune diseases, such as type 1 diabetes, celiac disease, and Addison disease, are at risk of also developing autoimmune hypothyroidism. Guidelines recommend periodic screening for thyroid dysfunction in children with type 1 diabetes [8].

As with congenital hypothyroidism, treatment is with levothyroxine, and dose varies by age. If profound hypothyroidism is present, children are at risk for pseudotumor cerebri with the initiation of treatment [9]. Therefore, in profound hypothyroidism, treatment doses can start at one-third to one-half of the typical dose and increased to the full dose over time. It is recommended that levothyroxine be administered at a consistent time in the day. Patients and their families should be advised that if they miss a dose of levothyroxine, they can "double-up" on their dose the next day. Studies have shown that taking the medication at bedtime is associated with higher T4 levels and lower TSH levels over the course of the day [10].

Subclinical Hypothyroidism

Subclinical hypothyroidism, also known as compensated hypothyroidism, describes normal circulating T4 and T3 levels with mild elevations of TSH (usually less than 10 μU/mL). This can result if adult reference ranges are applied to pediatric samples as patients may be falsely identified as having subclinical hypothyroidism [11]. Individuals with obesity can have slightly elevated TSH levels without decreased T4 levels [12]. TSH elevations can normalize with weight loss [13]. Slight elevations in TSH in children with obesity are physiologic and do not warrant therapy. Studies in children with mild TSH elevations (5–10 μU/mL) show that only a small fraction will progress to continued elevations above 10 μU/mL [14]. Children with TSH values 5–10 μU/mL do not exhibit benefits from treatment with levothyroxine [15]. Measurement of thyroid autoantibodies can be very useful in this population because the presence of thyroid autoimmunity and subclinical hypothyroidism can identify people more likely to progress to overt hypothyroidism.

Clinical Key:
Children with obesity may have slightly elevated TSH levels with normal T4 or free T4. This is physiologic and does not require treatment.

Central Hypothyroidism

Central hypothyroidism is the result of a decrease in the production of TSH or thyrotropin-releasing hormone (TRH). In central causes of hypothyroidism, there is a low serum T4 with a low or "inappropriately normal" TSH. This may be considered on the newborn screen if the T4 is low but the TSH is not elevated. It may also be missed in primary TSH newborn screens. While central hypothyroidism is rare, it can often be associated with additional hypothalamic, pituitary hormone deficiencies. In infants with central abnormalities such as cleft lip or palate, absent septum pellucidum or optic nerve hypoplasia, central endocrinopathies should be considered. Additionally, infants with poor growth, cholestasis, or hypoglycemia should also be evaluated for hypothalamic/pituitary hormone deficiencies. Frequently, infants who will eventually develop central hypothyroidism may initially have normal T4 and TSH at birth. Therefore, infants and children with concerns for central pituitary deficiencies should be screened over time. Nonthyroidal illness, prematurity, and differences in thyroid-binding globulin may manifest with a similar laboratory pattern. Thus, careful consideration of the clinical context is required to differentiate the cause of these laboratory test abnormalities.

Central hypothyroidism can also result from a traumatic brain injury, development, or treatment of brain tumors, meningitis, irradiation of the central nervous system, or other central malformations. Chemotherapeutic agents such as retinoid X receptor-selective ligands used in the treatment of lymphoma can also result in central hypothyroidism [16]. Children with a history of a central injury or malformation should be monitored for the development of central hypothyroidism.

Treatment includes replacement with levothyroxine. Children may need lower doses than primary hypothyroidism [17]. TSH levels are not helpful in guiding treatment and therefore free T4 should be monitored to adjust levothyroxine levels. A dose of 1.6 μg/kg/day is recommended to maintain the free T4 level in the upper half of the reference range [18]. Patients should be screened for central adrenal insufficiency before starting levothyroxine treatment for central hypothyroidism, as treatment of central hypothyroidism in the setting of adrenal insufficiency may precipitate an adrenal crisis.

References

1. Deladoey J, Ruel J, Giguere Y, Van Vliet G. Is the incidence of congenital hypothyroidism really increasing? A 20-year retrospective population-based study in Quebec. J Clin Endocrinol Metab. 2011;96(8):2422–9.
2. Haddow JE, Palomaki GE, Allan WC, Williams JR, Knight GJ, Gagnon J, et al. Maternal thyroid deficiency during pregnancy and subsequent neuropsychological development of the child. N Engl J Med. 1999;341(8):549–55.
3. Jonklaas J, Bianco AC, Bauer AJ, Burman KD, Cappola AR, Celi FS, et al. Guidelines for the treatment of hypothyroidism: prepared by the American Thyroid Association task force on thyroid hormone replacement. Thyroid. 2014;24(12):1670–751.
4. Bolton S. Bioequivalence studies for levothyroxine. AAPS J. 2005;7(1):E47–53.
5. Radetti G, Maselli M, Buzi F, Corrias A, Mussa A, Cambiaso P, et al. The natural history of the normal/mild elevated TSH serum levels in children and adolescents with Hashimoto's thyroiditis and isolated hyperthyrotropinaemia: a 3-year follow-up. Clin Endocrinol. 2012;76(3):394–8.
6. Foley TP Jr, Abbassi V, Copeland KC, Draznin MB. Brief report: hypothyroidism caused by chronic autoimmune thyroiditis in very young infants. N Engl J Med. 1994;330(7):466–8.
7. Hanna CE, LaFranchi SH. Adolescent thyroid disorders. Adolesc Med. 2002;13(1):13–35, v.
8. American Diabetes Association. 13. Children and adolescents: standards of medical care in diabetes-2019. Diabetes Care. 2019;42(Suppl 1):S148–S64.
9. Van Dop C, Conte FA, Koch TK, Clark SJ, Wilson-Davis SL, Grumbach MM. Pseudotumor cerebri associated with initiation of levothyroxine therapy for juvenile hypothyroidism. N Engl J Med. 1983;308(18):1076–80.
10. Bolk N, Visser TJ, Nijman J, Jongste IJ, Tijssen JG, Berghout A. Effects of evening vs morning levothyroxine intake: a randomized double-blind crossover trial. Arch Intern Med. 2010;170(22):1996–2003.
11. Lazar L, Frumkin RB, Battat E, Lebenthal Y, Phillip M, Meyerovitch J. Natural history of thyroid function tests over 5 years in a large pediatric cohort. J Clin Endocrinol Metab. 2009;94(5):1678–82.
12. Reinehr T. Thyroid function in the nutritionally obese child and adolescent. Curr Opin Pediatr. 2011;23(4):415–20.
13. Reinehr T, Isa A, de Sousa G, Dieffenbach R, Andler W. Thyroid hormones and their relation to weight status. Horm Res. 2008;70(1):51–7.
14. Rapa A, Monzani A, Moia S, Vivenza D, Bellone S, Petri A, et al. Subclinical hypothyroidism in children and adolescents: a wide range of clinical, biochemical, and genetic factors involved. J Clin Endocrinol Metab. 2009;94(7):2414–20.
15. Wasniewska M, Salerno M, Cassio A, Corrias A, Aversa T, Zirilli G, et al. Prospective evaluation of the natural course of idiopathic subclinical hypothyroidism in childhood and adolescence. Eur J Endocrinol. 2009;160(3):417–21.
16. Sherman SI, Gopal J, Haugen BR, Chiu AC, Whaley K, Nowlakha P, et al. Central hypothyroidism associated with retinoid X receptor-selective ligands. N Engl J Med. 1999;340(14):1075–9.
17. Carrozza V, Csako G, Yanovski JA, Skarulis MC, Nieman L, Wesley R, et al. Levothyroxine replacement therapy in central hypothyroidism: a practice report. Pharmacotherapy. 1999;19(3):349–55.
18. Slawik M, Klawitter B, Meiser E, Schories M, Zwermann O, Borm K, et al. Thyroid hormone replacement for central hypothyroidism: a randomized controlled trial comparing two doses of thyroxine (T4) with a combination of T4 and triiodothyronine. J Clin Endocrinol Metab. 2007;92(11):4115–22.

42 Overview and Initial Management: Hyperthyroidism

Christine E. Cherella

The terms "hyperthyroidism" and "thyrotoxicosis" are sometimes used interchangeably to describe conditions that lead to signs and symptoms of thyroid hormone excess. Hyperthyroidism is characterized by increased thyroid hormone synthesis and secretion from the thyroid gland. Thyrotoxicosis more generally describes conditions that lead to increased levels of circulating thyroid hormone (irrespective of the source). This section will review the causes of thyrotoxicosis, focusing on the pathophysiology of hyperthyroidism, and will discuss the management of pediatric Graves' disease and neonatal Graves' disease.

Etiology and Pathophysiology

Hyperthyroidism is an uncommon but serious condition in the pediatric population. The most common cause of hyperthyroidism in children and adolescents is Graves' disease (Table 42.1). While relatively rare in children, accounting for 1–5% of all patients with Graves' disease, it accounts for roughly 95% of hyperthyroidism in the pediatric population [1]. Graves' disease may occur at any age during childhood but increases in frequency with age – especially in postpubertal children, where the incidence is higher in girls than boys.

Graves' disease is an autoimmune disorder in which the body produces thyroid-stimulating hormone (TSH) receptor antibodies that mimic the action of TSH by binding directly to the TSH receptor. This leads to increased thyroid gland vascularity, follicular hyperplasia, and excessive production and secretion of thyroid hormone. The TSH-receptor-stimulating antibodies can also lead to the development of Graves' ophthalmopathy secondary to local inflammation, edema, and muscle swelling [2]. The underlying trigger for Graves' remains unclear, but it is thought to result from a combination of genetic, environmental, and immune factors [3]. Graves' disease is more common in children with other autoimmune conditions and/or family history of autoimmune diseases.

In newborns, the most common cause of hyperthyroidism is neonatal Graves' disease. This condition occurs when maternal TSH-receptor-stimulating antibodies cross the placenta and stimulate the TSH receptors of the neonate, leading

Table 42.1 Causes of thyrotoxicosis

Etiology	Mechanism
Thyrotoxicosis with hyperthyroidism (increased thyroid hormone production)	
Graves' disease	TSH-receptor stimulating antibodies
Neonatal Graves' disease	Maternal TSH-receptor-stimulating antibodies
Functioning adenoma/toxic multinodular goiter	Focus of functional autonomy
McCune–Albright syndrome	*GNAS* gene mutation
TSH-receptor-activating mutation	Activating mutation in TSHR
TSH-secreting pituitary adenoma	Pituitary adenoma
Thyrotoxicosis without hyperthyroidism (release of preformed thyroid hormone)	
Chronic lymphocytic thyroiditis ("Hashitoxicosis")	Thyrotoxic phase of autoimmune process
DeQuervain's thyroiditis (subacute)	Viral
Infectious (acute or chronic)	Bacterial or fungal
Silent thyroiditis	Painless
Drug effects	Drug-induced thyroiditis (amiodarone, lithium, iodine, interferon)
Mechanical insult	Follicle damage from manipulation
Extrathyroidal exposure	Excess exogenous thyroid hormone

Abbreviations: *TSH* thyroid-stimulating hormone, *TSHR* thyroid-stimulating hormone receptor

C. E. Cherella (✉)
Division of Endocrinology, Department of Pediatrics, Boston Children's Hospital, Boston, MA, USA
e-mail: Christine.Cherella@childrens.harvard.edu

T. Stanley, M. Misra (eds.), *Endocrine Conditions in Pediatrics*, https://doi.org/10.1007/978-3-030-52215-5_42

to transient neonatal hyperthyroidism. It affects approximately 2% of infants whose mothers have Graves' disease during pregnancy (about 0.2% of all pregnancies), and although antibodies are most prevalent in mothers with active Graves' disease treated with an antithyroid drug, they can also be present in mothers who have been treated for Graves' disease in the past with definitive therapy (i.e., surgery or radioactive iodine) [4]. It is therefore immensely important to obtain a thorough maternal medical history to clarify the underlying etiology of any possible thyroid disease prior to and during pregnancy.

Additional causes of hyperthyroidism include an autonomously functioning thyroid nodule ("hot" nodule) or multiple nodules (i.e., toxic multinodular goiter); while these etiologies are more common in the adult population, they are occasionally detected by a physical examination in children as well [5]. Less-common etiologies include McCune–Albright syndrome, which is caused by a somatic mutation of the *GNAS* gene and leads to constitutive activation of affected G-protein coupled receptors. Clinically, it is characterized by a classic triad of café-au-lait macules (with irregular boarders often compared to the "coast of Maine"), skeletal findings secondary to fibrous dysplasia, and peripheral precocious puberty (present in about 85% of cases). Not all elements of the triad may be present, however, and other endocrinopathies can occur, of which hyperthyroidism is the second most common after precocious puberty [6]. Rarely, isolated activating mutations in the TSH receptor gene can lead to familial non-autoimmune hyperthyroidism. Causes of hyperthyroidism associated with elevated TSH levels (i.e., from a brain tumor in pituitary gland making too much TSH, or pituitary resistance to thyroid hormone) are incredibly rare in the pediatric population.

Transient thyrotoxicosis (without hyperthyroidism) may result from the inflammation and subsequent destruction of thyroid follicular cells, perhaps secondary to an autoimmune process, infection, or medication, and leads to excess thyroid hormone leaking into the bloodstream. These symptoms usually resolve in about 2 months, as this is the approximate amount of thyroid hormone reserve that is maintained in the thyroid gland, though the hyperthyroid phase can be of variable duration in children [7]. Ingestion of exogenous thyroid hormone may also result in transient thyrotoxicosis, so it is important to obtain a history of possible exposure to prescription medication or thyroid supplements.

Diagnosis

The clinical signs and symptoms of thyrotoxicosis include stare/lid retraction and lid lag secondary to sympathetic hyperactivity, warm/moist skin, tachycardia, and widened pulse pressures with hyperdynamic precordium, tremor, and hyperreflexia. Children can present with growth changes and weight loss, although it is important to note that many have increased appetite which can cause unchanged or even increased weight [8]. Patients with Graves' disease may present with exophthalmos secondary to antibody stimulation causing inflammation, edema, and muscle swelling behind the eye.

Close examination of the thyroid gland may help in differentiating causes of thyrotoxicosis. In Graves' disease, the thyroid tends to be enlarged (minimally to maximally) and smooth with a spongy texture, and a bruit may be audible over the gland. Patients with a toxic nodule or multinodular goiter will present with palpable nodules. Patients with thyroiditis may have no to modest thyroid gland enlargement and, depending on the etiology, may or may not have pain with palpation.

In cases of primary hyperthyroidism, serum TSH levels are low or suppressed as a result of negative feedback of thyroid hormone levels on the anterior pituitary. Concurrent elevated serum-free T4 and/or total T3 levels help determine the degree of biochemical hyperthyroidism. Overt hyperthyroidism is characterized by low TSH concentrations with raised thyroid hormone concentrations (T4, T3, or both), whereas subclinical hyperthyroidism is characterized by low serum TSH with normal thyroid hormone levels. The ratio of total T3 to total T4 can also help determine the etiology, as a hyperactive thyroid gland produces more T3 than T4, whereas T4 is elevated more than T3 in thyrotoxicosis caused by thyroiditis [9].

Antibody studies further help clarify the underlying etiology of the hyperthyroidism (Table 42.2). TSH receptor antibodies (TRAbs) can be measured by competition assays or bioassays and are important in the diagnosis of Graves' disease. TRAbs measured by competition assay, also known as TSH-biding inhibitory immunoglobulin (or TBII) assays, detect all autoantibodies that compete for the TSH receptor (blocking and stimulating). Bioassays for thyroid-stimulating immunoglobulins (TSI) measure antibody activity that stimulates the TSH receptor. Newer antibody assays (both TBII and TSI) have very good sensitivity and specificity for Graves' disease [10]. Other thyroid autoantibodies, including thyroid peroxidase antibody or thyroglobulin antibody, can help in the diagnosis of autoimmune thyroiditis, though they may also be present in up to 10% of patients with Graves' disease [3].

Additional lab findings that may be present in a thyrotoxic state include abnormal cholesterol levels (low total, LDL, HDL); anemia and leukopenia; high alkaline phosphatase (suggesting increased bone turnover); mild elevation in liver function tests; and elevated glucose.

Importantly, some lab patterns may appear initially concerning for thyrotoxicosis, but are not secondary to hyperthyroidism (see also Chap. 25). These include binding protein abnormalities (i.e., in pregnancy or inherited forms like thyroxine-binding globulin (TBG) deficiency), or

Table 42.2 Diagnosis of hyperthyroidism

Diagnosis	Specific labs	TSH	Free T4	RAI/Tc99 uptake	Physical exam findings
Thyrotoxicosis with hyperthyroidism (increased thyroid hormone production)					
Graves' disease or neonatal Graves' disease	+TRAb (TBII/TSI)	↓	↑	Uniform ↑	Diffusely enlarged gland +/− eye findings
Functioning adenoma/toxic multinodular goiter		↓	↑	Focal or multifocal ↑	Palpable nodule(s)
McCune–Albright syndrome		↓	↑	↑	Variable thyroid; café au lait macules, fibrous dysplasia
TSH-receptor-activating mutation		↓	↑	↑	Normal thyroid or mildly enlarged
TSH-secreting pituitary adenoma		↑ or normal	↑	↑	Normal thyroid
Thyrotoxicosis without hyperthyroidism (release of preformed thyroid hormone)					
Autoimmune/chronic lymphocytic thyroiditis "Hashitoxicosis"	+TPO and/or thyroglobulin antibody	↓	↑	↓	Firm goiter
DeQuervain's thyroiditis (subacute) or infectious (acute or chronic)		↓	↑	↓	Painful to palpation
Silent thyroiditis	Occasional +TPO antibody	↓	↑	↓	Painless
Drug effects or mechanical insult		↓	↑	↓	Normal thyroid
Extrathyroidal exposure	Low thyroglobulin	↓	↑	↓	Normal thyroid

Abbreviations: *RAI* radioactive iodine, *Tc99* technetium, *TBII* TSH binding inhibitory immunoglobulin, *TPO* thyroid peroxidase, *TRAb* TSH receptor antibody, *TSI* thyroid-stimulating immunoglobulins

laboratory assay interference from heterophile antibodies or medications (most notably high-dose biotin, which is found in hair, skin, and nail supplements). TSH levels can also be low in the setting of critical illness (i.e., non-thyroidal illness or sick euthyroid) from a compensatory decrease in the hypothalamic–pituitary–thyroid axis, with concurrent normal or low thyroid hormone levels. It is vital to recognize the underlying clinical context in these scenarios, and if there is ever any question of the underlying etiology behind an abnormal lab pattern, discussion and review with a pediatric endocrinologist is appropriate.

If there remains any doubt about the causes of thyrotoxicosis, the use of thyroid scintigraphy may be helpful (see Chap. 38). Increased uptake in the setting of a suppressed TSH suggests increased thyroid hormone production. Additional isotope imaging is useful to differentiate between diffuse uptake as seen in Graves' disease versus focal uptake in the setting of one (or multiple) toxic adenomas. Low uptake is typically consistent with thyroiditis, as the thyrotoxicosis is secondary to the passive release of preformed thyroid hormone.

Initial Management of Hyperthyroidism

The initial approach to treating a child with hyperthyroidism consists of symptom control and measures aimed at decreasing thyroid hormone synthesis.

Symptom Control

Many of the systemic clinical features of hyperthyroidism (including tachycardia, hypertension, palpitations, and tremor) are secondary to the beta-adrenergic effects of catecholamines [11]. Accordingly, beta-blockers are effective in managing the symptoms present in a hyperthyroid state (including tachycardia and hypertension), especially because antithyroid medications may take several weeks to normalize thyroid hormone values. Assuming there are no contraindications to its use, a beta-blocker should be started in patients with thyrotoxicosis and symptoms of adrenergic overactivity as soon as the diagnosis is made. Atenolol can be administered once daily, and given its cardioselectivity, it is preferred in children with reactive airway disease; typical dosing ranges from 0.5 to 2 mg/kg/day. Propranolol can also be considered, as it has the potential benefit of decreasing T4 to T3 conversion; typical dosing ranges from 0.5 to 2 mg/kg/day divided three or four times daily.

Clinical Key:
For patients with newly diagnosed thyrotoxicosis who have hypertension and/or tachycardia, treatment with a beta-blocker can be initiated in the primary care setting and does not interfere with further diagnostic testing.

Decrease Thyroid Hormone Synthesis

For patients diagnosed with Graves' disease, there are three treatment options: medical therapy (i.e., antithyroid drugs or thionamides), radioactive iodine therapy, or surgery. All three options present distinct advantages and disadvantages, and the optimal approach depends on patient preference and clinical factors. However, most endocrinologists prefer a trial of antithyroid drugs as first-line therapy in pediatric patients.

Medical Therapy with Antithyroid Drugs

Thionamides inhibit thyroid peroxidase (TPO) oxidization of iodide (I-) to iodine (I2). In the United States and Canada, only methimazole (MMI, or Tapazole) is approved for the treatment of children and adolescents, as there is a black box warning for propylthiouracil (PTU) due to reports of fulminant hepatic necrosis and liver failure [12]. Starting doses of methimazole, depending on the level of severity of the hyperthyroidism, range from 0.25 to 1.0 mg/kg/day (maximal dose typically does not exceed 40 mg/day). It is available as 5 and 10 mg tablets. While administered doses are sometimes divided twice daily, there is improved compliance with daily dosing in adults [10]. Thyroid function tests should be followed closely (i.e., every 4 weeks at first), as dose reductions are often required as thyroid hormone values normalize to maintain a euthyroid state – though, importantly, TSH normalization may lag behind the normalization of circulating thyroid hormone by weeks/months [13].

Prior to initiation of antithyroid drug therapy, all adverse effects should be discussed at length with patients and their families and documented in the medical record. Minor side effects of methimazole include skin reactions (i.e., urticarial/macular rashes), arthralgias, and gastrointestinal complaints including reflux and nausea. These typically begin within the first few weeks of starting therapy and are usually dose-related. Mild rashes may resolve with continued therapy or with antihistamines but can be severe enough to require drug discontinuation.

Major side effects are rare but can be significant [14]. Agranulocytosis (i.e., absolute neutrophil count of <500/mm^3) can occur in 0.1–0.5% of patients, is dose-related to MMI, and, while it tends to present within the first 90 days of treatment, can reoccur upon re-exposure. A typical clinical presentation is fever with severe pharyngitis. All patients should be advised to seek medical attention if these symptoms develop and to have a complete blood count with differential checked in the setting of a fever. Hepatotoxicity, while more common with PTU (causing hepatocellular injury including fulminant hepatic failure), can also be seen with patients on MMI (more often cholestatic in nature). The overall frequency of hepatic dysfunction ranges from 0.1% to 0.2%, and usually occurs within the first few days to months of drug initiation with transaminase levels rising to over five times the normal limits. Importantly, as both leukopenia and transaminitis can be manifestations of Graves' disease, clinicians often obtain baseline white blood cell counts with an absolute neutrophil count, and liver function tests prior to starting therapy; however, monitoring labs throughout the disease process is more controversial. An ANCA vasculitis presenting as polyarthritis, renal dysfunction, and/or vasculitic rash can also be seen with medical treatment, more frequently after months to years of therapy, and again more commonly with PTU than MMI. Prompt drug discontinuation is of utmost importance if a patient presents with any major side effect, followed by a discussion with a pediatric endocrinologist about other treatment options. Lastly, adolescent females should be counseled about the risks of birth defects reported with antithyroid drug use during the first trimester of pregnancy, which include cutis aplasia, congenital heart defects, and omphalocele [15].

Newborns presenting with significant biochemical hyperthyroidism and/or clinical symptoms of neonatal Graves' disease may similarly require treatment with methimazole and/or beta-blockade to avoid complications. Potassium iodide therapy may also be used in conjunction with MMI in severe or refractory neonatal Graves'. Complications of neonatal Graves' include cardiac failure more acutely, and craniosynostosis and intellectual impairment in the long term. Because this is a transient process that usually resolves 1–3 months after birth, very close follow-up with a pediatric endocrinologist is encouraged. Typical starting doses of methimazole are 0.2–0.5 mg/kg/day divided twice daily, estimating 0.625 mg twice daily (0.4 mg/kg/day for a 3 kg newborn) [16]. Notably, transient hypothyroidism may also occur from prolonged TSH suppression, and in some situations, infants may require a short course of levothyroxine supplementation until TSH concentrations normalize.

Clinical Key:
Monitoring asymptomatic neonates in the context of maternal Graves'

- Most infants of mothers with Graves' disease will not have neonatal hyperthyroidism; however, neonates born to mothers with positive or unknown maternal TRAb levels in the second or third trimester should be considered high risk.
- Newborn screen should be sent as usual. For high-risk neonates, TRAb levels should be sent as soon as possible after birth if assay is available. Additionally, TSH and free T4 should be sent to a clinical laboratory between 3 and 5 days of life.
- In infants who remain asymptomatic, it is generally recommended to check TSH and free T4 once more at approximately 2 weeks of life.
- Because of waning antibody titers, infants of mothers with Graves' who do not present within the first few weeks of life are not likely to subsequently develop neonatal Graves'. Nonetheless, infants who develop possible signs or symptoms of hyperthyroidism at any point during the first 3–6 months of life should have TSH and free T4 checked urgently.

Thyroid Storm

Thyroid storm is a life-threatening condition and serious complication of hyperthyroidism that may be precipitated by an acute event. It is exceedingly rare in the pediatric population but is critical to recognize. The diagnosis is based on biochemical evidence of hyperthyroidism with severe symptoms including fevers, altered mental status, cardiovascular dysfunction, and gastrointestinal manifestations [17]. If there is ever any clinical suspicion for thyroid storm, immediate referral to an emergency room is recommended, as supportive therapy may be required in an intensive care unit.

Chronic Management and Considerations for Referral

After normalization of thyroid hormone levels and stabilization of ATD doses, labs (i.e., TSH and FT4) should be monitored every 3–4 months. Continuing on antithyroid drugs allows for a chance for permanent remission; however, the appropriate length of treatment of ATDs for children with Graves' disease remains a topic of controversy. Pediatric Graves' disease is more persistent than adult disease with remission rates estimated to be only 20–30% after 2 years of treatment [10] and reported relapse rates vary from 3% to 47% based on different studies [3]. Predictors of remission include older age, lower thyroid hormone levels at the time of diagnosis, and more rapid achievement of euthyroid status [18].

While long-term therapy with antithyroid drugs is possible, some patients elect for permanent therapy with either radioactive iodine (RAI) or surgery. The goal of both treatments is to induce hypothyroidism, which is then chronically treated with levothyroxine. RAI therapy has few acute adverse effects, and local radiation safety recommendations should be followed. While there are no long-term concerns about future infertility or congenital anomalies, there remain questions about the risk for secondary malignancy. Historically, these concerns have been based on increased incidence of thyroid neoplasms seen in children after natural disasters; more recently, however, there have been additional questions raised about the increased risk for secondary malignancies after RAI treatment in adults [19]. Surgical therapy is preferred for younger children <5 years of age, in addition to patients with toxic adenomas or multinodular goiters who are thyrotoxic. For patients with Graves' disease, a total or near-total thyroidectomy is recommended, and referral to an experienced pediatric thyroid surgeon is most important to reduce the risk of complications, which include transient or permanent hypoparathyroidism and vocal cord paralysis. Additional discussion about these definitive therapies, and the risks and benefits of each, should take place with a pediatric endocrinologist.

Conclusion

The clinical features of hyperthyroidism are important to recognize in children. The underlying etiology can be further clarified with an astute physical examination and the help of biochemical and antibody testing. Initial management of thyrotoxicosis consists of symptom control with beta-blockers, and for pediatric patients with Graves', medical treatments aimed at decreasing thyroid hormone synthesis. Definitive therapy should be reviewed with families as treatment options, with referral to an experienced pediatric endocrinologist for more in-depth discussions.

References

1. Leger J, Carel JC. Hyperthyroidism in childhood: causes, when and how to treat. J Clin Res Pediatr Endocrinol. 2013;5(Suppl 1):50–6.
2. Gogakos AI, Boboridis K, Krassas GE. Pediatric aspects in Graves' orbitopathy. Pediatr Endocrinol Rev. 2010;7(Suppl 2):234–44.
3. Srinivasan S, Misra M. Hyperthyroidism in children. Pediatr Rev. 2015;36(6):239–48.
4. Leger J. Management of fetal and neonatal Graves' disease. Horm Res Paediatr. 2017;87(1):1–6.
5. Ly S, Frates MC, Benson CB, Peters HE, Grant FD, Drubach LA, et al. Features and outcome of autonomous thyroid nodules in children: 31 consecutive patients seen at a single center. J Clin Endocrinol Metab. 2016;101(10):3856–62.
6. Brillante B, Guthrie L, Van Ryzin C. McCune-Albright Syndrome: an overview of clinical features. J Pediatr Nurs. 2015;30(5):815–7.
7. Nabhan ZM, Kreher NC, Eugster EA. Hashitoxicosis in children: clinical features and natural history. J Pediatr. 2005;146(4):533–6.
8. Nordyke RA, Gilbert FI Jr, Harada AS. Graves' disease. Influence of age on clinical findings. Arch Intern Med. 1988;148(3):626–31.
9. Carle A, Knudsen N, Pedersen IB, Perrild H, Ovesen L, Rasmussen LB, et al. Determinants of serum T4 and T3 at the time of diagnosis in nosological types of thyrotoxicosis: a population-based study. Eur J Endocrinol. 2013;169(5):537–45.
10. Ross DS, Burch HB, Cooper DS, Greenlee MC, Laurberg P, Maia AL, et al. 2016 American Thyroid Association guidelines for diagnosis and management of hyperthyroidism and other causes of thyrotoxicosis. Thyroid. 2016;26(10):1343–421.
11. Geffner DL, Hershman JM. Beta-adrenergic blockade for the treatment of hyperthyroidism. Am J Med. 1992;93(1):61–8.
12. Rivkees SA. 63 years and 715 days to the "boxed warning": unmasking of the propylthiouracil problem. Int J Pediatr Endocrinol. 2010;2010:658267.
13. Chung YJ, Lee BW, Kim JY, Jung JH, Min YK, Lee MS, et al. Continued suppression of serum TSH level may be attributed to TSH receptor antibody activity as well as the severity of thyrotoxicosis and the time to recovery of thyroid hormone in treated euthyroid Graves' patients. Thyroid. 2006;16(12):1251–7.
14. Cooper DS. Antithyroid drugs. N Engl J Med. 2005;352(9):905–17.
15. Yoshihara A, Noh J, Yamaguchi T, Ohye H, Sato S, Sekiya K, et al. Treatment of Graves' disease with antithyroid drugs in the first trimester of pregnancy and the prevalence of congenital malformation. J Clin Endocrinol Metab. 2012;97(7):2396–403.
16. van der Kaay DC, Wasserman JD, Palmert MR. Management of neonates born to mothers with Graves' disease. Pediatrics. 2016;137(4):e20151878.
17. Burch HB, Wartofsky L. Life-threatening thyrotoxicosis. Thyroid storm. Endocrinol Metab Clin N Am. 1993;22(2):263–77.
18. Glaser NS, Styne DM, Organization of Pediatric Endocrinologists of Northern California Collaborative Graves' Disease Study Group. Predicting the likelihood of remission in children with Graves' disease: a prospective, multicenter study. Pediatrics. 2008;121(3):e481–8.
19. Kitahara CM, Berrington de Gonzalez A, Bouville A, Brill AB, Doody MM, Melo DR, et al. Association of radioactive iodine treatment with cancer mortality in patients with hyperthyroidism. JAMA Intern Med. 2019;179(8):1034–42.

43 Precocious Puberty

Jia Zhu

Abbreviations

CNS	Central nervous system
CPP	Central precocious puberty
GnRHa	Gonadotropin-releasing hormone analogs
HPG	Hypothalamic–pituitary–gonadal
PP	Peripheral precocity

Overview

Precocious puberty is the onset of pubertal development at an age 2–2.5 standard deviations earlier than the mean for a population. In traditional clinical practice, this is defined as the development of secondary sexual characteristics prior to age 8 years for girls and 9 years for boys [1]. Based on this statistical definition, the expected prevalence of precocious puberty is approximately 2%. However, the reported prevalence is often higher and varies significantly based on the population studied, which likely reflects the more recent trend toward earlier pubertal timing in developed countries and differences in pubertal timing between racial and ethnic groups [2–13]. Precocious puberty is also more common in girls than boys, but it is unclear if this is due to referral bias or true differences in underlying biology [14]. Among numerous proposed environmental, physiologic, and genetic factors, increased body mass index (BMI) has been consistently associated with earlier pubertal onset in both girls and boys [13, 15].

J. Zhu (✉)
Division of Endocrinology, Department of Medicine, Boston Children's Hospital, Boston, MA, USA
e-mail: Jia.Zhu@childrens.harvard.edu

Etiology

The etiology of precocious puberty can broadly be classified into three categories based on the underlying pathophysiology (Fig. 43.1) [16, 17]. Central precocious puberty (CPP) occurs due to the early activation of the hypothalamic–pituitary–gonadal (HPG) axis with a subsequent normal pattern and timing of pubertal milestones that are congruent with the child's biological sex. Peripheral precocity (PP) is caused by the presence and/or production of sex hormones that occurs independently of the HPG axis and can be congruent or incongruent with the child's biological sex; sources of peripheral sex-steroids include the gonads, adrenal glands, tumors, and exogenous medication exposures. Variants of pubertal development can also initially present as precocious puberty but typically have a benign and/or nonprogressive course; these include conditions of apparent estrogen production (premature thelarche, isolated prepubertal vaginal bleeding) and conditions of apparent androgen production (premature adrenarche, pubic hair of infancy).

Central Precocious Puberty (CPP)

For the diagnosis of CPP, a basal LH level should be in the pubertal range with secondary sexual characteristics that are congruent with the biologic sex (Table 43.1). At the time of presentation, children typically have rapid linear growth acceleration and a bone age on X-ray >2 SD above chronological age. Although the onset of puberty is early in CPP, the subsequent timing and order of pubertal milestones are typically normal [16, 17].

CPP is idiopathic in the majority of cases, and idiopathic CPP is notably more common in girls than boys [18]. In case series, up to 90% of girls with CPP are diagnosed with an idiopathic cause compared to 25–60% of boys [19–22]. In both familial and sporadic cases of idiopathic CPP, rare genetic mutations in genes (*MKRN3*, *DLK1*, *KISS1*, *KISS1R*) that influence pubertal timing have been reported [23–27].

T. Stanley, M. Misra (eds.), *Endocrine Conditions in Pediatrics*, https://doi.org/10.1007/978-3-030-52215-5_43

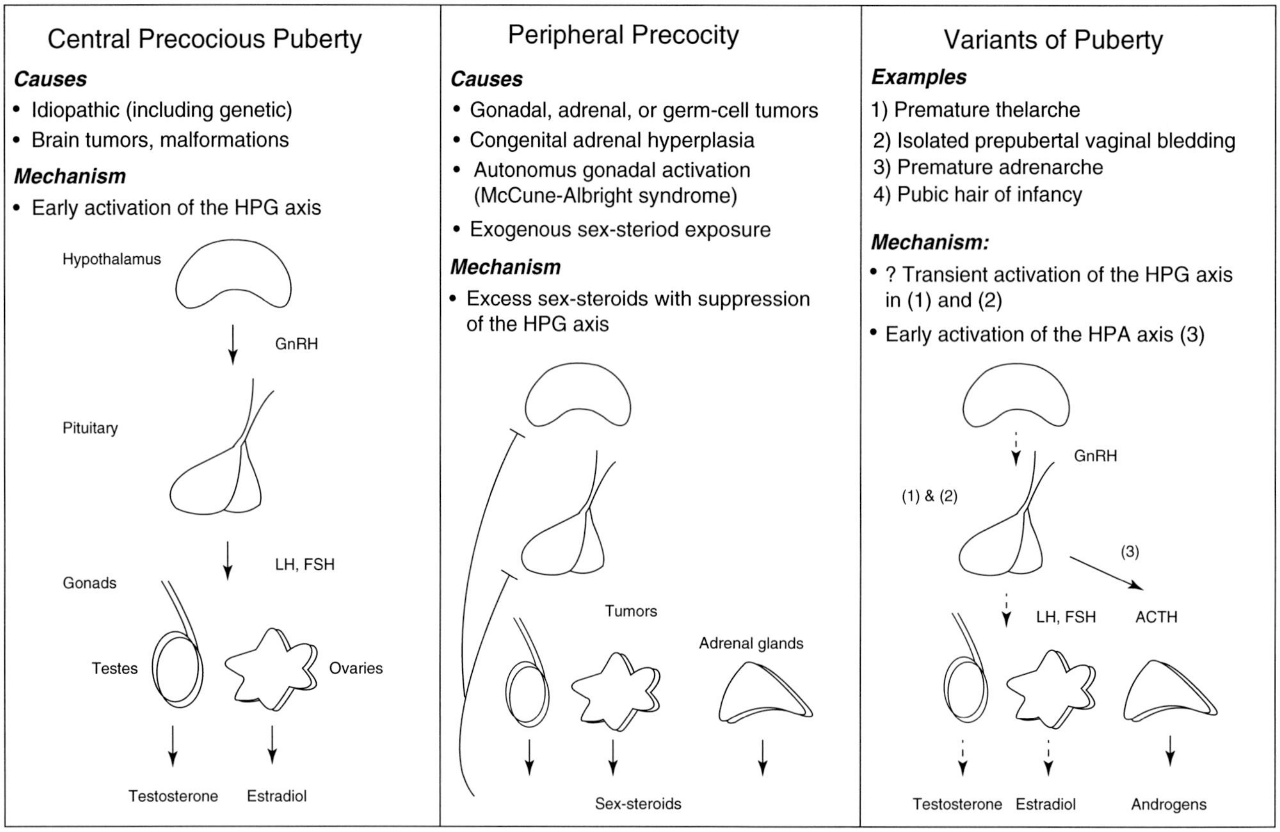

Fig. 43.1 Key pathophysiology

Table 43.1 Items required and supporting diagnosis

	Required for diagnosis	Supporting diagnosis
Central precocious puberty	LH level in pubertal range on AM measurement or GnRH stimulation test Secondary sexual characteristics congruent with biologic sex	Advanced bone age >2 SD above chronological age Rapid linear growth acceleration Subsequent normal sequence and timing of pubertal milestones
Idiopathic	Absence of CNS pathology (diagnosis of exclusion)	Family history of precocious puberty No evidence of significant abnormality on brain MRI
Non-idiopathic	Tumor or malformation on brain MRI or history of CNS injury	Signs/symptoms of increased ICP Additional pituitary hormone deficiencies (i.e., GH, TSH)
Peripheral precocity	Elevated sex steroids with suppression of gonadotropins	Advanced bone age >2 SD above chronological age Rapid linear growth acceleration Secondary sexual characteristics *incongruent* with biological sex Abnormal sequence and timing of pubertal milestones Very high levels of sex steroids
Variants of puberty	Negative evaluation for above etiologies	
Premature adrenarche	Clinical and/or biochemical evidence of adrenal androgen production (i.e., DHEAS) prior to 8 years in girls and 9 years in boys	Overweight Advanced bone age typically within 2 SD of chronological age *Gradual* linear growth acceleration
Other	Transient or nonprogressive	Early/mild physical exam, typically not exceeding Tanner stage 3

Abbreviations: *CNS* central nervous system, *SD* standard deviation, *ICP* intracranial pressure, *GH* growth hormone, *TSH* thyroid-stimulating hormone

As these rare mutations are an uncommon cause of precocious puberty, routine genetic testing is not recommended in the absence of an extensive family history of the condition. Less commonly, CPP can be caused by a congenital or acquired central nervous system (CNS) structural abnormality or injury, such as hypothalamic hamartomas, tumors, trauma, irradiation, and seizures, as well as environmental factors, including international adoption thought to be due to nutritional factors [18]. In cases where a CNS pathology is suspected, a brain MRI should be urgently obtained.

Peripheral Precocity (PP)

For the diagnosis of PP, basal sex-steroid levels should be elevated with suppression of gonadotropins (Table 43.1). Similar to CPP, children at presentation typically have rapid linear growth acceleration and a bone age on X-ray >2 SD above chronological age. However, the order and progression of pubertal milestones are often abnormal depending on the underlying cause [16, 17, 28]. For example, children with McCune–Albright syndrome, a form of autonomous gonadal activation due to somatic activating mutations of the alpha subunit of the Gs protein, can present initially with vaginal bleeding rather than thelarche. Boys with PP from familial male limited precocious puberty (caused by activating mutations of the LH receptor) and children with PP from germ cell tumors (due to hCG secretion and activation of the LH receptor in gonadal tissue) can undergo a rapid pubertal course due to unregulated production of very high levels of sex steroids [28]. Depending on the cause, secondary sexual characteristics can be congruent or incongruent with the child's biological sex. For example, girls with adrenal sources of excess androgens, such as nonclassical congenital adrenal hyperplasia or adrenal tumors, can present with excessive virilization, including hirsutism, voice deepening, and clitoromegaly [17, 28]. Any child with a laboratory pattern suggestive of PP should undergo an urgent multidisciplinary evaluation to identify an etiology, and in particular, assessment for an underlying tumor.

Variants of Pubertal Development

Numerous variants of pubertal development have been described and include premature thelarche and isolated prepubertal vaginal bleeding in girls and premature adrenarche and pubic hair of infancy in both girls and boys. The underlying pathophysiology of these variants is unknown. Transient and/or intermittent activation of the HPG axis has been proposed to play a role in premature thelarche and isolated prepubertal vaginal bleeding, and early activation of the hypothalamic–pituitary–adrenal (HPA) axis leads to premature adrenarche (Fig. 43.1). Children with a variant of pubertal development typically present with only the early stages of puberty, generally not greater than Tanner 3 for breast or pubic hair staging, and the key distinguishing characteristic of these variants is a benign and/or nonprogressive course (Table 43.1) [16, 17]. As the clinical course can only be determined after a period of observation, children who present with the early development of secondary sexual characteristics should undergo a clinical evaluation to assess for other etiologies of precocious puberty.

Premature adrenarche is the most common variant of pubertal development and is characterized by clinical or biochemical evidence of adrenal androgen production (i.e., DHEAS) prior to age 8 years in girls and 9 years in boys [29, 30]. In cases of isolated premature adrenarche, children present with body odor and axillary and pubic hair with no signs of central puberty (i.e., breast development in girls and testicular growth in boys). The condition is frequently associated with childhood obesity, and children with premature adrenarche are typically taller than expected for their mid-parental height. Linear growth is notable for a gradual acceleration often with a mirroring pattern of weight gain, and the bone age is frequently advanced but within 2 SD of the chronological age (Table 43.1).

Urgent or Emergent Considerations and Initial Management

The immediate concern in the evaluation of a child presenting with precocious puberty is an underlying CNS or peripheral tumor. Following diagnosis, initial management should be tailored to assess for the presence of a malignant or benign tumor that could have emergent life-threatening complications while facilitating urgent referral to pediatric endocrinology and other subspecialists as indicated.

Clinical Key:
The "cannot miss" condition in a child presenting with precocious puberty is an underlying CNS or peripheral tumor. In addition to careful history and physical at presentation, close clinical follow-up within 4–6 months is advised to assess for rapid progression of pubertal changes, which raises concern for such pathology and should prompt further testing or endocrine referral.

Central Precocious Puberty

Any child with symptoms of increased intracranial pressure by history or physical examination, such as early morning headaches, nausea, vomiting, seizures, and/or changes in vision, should undergo an urgent brain MRI to assess for CNS pathology. In addition, a brain MRI should be obtained in all asymptomatic boys with CPP and in girls who present with CPP before 6 years of age due to the high rate of intracranial pathology in these groups. In contrast, there is an ongoing debate about the utility of brain MRI in girls who present after 6 years of age without overt symptoms of CNS pathology [31, 32]. Potential consequences of unnecessary brain MRIs include incidental findings that require follow-up, costs to the healthcare system, and patient and family anxiety [31]. In general, a younger age at presentation increases the concern for CNS pathology, whereas the presence of known factors associated with earlier pubertal timing, such as a higher BMI, family history of precocious puberty, or being a member of a racial and/or ethnic group that tends to have earlier pubertal timing, can decrease the level of concern. The decision to obtain a brain MRI in a girl presenting with CPP after 6 years of age should weigh these risk factors with parental preferences and can be made in conjunction with an endocrinologist.

Peripheral Precocity

Peripheral precocity can be categorized into genetic or acquired disorders. Acquired disorders include hormone-secreting tumors, which require urgent workup and referral to a multidisciplinary specialty team to expedite diagnosis and formulation of a treatment plan. Girls with a laboratory pattern suggestive of peripheral precocity should undergo a pelvic ultrasound to assess for the presence of an ovarian tumor or cyst. Boys with evidence of peripheral precocity should undergo an ultrasound of the testes to assess for the presence of a gonadal tumor, such as a Leydig cell tumor. For any child with a history of rapid and progressive virilization and elevated adrenal androgens (i.e., DHEA, DHEAS), an abdominal ultrasound should be obtained as an initial assessment for an adrenal tumor.

Variants of Pubertal Development

An early presentation of an adrenal tumor may initially masquerade as a variant of pubertal development, including pubic hair of infancy and premature adrenarche. Unlike these variants, the virilization associated with adrenal tumors is progressive. Thus, any change in the tempo or degree of virilization in a child previously thought to have a variant of pubertal development should prompt urgent clinical and laboratory reevaluation, and an abdominal ultrasound should be considered to assess for the presence of an adrenal tumor.

Chronic Management and Considerations for Referral

The long-term management of precocious puberty depends on the underlying etiology. All cases of peripheral precocity should be urgently referred to an endocrinologist and appropriate other subspecialists for further workup and treatment of the underlying cause. For central precocious puberty, referral to a pediatric endocrinologist should be considered to discuss treatment to temporarily halt puberty. In children with a suspected variant of pubertal development, the decision to refer to an endocrinologist often depends on the age at presentation and the comfort level of the provider and family.

Central Precocious Puberty

The main goals of treatment for central precocious puberty are to preserve height potential and limit the psychosocial distress that may be associated with early pubertal maturation. Gonadotropin-releasing hormone analogs (GnRHa) are a safe and effective treatment for CPP and can achieve the goals of treatment in select children [31, 33]. Continuous exposure to GnRH (as opposed to physiologic pulsatile secretion) leads to suppression of the gonadotropins and a subsequent decrease in sex-steroid production. The decision to initiate treatment depends on the individual child's age, tempo of pubertal progression, height velocity, estimated adult height from a bone age, and psychosocial adjustment. The greatest benefit in adult height gain has been reported in girls with CPP who are treated prior to 6 years of age [34]. More variable results have been reported in girls who are treated between 6 and 8 years, and there appears to be limited benefit in girls who are treated after 8 years of age. For boys, data are limited, but treatment is considered reasonable for those presenting prior to 9 years of age [31, 33, 34]. The psychosocial consequences of precocious puberty are less clear with conflicting conclusions, and thus, the decision to treat should not be solely based on psychosocial concerns [31, 33].

If GnRHa treatment is initiated, regular pediatric endocrinology follow-up is recommended to monitor for adequate suppression of the HPG axis through clinical and laboratory parameters. The decision on when to discontinue treatment is tailored to the individual patient based on growth, predicted adult height, chronological and bone age, and psychosocial considerations [31, 33].

While referral to a pediatric endocrinologist for all children with CPP should be considered to discuss treatment with a GnRHa, treatment is less likely to be recommended after the age of 8 years in girls with idiopathic CPP [31, 33]. Thus, for girls with a clear diagnosis of idiopathic CPP (i.e., factors associated with earlier pubertal timing, no CNS concerns) who present around 8 years of age, a pediatric endocrinology referral may not be necessary in all cases. However, this depends on the certainty of the diagnosis and the comfort level of the primary provider and the family.

Peripheral Precocity

For cases of PP due to hormone-secreting tumors, the treatment of the underlying tumor results in the rapid decrease of sex hormone levels and regression of secondary sexual characteristics. In some cases, children with a history of PP can develop secondary CPP due to the release of the inhibition of the sex steroids on the prematurely matured HPG axis [35]. Thus, all children with a history of treated PP should undergo regular surveillance by a pediatric endocrinologist to assess for secondary CPP and consideration of GnRHa therapy if indicated.

For genetic causes of PP, the treatment is tailored to the specific etiology and should be instituted and monitored closely by a pediatric endocrinologist. For McCune–Albright syndrome, medical therapy is typically reserved for girls with frequent episodes of vaginal bleeding and advanced bone age with compromised adult height. Treatment options include an aromatase inhibitor (commonly letrozole) or a blocker of estrogen action (i.e., tamoxifen). In boys, the data on treatment outcomes in McCune–Albright syndrome are limited, and combination therapy with an aromatase inhibitor (anastrozole) and an antiandrogen (bicalutamide) has been successful in case reports [28]. In familial male limited precocious puberty, combination therapy with anastrozole and bicalutamide is frequently used [36]. In cases of non-classical congenital adrenal hyperplasia, glucocorticoid replacement therapy may be considered in cases with significant virilization and/or bone age advancement to suppress adrenal androgen production [28].

Variants of Pubertal Development

If the initial evaluation in a child presenting with early-onset secondary sexual characteristics suggests a variant of pubertal development, the mainstay of management is observation to confirm the suspected diagnosis. In premature thelarche, the breast development is not progressive and often regresses with age. Pubic hair of infancy also self-resolves in a period of several months. As discussed previously, children with premature adrenarche typically have a history of gradual growth acceleration with weight gain and mild advancement of bone age without evidence of rapid or advanced virilization.

As variants of pubertal development can only be confirmed in retrospect after a period of clinical observation, there are no guidelines on if and when to refer these suspected cases to pediatric endocrinology. Referral often depends on the comfort level of the provider, as well as risk factors for alternative diagnoses. Indications that should prompt an immediate referral to a pediatric endocrinologist include vaginal bleeding, rapid growth acceleration, advanced bone age >2 SD above chronological age, and significant virilization (clitoromegaly, facial hair, voice deepening), as these features may indicate an alternative diagnosis.

References

1. Boepple P, Crowley WF Jr. Precocious puberty. In: Adashi EY, Rock JA, Rosenwaks Z, editors. Reproductive endocrinology, surgery, and technology, vol. 1. Philadelphia: Lippincott-Raven; 1996. p. 989.
2. Herman-Giddens ME, Slora EJ, Wasserman RC, Bourdony CJ, Bhapkar MV, Koch GG, et al. Secondary sexual characteristics and menses in young girls seen in office practice: a study from the Pediatric Research in Office Settings network. Pediatrics. 1997;99(4):505–12.
3. Liu YX, Wikland KA, Karlberg J. New reference for the age at childhood onset of growth and secular trend in the timing of puberty in Swedish. Acta Paediatr. 2000;89(6):637–43.
4. Sun SS, Schubert CM, Chumlea WC, Roche AF, Kulin HE, Lee PA, et al. National estimates of the timing of sexual maturation and racial differences among US children. Pediatrics. 2002;110(5):911–9.
5. Wu T, Mendola P, Buck GM. Ethnic differences in the presence of secondary sex characteristics and menarche among US girls: the Third National Health and Nutrition Examination Survey, 1988–1994. Pediatrics. 2002;110(4):752–7.
6. Anderson SE, Must A. Interpreting the continued decline in the average age at menarche: results from two nationally representative surveys of U.S. girls studied 10 years apart. J Pediatr. 2005;147(6):753–60.
7. Sorensen K, Aksglaede L, Petersen JH, Juul A. Recent changes in pubertal timing in healthy Danish boys: associations with body mass index. J Clin Endocrinol Metab. 2010;95(1):263–70.
8. Susman EJ, Houts RM, Steinberg L, Belsky J, Cauffman E, Dehart G, et al. Longitudinal development of secondary sexual characteristics in girls and boys between ages 91/2 and 151/2 years. Arch Pediatr Adolesc Med. 2010;164(2):166–73.
9. Goldstein JR. A secular trend toward earlier male sexual maturity: evidence from shifting ages of male young adult mortality. PLoS One. 2011;6(8):e14826.
10. Ma HM, Chen SK, Chen RM, Zhu C, Xiong F, Li T, et al. Pubertal development timing in urban Chinese boys. Int J Androl. 2011;34(5 Pt 2):e435–45.
11. Monteilh C, Kieszak S, Flanders WD, Maisonet M, Rubin C, Holmes AK, et al. Timing of maturation and predictors of Tanner stage transitions in boys enrolled in a contemporary British cohort. Paediatr Perinat Epidemiol. 2011;25(1):75–87.
12. Herman-Giddens ME, Steffes J, Harris D, Slora E, Hussey M, Dowshen SA, et al. Secondary sexual characteristics in boys: data

from the Pediatric Research in Office Settings Network. Pediatrics. 2012;130(5):e1058–68.
13. Biro FM, Greenspan LC, Galvez MP, Pinney SM, Teitelbaum S, Windham GC, et al. Onset of breast development in a longitudinal cohort. Pediatrics. 2013;132(6):1019–27.
14. Kaplowitz P. Clinical characteristics of 104 children referred for evaluation of precocious puberty. J Clin Endocrinol Metab. 2004;89(8):3644–50.
15. Lee JM, Wasserman R, Kaciroti N, Gebremariam A, Steffes J, Dowshen S, et al. Timing of puberty in overweight versus obese boys. Pediatrics. 2016;137(2):e20150164.
16. Harrington J, Palmert MR, Hamilton J. Use of local data to enhance uptake of published recommendations: an example from the diagnostic evaluation of precocious puberty. Arch Dis Child. 2014;99(1):15–20.
17. Eugster EA. Update on precocious puberty in girls. J Pediatr Adolesc Gynecol. 2019;32(5):455–9.
18. Cantas-Orsdemir S, Eugster EA. Update on central precocious puberty: from etiologies to outcomes. Expert Rev Endocrinol Metab. 2019;14(2):123–30.
19. Cisternino M, Arrigo T, Pasquino AM, Tinelli C, Antoniazzi F, Beduschi L, et al. Etiology and age incidence of precocious puberty in girls: a multicentric study. J Pediatr Endocrinol Metab. 2000;13(Suppl 1):695–701.
20. Pedicelli S, Alessio P, Scire G, Cappa M, Cianfarani S. Routine screening by brain magnetic resonance imaging is not indicated in every girl with onset of puberty between the ages of 6 and 8 years. J Clin Endocrinol Metab. 2014;99(12):4455–61.
21. Choi KH, Chung SJ, Kang MJ, Yoon JY, Lee JE, Lee YA, et al. Boys with precocious or early puberty: incidence of pathological brain magnetic resonance imaging findings and factors related to newly developed brain lesions. Ann Pediatr Endocrinol Metab. 2013;18(4):183–90.
22. De Sanctis V, Corrias A, Rizzo V, Bertelloni S, Urso L, Galluzzi F, et al. Etiology of central precocious puberty in males: the results of the Italian Study Group for Physiopathology of Puberty. J Pediatr Endocrinol Metab. 2000;13(Suppl 1):687–93.
23. Abreu AP, Dauber A, Macedo DB, Noel SD, Brito VN, Gill JC, et al. Central precocious puberty caused by mutations in the imprinted gene MKRN3. N Engl J Med. 2013;368(26):2467–75.
24. Dauber A, Cunha-Silva M, Macedo DB, Brito VN, Abreu AP, Roberts SA, et al. Paternally inherited DLK1 deletion associated with familial central precocious puberty. J Clin Endocrinol Metab. 2017;102(5):1557–67.
25. Silveira LG, Noel SD, Silveira-Neto AP, Abreu AP, Brito VN, Santos MG, et al. Mutations of the KISS1 gene in disorders of puberty. J Clin Endocrinol Metab. 2010;95(5):2276–80.
26. Teles MG, Bianco SD, Brito VN, Trarbach EB, Kuohung W, Xu S, et al. A GPR54-activating mutation in a patient with central precocious puberty. N Engl J Med. 2008;358(7):709–15.
27. Zhu J, Kusa TO, Chan YM. Genetics of pubertal timing. Curr Opin Pediatr. 2018;30(4):532–40.
28. Haddad NG, Eugster EA. Peripheral precocious puberty including congenital adrenal hyperplasia: causes, consequences, management and outcomes. Best Pract Res Clin Endocrinol Metab. 2019;33(3):101273.
29. Utriainen P, Laakso S, Liimatta J, Jaaskelainen J, Voutilainen R. Premature adrenarche – a common condition with variable presentation. Horm Res Paediatr. 2015;83(4):221–31.
30. Voutilainen R, Jaaskelainen J. Premature adrenarche: etiology, clinical findings, and consequences. J Steroid Biochem Mol Biol. 2015;145:226–36.
31. Eugster EA. Treatment of central precocious puberty. J Endocr Soc. 2019;3(5):965–72.
32. Cantas-Orsdemir S, Garb JL, Allen HF. Prevalence of cranial MRI findings in girls with central precocious puberty: a systematic review and meta-analysis. J Pediatr Endocrinol Metab. 2018;31(7):701–10.
33. Bangalore Krishna K, Fuqua JS, Rogol AD, Klein KO, Popovic J, Houk CP, et al. Use of gonadotropin-releasing hormone analogs in children: update by an international consortium. Horm Res Paediatr. 2019;91(6):357–72.
34. Lazar L, Padoa A, Phillip M. Growth pattern and final height after cessation of gonadotropin-suppressive therapy in girls with central sexual precocity. J Clin Endocrinol Metab. 2007;92(9):3483–9.
35. Partsch CJ, Sippell WG. Pathogenesis and epidemiology of precocious puberty. Effects of exogenous oestrogens. Hum Reprod Update. 2001;7(3):292–302.
36. Reiter EO, Mauras N, McCormick K, Kulshreshtha B, Amrhein J, De Luca F, et al. Bicalutamide plus anastrozole for the treatment of gonadotropin-independent precocious puberty in boys with testotoxicosis: a phase II, open-label pilot study (BATT). J Pediatr Endocrinol Metab. 2010;23(10):999–1009.

Delayed Puberty

44

Jessica Schmitt and Paul Boepple

Part 1: Overview of Delayed Puberty

Delayed puberty affects 2–3% of the population [3] and is a condition the general practitioner can expect to see with regularity. Please refer to Chap. 11 to determine in which patients a diagnosis of delayed puberty should be considered and Chaps. 24, 27, and 36 to review the interpretation of the initial laboratory and imaging workup of delayed puberty.

Features of delayed pubertal development can include a complete lack of sexual development, "stalled" sexual development where puberty begins but fails to progress as expected, and "incomplete" pubertal development. The latter may present with signs of estrogen effects but not those of androgen exposure or vice versa. In addition, adolescent girls may present with normal secondary sexual development but failure to attain menarche by the expected age. Anything affecting the hypothalamic–pituitary–gonadal (HPG) axis can present with delayed or stalled pubertal development. Hypergonadotropic hypogonadism results when there is primary gonadal (testicular or ovarian) failure or dysfunction. Hypogonadotropic hypogonadism occurs when there is dysfunction at the level of the pituitary or hypothalamus and can be permanent or transient (functional) (see Reference Box). Anatomic differences in the development of the uterus and vagina can present with isolated delayed menarche (primary amenorrhea) in females.

Reference Box: Pathophysiology of Delayed Pubertal Development

Hypergonadotropic hypogonadism	*Defect/dysfunction of the testicle or ovary*: Includes acquired and congenital causes of gonadal dysfunction. Can be related to gonadal dysgenesis, testicular hypoplasia, disorders of gonadal steroidogenesis, autoimmune destruction, and chemotherapy/radiation injury
Transient hypogonadotropic hypogonadism	*Temporary pituitary or hypothalamic dysfunction*: Includes functional hypogonadotropic hypogonadism and constitutional delay of growth and puberty
Permanent hypogonadotropic hypogonadism	*Permanent dysfunction of hypothalamic or pituitary*: Includes isolated GnRH or gonadotropin deficiency, multiple pituitary hormone deficiency, and CNS structural abnormalities

While there are many causes of delayed puberty, among children with no significant medical history, the most common cause is the constitutional delay of growth and puberty (CDGP), followed by functional hypogonadotropic hypogonadism, permanent hypogonadotropic hypogonadism, and finally hypergonadotropic hypogonadism [3, 49]. History, physical, and initial laboratory workup can help distinguish these conditions (see Table 44.1). In adolescent girls with thelarche (breast development), but delayed menarche, causes include disorders of Müllerian structure development (including that associated with complete androgen insensitivity), disorders of urogenital sinus development, polycystic ovarian syndrome, and acquired hypogonadotropic hypogonadism [44].

J. Schmitt (✉)
University of Alabama at Birmingham, Birmingham, AL, USA
e-mail: jessicaschmitt@uabmc.edu

P. Boepple
MassGeneral Hospital for Children, Boston, MA, USA
e-mail: Boepple.Paul@mgh.harvard.edu

T. Stanley, M. Misra (eds.), *Endocrine Conditions in Pediatrics*, https://doi.org/10.1007/978-3-030-52215-5_44

Table 44.1 Features associated with specific causes of delayed puberty

Constitutional delay of growth and puberty (also called constitutional delay of growth and development)	Required: Normal growth velocity for bone age Normal karyotype (if obtained) Normal external genitalia Supporting: Family history of delayed puberty Delayed adrenarche Self-resolving Delayed bone age Normal inhibin B and AMH concentration
Functional hypogonadotropic hypogonadism	Required: Low-normal or low gonadotropins for age/pubertal stage Recovery of HPG axis after underlying cause is addressed Supporting: History of chronic illness Recent weight loss Under 80% of ideal body weight High physical activity levels Restrictive eating habits
Permanent isolated hypogonadotropic hypogonadism	Required: Prepubertal gonadotropins Prepubertal response to GnRH stimulation Normal karyotype Supporting: Microphallus or cryptorchidism in boys Anosmia Delayed bone age Normal stature for family potential in early childhood with decline in height percentiles when pubertal growth spurt is absent Normal adrenarche
Hypergonadotropic hypogonadism	Required: Elevated gonadotropins with low sex steroids (testosterone, estradiol) Supporting: Depending on underlying etiology can have abnormal karyotype, history of radiation/ chemotherapy, short (Turners) or tall (Klinefelter) stature Normal adrenarche

Constitutional Delay of Growth and Puberty

CDGP, also called constitutional delay of growth and development, affects 50–70% of healthy children presenting for delayed puberty [3, 48, 61] and is more commonly diagnosed in boys than in girls [49, 61]. Population-based studies, as opposed to subspecialty clinic case series, suggest that the male predominance may, in large part, reflect a referral bias with male children more likely to be referred than females [63]. Children with CDGP represent the "extreme end" of normal pubertal development [30]. Puberty is expected to progress typically but at an older age than the general population. While 2% of boys are prepubertal at age 14, by age 15, only 0.4% remain prepubertal [56].

Approximately 60–80% of the variation in the timing of pubertal onset is genetic [40]. Over half of children with CDGP have a family history of delayed puberty [4, 7, 48, 49]. The inheritance pattern of CDGP is variable, with autosomal dominant with complete penetrance, autosomal dominant with incomplete penetrance, autosomal recessive, X-linked, paternally imprinted, and sporadic inheritance patterns reported [4, 30, 48, 63]. Genetic testing has increased understanding of the genetic components regulating puberty; however, the absolute impact of each individual genetic variation may be minimal. For example, analysis of over 350,000 women found 389 candidate genes, each impacting age of menarche (time of first menses) by 1 week to 5 months, but in total, all 389 genes accounted for only 25% of the estimated heritability of variation of age at menarche [18].

Children with CDGP tend to have delayed gonadarche (gonadotropin-stimulated gonadal maturation resulting in testicular enlargement in boys and breast development in girls) in addition to delayed pubarche (axillary and pubic hair growth, typically representing a delay in the maturation of adrenal androgen secretion) [48]. This can help distinguish them from children with isolated hypogonadotropic hypogonadism (IHH) in whom pubarche tends to occur at the typical time [16, 54]. Please see Chaps. 24, 27, and 26 and Table 44.1 for further labs and imaging results suggestive of CDGP.

Functional Hypogonadotropic Hypogonadism

Functional hypogonadotropic hypogonadism (FHH), the second most common cause of delayed puberty, affects approximately 20% of children presenting with delayed puberty [3, 49, 61]. Any chronic illness or state of undernutrition, if severe enough for long enough, can suppress the HPG axis and cause FHH [7]. Children with delayed pubertal development due to FHH tend to have lower height, weight, and BMI z-scores [49]. Boys, but not girls, with FHH tend to have a lower growth velocity than those with delayed puberty due to other causes [61].

Low-Weight Status Adequate nutrition is required for the normal HPG axis function. Both intentional and unintentional weight loss can cause FHH by contributing to hypothalamic dysfunction [36] including suppressed gonadotropin-releasing hormone (GnRH) release and thus reduced luteinizing hormone [9] secretion [60, 62]. Decreased body fat results in decreased leptin, causing a reversible hypogonadotropic hypogonadism (HH) [31]. While this is more often described in females than in males, likely due to the increased frequency of anorexia nervosa in females combined with the loss and regain of menses as a clinical indicator of function of the HPG axis, underweight males may also exhibit reversible HH [21].

Weight regain improves function of the HPG axis and typically allows for pubertal development in those who were prepubertal, continuing pubertal development in those with stalled puberty, and resumption of menses in those who were postmenarchal. The timing of weight regain and recovery of the HPG axis varies significantly between individuals [62]. While there is individual variation, in general, a minimum of 19% body fat is required for menarche, and 22% body fat is needed for the maintenance of menses [24].

Anorexia Nervosa In postmenarchal women, secondary amenorrhea is a cardinal feature of anorexia nervosa [36], and, until the Diagnostic and Statistical Manual of Mental Disorders V, amenorrhea was required for the diagnosis [35]. In general, women who become amenorrheic as a result of weight loss due to anorexia nervosa resume menses at a *higher* weight than they were when they became amenorrheic [24]. Although there is large individual variation, it can take up to 6 months after weight regain to resume menses [36].

Athleticism with Normal Weight Status Demanding physical activity prior to menarche has been associated with delayed menarche, presumably due to suboptimal energy balance. Specifically, female athletes, who started competitive rowing, swimming, or running *before* menarche, started menses on average 1–2 years after those who started competitive athletics *after* menses [15, 23]. Additionally, postmenarchal females with normal weight who engage in extended periods of strenuous activity on a near-daily basis (e.g., running several miles every day) may develop secondary amenorrhea, also presumably due to nutritional imbalance.

Chronic Diseases In addition to undernutrition, chronic disease itself can contribute to hypothalamic dysfunction and HPG axis suppression. Common underlying causes of FHH include sickle cell disease, chronic renal failure, inflammatory bowel disease, cystic fibrosis, untreated celiac disease, rheumatoid arthritis, eating disorders, female athlete triad, and even severe asthma [31]. Delayed menarche has been well described in hemoglobinopathies [51], acquired immunodeficiency syndrome [13], and cystic fibrosis [8]. Severity of disease generally correlates with severity of pubertal delay [8, 13, 51].

Permanent Hypogonadotropic Hypogonadism

Permanent hypogonadotropic hypogonadism affects approximately 10% of patients referred for delayed puberty [3, 49, 61]. Dysfunction at the level of the hypothalamus and/or pituitary results in low (or low-normal) gonadotropins (FSH and LH) and lack of gonadal stimulation with subsequent low estradiol (in females) or testosterone (in males). This causes delayed puberty. While not required for diagnosis, boys may have a history of cryptorchidism and/or microphallus stemming from androgen deficiency in utero [43, 61]. Etiology of permanent hypogonadotropic hypogonadism is extensive. It can be congenital or acquired, isolated, or associated with multiple pituitary insufficiencies. In most children with permanent hypogonadotropic hypogonadism, it is an isolated finding not associated with other pituitary deficiencies [19].

Acquired Hypogonadotropic Hypogonadism Hypogonadotropic hypogonadism can occur after surgery to the hypothalamic–pituitary region [53] or radiotherapy [14, 53]. Up to 11% of childhood cancer survivors with a history of cranial radiation therapy develop hypogonadotropic hypogonadism [14]. The risk of developing hypogonadotropic hypogonadism increases with higher doses of radiation [14, 53], longer duration of radiotherapy, longer time since radiation treatment [53], and presence of other pituitary insufficiencies [53]. Depending on the age and developmental stage at presentation, patients can present with delayed puberty, stalled pubertal development, amenorrhea, or oligomenorrhea.

Congenital Permanent Hypogonadotropic Hypogonadism

Isolated or idiopathic hypogonadotropic hypogonadism (IHH) in otherwise healthy children: IHH can be difficult to distinguish from CDGP due to significant phenotypic overlap. Classically, both conditions present in otherwise healthy children with delayed puberty who have a normal growth velocity for pubertal stage and often have a family history of delayed puberty [43]. Close evaluation of growth charts can help distinguish the two. In general, children with CDGP grow at a lower height percentile than expected for their genetic potential throughout early childhood. In IHH, children typically grow at the expected height percentile for genetic potential until adolescence, when their growth velocity slows due to the lack of pubertal growth spurt.

Relative to their peers with CDGP, boys with IHH tend to have an older bone age, lower testosterone, and lower gonadotropins [19], but there is a significant overlap [17]. Researchers have investigated other potential biochemical markers to distinguish CDGP and IHH. Anti-Müllerian hormone (AMH) and inhibin B (INHB), both made by testicular

Sertoli cells, have been investigated as potential biomarkers. Although both tend to be lower in males with IHH compared to those with CDGP [17, 42, 61], an INHB <35 pg/mL, particularly when associated with small testicular volume, appears to reasonably distinguish IHH from CDGP [17, 61] although further work is needed to validate this threshold.

IHH can be complete or partial [42]. Partial IHH can be particularly difficult to diagnose as it might present with normal timing of pubertal onset but lack of completion of sexual development [17, 43]. IHH can be associated with anosmia (decreased sense of smell) or with a normal sense of smell. The frequency of anosmic and normosmic IHH is similar [10]. While several causative genes have been found, less than 50% of children with IHH have a genetic cause identified [10, 42]. Even among children with the same genetic mutation, there is significant genotype–phenotype variation [29, 47, 50].

Clinical Key
Distinguishing between CDGP and IHH is challenging, and the current "gold standard" is observation through age 18 years, at which time persistent lack of pubertal progression is diagnosed as IHH. For both psychosocial and medical reasons, however, treatment is often warranted before age 18 years. For this reason, prepubertal children age 14–16 years old should be referred to a pediatric endocrinologist.

Anosmic IHH Anosmic IHH, also called Kallmann syndrome, affects 1 in 10,000 men and 1 in 50,000 women [11]. It is associated with aplasia of GnRH neurons and olfactory bulbs [10]. Kallmann syndrome affects males more often than females in part because one of the commonly affected genes, *KAL1* (now called *ANOS1*), is on the X-chromosome [47]. In addition to X-linked inheritance, autosomal dominant and autosomal recessive forms exist [10, 43, 47].

Normosmic IHH Normosmic IHH is not associated with deficits in olfactory bulb formation, so the sense of smell is intact in these patients. Patients with normosmic IHH have a higher rate of partial IHH than those with anosmic IHH [42]. Mutations affecting proteins involved in GnRH signaling and LH or FSH production have all been associated with normosmic IHH [5, 10, 30, 50, 57, 65].

Syndromic Hypogonadotropic Hypogonadism

Syndromic hypogonadotropic hypogonadism is seen in clinical syndromes in which IHH is a characteristic feature and in children with deficiencies in multiple pituitary hormones. For example, IHH without other significant pituitary insufficiencies is a characteristic feature of CHARGE syndrome associated with CHD7 mutations [10], Prader–Willi syndrome [19], leptin or leptin receptor deficiencies [43, 47], and X-linked adrenal hypoplasia congenita [50]. In patients with atypical pituitary development, FSH and LH deficiency can be seen as one of several pituitary insufficiencies [22, 30, 64]. In these children, delayed puberty is rarely the initial finding as growth hormone and TSH insufficiency are usually noted earlier in childhood [22].

Hypergonadotropic Hypogonadism

Hypergonadotropic hypogonadism is seen in up to 4% of previously healthy children with delayed puberty [3], but it is seen in up to 13% when children with a significant medical history are included [49]. In hypergonadotropic hypogonadism, pituitary function is normal, but the gonads (testes/ovaries) are nonfunctional or dysfunctional. Leading causes of hypergonadotropic hypogonadism are long-term effects of cancer treatment (chemotherapy, radiation, and surgery), idiopathic gonadal failure, and sex chromosome disorders such as Klinefelter and Turner syndromes [49, 56, 61]. Less common causes include disorders of sex steroidogenesis [32], vanishing testes syndrome [27], and autoimmunity [1]. For discussions on Turner syndrome, Klinefelter syndrome, and genital ambiguity, please see Chaps. 47, 48, and 46, respectively.

Gonadal Dysfunction

Postoncologic Treatment Childhood cancer survivors with a history of pelvic/gonadal radiation [52, 53] and/or specific chemotherapeutic agents, particularly alkylating agents [52], are at risk of gonadal dysfunction. These children should be followed by a team with experience in monitoring for delayed endocrine effects of cancer treatment.

Premature Ovarian Insufficiency (POI) POI is the premature loss of ovarian follicles and function prior to age 40 [1, 31] and results in hypergonadotropic hypogonadism. Depending on the age of presentation, women can present with complete lack of thelarche (breast development), delayed onset of menarche (primary amenorrhea), secondary amenorrhea, or irregular menses. Adrenarche is unaffected. Unfortunately, a cause is unidentified in up to 90% of affected patients [38]. In 46,XX females with no medical history, if a cause is found, it is typically due to Fragile X permutation state or autoimmunity [1, 38]. Women with galactosemia should be closely followed, as POI is common in this condition [45].

Gonadal Absence While usually diagnosed in young childhood and infancy, testicular regression syndrome (also known as vanishing testes syndrome or congenital anorchia) has been diagnosed in the peripubertal age during evaluation for nonpalpable testicles or delayed puberty [27, 31]. In testicular regression, external genitalia can vary from mildly undervirilized to typical male depending on the timing of testicular loss in utero.

Primary Amenorrhea

Girls with appropriate breast development who do not have menses by age 15 meet the definition of primary amenorrhea. While all of the previously discussed conditions can cause primary amenorrhea and delayed thelarche, there are additional conditions that can cause primary amenorrhea alone that warrant discussion. After excluding previously discussed conditions, the most common causes of primary amenorrhea are disorders of Müllerian structure development, disorders of urogenital sinus development, polycystic ovarian syndrome, and acquired hypogonadotropic hypogonadism [34, 39, 44]. In all of these conditions, breast development typically occurs at the expected time. For a discussion of polycystic ovarian syndrome, please see Chap. 45.

Disorders of Müllerian Development During female fetal development, Müllerian ducts give rise to the uterus, cervix, upper vagina, and part of the fallopian tubes. In male fetuses, anti-Müllerian hormone (AMH) induces regression of these structures.

In 46,XY females with complete androgen insensitivity, testes form and secrete testosterone, but a nonfunctioning androgen receptor prevents masculinization of external genitalia. The testes also produce AMH, which causes regression of the Müllerian ducts and lack of development of the uterus, cervix, and upper vagina. A common presentation of complete androgen insensitivity, therefore, is in young women with primary amenorrhea [9].

In 46,XX women, Müllerian duct agenesis can also cause primary amenorrhea. This condition, commonly called Mayer–Rokitansky–Küster–Hauser (MRKH) syndrome, is seen in approximately 1 in 4000–5000 births and is diagnosed when there is aplasia or hypoplasia of the uterus and upper vagina [28, 58]. Ovarian function is normal, so breast development typically occurs at the expected age.

Defect in Urogenital Sinus Development In female fetuses, the urogenital sinus gives rise to the lower vagina, bladder, urethra, and hymen. Atypical development can result in vaginal septum, vaginal stenosis, vaginal agenesis, and imperforate hymen. These structural anomalies cause primary amenorrhea due to outflow tract obstruction. History may reveal cyclical abdominal pain, urinary retention, and a feeling of rectal fullness [2]. These developmental defects are characterized by normal gonadotropin secretion and normal ovarian function.

Acquired Hypogonadotropic Hypogonadism Rarely, patients can develop acquired hypogonadotropic hypogonadism after breast development (thelarche) has started. In this case, young women will present with a history of thelarche but no menses. Acquired hypogonadotropic hypogonadism can be a presenting symptom of hyperprolactinemia, CNS tumor, hypothyroidism, or glucocorticoid excess [39].

Part 2: Urgent and Emergent Considerations in Children with Delayed Puberty

While all children with delayed puberty can reasonably warrant a referral to endocrinology, some conditions warrant additional evaluation while awaiting referral. Please see Chap. 27 for interpretation of labs assessing the HPG axis and Chap. 36 for interpretation of bone ages. In children with presumed FHH, the general practitioner's primary goal should be identifying the underlying cause. Whether general screening labs such as complete blood counts, celiac screen, renal panel, and liver function are likely to yield a diagnosis is an area of debate [3, 39, 45], and initial workup should be tailored to the patient's symptoms [59].

In children with syndromic IHH, referrals and workup should be tailored to the underlying diagnosis. Depending on the genetic cause, anosmic IHH (Kallmann syndrome) can be associated with developmental delay, ichthyosis, renal anomalies, dental agenesis, cleft palate, and ocular albinism, so dermatology, ophthalmology, nephrology, and developmental referrals should be considered if these conditions are noted [11, 42, 47].

In females with disorders of Müllerian duct or urogenital sinus development, renal, vertebral, and cardiac anomalies can be seen; screening imaging studies are warranted [2, 28, 58]. In women with obstruction of the vaginal outflow tract, acute urinary retention and infection can be indications for more urgent surgical intervention [2].

In all patients with prolonged insufficient gonadal (testicular or ovarian) function, decreased bone mineral density is a concern. A dietary history to assess adequate calcium and vitamin D intake is reasonable. Assessment of vitamin D status and dual-energy X-ray absorptiometry (DXA) can be considered, particularly in those with a fracture history or more severe pubertal delay.

Part 3: Chronic Management and Considerations for Referral

By definition, those with an onset of puberty two standard deviations later than the mean of the population have delayed puberty. Using this statistical definition, 2–3% of the population will have delayed puberty. Patients who are the most "out of bounds" in terms of age warrant more comprehensive evaluations and referral, while those "on the borderline" might reasonably be observed by their primary practitioner after an initial workup. For all adolescents with delayed puberty, goals of management include promoting typical development of secondary sexual characteristics, supporting psychosocial development, reaching optimal final adult height, and optimizing bone health [26, 59].

Treatment in Constitutional Delay of Growth and Puberty Children with CDGP will eventually undergo typical pubertal development, with a longer period of growth than their unaffected peers have, and their final adult height is usually consistent with their genetic height potential [31]. Depending on the child and family's level of distress, an initial observation period of 6–12 months can be an appropriate first step, with referral to endocrinology if puberty does not begin [59]. Factors to consider when deciding on the timing of endocrinology referral are the age of the patient, family history of pubertal delay, and family/child preferences.

If medical intervention is desired by the patient and family, one can "prime" the HPG axis with low doses of testosterone or estrogen. It is not clear if treatment impacts bone health in the long term, and impact on adult height is not expected. Despite these limitations, young men tolerate the treatment [12, 46, 55] and may benefit psychologically [31, 55]. There are less data available on the treatment of CDGP in young women.

Treatment in Functional Hypogonadotropic Hypogonadism As mentioned previously, treatment of FHH centers on treating the underlying condition. With prolonged FHH, risks include infertility and decreased bone mineral density [25]. Referral to endocrinology should be considered in those with FHH, particularly in those with decreased bone mineral density, history of fracture, older age, or secondary amenorrhea.

Treatment in Permanent Hypogonadism *Including hyper- and hypogonadotropic hypogonadism*: All patients with permanent hypogonadism should be referred to endocrinology for pubertal induction and maintenance. Management centers upon mimicking typical puberty with escalating doses of sex steroids. Young men are typically given testosterone injections, with a dose increase every 3–6 months until they reach adult dosing. In addition to transdermal preparations (i.e., patches and gels), as of 2019, there is an oral testosterone option for men over 18 years old for maintenance therapy. For young women, transdermal as opposed to oral estradiol is preferred for pubertal induction [26, 33] with addition of progesterone after 2 years or once breakthrough bleeding occurs, whichever is first [26]. After pubertal development is complete, one should consider the use of transdermal estradiol and additional progesterone for hormonal replacement therapy due to thrombotic risk of oral estrogen replacements [37] and effects on bone density [6]; however, patients may prefer oral estrogen and oral progesterone or combination oral contraceptive pills due to ease of use [33].

Treatment and Referral in Women with Primary Amenorrhea Treatment options depend upon the underlying cause. In women with CAIS, a discussion of risk and benefits of testicular removal is paramount, given the increased risk of germ cell tumors [9, 20]. If gonadectomy is *not* done, hormonal replacement therapy is unnecessary, as testosterone is aromatized to estrogen, producing normal pubertal development and normal adult estrogen levels. If gonadectomy is preformed, sex hormones must be replaced.

In women with MRKH syndrome and other outflow tract disorders, referral to a pediatric gynecologist with experience in these conditions is warranted. Mainstays of treatment include vaginal dilators and surgical vaginoplasty [2, 41]. While awaiting intervention in outflow tract conditions, menstrual suppression with combination oral contraceptive pills, progestin-only pills, depot medroxyprogesterone acetate, or GnRH agonist injection with supplemental hormonal replacement can be used to alleviate pain [2].

References

1. Committee opinion no. 605: primary ovarian insufficiency in adolescents and young women. Obstet Gynecol. 2014;124(1):193–7.
2. Management of acute obstructive uterovaginal anomalies: ACOG Committee opinion, number 779. Obstet Gynecol. 2019;133(6):e363–e71.
3. Abitbol L, Zborovski S, Palmert MR. Evaluation of delayed puberty: what diagnostic tests should be performed in the seemingly otherwise well adolescent? Arch Dis Child. 2016;101(8):767–71.
4. Abreu AP, Dauber A, Macedo DB, Noel SD, Brito VN, Gill JC, et al. Central precocious puberty caused by mutations in the imprinted gene MKRN3. N Engl J Med. 2013;368(26):2467–75.
5. Achermann JC, Gu WX, Kotlar TJ, Meeks JJ, Sabacan LP, Seminara SB, et al. Mutational analysis of DAX1 in patients with hypogonadotropic hypogonadism or pubertal delay. J Clin Endocrinol Metab. 1999;84(12):4497–500.
6. Ackerman KE, Singhal V, Baskaran C, Slattery M, Campoverde Reyes KJ, Toth A, et al. Oestrogen replacement improves bone mineral density in oligo-amenorrhoeic athletes: a randomised clinical trial. Br J Sports Med. 2019;53(4):229–36.

7. Argente J. Diagnosis of late puberty. Horm Res. 1999;51(Suppl 3):95–100.
8. Arrigo T, De Luca F, Lucanto C, Lombardo M, Rulli I, Salzano G, et al. Nutritional, glycometabolic and genetic factors affecting menarcheal age in cystic fibrosis. Diabetes Nutr Metab. 2004;17(2):114–9.
9. Batista RL, Costa EMF, Rodrigues ADS, Gomes NL, Faria JA, Nishi MY, et al. Androgen insensitivity syndrome: a review. Arch Endocrinol Metab. 2018;62(2):227–35.
10. Beate K, Joseph N, de Nicolas R, Wolfram K. Genetics of isolated hypogonadotropic hypogonadism: role of GnRH receptor and other genes. Int J Endocrinol. 2012;2012:147893.
11. Berges-Raso I, Gimenez-Palop O, Gabau E, Capel I, Caixas A, Rigla M. Kallmann syndrome and ichthyosis: a case of contiguous gene deletion syndrome. Endocrinol Diabetes Metab Case Rep. 2017;2017:EDM170083.
12. Brown DC, Butler GE, Kelnar CJ, Wu FC. A double blind, placebo controlled study of the effects of low dose testosterone undecanoate on the growth of small for age, prepubertal boys. Arch Dis Child. 1995;73(2):131–5.
13. Buchacz K, Rogol AD, Lindsey JC, Wilson CM, Hughes MD, Seage GR 3rd, et al. Delayed onset of pubertal development in children and adolescents with perinatally acquired HIV infection. J Acquir Immune Defic Syndr. 2003;33(1):56–65.
14. Chemaitilly W, Li Z, Huang S, Ness KK, Clark KL, Green DM, et al. Anterior hypopituitarism in adult survivors of childhood cancers treated with cranial radiotherapy: a report from the St Jude Lifetime Cohort study. J Clin Oncol. 2015;33(5):492–500.
15. Claessens AL, Bourgois J, Beunen G, Philippaerts R, Thomis M, Lefevre J, et al. Age at menarche in relation to anthropometric characteristics, competition level and boat category in elite junior rowers. Ann Hum Biol. 2003;30(2):148–59.
16. Counts DR, Pescovitz OH, Barnes KM, Hench KD, Chrousos GP, Sherins RJ, et al. Dissociation of adrenarche and gonadarche in precocious puberty and in isolated hypogonadotropic hypogonadism. J Clin Endocrinol Metab. 1987;64(6):1174–8.
17. Coutant R, Biette-Demeneix E, Bouvattier C, Bouhours-Nouet N, Gatelais F, Dufresne S, et al. Baseline inhibin B and anti-Mullerian hormone measurements for diagnosis of hypogonadotropic hypogonadism (HH) in boys with delayed puberty. J Clin Endocrinol Metab. 2010;95(12):5225–32.
18. Day FR, Thompson DJ, Helgason H, Chasman DI, Finucane H, Sulem P, et al. Genomic analyses identify hundreds of variants associated with age at menarche and support a role for puberty timing in cancer risk. Nat Genet. 2017;49(6):834–41.
19. Degros V, Cortet-Rudelli C, Soudan B, Dewailly D. The human chorionic gonadotropin test is more powerful than the gonadotropin-releasing hormone agonist test to discriminate male isolated hypogonadotropic hypogonadism from constitutional delayed puberty. Eur J Endocrinol. 2003;149(1):23–9.
20. Döhnert U, Wünsch L, Hiort O. Gonadectomy in complete androgen insensitivity syndrome: why and when? Sex Dev. 2017;11(4):171–4.
21. Dwyer AA, Chavan NR, Lewkowitz-Shpuntoff H, Plummer L, Hayes FJ, Seminara SB, et al. Functional hypogonadotropic hypogonadism in men: underlying neuroendocrine mechanisms and natural history. J Clin Endocrinol Metab. 2019;104(8):3403–14.
22. Fluck C, Deladoey J, Rutishauser K, Eble A, Marti U, Wu W, et al. Phenotypic variability in familial combined pituitary hormone deficiency caused by a PROP1 gene mutation resulting in the substitution of Arg-->Cys at codon 120 (R120C). J Clin Endocrinol Metab. 1998;83(10):3727–34.
23. Frisch RE, Gotz-Welbergen AV, McArthur JW, Albright T, Witschi J, Bullen B, et al. Delayed menarche and amenorrhea of college athletes in relation to age of onset of training. JAMA. 1981;246(14):1559–63.
24. Frisch RE, McArthur JW. Menstrual cycles: fatness as a determinant of minimum weight for height necessary for their maintenance or onset. Science. 1974;185(4155):949–51.
25. Gordon CM, Ackerman KE, Berga SL, Kaplan JR, Mastorakos G, Misra M, et al. Functional hypothalamic amenorrhea: an Endocrine Society clinical practice guideline. J Clin Endocrinol Metab. 2017;102(5):1413–39.
26. Gravholt CH, Andersen NH, Conway GS, Dekkers OM, Geffner ME, Klein KO, et al. Clinical practice guidelines for the care of girls and women with Turner syndrome: proceedings from the 2016 Cincinnati International Turner Syndrome Meeting. Eur J Endocrinol. 2017;177(3):G1–g70.
27. Heksch RA, Matheson MA, Tishelman AC, Swartz JM, Jayanthi VR, Diamond DA, et al. Testicular regression syndrome: practice variation in diagnosis and management. Endocr Pract. 2019;25(8):779–86.
28. Herlin M, Bjørn A-MB, Rasmussen M, Trolle B, Petersen MB. Prevalence and patient characteristics of Mayer–Rokitansky–Küster–Hauser syndrome: a nationwide registry-based study. Hum Reprod. 2016;31(10):2384–90.
29. Hipkin LJ, Casson IF, Davis JC. Identical twins discordant for Kallmann's syndrome. J Med Genet. 1990;27(3):198–9.
30. Howard SR, Dunkel L. The genetic basis of delayed puberty. Neuroendocrinology. 2018;106(3):283–91.
31. Kaplowitz PB. Delayed puberty. Pediatr Rev. 2010;31(5):189–95.
32. Kardelen AD, Toksoy G, Bas F, Yavas Abali Z, Gencay G, Poyrazoglu S, et al. A rare cause of congenital adrenal hyperplasia: clinical and genetic findings and follow-up characteristics of six patients with 17-hydroxylase deficiency including two novel mutations. J Clin Res Pediatr Endocrinol. 2018;10(3):206–15.
33. Klein KO, Rosenfield RL, Santen RJ, Gawlik AM, Backeljauw PF, Gravholt CH, et al. Estrogen replacement in Turner syndrome: literature review and practical considerations. J Clin Endocrinol Metab. 2018;103(5):1790–803.
34. Kriplani A, Goyal M, Kachhawa G, Mahey R, Kulshrestha V. Etiology and management of primary amenorrhoea: a study of 102 cases at tertiary centre. Taiwan J Obstet Gynecol. 2017;56(6):761–4.
35. Marks A. The evolution of our understanding and treatment of eating disorders over the past 50 years. J Clin Psychol. 2019;75(8):1380–91.
36. Misra M, Klibanski A. Neuroendocrine consequences of anorexia nervosa in adolescents. Endocr Dev. 2010;17:197–214.
37. Mohammed K, Abu Dabrh AM, Benkhadra K, Al Nofal A, Carranza Leon BG, Prokop LJ, et al. Oral vs transdermal estrogen therapy and vascular events: a systematic review and meta-analysis. J Clin Endocrinol Metab. 2015;100(11):4012–20.
38. Nelson LM. Clinical practice. Primary ovarian insufficiency. N Engl J Med. 2009;360(6):606–14.
39. Palmert MR, Dunkel L. Clinical practice. Delayed puberty. N Engl J Med. 2012;366(5):443–53.
40. Parent AS, Teilmann G, Juul A, Skakkebaek NE, Toppari J, Bourguignon JP. The timing of normal puberty and the age limits of sexual precocity: variations around the world, secular trends, and changes after migration. Endocr Rev. 2003;24(5):668–93.
41. Perlman S, Hertweck SP. Vaginal agenesis: an opinion on the surgical management. J Pediatr Adolesc Gynecol. 2000;13(3):143–4.
42. Pitteloud N, Hayes FJ, Boepple PA, DeCruz S, Seminara SB, MacLaughlin DT, et al. The role of prior pubertal development, biochemical markers of testicular maturation, and genetics in elucidating the phenotypic heterogeneity of idiopathic hypogonadotropic hypogonadism. J Clin Endocrinol Metab. 2002;87(1):152–60.
43. Raivio T, Falardeau J, Dwyer A, Quinton R, Hayes FJ, Hughes VA, et al. Reversal of idiopathic hypogonadotropic hypogonadism. N Engl J Med. 2007;357(9):863–73.

44. Reindollar RH, Byrd JR, McDonough PG. Delayed sexual development: a study of 252 patients. Am J Obstet Gynecol. 1981;140(4):371–80.
45. Rosen DS, Foster C. Delayed puberty. Pediatr Rev. 2001;22(9):309–15.
46. Rosenfeld RG, Northcraft GB, Hintz RL. A prospective, randomized study of testosterone treatment of constitutional delay of growth and development in male adolescents. Pediatrics. 1982;69(6):681–7.
47. Sato N, Katsumata N, Kagami M, Hasegawa T, Hori N, Kawakita S, et al. Clinical assessment and mutation analysis of Kallmann syndrome 1 (KAL1) and fibroblast growth factor receptor 1 (FGFR1, or KAL2) in five families and 18 sporadic patients. J Clin Endocrinol Metab. 2004;89(3):1079–88.
48. Sedlmeyer IL, Hirschhorn JN, Palmert MR. Pedigree analysis of constitutional delay of growth and maturation: determination of familial aggregation and inheritance patterns. J Clin Endocrinol Metab. 2002;87(12):5581–6.
49. Sedlmeyer IL, Palmert MR. Delayed puberty: analysis of a large case series from an academic center. J Clin Endocrinol Metab. 2002;87(4):1613–20.
50. Seminara SB, Achermann JC, Genel M, Jameson JL, Crowley WF Jr. X-linked adrenal hypoplasia congenita: a mutation in DAX1 expands the phenotypic spectrum in males and females. J Clin Endocrinol Metab. 1999;84(12):4501–9.
51. Serjeant GR, Hambleton I, Thame M. Fecundity and pregnancy outcome in a cohort with sickle cell-haemoglobin C disease followed from birth. BJOG. 2005;112(9):1308–14.
52. Skinner R, Mulder RL, Kremer LC, Hudson MM, Constine LS, Bardi E, et al. Recommendations for gonadotoxicity surveillance in male childhood, adolescent, and young adult cancer survivors: a report from the International Late Effects of Childhood Cancer Guideline Harmonization Group in collaboration with the PanCareSurFup Consortium. Lancet Oncol. 2017;18(2):e75–90.
53. Sklar CA, Antal Z, Chemaitilly W, Cohen LE, Follin C, Meacham LR, et al. Hypothalamic-pituitary and growth disorders in survivors of childhood cancer: an Endocrine Society clinical practice guideline. J Clin Endocrinol Metab. 2018;103(8):2761–84.
54. Sklar CA, Kaplan SL, Grumbach MM. Evidence for dissociation between adrenarche and gonadarche: studies in patients with idiopathic precocious puberty, gonadal dysgenesis, isolated gonadotropin deficiency, and constitutionally delayed growth and adolescence. J Clin Endocrinol Metab. 1980;51(3):548–56.
55. Soliman AT, Khadir MM, Asfour M. Testosterone treatment in adolescent boys with constitutional delay of growth and development. Metab Clin Exp. 1995;44(8):1013–5.
56. Styne DM, Grumbach MM. Puberty: ontogeny, neuroendocrinology, physiology, and disorders. In: Kronenberg H, editor. Williams textbook of endocrinology. 11th ed. Philadelphia: Elsevier Health Sciences; 2007. p. 969–1166.
57. Tabarin A, Achermann JC, Recan D, Bex V, Bertagna X, Christin-Maitre S, et al. A novel mutation in DAX1 causes delayed-onset adrenal insufficiency and incomplete hypogonadotropic hypogonadism. J Clin Invest. 2000;105(3):321–8.
58. Thomas E, Shetty S, Kapoor N, Paul TV. Mayer-Rokitansky-Kuster-Hauser syndrome. BMJ Case Rep. 2015;2015:bcr2015210187-b.
59. Trotman GE. Delayed puberty in the female patient. Curr Opin Obstet Gynecol. 2016;28(5):366–72.
60. van Binsbergen CJ, Coelingh Bennink HJ, Odink J, Haspels AA, Koppeschaar HP. A comparative and longitudinal study on endocrine changes related to ovarian function in patients with anorexia nervosa. J Clin Endocrinol Metab. 1990;71(3):705–11.
61. Varimo T, Miettinen PJ, Kansakoski J, Raivio T, Hero M. Congenital hypogonadotropic hypogonadism, functional hypogonadotropism or constitutional delay of growth and puberty? An analysis of a large patient series from a single tertiary center. Hum Reprod. 2017;32(1):147–53.
62. Vigersky RA, Andersen AE, Thompson RH, Loriaux DL. Hypothalamic dysfunction in secondary amenorrhea associated with simple weight loss. N Engl J Med. 1977;297(21):1141–5.
63. Wehkalampi K, Widen E, Laine T, Palotie A, Dunkel L. Patterns of inheritance of constitutional delay of growth and puberty in families of adolescent girls and boys referred to specialist pediatric care. J Clin Endocrinol Metab. 2008;93(3):723–8.
64. Wu W, Cogan JD, Pfaffle RW, Dasen JS, Frisch H, O'Connell SM, et al. Mutations in PROP1 cause familial combined pituitary hormone deficiency. Nat Genet. 1998;18(2):147–9.
65. Zhang Z, Feng Y, Ye D, Li CJ, Dong FQ, Tong Y. Clinical and molecular genetic analysis of a Chinese family with congenital X-linked adrenal hypoplasia caused by novel mutation 1268delA in the DAX-1 gene. J Zhejiang Univ Sci B. 2015;16(11):963–8.

Polycystic Ovary Syndrome

45

Sungeeta Agrawal

Overview

Polycystic ovary syndrome (PCOS) is a complex disorder that affects ovarian function and results in anovulatory menstrual cycles, hyperandrogenism, and/or polycystic ovarian morphology. PCOS affects approximately 5–20% of women worldwide, depending on the population and definition criteria used [1–3]. Genetics, insulin resistance, and environmental factors such as obesity are all thought to play a role in the development of PCOS [4, 5]. In most cases, the origin of androgen excess is ovarian, though adrenal androgen excess can also contribute to the manifestations of PCOS [6, 7].

Pathophysiology

In normal ovaries, the gonadotropins follicle-stimulating hormone (FSH) and luteinizing hormone (LH) stimulate follicular growth and estrogen production [8]. In the follicle, LH stimulates the theca cells to produce androstenedione. Androstenedione then diffuses to the granulosa cells [9], and FSH, through increased expression of aromatase, stimulates the conversion of androstenedione to estrone. Estrone is further catalyzed to estradiol. In patients with PCOS, there is often increased LH secretion, resulting in excess androgen production [6]. Insufficient FSH secretion results in failure to convert androstenedione to estradiol and results in follicular arrest. Follicular arrest results in the polycystic appearance of the ovaries.

Etiology

The etiology of PCOS is multifactorial. There is likely a genetic component, as one study found that in women with PCOS, 24% of their mothers and 32% of their sisters also had the diagnosis [9, 10]. Through multiple studies, over 100 potential genes have been identified as possibly playing a role in the development of PCOS [5, 6, 8]. These genes are related to steroidogenesis, chronic inflammation, metabolism, and the hypothalamic-pituitary-gonadal axis.

Insulin resistance, while not part of the diagnostic criteria, is also believed to play a major role in the pathophysiology of PCOS [8]. Even lean patients with PCOS have an increased incidence of insulin resistance, compared to BMI-matched controls. In one study, insulin resistance was present in 75% of lean and 95% of overweight patients with PCOS [11]. Furthermore, studies have shown that those with conditions associated with insulin resistance are at increased risk of developing PCOS during adolescence [5]. These conditions include intrauterine growth restriction (IUGR), small for gestational age (SGA), premature adrenarche, and obesity [5, 12–14].

There are a couple of ways that insulin resistance can contribute to PCOS. Increased insulin levels reduce levels of sex hormone–binding globulin (SHBG), a glycoprotein that binds to sex steroids [8, 15]. Lower levels of SHBG result in an increase in bioavailable estrogen and androgens. Obesity is also associated with a decrease in SHBG levels and, independent of fasting insulin, can further increase free testosterone levels [16]. Insulin also accentuates LH action in theca cells to increase androgen production [6, 9]. Of note, during puberty both insulin secretion and resistance increase, especially in girls [17, 18], and this may contribute to the clinical signs of hyperandrogenism during puberty.

S. Agrawal (✉)
Division of Pediatric Endocrinology, Floating Hospital for Children at Tufts Medical Center/Tufts University School of Medicine, Boston, MA, USA
e-mail: SAgrawal1@tuftsmedicalcenter.org

T. Stanley, M. Misra (eds.), *Endocrine Conditions in Pediatrics*, https://doi.org/10.1007/978-3-030-52215-5_45

Reference Box: Key Pathophysiology

- Excess LH and insufficient FSH secretion lead to increased androgen production.
- The imbalance between LH and FSH results in follicular arrest, which leads to the polycystic appearance of ovaries.
- Insulin resistance and obesity lower SHBG levels, which results in elevated free androgens.

Diagnosis

In 1990 the National Institutes of Health (NIH) diagnosed PCOS based on the presence of hyperandrogenism, oligo-ovulation, and exclusion of other disorders [5, 9]. In 2003 the Rotterdam criteria were established, which stated that any two of the following three criteria needed to be met in order to diagnose PCOS: oligo-anovulation, clinical and/or biochemical hyperandrogenism, and polycystic ovaries [19]. Biochemical hyperandrogenism may include elevated total testosterone, free testosterone, androstenedione, or dehydroepiandrosterone sulfate (DHEAS), though free testosterone levels are thought to be the most sensitive marker for hyperandrogenism [8]. Polycystic ovaries are defined as ovaries with an excess of small (antral) follicles, measuring 2–9 mm, arrested in development prior to the follicular stage [8]. Twelve or more such follicles in at least one ovary, or ovarian volume of more than 10 cm^3 (on transvaginal ultrasound), are required to meet criteria for polycystic ovaries [20].

In addition to meeting requirements of the Rotterdam criteria, in order to establish the diagnosis of PCOS, other causes of irregular menses or hyperandrogenism need to be ruled out with laboratory studies. These include pregnancy, non-classical congenital adrenal hyperplasia (NCCAH), thyroid disease, hyperprolactinemia, premature ovarian insufficiency, and ovarian/adrenal tumors. Systemic illnesses and conditions associated with low weight, excessive exercise, and increased stress may also cause irregular or absent periods, but should not cause hirsutism. Distinguishing between PCOS and NCCAH can be challenging, as there is overlap of signs and symptoms [5]. NCCAH is relatively common with a prevalence of 1 in 1000. Additionally, polycystic ovaries can be found in patients with untreated non-classical CAH [9]. A morning 17-hydroxyprogesterone (17-OHP) level ≥200 ng/dl, drawn during the follicular phase if the patient is having regular cycles [21] or at any time in those with amenorrhea, is suggestive of NCCAH, though one study found ~20% of women with PCOS also met this criteria [5, 22]. In women with an elevated 17-OHP, a corticotropin (ACTH) stimulation test can help distinguish between NCCAH and PCOS [23].

The Endocrine Society recommends using the Rotterdam Criteria to establish the diagnosis of PCOS in adults [24]. PCOS symptoms can start around the time of menarche [9, 25], and premature pubarche in young girls may be an early sign of PCOS [12]. The diagnosis of PCOS in adolescents is more challenging than in adults, as there is overlap between normal adolescent physiology and the symptoms of PCOS [5]. Approximately 85% of cycles may be anovulatory in the first year after menarche [8, 24], and cycles can remain anovulatory for the first two postmenarchal years. Acne, a clinical sign of hyperandrogenism, also affects the majority of teenagers during puberty and is often associated with normal androgen levels [26]. Further, testosterone levels can be transiently elevated in normal adolescent girls shortly after attaining menarche, particularly in those with anovulatory cycles [5].

Imaging in adolescents also presents challenges. Subjecting an adolescent to a transvaginal ultrasound may not be ideal, especially if they have not yet had intercourse. Transabdominal ultrasound may not visualize pelvic anatomy optimally, especially in patients with obesity. One study did find transabdominal ultrasound in adolescent females to be useful in detecting polycystic ovarian morphology, with a higher occurrence of this finding in girls with menstrual irregularities and clinical and/or biochemical hyperandrogenism compared to girls without these signs and symptoms (65% vs. 11%) [27]. However, a multicystic appearance of the ovaries in this age group can be completely normal [8, 27].

Given the overlap between signs/symptoms of PCOS and normal adolescent puberty, the Endocrine Society advises not using the Rotterdam criteria to establish PCOS diagnosis in this age group. Instead, they recommend that diagnosis in adolescents only be made if there is both persistent oligomenorrhea (cycles longer than 45 days) and biochemical and/or clinical hyperandrogenism (Table 45.1) [6, 24]. The Pediatric Endocrine Society expands the definition to include other forms of irregular menses, in addition to persistent oligomenorrhea [6]. After a year of menarche, signs of menstrual irregularity in adolescents can include cycles less than 21 days, secondary amenorrhea (3 months without menstrua-

Table 45.1 Symptoms and signs required for the diagnosis of PCOS in adolescents

Hyperandrogenism		
Clinical signs	Biochemical markers	Irregular menses
Acne	↑ Total and/or free testosterone	Cycles >45 days[a]
Hirsutism	↑ DHEAS	Cycles <21 days[a]
Male pattern balding	↑ Androstenedione	Primary amenorrhea
–	–	Secondary amenorrhea

[a]In girls who have had menses for at least 1 year
DHEAS dehydroepiandrosterone sulfate

tion), or primary amenorrhea (defined as no menses by 15 years of age or 3 years after breast development) [28]. As in adults, other causes of irregular menses/hyperandrogenism need to be ruled out to establish the diagnosis of PCOS.

Management and Treatment

The majority of patients with PCOS are either overweight or obese [8]. They have an increased incidence of metabolic syndrome, which includes insulin resistance, hyperlipidemia, and hypertension [5, 9]. For these reasons, the Endocrine Society recommends that both adolescents and adult women with PCOS be monitored regularly for obesity and the metabolic syndrome [28]. They should be screened for prediabetes/type 2 diabetes mellitus with an oral glucose tolerance test [24].

Given the risk of obesity and metabolic syndrome, lifestyle modifications are an important component of PCOS treatment for those who are overweight/obese [6, 8, 24]. These modifications include a healthy diet with the goal of weight loss, as well as regular exercise. Studies have shown that these lifestyle modifications can help decrease testosterone levels, improve the metabolic profile, and regulate menses [6, 29].

In addition to lifestyle modifications, the Endocrine Society recommends hormonal contraceptives as the first-line treatment for irregular menses and hyperandrogenism [24]. These can include oral contraceptive pills (OCPs) or ethinyl estradiol and progestin-releasing patches/rings. For adolescents, the Pediatric Endocrine Society recommends using OCPs [6]. Estrogen reduces free androgen levels through an increase in SHBG and suppression of LH, resulting in improved acne and sometimes improved hirsutism. Progesterone helps prevent endometrial hyperplasia. Hormonal contraceptives do increase the risk of blood clots, and can sometimes lead to greater insulin resistance and hyperlipidemia [5]. Contraindications to hormonal contraceptives include hypercoagulable states, such as protein C deficiency, Protein S deficiency, or Factor V Leiden mutation [9]. Migraines and hypertension are relative contraindications, given the increased risk of stroke when using OCPs in these conditions [30]. When OCPs are contraindicated, progestin-only contraceptives, including progestin-releasing intrauterine devices (IUD), that prevent endometrial hyperplasia may be considered. However, progestin-only contraceptives do not always reduce free testosterone levels (particularly the progestin-releasing IUD), and thus may not improve features of hyperandrogenism.

For those girls with significant hyperandrogenism, particularly hirsutism, anti-androgens can also be used. Spironolactone, an androgen receptor blocker, is the drug most commonly used in adolescents [6]. Spironolactone is usually well tolerated with a low side-effect profile, although it can cause hyperkalemia, orthostatic hypotension, headaches, or fatigue [9]. Electrolytes should be monitored periodically in patients on spironolactone [28]. It is recommended that spironolactone be used with OCPs for maximal effect and because spironolactone is teratogenic and can cause under-virilization in a male fetus. Spironolactone, without concomitant OCP use, has also been associated with irregular menses with heavy or variable flow. When OCPs are contraindicated, a progestin-only contraceptive may be considered with spironolactone. For those with hirsutism, as medications generally only slow hair growth, cosmetic treatments are also often necessary. These can include electrolysis, laser hair removal, waxing, depilatory creams, or shaving [28].

Metformin is often used in PCOS, particularly in those with impaired glucose tolerance or type 2 diabetes mellitus. It can be used in conjunction with OCPs, or sometimes as a second-line treatment if OCPs are contraindicated. Studies in adolescents have shown some improvement in BMI and menstrual regularity with metformin [6], and it has the advantage of not causing hyperlipidemia. However, one met-analysis showed that OCPs were better at achieving menstrual regularity than metformin [4]. Metformin use is also associated with improved ovulation in patients with PCOS [5]; therefore, this is best used with hormonal or other contraceptives. Further studies are needed before clear recommendations can be made on the utility of metformin in adolescents with PCOS [6].

Summary

PCOS is a relatively common disorder of ovarian dysfunction that can result in anovulatory cycles, hyperandrogenism, and polycystic ovaries. Genetics, environmental factors, and insulin resistance likely all play a role in its etiology. Patients with PCOS should be monitored for obesity and associated comorbidities, especially type 2 diabetes mellitus. Treatment includes lifestyle modifications, along with OCPs, and/or spironolactone, and/or metformin.

References

1. Yildiz BO, Bozdag G, Yapici Z, Esinler I, Yarali H. Prevalence, phenotype and cardiometabolic risk of polycystic ovary syndrome under different diagnostic criteria. Hum Reprod. 2012;27(10):3067–73.
2. Azziz R, Carmina E, Chen Z, Dunaif A, Laven JS, Legro RS, et al. Polycystic ovary syndrome. Nat Rev Dis Primers. 2016;2:16057.
3. Lizneva D, Suturina L, Walker W, Brakta S, Gavrilova-Jordan L, Azziz R. Criteria, prevalence, and phenotypes of polycystic ovary syndrome. Fertil Steril. 2016;106(1):6–15.
4. Al Khalifah RA, Florez ID, Dennis B, Thabane L, Bassilious E. Metformin or oral contraceptives for adolescents with polycystic ovarian syndrome: a meta-analysis. Pediatrics. 2016;137(5)

5. Witchel SF, Roumimper H, Oberfield S. Polycystic ovary syndrome in adolescents. Endocrinol Metab Clin N Am. 2016;45(2):329–44.
6. Ibanez L, Oberfield SE, Witchel S, Auchus RJ, Chang RJ, Codner E, et al. An international consortium update: pathophysiology, diagnosis, and treatment of polycystic ovarian syndrome in adolescence. Horm Res Paediatr. 2017;88(6):371–95.
7. Rosenfield RL, Ehrmann DA, Littlejohn EE. Adolescent polycystic ovary syndrome due to functional ovarian hyperandrogenism persists into adulthood. J Clin Endocrinol Metab. 2015;100(4):1537–43.
8. Rothenberg SS, Beverley R, Barnard E, Baradaran-Shoraka M, Sanfilippo JS. Polycystic ovary syndrome in adolescents. Best Pract Res Clin Obstet Gynaecol. 2018;48:103–14.
9. Lifshitz F. Pediatric endocrinology. 5th ed; 2006. p. 325–48.
10. Kahsar-Miller MD, Nixon C, Boots LR, Go RC, Azziz R. Prevalence of polycystic ovary syndrome (PCOS) in first-degree relatives of patients with PCOS. Fertil Steril. 2001;75(1):53–8.
11. Stepto NK, Cassar S, Joham AE, Hutchison SK, Harrison CL, Goldstein RF, et al. Women with polycystic ovary syndrome have intrinsic insulin resistance on euglycaemic-hyperinsulaemic clamp. Hum Reprod. 2013;28(3):777–84.
12. Ibanez L, Dimartino-Nardi J, Potau N, Saenger P. Premature adrenarche–normal variant or forerunner of adult disease? Endocr Rev. 2000;21(6):671–96.
13. Neville KA, Walker JL. Precocious pubarche is associated with SGA, prematurity, weight gain, and obesity. Arch Dis Child. 2005;90(3):258–61.
14. Anderson AD, Solorzano CM, McCartney CR. Childhood obesity and its impact on the development of adolescent PCOS. Semin Reprod Med. 2014;32(3):202–13.
15. Aydin B, Winters SJ. Sex hormone-binding globulin in children and adolescents. J Clin Res Pediatr Endocrinol. 2016;8(1):1–12.
16. McCartney CR, Prendergast KA, Chhabra S, Eagleson CA, Yoo R, Chang RJ, et al. The association of obesity and hyperandrogenemia during the pubertal transition in girls: obesity as a potential factor in the genesis of postpubertal hyperandrogenism. J Clin Endocrinol Metab. 2006;91(5):1714–22.
17. Moran A, Jacobs DR Jr, Steinberger J, Hong CP, Prineas R, Luepker R, et al. Insulin resistance during puberty: results from clamp studies in 357 children. Diabetes. 1999;48(10):2039–44.
18. Caprio S, Plewe G, Diamond MP, Simonson DC, Boulware SD, Sherwin RS, et al. Increased insulin secretion in puberty: a compensatory response to reductions in insulin sensitivity. J Pediatr. 1989;114(6):963–7.
19. EA-SPCWG R. Revised 2003 consensus on diagnostic criteria and long-term health risks related to polycystic ovary syndrome. Fertil Steril. 2004;81(1):19–25.
20. Balen AH, Laven JS, Tan SL, Dewailly D. Ultrasound assessment of the polycystic ovary: international consensus definitions. Hum Reprod Update. 2003;9(6):505–14.
21. Witchel SF, Azziz R. Nonclassic congenital adrenal hyperplasia. Int J Pediatr Endocrinol. 2010;2010:625105.
22. Pall M, Azziz R, Beires J, Pignatelli D. The phenotype of hirsute women: a comparison of polycystic ovary syndrome and 21-hydroxylase-deficient nonclassic adrenal hyperplasia. Fertil Steril. 2010;94(2):684–9.
23. Escobar-Morreale HF, Sanchon R, San Millan JL. A prospective study of the prevalence of nonclassical congenital adrenal hyperplasia among women presenting with hyperandrogenic symptoms and signs. J Clin Endocrinol Metab. 2008;93(2):527–33.
24. Legro RS, Arslanian SA, Ehrmann DA, Hoeger KM, Murad MH, Pasquali R, et al. Diagnosis and treatment of polycystic ovary syndrome: an Endocrine Society clinical practice guideline. J Clin Endocrinol Metab. 2013;98(12):4565–92.
25. Franks S. Adult polycystic ovary syndrome begins in childhood. Best Pract Res Clin Endocrinol Metab. 2002;16(2):263–72.
26. Olutunmbi Y, Paley K, English JC 3rd. Adolescent female acne: etiology and management. J Pediatr Adolesc Gynecol. 2008;21(4):171–6.
27. Youngster M, Ward VL, Blood EA, Barnewolt CE, Emans SJ, Divasta AD. Utility of ultrasound in the diagnosis of polycystic ovary syndrome in adolescents. Fertil Steril. 2014;102(5):1432–8.
28. Witchel SF, Oberfield SE, Pena AS. Polycystic ovary syndrome: pathophysiology, presentation, and treatment with emphasis on adolescent girls. J Endocr Soc. 2019;3(8):1545–73.
29. Lass N, Kleber M, Winkel K, Wunsch R, Reinehr T. Effect of lifestyle intervention on features of polycystic ovarian syndrome, metabolic syndrome, and intima-media thickness in obese adolescent girls. J Clin Endocrinol Metab. 2011;96(11):3533–40.
30. Curtis KM, Chrisman CE, Peterson HB, WHOPfMBPiR H. Contraception for women in selected circumstances. Obstet Gynecol. 2002;99(6):1100–12.

Disorders of Sex Development

46

Rebecca M. Harris

Overview

Disorders of sex development (DSDs) are a heterogeneous group of conditions where genetic, gonadal, and phenotypic sex are discordant. DSDs are often diagnosed soon after birth due to variation in genital appearance on newborn exam. With the invention of noninvasive prenatal testing (NIPT), DSDs are increasingly diagnosed prenatally when sex chromosome complement is altered or found to be discordant from phenotypic sex. Fetal imaging alone may identify genital ambiguity, sometimes prompting further workup prenatally. DSDs that are not diagnosed prenatally or in infancy may be diagnosed later in life due to pubertal abnormalities (e.g., primary amenorrhea, progressive virilization in a phenotypic female, etc.) or infertility.

DSDs can be divided into three categories: 46,XX, 46,XY [1], and sex chromosome DSDs [2, 3]. Sex chromosome DSDs involve changes in the number of sex chromosomes, such as in Turner syndrome (45,X), Klinefelter syndrome (47,XXY), and mixed gonadal dysgenesis (MGD) (45,X/46,XY). Individuals with 46,XX DSDs demonstrate virilization on exam, and individuals with 46,XY DSDs are under-virilized. Alteration in virilization can be due to aberrant gonadal development, abnormal androgen synthesis or action, or in utero exposure to exogenous compounds. The ability to make a molecular diagnosis varies widely based on type of DSD [1] and also specific underlying etiology (80–90% in complete androgen insensitivity syndrome (CAIS) compared with ~20% in gonadal dysgenesis) [4]. Currently, there are gene panels that are used to diagnose DSDs clinically, and there is ongoing research using whole exome and genome sequencing [5]. The incidence of DSDs varies widely based on the underlying etiology, but it has been estimated that the incidence of ambiguous genitalia in infants is 1 in 5500 [6].

In 2006, the American Academy of Pediatrics, the Pediatric Endocrine Society, and the European Society for Paediatric Endocrinology released a joint consensus statement on the management of DSDs. While the title of the article used the term "intersex," the groups noted the controversial nature of such terminology (e.g., intersex, hermaphroditism, etc.) and recommended using "disorders of sex development" [2, 7]. However, even this term remains somewhat controversial, and some prefer the term "differences in sex development" [8].

The consensus statement highlighted the importance of a supportive initial interaction between medical personnel, the patient (depending on the age), and the family [2]. Oftentimes, it is the primary care physician who makes the diagnosis of a DSD, and that first interaction is crucial to setting the stage for future interactions. In the case of newborns, it is recommended that gender assignment occur after evaluation at a center with a multidisciplinary team comprised of pediatric subspecialists (endocrinology, urology/surgery, and psychology/psychiatry). Additionally, there must be good communication between the multidisciplinary team and the primary care provider. All members of the medical team must respect the family's desire for privacy and work together to support the family's needs and provide information to assist the family in medical decision-making [2]. Additionally, many families find support and advocacy groups to be a helpful resource. An update to the 2006 consensus statement published in 2016 included an extensive, international list of DSD support and advocacy groups [9].

Clinical Key
Making a gender assignment should not be considered an "emergency," nor should performing genital surgery (unless there is an urgent indication). Consensus recommendations suggest a multidisciplinary approach with multiple discussions between the family and providers to discuss gender assignment and timing of genital surgery.

R. M. Harris (✉)
Department of Pediatrics, Division of Endocrinology, Boston Children's Hospital, Boston, MA, USA
e-mail: rebecca.harris@childrens.harvard.edu

T. Stanley, M. Misra (eds.), *Endocrine Conditions in Pediatrics*, https://doi.org/10.1007/978-3-030-52215-5_46

Urgent/Emergent Considerations and Initial Management

Critical first steps in communication and management for an infant with a DSD are shown in Table 46.1, and recommended initial laboratory evaluation is shown in Table 46.2. From a medical perspective, the one emergent issue is salt-wasting congenital adrenal hyperplasia (CAH). Salt-wasting CAH can be caused by deficiency of steroid acute regulatory (StAR) protein, 3ß-hydroxysteroid dehydrogenase (3ß-HSD), or 21-hydroxylase (21-OHD) (see Chap. 49) [10]. Salt-wasting, due to mineralocorticoid deficiency, results in hyperkalemia and hyponatremia between a few days to a few weeks after birth [10]. Once CAH is suspected, a pediatric endocrinologist should be contacted immediately to discuss workup, monitoring, and management. Electrolytes should be monitored daily, and medical management with hydrocortisone, fludrocortisone, and, if needed, sodium supplementation should be initiated.

When evaluating an infant for a DSD, it is important to obtain a thorough prenatal history, including maternal medical conditions, medication use during pregnancy, exposures, maternal virilization during pregnancy, and results of prenatal testing [10]. A family history should also be obtained, including consanguinity, genetic conditions, infertility, lack of menstruation, ambiguous genitalia, and unexplained deaths [10]. A physical exam should be completed, including vital signs (particularly blood pressure), anthropomorphic measurements, evaluation for dysmorphology, and assessment of the genitals. In cases where the karyotype is unknown and the genital anatomy is ambiguous, it may be appropriate to use non-gendered terms such as "labioscrotal" instead of "labial" or "scrotal." A complete genital examination includes assessing the length and width of the clitorophallus, palpation for phallic tissue, assessing labioscrotal fusion, labioscrotal hyperpigmentation, presence of inguinal/labioscrotal masses, location of the urethral meatus, and Prader or Quigley staging [11]. Anogenital length was previously used as a metric of androgen action, but insufficient normative data have made this measurement less useful [12]. Quantitative scoring systems, such as the external masculinization score, have also been developed to standardize the assessment of ambiguous genitalia in infants [13].

Table 46.1 Initial steps in communication and management for newborns with DSD

Diagnostic priorities
The medical priority is to ensure the absence of salt-wasting CAH, which causes electrolyte abnormalities and virilization in 46,XX infants. This is done with assessment of 17-hydroxyprogesterone and serial electrolyte measurements.
If hypopituitarism is suspected, additional pituitary hormones should be assessed, and testing performed for hypoglycemia.
Beyond these two issues, the diagnostic evaluation should be expedited to provide parents with additional information as soon as possible, but this is not emergent.
Communication priorities
Acknowledge the difficulty of the situation while providing reassurance to families regarding the infant's overall health when appropriate.
Discourage premature decisions about gender assignment and naming until all necessary diagnostic information is available.
Provide the family with vetted information regarding online support groups for DSD.
Enlist specialist consultation from a pediatric endocrinologist, mental health professional (psychiatrist, psychologist, and/or social worker), pediatric urologist and/or pediatric surgeon, and, when possible, a geneticist, gynecologist, and neonatologist.

Table 46.2 Initial laboratory management of an infant with ambiguous genitalia

Laboratory testing	
Test	*Comments*
Karyotype	Call lab to request expedited testing
17-hydroxyprogesterone	Elevated in the most common forms of CAH (21-hydroxylase deficiency, 11-hydroxylase deficiency, and 3β-HSD deficiency). For newborn screening values, interpret and manage based on gestational age and algorithms provided by screening programs. Note that the reference units used by the newborn screen may be different than those used by the hospital laboratory.
Gonadotropins (luteinizing hormone (LH) and follicle stimulating hormone (FSH))	Helpful in differentiating primary (high LH and FSH) vs. secondary/tertiary (inappropriately low LH and FSH) gonadal dysfunction.
Total testosterone	Testosterone peaks around day 1 of life, and then there is a physiologic nadir during the first week of life. Testosterone should ideally be measured after 1 week of life. Low values during the first week of life should be verified with subsequent measurement.
Anti-Mullerian hormone (AMH)	Produced by Sertoli cells in response to FSH; values in the male range indicate functioning testicular tissue.
Electrolytes (sodium and potassium)	In infants with salt-wasting forms of CAH, electrolytes may be normal during the first 1–3 weeks of life and should be followed every 1–3 days as long as CAH remains on the differential.

If the patient is peri- or postpubertal, a history of pubertal development, menstrual history, and surgeries (e.g., repair of an inguinal hernia) should be obtained. The exam may include anthropomorphic measurements, vital signs (particularly blood pressure), evaluation for dysmorphic features, Tanner staging [14, 15], measurement of gonadal volume using an orchidometer, virilization status (e.g., Ferriman-Gallway scale [16]), evaluation for inguinal hernias, and evaluation for breast tissue in designated males.

In newborns, initial laboratory evaluation includes a karyotype and levels of 17-hydroxyprogesterone, gonadotropins, testosterone, anti-Mullerian hormone, and electrolytes (Table 46.1) [10]. Measurement of 17-hydroxyprogesterone should occur at least 36 hours after birth as there is a surge immediately after birth, which may result in a false positive [9]. Abdominal and pelvic ultrasound is useful to evaluate internal structures and gonads. Depending on the results, further evaluation in the subspecialty clinic can occur. Before obtaining laboratory and imaging studies, it is beneficial to contact a pediatric endocrinologist to discuss testing recommendations and to determine if testing should be sent by the primary care physician or the subspecialist as different laboratories use different assays, and some laboratories may process specimens more emergently.

While not medically urgent, the issue of sex designation in an infant with ambiguous genitalia can instill a sense of psychosocial urgency [4]. It can be very stressful when families are confronted with the diagnosis of a DSD, calling into question the sex of the baby. Additionally, recommending that families wait to designate the infant's sex until after the medical workup has been completed can be very difficult for families. Multidisciplinary teams in dedicated DSD clinics can provide assistance navigating such interactions, but the initial interaction between a family and their primary care provider is critical. Refraining from the use of gendered-pronouns (he/his or she/her) and instead using gender-neutral terms such as "your child" or "your baby" may be helpful. It may also be appropriate to ask parents what pronouns they prefer.

Historically, several factors contributed to the designation of sex, including the type of DSD, degree of virilization, surgical options, future fertility, and familial beliefs/culture [2]. Over time, the relative contributions of some of these factors have shifted, but it is still important to discuss each factor with the family. While many physicians wish they could provide a definitive answer regarding sex of rearing based on the underlying etiology of the DSD, there remain insufficient data on the affirmed genders of individuals with DSDs. As each type of DSD is distinct, gender outcomes cannot be studied in aggregate, and some DSD subtypes are rare. The two DSD diagnoses with the most data on gender outcomes are 46,XY CAIS and 46,XX CAH. In these conditions, the vast majority of individuals affirm a female gender, but there remain individuals who affirm a male gender or lie somewhere along the gender spectrum. Part of the job of the multidisciplinary DSD team is to discuss what is known about gender outcomes based on the underlying diagnosis but also to explain that there is always a degree of uncertainty.

Surgery and Considerations for Referral

The question of surgery is often one of the most ethically complex issues in the care of individuals with DSDs [17]. There are different types of surgeries depending on the underlying diagnosis and genital appearance, including genitoplasty (i.e., clitoroplasty, vaginoplasty, and phalloplasty), urogenital sinus mobilization, hypospadias repair, and gonadectomy. Some surgeries are indicated to prevent malignancy, such as gonadectomy in the case of gonadal dysgenesis with Y-chromosome material. Other surgeries, such as hypospadias repair, are generally agreed upon to maintain function. However, many surgeries are elective and may not have sufficient data on long-term outcomes such as rates of additional surgeries or complications [18]. There has been a shift away from performing surgery solely for cosmesis and toward preserving function and innervation. There has also been a shift toward delaying surgery until the individual with a DSD has affirmed their gender identity or attained decisional capacity to engage in discussions regarding surgery.

Regardless of age, all individuals with a DSD should be referred to a multidisciplinary DSD clinic. The needs of an individual with a DSD and the family will change over time [3], and having access to a team of knowledgeable subspecialty providers to help navigate the medical and psychosocial decisions is key. Issues such as whether or when to undergo surgery, what type of surgery should be undertaken, assistance with progression through puberty, and questions about future fertility may arise over time. Discussions surrounding these issues need to be tailored to the specific diagnosis and circumstances, again requiring the input from multiple subspecialists working together with the primary care provider.

Bibliography

1. Wisniewski AB, Batista RL, Costa EMF, Finlayson C, Sircili MHP, Dénes FT, et al. Management of 46,XY differences/disorders of sex development (DSD) throughout life. Endocr Rev. 2019;40(6):1547–72.
2. Lee PA, Houk CP, Ahmed SF, Hughes IA. Consensus statement on management of intersex disorders. Pediatrics. 2006;118(2):e488–500.
3. Cools M, Nordenström A, Robeva R, Hall J, Flück C, Köhler B, et al. Caring for individuals with a difference of sex development (DSD): a consensus statement. Nat Rev Endocrinol. 2018;14(7):415–29.

4. Hughes IA. Disorders of sex development: a new definition and classification. Best Pract Res Clin Endocrinol Metab. 2008;22(1):119–34.
5. Arboleda VA, Sandberg DE, Vilain E. DSDs: genetics, underlying pathologies and psychosexual differentiation. Nat Rev Endocrinol. 2014;10(10):603–15.
6. Sax L. How common is intersex? A response to Anne Fausto-Sterling. J Sex Res. 2002;39(3):174–8.
7. Hughes IA, Houk C, Ahmed SF, Lee PA. Consensus statement on management of intersex disorders. J Pediatr Urol. 2006;2(3):148–62.
8. Lin-su K, Lekarev O, Poppas DP, Vogiatzi MG. Congenital adrenal hyperplasia patient perception of ' disorders of sex development ' nomenclature. Int J Pediatr Endocrinol. 2015;1(9):1–7.
9. Lee PA, Nordenström A, Houk CP, Ahmed SF, Auchus R, Baratz A, et al. Global disorders of sex development update since 2006: perceptions, approach and care. Horm Res Paediatr. 2016;85(3):158–80.
10. Ogilvy-Stuart AL, Brain CE. Early assessment of ambiguous genitalia. Arch Dis Child. 2004;89(5):401–7.
11. Prader A. Genital findings in the female pseudo-hermaphroditism of the congenital adrenogenital syndrome; morphology, frequency, development and heredity of the different genital forms. Helv Paediatr Acta. 1954;9(3):231–48.
12. Dean A, Sharpe RM. Anogenital distance or digit length ratio as measures of fetal androgen exposure: relationship to male reproductive development and its disorders. J Clin Endocrinol Metab. 2013;98(6):2230–8.
13. Ahmed SF, Khwaja O, Hughes IA. The role of a clinical score in the assessment of ambiguous genitalia. BJU Int. 2000;85:120–4.
14. Marshall W, Tanne J. Variations in the pattern of pubertal changes in girls. Arch Dis Child. 1969;44(235):291–303.
15. Marshall W, Tanner J. Variations in the pattern of pubertal changes in boys. Arch Dis Childhood. 1970;45(239):13.
16. Hatch R, Rosenfield R, Kim M, Tredway D. Hirsutism: implications, etiology, and management. Am J Obes Gynecol. 1981;140(7):815–30.
17. Harris RM, Chan Y-M. Ethical issues with early genitoplasty in children with disorders of sex development. Curr Opin Endocrinol Diabetes Obes. 2019;26(1):49–53.
18. Lee P, Schober J, Nordenström A, Hoebeke P, Houk C, Looijenga L, et al. Review of recent outcome data of disorders of sex development (DSD): emphasis on surgical and sexual outcomes. J Pediatr Urol. 2012;8(6):611–5.

Turner Syndrome

47

Lynne L. Levitsky

Overview

Turner syndrome is a relatively common sex chromosome disorder, found in 1 in 2000–4000 phenotypically female newborns. It is the result of the loss of all or part of the genetic material of one of the X chromosomes in some or all cells in the body (complete or partial monosomy X). Turner syndrome may be diagnosed prenatally because of chromosome studies (karyotype) performed because of advanced maternal age or in vitro fertilization, or because findings on ultrasound including an enhanced nuchal fold, cystic hygroma, or left-sided heart disease prompt a genetic evaluation. Postnatally, congenital cardiac disease (most commonly involving the left heart and vessels), neck webbing with redundant posterior neck skin, or lymphedema of the feet and hands may suggest the need for karyotype studies for Turner syndrome. Because girls with Turner syndrome who lack the short arm of an X chromosome (Xp) have a deletion in the SHOX gene important for growth, slow postnatal linear growth often triggers a genetic study for Turner syndrome. Absence of the SHOX gene, which encodes a protein necessary for continued growth at the growth plate, leads to short stature, abnormal development of facial bones, and other bony abnormalities such as short fourth metacarpals, Madelung deformity, and cubitus valgus with relatively short limbs compared with the trunk. Other genes affecting ovarian development, found mostly on the long arm of the X chromosome (Xq), lead to maldevelopment of the ovaries or early ovarian failure. During adolescence, girls are commonly diagnosed because they do not have breast development or reach menarche, although they may have pubic hair. Occasionally women are diagnosed only as adults during evaluations for infertility. Associated renal problems related to loss of X chromosome genes include horseshoe kidney or other renal malformations. Cardiac malformations can range from bicuspid aortic valve to left heart hypoplasia. Progressive aortic dilatation and aortic arch dissection may occur. Lymphedema of the feet and legs may persist into adulthood. Girls and young women with Turner syndrome are more prone to develop various autoimmune endocrine disorders including chronic lymphocytic thyroiditis and hypothyroidism, as well as hyperthyroidism and type 1 diabetes. They may also develop other autoimmune disorders including vitiligo, celiac disease, and inflammatory bowel disease. Conductive as well as sensorineural hearing loss is more common, as is strabismus and hyperopia. Specific problems with learning may manifest, particularly at school age.

The loss of X chromosomal material during early development seems to occur randomly and is not related to older maternal or paternal age.

L. L. Levitsky (✉)
Harvard Medical School, Boston, MA, USA

Massachusetts General Hospital, Boston, MA, USA
e-mail: Lynne.Levitsky@mgh.harvard.edu

Reference Box: Key Pathophysiology (Clinical Findings): (Modified from Data in Ref. [1])

All Ages

Congenital heart disease (50%)—usually left heart
Renal malformations (10–20%), often horseshoe kidney (10%)

Infancy

Redundant neck skin folds (25%)
Low posterior hairline (40%)
Small mandible (60%)
High-arched palate; trouble latching on to breastfeed (35%)
Puffy hands and feet (lymphedema of dorsal surface) (25%)

Childhood

Slow growth or short stature (95%)
Neck webbing with low posterior hairline (25–40%)

T. Stanley, M. Misra (eds.), *Endocrine Conditions in Pediatrics*, https://doi.org/10.1007/978-3-030-52215-5_47

Classic facial appearance (60 + %)
Broad, "shield-shaped" chest with appearance of widely spaced nipples (30%)
Madelung deformity (5%)
Short fourth metacarpals (35%)
Cubitus valgus (50%)
Ear infections (60%)
Hearing deficits (30%)

Adolescence
Short stature (95%)
Incomplete puberty:
  Lack of breast development (70%)
  Amenorrhea (90%)
  Normal pubic and axillary hair (+/−100%)

Making the Diagnosis

Required for Diagnosis

Abnormal karyotype demonstrating partial or complete monosomy X in some or all of the cells examined in association with one or more classic clinical findings.

Supporting the Diagnosis

Some or all of the clinical features of Turner syndrome including short stature, congenital heart disease, kidney abnormalities, and primary ovarian failure.

Urgent or Emergent Considerations and Initial Management Vary Depending upon Age at Diagnosis

Prenatal

When the diagnosis is made by karyotype prenatally, a geneticist can assess the severity of the findings and offer the parents a guarded picture of their daughter's future health and functioning. Prenatal counselling can assist the parents with decision-making and planning. Approximately 50% of Turner syndrome girls have X monosomy in all cells studied. The remainder have mosaicism (45,X/46,XX or other karyotypes). Many monosomy X fetuses do not survive and are relatively early spontaneous abortions. However, girls with Turner syndrome diagnosed prenatally because of an abnormal mosaic karyotype tend to have a milder phenotype than those diagnosed later because of phenotype. Most girls with Turner syndrome are intellectually normal, although some may have specific nonverbal learning disabilities and an increased risk of anxiety, obsessive thoughts, and behaviors. Some may have poor interpersonal skills. They tend to score higher in language than in mathematical skills and can have specific problems with spatial relationships. Girls with a very large X chromosome deletion, as in a ring chromosome X, may have more severe intellectual disability and function on the autism spectrum.

Ultrasound findings may also contribute to the decision-making process by identifying anatomic problems incompatible with long-term survival. Severe congenital heart disease diagnosed prenatally can lead to emergent or urgent delivery and treatment.

Infancy

Urgent management is required if there is severe cardiac disease. Redundant neck folds, puffy hands and feet because of lymphedema, a high-arched palate, and a classic facies may lead to a clinical diagnosis confirmed by karyotype in the newborn period. Appropriate subspecialty consultation, an echocardiogram, and a renal ultrasound are important to evaluate cardiac and renal anatomy. A high-arched palate may interfere with the ability to breastfeed. In addition, short and angled Eustachian tubes may prevent good drainage, increasing the risk of ear infection and hearing loss.

Rarely, there may be Y chromosome material present in some cells studied. The presence of Y chromosomal genetic material increases the risk of development of gonadal tumors during growth and development and in adulthood. Depending on the amount and location of Y chromosome material, close surveillance or early gonadectomy might be recommended.

Childhood

Girls are usually diagnosed in middle childhood because of slow growth rate and short stature. A peripheral blood karyotype should be part of all evaluations for short stature and slow growth in girls, without another obvious diagnosis. When the diagnosis of Turner syndrome is made in school-age children before the normal age of puberty, evaluation with cardiac and renal ultrasound, studies of thyroid function, tests for celiac disease, and a hearing evaluation comprise much of the initial clinical management. Parental counselling with age-appropriate counselling for the child is very important.

Adolescence

This diagnosis with its likelihood of infertility can be quite psychologically devastating to an adolescent, and psychological support may be very important, in parallel with the medical evaluation, as at other ages. Assessment of potential for ovarian function can be made by measurement of pituitary gonadotropin levels and anti-Müllerian hormone (see Chap. 27). Elevated gonadotropin levels measured as part of an evaluation for delayed puberty or amenorrhea should lead to karyotype analysis. If the X chromosome which is partially monosomic is deleted only distal to the long arm marker Xq24, then ovarian failure but not true Turner syndrome is likely, and this may be confirmed by other largely normal physical findings.

After the diagnosis of Turner syndrome, evaluation for other medical complications, counselling in regard to fertility, and plans for medical treatment should be developed.

Chronic Management and Considerations for Referral

During Childhood

At each physical examination at 4–6-month intervals after infancy, careful measurement of height and weight, observation for clinical history or physical findings of chronic illness, and pubertal progression should be made. Findings such as thyroid enlargement, failure to gain weight, abdominal pain, and changes in bowel habits should be evaluated. Poor eating habits and inactivity may lead to obesity, hypertension, and abnormal liver function studies, as well as hyperlipidemia. Type 2 diabetes may be a long-term outcome. Health maintenance includes yearly blood studies checking for autoimmune thyroid dysfunction (free thyroxine, thyroid stimulating hormone), lipid panel, comprehensive metabolic profile, complete blood count, a sedimentation rate or C-reactive protein looking for undiagnosed inflammatory bowel disease, and a hemoglobin A1C looking for glucose intolerance or frank diabetes. Because of concerns about bone density, 25-hydroxyvitamin D level should also be assessed yearly and vitamin D supplementation provided to maintain vitamin D in the normal range. Celiac disease antibody measurements should be performed every 2 years. Assessment of school and social functioning is equally important and may lead to appropriate referrals for focused evaluation.

All girls diagnosed with Turner syndrome should have the advantage of follow-up by a geneticist and an endocrinologist. Other subspecialists are important if associated comorbidities such as cardiac disease, hearing loss, or other neuropsychiatric problems become an issue. Diagnostic and management guidelines developed by an international consensus group in 2016 have been supported by multiple stakeholder societies (1, 2). It is important to follow these recommendations to maintain Turner syndrome patients in the best of health.

Subspecialty referrals should include the following.

Genetics

Diagnostic guidelines in children include complete X chromosome monosomy with loss of the other sex chromosome, or partial X chromosome monosomy with deletion of X chromosomal material on both the short arm (Xp) and long arm (Xq) of the X chromosome. Geneticists may sometimes recommend more specialized testing in other tissues to quantitate the nature of the monosomy. This is particularly important if there is unusual mosaicism, only low-level mosaicism in peripheral blood lymphocytes, or identification of Y chromosomal material. In some centers, geneticists will also maintain long-term follow-up of certain aspects of chronic care and work to ensure that Turner syndrome girls receive appropriate studies for health maintenance. Geneticists may also assist in counselling in regard to potential egg-saving techniques to enhance future fertility in some girls with mosaicism.

Endocrinology

The endocrinologist usually focuses on physical growth and development in girls with Turner syndrome. In some centers, the endocrinologist serves as the point person for many health maintenance activities as described above. In others, these activities are shared with the generalist, or with the geneticist. The endocrinologist will usually be responsible for growth- and development-related drug treatments, including the following.

Growth Hormone [3]

The mean adult height of untreated girls with Turner syndrome in the United States is 56 inches. Girls who come from shorter families will often be much shorter than this. Girls with Turner syndrome are not growth hormone deficient, but daily injections of growth hormone have been demonstrated to increase adult height by several inches. The earlier growth hormone is started, the greater height increase may be expected. In general, growth hormone therapy is initiated by 4–6 years of age, particularly in girls who have decreased growth velocity or come from families with short stature. Girls diagnosed later in childhood are often started on growth hormone soon after diagnosis. Growth hormone is ineffective after growth plate fusion and works best the earlier it is started. Most families opt for growth hormone therapy for their children, but others decide they would prefer not to treat. Growth hormone is discontinued when an adult height which the patient and her family deem appropriate is reached, or when the child reaches epiphyseal fusion. During the time growth hormone is administered, it is important to monitor for glucose intolerance with a hemoglobin A1c, and with an IGF-1 to assure that the circulating levels of IGF-1 do not become too high during growth hormone treatment. Studies should be obtained yearly and after dose increases. Careful physical examination and history, looking for physical side effects of growth hormone, including slipped capital femoral epiphysis, a rare result of rapid growth, increased intracranial pressure, manifested as headaches and blurred vision, as well as the development of other chronic illness, is important at each 4–6-month visit.

Oxandrolone

Oxandrolone is a weak androgen which cannot be converted to estrogen, so it is felt not to advance bone age. Some girls will receive this with growth hormone to enhance their height potential. It can be associated with mild androgen side effects such as a change in voice, slight hirsutism, or clitoromegaly.

Estrogen [4]

Estrogen is required at the age of normal puberty in girls who do not have sufficient ovarian function (95% of girls with Turner syndrome). About 30% of girls, largely with mosaic Turner syndrome, may have initial spontaneous puberty, but only a few maintain normal fertile ovarian cycles. Presently, very-low-dose estrogen therapy using an estradiol patch is recommended beginning between 11 and 12 years of age. The amount of estrogen is gradually increased, with the intent of inducing menarche with the addition of progesterone after 2–3 years. Because estrogen exposure leads to fusion of the epiphyseal growth plates, estrogen treatment is usually begun in a slow and judicious manner, in order to enhance adult height. Estrogen can also be provided as an oral medication, but most studies suggested that the patch has an improved safety profile and better outcomes in terms of increased bone density. Bone density should be checked at puberty and followed every 5 years, or more often, if there is reason for concern.

Progesterone

Oral progesterone is administered for 10–12 days out of every month once close-to-adult estrogen effect has been reached, in order to complete breast development, contribute to regular shedding of the endometrium, and decrease the risk of erratic bleeding and endometrial malignancy.

Estrogen–Progesterone Combinations

Once an adult pattern of "menstrual cycling" (withdrawal bleeding) has been established, many girls opt for a treatment that permits them to have menses only once every 3 months, using either patches and oral progesterone, an oral contraceptive medication, or some other effective combination of estrogen and progesterone.

Cardiology

All girls should have cardiology consultations and initial echocardiograms at diagnosis and, if these are normal, should have repeat studies at 5-year intervals. In later adolescence, cardiac magnetic resonance imaging (MRI) is recommended. Because of the risk of aortic enlargement and aortic dissection, depending upon the severity of findings, closer follow-up may be necessary.

Nephrology

Initial nephrology consultation and renal ultrasound will determine the nature and significance of renal abnormalities. If kidneys are anatomically normal, no further follow-up is indicated, unless a urinary tract infection, hypertension, or other issues develop. Hypertension is more common in these girls, particularly in association with obesity and inactivity. Children with horseshoe kidneys need to be counselled about avoidance of contact sports, including karate and horseback riding.

Audiology/Otolaryngology

Hearing should be assessed initially and then at 3–5-year intervals—more often in children with frequent ear infections. Otitis media should be treated aggressively to preserve hearing.

Child Development/Neuropsychology

Girls with Turner syndrome have an increased frequency of specific nonverbal learning disabilities and should be evaluated for these as is age appropriate so that they may have access to appropriate resources. Girls with larger deletions of X chromosome material (ring chromosome X) may have more severe learning and developmental issues and are more likely to present with an autism-spectrum disorder.

Child Psychiatry/Psychology/Counselling

Turner syndrome is associated with a higher prevalence of anxiety disorders, obsessive compulsive behaviors, and depression than in the general population. Access to therapists who can assist with these issues is most important. Both medication and cognitive behavioral therapy are very useful.

Other Commonly Needed Specialty Referrals

Girls with Turner syndrome should be seen by a dermatologist on a yearly basis because of a higher-than-usual number of nevi and a small risk of malignancy, by a vascular/lymphedema specialist if lymphedema is a persistent problem, by ophthalmology on a regular basis if esotropia or hyperopia needs treatment, and by orthopedics should there be evidence of scoliosis or a need to correct Madelung deformity interfering with function.

Transition to Adult Care

Comprehensive care should not cease at the end of adolescence. These young women will require specialized care for their multiple medical and psychological needs throughout life. Like other individuals with chronic conditions, their transition to adulthood is difficult, and transition to adult medical care must be carefully modeled and planned so that continuity of care is achieved. The generalist should facilitate and ensure this transition.

References

1. Gravholt CH, Andersen NH, Conway GS, et al; International Turner Syndrome Consensus Group. Clinical practice guidelines for the care of girls and women with Turner syndrome: proceedings from the 2016 Cincinnati International Turner Syndrome Meeting Eur J Endocrinol. 2017;177(3):G1–G70. https://doi.org/10.1530/EJE-17-0430. PMID: 28705803.
2. Lin AE, Prakash SK, Andersen NH, et al. Recognition and management of adults with Turner syndrome: from the transition of adolescence through the senior years. Am J Med Genet A. 2019;179(10):1987–2033. https://doi.org/10.1002/ajmg.a.61310. PMID: 31418527.
3. Los E, Rosenfeld RG. Growth and growth hormone in Turner syndrome: looking back, looking ahead. Am J Med Genet C Semin Med Genet. 2019;181(1):86–90. https://doi.org/10.1002/ajmg.c.31680. PMID: 30811776.
4. Klein KO, Rosenfield RL, Santen RJ, et al. Estrogen replacement in Turner syndrome: literature review and practical considerations. J Clin Endocrinol Metab. 2018;103(5):1790–803. https://doi.org/10.1210/jc.2017-02183x. PMID: 29438552.

48 Klinefelter Syndrome

Jordan S. Sherwood

Overview

Klinefelter syndrome is the most prevalent sex chromosomal disorder in the male population, with an estimated incidence of about 1:650 men [1]. The most common underlying etiology is XXY aneuploidy, but other rarer causes include 46,XY/47,XXY mosaicism, 48,XXXY, and 49,XXXXY [2, 3]. The additional X chromosome can be inherited from either parent due to nondisjunction during meiosis. The phenotypical presentation of Klinefelter syndrome is variable, ranging from mildly affected individuals to those with more severe presentations. The severity of presentation is more pronounced with an increased number of X chromosomes present [4, 5]. Given the phenotypic variability, Klinefelter syndrome is often diagnosed later in life, with an average age of diagnosis of 21 years [6]. However, with the increasing frequency of noninvasive prenatal genetic testing (NIPT) via cell-free fetal DNA, there may be a growing number of cases diagnosed prior to birth [7].

The primary feature of Klinefelter syndrome is hypergonadotropic hypogonadism related to underlying testicular dysfunction [8, 9]. Signs of hypogonadism may be present at birth, with microphallus and cryptorchidism, or during adolescence, with incomplete progression of puberty, or in adulthood, with infertility. Delayed puberty per se is not a typical feature of Klinefelter syndrome. Nearly all patients with Klinefelter syndrome will have underlying infertility [10]. Many cases of Klinefelter syndrome are diagnosed in the process of evaluation for difficulty conceiving [11]. Adults with Klinefelter syndrome will have small, firm testes and elevated gonadotropins (luteinizing hormone and follicle stimulating hormone) with low or low-normal testosterone levels. Other physical stigmata of Klinefelter syndrome include taller-than-average height, increased arm span and gynecomastia [12]. Patients with Klinefelter syndrome also have a higher frequency of obesity, insulin resistance, type 2 diabetes, and metabolic syndrome [13]. Furthermore, those with Klinefelter syndrome are at risk for decreased bone mineral density [14]. Individuals with Klinefelter syndrome may have learning difficulty, specifically in the area of speech and language development [15]. Most studies demonstrate that cognitive ability of patients with Klinefelter's is generally in the normal range [16–18]. Comorbid psychiatric conditions such as depression and anxiety are also common in Klinefelter's, as are attention-deficit/hyperactivity disorder (ADHD) and autism spectrum disorder [19]. Testosterone replacement therapy is the primary medical treatment. The care team for patients with Klinefelter's may include medical genetics, endocrinology, reproductive endocrinology, and psychiatry/neuropsychology.

Key Pathophysiology

The underlying pathology in Klinefelter syndrome is related to the aneuploidy of the extra X chromosome, typically due to nondisjunction [2, 3]. This aneuploidy results in dysfunction of Sertoli and Leydig cells, which leads to impaired testosterone synthesis, as well as diminished spermatogenesis (oligospermia or azoospermia), resulting in hypogonadism and infertility [20]. Hypogonadism may have variable presentation depending on age. In infancy, hypogonadism may present with signs of under-virilization such as microphallus and/or cryptorchidism. In adolescence, hypogonadism may present with incomplete pubertal progression or, much less commonly, delayed puberty. In adulthood, infertility is nearly universal, and testicular sperm extraction (TESE) has variable success in achieving sperm retrieval for fertility [21–24]. As in other etiologies of hypergonadotropic hypogonadism, gonadotropins (LH and FSH) are elevated, with low or low-normal testosterone levels, as well as low inhibin B and AMH (makers of Sertoli cell reserve/function) [25].

Hypogonadism is also thought to be one of the contributing etiologies of other clinical features seen in Klinefelter

J. S. Sherwood (✉)
Massachusetts General Hospital, Boston, MA, USA
e-mail: jssherwood@partners.org

T. Stanley, M. Misra (eds.), *Endocrine Conditions in Pediatrics*, https://doi.org/10.1007/978-3-030-52215-5_48

syndrome, such as gynecomastia, increased adiposity, decrease in lean muscle mass, insulin resistance, and metabolic syndrome. Low bone mineral density has been reported in individuals with Klinefelter syndrome, potentially predisposing patients to increased fracture risk [26].

Gynecomastia may present in the adolescent age group and persist into adulthood. Severe gynecomastia may require surgical referral for treatment. An elevated risk of breast cancer in men with Klinefelter syndrome compared to individuals with 46,XY karyotype has been described. However, the overall lifetime breast cancer risk is lower than that of women [27]. Additionally, there has been a reported increased incidence of other cancers, particularly mediastinal germ cell tumors, in those with Klinefelter syndrome [28].

Increased risk for autoimmune disorders, compared to the general population, has also been reported in patients with Klinefelter syndrome; increased prevalence of hypothyroidism, type 1 diabetes, adrenal insufficiency, and systemic lupus erythematosus has been described [29].

Other features of Klinefelter syndrome are thought to be related to increased gene expression from the extra X chromosome due to altered X-inactivation [12]. For example, the SHOX gene (short-stature-homeobox-containing gene), a transcription factor expressed in bone, is located and expressed on a pseudoautosomal region of the X chromosome. Mutations of the SHOX gene and its under-expression in Turner syndrome (45X) have been shown to result in short stature [30]. Overexpression of this gene due to an extra copy in patients with 47,XXY is thought to be the cause of tall stature [31].

Diagnosis

Klinefelter syndrome is a genetic diagnosis achieved by karyotyping. Findings common to Klinefelter syndrome that should prompt consideration of testing are shown in Table 48.1.

Table 48.1 Findings supporting the diagnosis of Klinefelter syndrome

History/physical findings	Tall stature
	Increased arm span
	Increased leg length
	Gynecomastia
	Microphallus
	Cryptorchidism
	Hypospadias
	Small and firm testes (adults/adolescents)
	Low bone mineral density
	Obesity
	Learning difficulties
	Anxiety/depression
Laboratory findings	↓ Testosterone
	↓ Inhibin B
	↓ Anti-Müllerian hormone (AMH)
	↑ Luteinizing hormone (LH)
	↑ Follicle stimulating hormone (FSH)
	Azoospermia/oligospermia
Confirmatory testing	Genetic testing (karyotype)

Urgent or Emergent Considerations and Initial Management

Consideration must be given regarding the disclosure of the diagnosis of Klinefelter syndrome to families when patients are in the pediatric age group [32]. Especially with the advancement and increasing uptake of non-invasive prenatal genetic testing, early diagnosis may become more frequent. There are no specific guidelines regarding disclosing the diagnosis of Klinefelter syndrome. Involvement of a genetic counselor or geneticist when possible may improve families' experiences. Information provided should be age-appropriate and provided in consultation with families.

The initial management of those with Klinefelter syndrome is ensuring that patients are screened for known sequalae and referred to appropriate subspecialties as needed.

Hypogonadism: Screening for hypogonadism includes obtaining gonadotropins (LH and FSH), as well as total testosterone levels. Other markers of testicular reserve can also be obtained, including anti-Müllerian hormone and inhibin B. Treatment of hypogonadism is accomplished with testosterone replacement therapy. There is limited evidence that suggests a course of androgen replacement in childhood may help improve neurocognitive outcomes [33]. During adolescence or adulthood, testosterone replacement can be given either via injection or transdermal preparations. The Endocrine Society has published guidelines regarding testosterone replacement for the treatment of primary hypogonadism [34].

Dyslipidemia: A lipid profile should be obtained given the increased risk of hyperlipidemia in this population. Treatment with lifestyle therapy and medical intervention can be initiated per American Heart Association guidelines [35].

Diabetes: Given the increased risk of metabolic syndrome and insulin resistance, screening for type 2 diabetes should be performed per American Diabetes Association recommendations. Screening for diabetes may be conducted with either a hemoglobin A1c, fasting plasma glucose, or a 2-hour oral glucose tolerance test [36].

Bone Density: Those with Klinefelter syndrome are at high risk for low bone mineral density. Optimization of calcium and vitamin D intake is per age- and sex-specific recommended dietary intake. A dual-energy X-ray absorptiometry scan (DXA) can be considered for patients with history of recurrent fracture or history of low back pain concerning for vertebral fracture.

Autoimmune Disease: Thyroid function testing (see Chap. 25) can be performed to evaluate for autoimmune chronic lymphocytic thyroiditis (Hashimoto's hypothyroidism). Screening for other specific autoimmune disorders can be conducted based on symptomology and clinical suspicion.

Chronic Management and Considerations for Referral

Chronic management of patients with Klinefelter syndrome entails tailoring therapy based on individual need. Detailed history and physical findings should prompt screening and testing based on conditions known to present with increased frequency in those with Klinefelter syndrome. Referrals to the following subspecialists should be considered.

Genetics: Patients can be referred to a medical genetic specialist for genetic counseling and discussion of risks associated with the syndrome.

Endocrinology/Urology: Referral to a specialist can be considered for management of androgen replacement therapy for treatment of hypogonadism. Reproductive endocrinology/urology referral should be offered for discussion of fertility preservation. Testicular sperm extraction has been performed successfully in patients with Klinefelter syndrome.

Cognitive Behavioral Specialist/Neuropsychologist: Impaired verbal functioning is the most common neurodevelopmental issue. This may manifest with delayed language acquisition, as well as difficulty with reading, spelling, and expressive speech. Patients can be referred for neurocognitive testing to assess cognitive function to help guide treatment. Anxiety and depression are also prevalent; thus, it is important to screen for possible comorbid psychiatric conditions and refer to a mental health specialist if warranted.

References

1. Kronenberg H, Williams RH. Williams textbook of endocrinology. 11th ed. Philadelphia: Saunders/Elsevier; 2008. xix, 1911 pp.
2. Bojesen A, Juul S, Gravholt CH. Prenatal and postnatal prevalence of Klinefelter syndrome: a national registry study. J Clin Endocrinol Metab. 2003;88(2):622–6.
3. Tartaglia N, Ayari N, Howell S, D'Epagnier C, Zeitler P. 48,XXYY, 48,XXXY and 49,XXXXY syndromes: not just variants of Klinefelter syndrome. Acta Paediatr. 2011;100(6):851–60.
4. Close S, Fennoy I, Smaldone A, Reame N. Phenotype and adverse quality of life in boys with Klinefelter syndrome. J Pediatr. 2015;167(3):650–7.
5. Visootsak J, Graham JM Jr. Social function in multiple X and Y chromosome disorders: XXY, XYY, XXYY, XXXY. Dev Disabil Res Rev. 2009;15(4):328–32.
6. Visootsak J, Ayari N, Howell S, Lazarus J, Tartaglia N. Timing of diagnosis of 47,XXY and 48,XXYY: a survey of parent experiences. Am J Med Genet A. 2013;161A(2):268–72.
7. Zhang B, Lu BY, Yu B, Zheng FX, Zhou Q, Chen YP, et al. Noninvasive prenatal screening for fetal common sex chromosome aneuploidies from maternal blood. J Int Med Res. 2017;45(2):621–30.
8. Bonomi M, Rochira V, Pasquali D, Balercia G, Jannini EA, Ferlin A, et al. Klinefelter syndrome (KS): genetics, clinical phenotype and hypogonadism. J Endocrinol Investig. 2017;40(2):123–34.
9. Chang S, Skakkebaek A, Gravholt CH. Klinefelter syndrome and medical treatment: hypogonadism and beyond. Hormones (Athens). 2015;14(4):531–48.
10. Groth KA, Skakkebaek A, Host C, Gravholt CH, Bojesen A. Clinical review: Klinefelter syndrome--a clinical update. J Clin Endocrinol Metab. 2013;98(1):20–30.
11. Flannigan R, Schlegel PN. Genetic diagnostics of male infertility in clinical practice. Best Pract Res Clin Obstet Gynaecol. 2017;44:26–37.
12. Lanfranco F, Kamischke A, Zitzmann M, Nieschlag E. Klinefelter's syndrome. Lancet. 2004;364(9430):273–83.
13. Lizarazo AH, McLoughlin M, Vogiatzi MG. Endocrine aspects of Klinefelter syndrome. Curr Opin Endocrinol Diabetes Obes. 2019;26(1):60–5.
14. Breuil V, Euller-Ziegler L. Gonadal dysgenesis and bone metabolism. Joint Bone Spine. 2001;68(1):26–33.
15. Kanakis GA, Nieschlag E. Klinefelter syndrome: more than hypogonadism. Metabolism. 2018;86:135–44.
16. Fales CL, Knowlton BJ, Holyoak KJ, Geschwind DH, Swerdloff RS, Gonzalo IG. Working memory and relational reasoning in Klinefelter syndrome. J Int Neuropsychol Soc. 2003;9(6):839–46.
17. Bender BG, Linden MG, Harmon RJ. Neuropsychological and functional cognitive skills of 35 unselected adults with sex chromosome abnormalities. Am J Med Genet. 2001;102(4):309–13.
18. Ross JL, Roeltgen DP, Stefanatos G, Benecke R, Zeger MP, Kushner H, et al. Cognitive and motor development during childhood in boys with Klinefelter syndrome. Am J Med Genet A. 2008;146A(6):708–19.
19. Skakkebaek A, Moore PJ, Pedersen AD, Bojesen A, Kristensen MK, Fedder J, et al. Anxiety and depression in Klinefelter syndrome: the impact of personality and social engagement. PLoS One. 2018;13(11):e0206932.
20. Van Saen D, Vloeberghs V, Gies I, Mateizel I, Sermon K, De Schepper J, et al. When does germ cell loss and fibrosis occur in patients with Klinefelter syndrome? Hum Reprod. 2018;33(6):1009–22.
21. Rives N, Milazzo JP, Perdrix A, Castanet M, Joly-Helas G, Sibert L, et al. The feasibility of fertility preservation in adolescents with Klinefelter syndrome. Hum Reprod. 2013;28(6):1468–79.
22. Plotton I, Giscard d'Estaing S, Cuzin B, Brosse A, Benchaib M, Lornage J, et al. Preliminary results of a prospective study of testicular sperm extraction in young versus adult patients with nonmosaic 47,XXY Klinefelter syndrome. J Clin Endocrinol Metab. 2015;100(3):961–7.
23. Mehta A, Bolyakov A, Roosma J, Schlegel PN, Paduch DA. Successful testicular sperm retrieval in adolescents with Klinefelter syndrome treated with at least 1 year of topical testosterone and aromatase inhibitor. Fertil Steril. 2013;100(4):970–4.

24. Corona G, Pizzocaro A, Lanfranco F, Garolla A, Pelliccione F, Vignozzi L, et al. Sperm recovery and ICSI outcomes in Klinefelter syndrome: a systematic review and meta-analysis. Hum Reprod Update. 2017;23(3):265–75.
25. Rohayem J, Fricke R, Czeloth K, Mallidis C, Wistuba J, Krallmann C, et al. Age and markers of Leydig cell function, but not of Sertoli cell function predict the success of sperm retrieval in adolescents and adults with Klinefelter's syndrome. Andrology. 2015;3(5):868–75.
26. Swerdlow AJ, Higgins CD, Schoemaker MJ, Wright AF, Jacobs PA, United Kingdom Clinical Cytogenetics G. Mortality in patients with Klinefelter syndrome in Britain: a cohort study. J Clin Endocrinol Metab. 2005;90(12):6516–22.
27. Ferzoco RM, Ruddy KJ. The epidemiology of male breast cancer. Curr Oncol Rep. 2016;18(1):1.
28. Ji J, Zoller B, Sundquist J, Sundquist K. Risk of solid tumors and hematological malignancy in persons with Turner and Klinefelter syndromes: A national cohort study. Int J Cancer. 2016;139(4):754–8.
29. Seminog OO, Seminog AB, Yeates D, Goldacre MJ. Associations between Klinefelter's syndrome and autoimmune diseases: English national record linkage studies. Autoimmunity. 2015;48(2):125–8.
30. Oliveira CS, Alves C. The role of the SHOX gene in the pathophysiology of Turner syndrome. Endocrinol Nutr. 2011;58(8):433–42.
31. Berletch JB, Yang F, Disteche CM. Escape from X inactivation in mice and humans. Genome Biol. 2010;11(6):213.
32. Dennis A, Howell S, Cordeiro L, Tartaglia N. "How should I tell my child?" Disclosing the diagnosis of sex chromosome aneuploidies. J Genet Couns. 2015;24(1):88–103.
33. Ross JL, Kushner H, Kowal K, Bardsley M, Davis S, Reiss AL, et al. Androgen treatment effects on motor function, cognition, and behavior in boys with Klinefelter syndrome. J Pediatr. 2017;185:193–9 e4.
34. Bhasin S, Brito JP, Cunningham GR, Hayes FJ, Hodis HN, Matsumoto AM, et al. Testosterone therapy in men with hypogonadism: an endocrine society clinical practice guideline. J Clin Endocrinol Metab. 2018;103(5):1715–44.
35. Bittner VA. The new 2019 ACC/AHA guideline on the primary prevention of cardiovascular disease. Circulation. 2019;
36. American Diabetes A. 2. Classification and diagnosis of diabetes: standards of medical care in diabetes-2019. Diabetes Care. 2019;42(Suppl 1):S13–28.

Adrenal Insufficiency

49

Aluma Chovel-Sella and Alyssa Halper

Overview

Adrenal Insufficiency Overview [1, 2]

Adrenal insufficiency (AI) is characterized by inadequate glucocorticoid production with or without aldosterone deficiency. It can be classified either as primary adrenal insufficiency (PAI) or secondary adrenal insufficiency (SAI). PAI results from congenital causes or one of various processes that cause the destruction of the adrenal cortex, whereas SAI is primarily due to pituitary or hypothalamic disease. Aldosterone deficiency leads to hyponatremia, hyperkalemia, and metabolic acidosis. Adrenal insufficiency can be life-threatening due to the central roles that cortisol and aldosterone play in energy and salt and fluid homeostasis and is therefore important to diagnose quickly and accurately.

In children, typical symptoms include fatigue, muscle weakness, vomiting, abdominal pain, diarrhea, weight loss, slow growth, and salt craving. Physical exam findings for PAI may include darkening of the skin, especially in areas such as the buccal mucosa, gumline, nipples, or scrotum due to the elevated adrenocorticotropin (ACTH) secretion, as described below in the *Key Pathophysiology* section. However, infants may present with more non-specific symptoms, including dehydration, poor feeding, weight loss, lethargy, hyponatremia, hyperkalemia, and hypoglycemia, as cortisol is an important counterregulatory hormone for glucose homeostasis.

Primary Adrenal Insufficiency (PAI)

PAI is a rare disease, with a prevalence of 100–140:1,000,000. The main etiologies for PAI include the following [1–3]:

1. Congenital
   A. Enzyme deficiencies: *congenital adrenal hyperplasia (CAH)* is the most common cause of PAI in children (70% of cases). Please see below for description.
   B. Peroxisomal disorders: *adrenoleukodystrophy (ALD)* – please see below for description; Zellweger syndrome.
   C. Abnormal adrenal development: congenital adrenal hypoplasia.
   D. Inherited ACTH unresponsiveness syndromes: familial glucocorticoid deficiency, triple A syndrome (Allgrove).
2. Adrenal damage
   A. Autoimmunity: typically called *Addison's disease* (15% of cases). Note: About 50% of patients with autoimmune PAI also have autoimmune destruction of other endocrine glands, so it may be beneficial to screen for thyroid disease, type 1 diabetes, and/or hypoparathyroidism (as seen with Autoimmune Polyglandular Syndrome [APS] 1 or 2).
   B. Other causes: infections (TB, fungal, HIV), hemorrhage.
3. Drugs that interfere with adrenal steroid synthesis (e.g., ketoconazole)

Congenital adrenal hyperplasia (CAH) is an autosomal recessive disorder most commonly related to a deficiency of the 21-hydroxylase enzyme (>90% of cases), leading to deficiencies of cortisol with or without aldosterone [4]. Due to the 21-hydroxylase enzyme deficiency, accumulation of

A. Chovel-Sella · A. Halper (✉)
Massachusetts General Hospital, Boston, MA, USA
e-mail: asella@mgh.harvard.edu; ahalper@mgh.harvard.edu

T. Stanley, M. Misra (eds.), *Endocrine Conditions in Pediatrics*, https://doi.org/10.1007/978-3-030-52215-5_49

cortisol and aldosterone precursors including 17-hydroxyprogesterone (17OHP) and progesterone are diverted into sex hormone synthesis. Thus, cardinal symptoms include virilization and ambiguous genitalia of newborn females (enlarged clitoris, rugation of the labia, partly fused labia majora, and common urogenital sinus). Fortunately, in many states, 21-hydroxylase CAH is on the newborn screen, through measurement of 17OHP, but cases can be missed [5].

There are two main types of CAH (classic vs. non-classic) and three main phenotypes within the two types, depending on the degree of the enzyme's deficiency:

1. Classic CAH:
   A. *Salt-wasting CAH* is the most severe phenotype, accounting for 75% of the classic cases [4]. These children have both cortisol and aldosterone deficiency. Symptoms include failure to thrive (FTT), potential life-threatening hypovolemia, hyperkalemia, hyponatremia, hypotension, weight loss, and seizures within the first 1–4 weeks of life. Boys are more likely to be misdiagnosed at birth, because they do not have ambiguous genitalia [4].
   B. *Simple virilizing CAH* accounts for 25% of the classic cases [4]. These children have 1–2% of the 21-hydroxylase enzyme activity present, so they cannot produce cortisol but may have sufficient aldosterone production. These children may present at 2–4 years of age with early virilization (pubic hair, adult body odor, growth spurt, and/or advanced bone age) [4].
2. *Non-classic or late-onset CAH* has a prevalence as high as 1 in 1000 to 1 in 100, and even higher among Mediterranean, Hispanics, and Eastern European Jews [6, 7]. These children have about 20–50% of the 21-hydroxylase enzyme activity present, so they may have enough cortisol and aldosterone to maintain normal vital signs. While some with sufficient cortisol production may not present with signs/symptoms, some young women present with hirsutism and menstrual irregularities, and some school-age children present with early adrenarche, sexual precocity, or growth acceleration. If signs of growth acceleration and early adrenarche are seen, it is important to screen for non-classic CAH with a morning 17-hydroyprogesterone level [6, 7].

Adrenoleukodystrophy disease (ALD) is an X-linked peroxisomal disorder. Males are most often affected; however, women may be carriers and have milder forms of the disease. The incidence is estimated at 1:14,700 but may be found to be higher now that ALD is on the newborn screen in many states. It is caused by mutation at the ABCD1 transporter, which helps channel very long chain fatty acids (VLCFAs) to the peroxisome. The VLCFAs accumulate in the brain, adrenal cortex, and Leydig cells of the testes [8]. The accumulation in the brain may lead to declining school performance, and some boys may be misdiagnosed as having ADHD. The accumulation in the adrenal cortex leads to *primary* adrenal insufficiency. Thus, darkening of the skin may be an early sign as well [8].

Key Pathophysiology

Primary adrenal insufficiency (PAI):

1. *Autoimmune adrenalitis* – serum antibodies against the steroidogenic enzyme, CYP21A2 [3].
2. *CAH* – most commonly related to 21-hydroxylase deficiency → a defective conversion of 17-hydroxyprogesterone to 11-deoxycortisol in the steroidogenesis pathway → ↓cortisol +/– aldosterone and ↑androgens [7].
3. *X-linked ALD* – mutations in ABCD1, a peroxisomal transmembrane protein involved in the transport of VLCFAs into the peroxisome → accumulation of VLCFA in CNS, Leydig cells of the testes, and the adrenal cortex [8].

Note: Hyperpigmentation and salt wasting are only present in PAI. Hyperpigmentation results from excessive production of the precursor to ACTH, pro-opiomelanocortin, which can be cleaved into ACTH, as well as melanocyte stimulating hormones (MSH). MSH bind to the melanocortin receptors in the skin, and ACTH may bind these receptors as well [9].

Secondary adrenal insufficiency (SAI): damage to the hypothalamus/pituitary → ↓adrenocorticotropin (ACTH) signal from the pituitary → ↓cortisol

Diagnosis

	Concerning signs and symptoms	Supporting labs	Etiologies	Tests for confirmation of etiology
PAI	Dehydration Hypotension Hyperpigmentation Abdominal pain Vomiting Fever Fatigue	↓ 8 a.m. cortisol[a] ↑ 8 a.m. ACTH ↓ Glucose ↓ Na[b] ↑ K[b] ↑ Renin[b] *Diagnostic test* – high-dose ACTH stimulation test	Addison's	21-hydroxylase antibodies
			CAH	↑ 8 a.m. 17-hydroxyprogesterone (17OHP) Classic: 17OHP usually >3500 ng/dL, always >1000 ng/dL Non-classic:17OHP >1000 ng/dL If 17OHP 200–1000 ng/dL, proceed with high-dose ACTH stimulation test (see testing section for more information) For borderline cases or genetic counseling of CAH test for *CYP21A2* genotype [4]
			X-linked ALD	↑ VLCFA level ABCD1 gene analysis Brain MRI if elevated VLCFA or ABCD1 mutation found
SAI	Fatigue Weakness Abdominal pain Vomiting Fever Same as PAI without hyperpigmentation and symptoms of mineralocorticoid deficiency.	↓ 8 a.m. cortisol ↓ 8 a.m. ACTH *Diagnostic test* – low-dose ACTH stimulation test		

[a]Timing is important for the cortisol level, as cortisol follows a circadian rhythm and will be the highest around 8 a.m.
[b]If aldosterone pathway affected

Urgent Considerations

We recommend a low threshold for testing children for AI, as it can be life-threatening and signs and symptoms may not be specific.

When to test:

1. Unexplained signs and symptoms of dehydration, hypotension, hyperpigmentation, abdominal pain, vomiting, fever, and fatigue, especially in an acutely ill child and/or a child with unexplained weight loss
2. Unexplained hyponatremia, hyperkalemia (may be masked by vomiting), or hypoglycemia
3. Positive family history of adrenal insufficiency

Initial Management

What to obtain: Vitals, basic metabolic panel, 8 a.m. cortisol and ACTH levels, +/− 8 a.m. 17OHP (if any genital ambiguity or suspected CAH). Note that an 8 a.m. cortisol of >10 mcg/dL is generally considered normal, whereas <5 mcg/dL generally should further raise suspicion. Infants may not yet have established a circadian rhythm and may have lower cortisol-binding globulin, both of which may complicate interpretation of the 8 a.m. cortisol.

Next steps: If 8 a.m. cortisol <5 mcg/dL and/or ACTH >2 × upper limit of normal, consider urgent phone call to pediatric endocrinology for next steps (likely PAI).

- If both 8 a.m. cortisol and ACTH levels are low and a central process is suspected, consider urgent phone referral to pediatric endocrinology (likely SAI).
- If low Na, high K, and/or hypoglycemia and hypotension in the setting of suspected AI, please send to the emergency department and call pediatric endocrinology.
- If any genital ambiguity or 17OHP >1000 ng/dL, please consult pediatric endocrinology emergently.
- For borderline cases, including 8 a.m. cortisol between 5 and 10 mcg/dL with clinical suspicion, ACTH stimulation testing may be a necessary next step. Please see the section on ACTH stimulation testing (Chap. 29) for further information.

Chronic Management

1. Glucocorticoid replacement – typically three times per day dosing with hydrocortisone in a growing child (~6–10 mg/m^2/day, which is approximate physiologic dosing) [10]. Patients with CAH usually require a higher dose of hydrocortisone (~10–15 mg/m^2/day) in order to suppress the excessive androgen production [1].

   Note: Dexamethasone and prednisone are not recommended in a growing child due to suppression of growth and significant weight gain; however, these glucocorticoids may be used in an older child who has completed growth [1, 11].

   Stress dosing: A higher dose of hydrocortisone, fluids, and electrolytes are needed during illness, injury, and surgery to avoid a life-threatening adrenal crisis. Typically about 30–50 mg/m^2/day of hydrocortisone is needed for mild to moderate stress, and 100 mg/m^2/day during significant stress such as major surgery or critical illness.

   - In an emergency, when a patient's weight or height may not be available, a quick, simple age-based dosing guide can be used:
     - 25 mg IV/IM hydrocortisone for 0–3 years
     - 50 mg IV/IM hydrocortisone for 3–12 years
     - 100 mg IV/IM hydrocortisone for ≥12 years.
2. Mineralocorticoid replacement (if needed) – typically with 1–2 times per day dosing with fludrocortisone [1]. Please note this is only relevant for patients with PAI, as children with SAI typically only require cortisol replacement.
3. Salt supplementation (1–2 mg/day of sodium chloride) should also be provided to infants up to 8–12 months who require mineralocorticoid replacement due to the low salt content in breast milk and formulas and the kidney's decreased responsiveness to mineralocorticoid at this age [4].
4. Monitoring growth velocity, weight, blood pressure, physical examination, and labs for electrolytes [1].

Please note that in a patient who is identified to have ALD based on newborn screening, screening for PAI will occur at regular intervals based on the ALD guidelines [10].

Considerations for Urgent/Emergent Referral

1. A positive newborn screening for CAH or ALD
2. A newborn baby with ambiguous genitalia/virilization
3. Unexplained signs and symptoms of dehydration, hypotension, hyperpigmentation abdominal pain, vomiting, fever, and fatigue, especially in an acutely ill child
4. Unexplained hyponatremia, hyperkalemia (can be masked by vomiting), or hypoglycemia
5. Positive family history of adrenal insufficiency

Take-Home Messages

1. If adrenal insufficiency is suspected, it is important to screen right away with an 8 a.m. cortisol and ACTH level with or without electrolytes. Please note that timing is important, because cortisol follows a circadian rhythm.
2. If CAH is expected, an 8 a.m. 17-hydroxyprogesterone level should also be sent. This is an *urgent* pediatric endocrine referral.
3. If ALD is expected, an 8 a.m. cortisol and ACTH level will suffice, but this is also an *urgent* pediatric endocrine referral if ACTH is elevated.

References

1. Bornstein SR, Allolio B, Arlt W, et al. Diagnosis and treatment of primary adrenal insufficiency: an endocrine society clinical practice guideline. J Clin Endocrinol Metab. 2016;101(2):364–89. https://doi.org/10.1210/jc.2015-1710.
2. Bowden SA, Henry R. Pediatric adrenal insufficiency: diagnosis, management, and new therapies. Int J Pediatr. 2018;2018:1739831. https://doi.org/10.1155/2018/1739831.
3. Falorni A, Chen S, Zanchetta R, et al. Measuring adrenal autoantibody response: interlaboratory concordance in the first international serum exchange for the determination of 21-hydroxylase autoantibodies. Clin Immunol (Orlando, FL). 2011;140(3):291–9. https://doi.org/10.1016/j.clim.2011.04.012.
4. Speiser PW, Arlt W, Auchus RJ, et al. Congenital adrenal hyperplasia due to steroid 21-hydroxylase deficiency: an endocrine society clinical practice guideline. J Clin Endocrinol Metab. 2018;103(11):4043–88. https://doi.org/10.1210/jc.2018-01865.
5. Sarafoglou K, Gaviglio A, Hietala A, et al. Comparison of newborn screening protocols for congenital adrenal hyperplasia in preterm infants. J Pediatr. 2014;164(5):1136–40. https://doi.org/10.1016/j.jpeds.2014.01.038.
6. Extensive clinical experience: nonclassical 21-hydroxylase deficiency. – PubMed – NCBI. https://www.ncbi.nlm.nih.gov/pubmed?term=16912124. Accessed 4 Jan 2020.
7. Merke DP, Bornstein SR. Congenital adrenal hyperplasia. Lancet (Lond Engl). 2005;365(9477):2125–36. https://doi.org/10.1016/S0140-6736(05)66736-0.
8. Kemp S, Wanders R. Biochemical aspects of X-linked adrenoleukodystrophy. Brain Pathol Zurich Switz. 2010;20(4):831–7. https://doi.org/10.1111/j.1750-3639.2010.00391.x.
9. Sperling M. Pediatric endocrinology. 4th ed: Saunders; 2014.
10. Regelmann MO, Kamboj MK, Miller BS, et al. Adrenoleukodystrophy: guidance for adrenal surveillance in males identified by newborn screen. J Clin Endocrinol Metab. 2018;103(11):4324–31. https://doi.org/10.1210/jc.2018-00920.
11. Bonfig W, Bechtold S, Schmidt H, Knorr D, Schwarz HP. Reduced final height outcome in congenital adrenal hyperplasia under prednisone treatment: deceleration of growth velocity during puberty. J Clin Endocrinol Metab. 2007;92(5):1635–9. https://doi.org/10.1210/jc.2006-2109.

Overview and Initial Management of Cushing Syndrome

50

Soundos Youssef and Vibha Singhal

Definition and Etiology

Cushing syndrome (CS) is a metabolic and endocrine disorder, characterized by excessive exposure to endogenous or exogenous glucocorticoids.

I. *Exogenous CS (iatrogenic from prolonged use of supra-physiological doses of glucocorticoids such as (but not limited to) hydrocortisone, prednisone, prednisolone, methyl prednisolone, and dexamethasone)*
II. *Endogenous CS secondary to:*
   (a) ACTH-independent CS from an adrenal tumor (primary CS)
   (b) ACTH-dependent CS from a pituitary tumor (Cushing disease (CD)), or from an ectopic site of ACTH production (ectopic ACTH secretion (EAS))

The incidence of CS is variable (Fig. 50.1), with most reports underestimating the frequency of iatrogenic CS and failing to capture mild endogenous hypercortisolism [23]. Exogenous CS is the most common cause overall of CS in all age groups.

- Exogenous (Iatrogenic) CS
  - *Pathophysiology:* Exogenous glucocorticoids administered via topical, inhalation, subcutaneous, intramuscular, or intra-articular (chronic or pulsatile) routes in supra-physiologic doses for prolonged durations result in exogenous or iatrogenic CS. Rarely, this is due to exogenous ACTH administration, as in myoclonic epilepsy [1–3, 23].
  - *Epidemiology:* Nearly 10,000,000 Americans are prescribed therapeutic glucocorticoids every year, making iatrogenic CS the leading cause of CS overall in adult and pediatric populations; however, this remains underreported [3, 23].
  - *Effect on Hypothalamic-Pituitary-Adrenal (HPA) Axis:* Exogenous glucocorticoids decrease corticotropin-releasing hormone (CRH) and ACTH secretion from the hypothalamus and pituitary gland, respectively, because of increased negative feedback, which in turn results in bilateral adrenal atrophy. Hence, an individual on exogenous glucocorticoids can have CS while taking the medication but develop adrenal insufficiency if they suddenly discontinue glucocorticoids because of their atrophied adrenal glands [2, 3].
- Cushing Disease (ACTH-Dependent)
  - *Pathophysiology:* ACTH-secreting anterior pituitary adenoma. This is usually a benign microadenoma (less than 1 cm) but can less commonly be a macroadenoma (more than 1 cm) or very rarely a malignant tumor (with evidence of metastasis).
  - *Epidemiology*: ACTH-secreting microadenomas account for 10–15% of all pituitary adenomas. They are the second most common cause of CS in adults (after exogenous CS) (accounting for >70% of endogenous CS) as well as in children more than 7 years of age (accounting for 75–90% of endogenous CS) [4–6]. Adult CD has a female predilection (female to male ratio of 3–4:1). Pediatric CD has a male preponderance before puberty, an even gender distribution during puberty, and a female preponderance in late puberty [4].
  - *Effect on HPA Axis:* Inappropriately increased ACTH causes bilateral adrenal hyperplasia, which leads to increased adrenal secretion of cortisol.

S. Youssef (✉)
Neuroendocrine Unit, Massachusetts General Hospital, Boston, MA, USA
e-mail: SYOUSSEF@mgh.harvard.edu

V. Singhal
Neuroendocrine Unit, Massachusetts General Hospital, Boston, MA, USA

Division of Pediatric Endocrinology, Pediatrics, Massachusetts General Hospital, Harvard Medical School, Boston, MA, USA
e-mail: VSINGHAL1@mgh.harvard.edu

T. Stanley, M. Misra (eds.), *Endocrine Conditions in Pediatrics*, https://doi.org/10.1007/978-3-030-52215-5_50

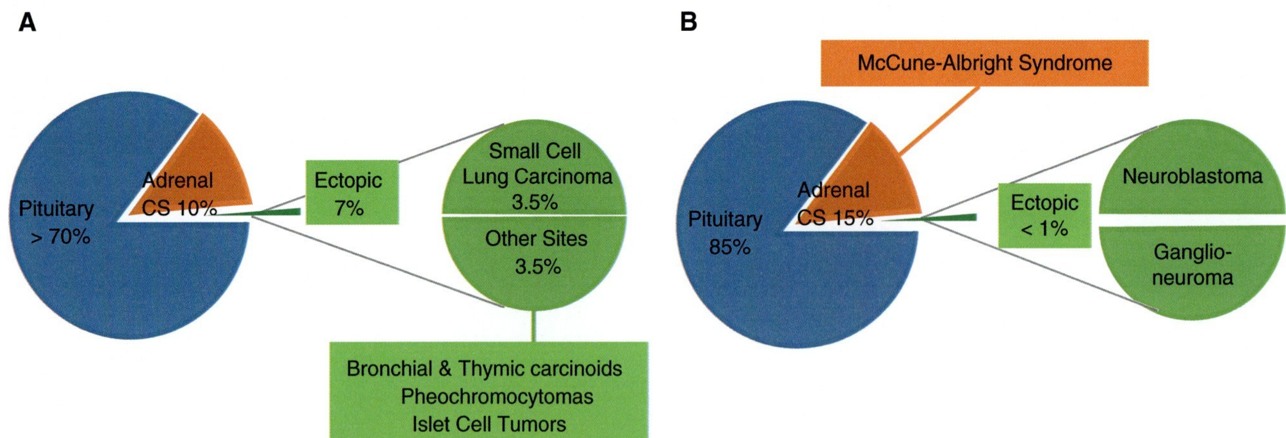

Fig. 50.1 Distribution of main etiologies of endogenous Cushing syndrome in adult (**a**) and in pediatric (**b**) populations

- Ectopic Source of ACTH (ACTH-Dependent)
  - *Pathophysiology:* ACTH (or rarely CRH) secretion from a non-pituitary source causes ectopic CS. This condition results from paraneoplastic cortisol release from a tumor at a site other than the pituitary or the adrenal glands. Small-cell lung carcinoma accounts for almost half of the cases, followed by carcinoids, islet cell tumors, and pheochromocytomas [2, 3]. A neuroblastoma or ganglioneuroma may be the site of ectopic ACTH secretion in young infants [3, 7].
  - *Epidemiology:* Very rare in pediatrics (<1% of adolescent CS); 7–15% of all endogenous CS in adults [2, 3] with a male preponderance.
  - *Effect on HPA Axis:* Similar to other ACTH-dependent etiologies [7]. Bilateral adrenal hyperplasia occurs due to excessive ACTH secretion leading to increased adrenal secretion of cortisol [7]. The rare CRH-secreting ectopic tumors also cause corticotrope hyperplasia.
- Primary Adrenal Hypercortisolism (ACTH-Independent)
  - *Pathophysiology:* Adrenal adenoma, unilateral or bilateral hyperplasia, or carcinoma. Adrenal hyperplasia is seen in children with McCune-Albright syndrome (Gsα mutation which constitutively activates ACTH signaling pathway) [8], primary bilateral macronodular adrenal hyperplasia (BMAH), and primary pigmented nodular adrenocortical disease (PPNAD), which could be sporadic or familial (e.g., Carney complex) [9].
  - *Epidemiology:* Accounts for about 15% of all cases of endogenous CS in children and adolescents (this is the most common cause of endogenous CS in children <7 years old) [2, 3]. Adrenal carcinoma has a bimodal age distribution, peaking first at 3 years of age, and then in the fourth and fifth decades [20]. Cortisol-secreting adrenal malignancies account for 0.6% of all childhood tumors. A third of pediatric adrenal lesions occurring before 5 years of age are associated with CS, especially in females. The different types of hyperplasia are more frequently implicated in childhood CS than in adult CS [5].
  - *Effect on HPA Axis:* Atrophy occurs of the contralateral, uninvolved adrenal gland if the etiology is unilateral. Autonomous cortisol secretion from the affected adrenal gland causes decreased ACTH secretion from increased negative feedback at the hypothalamic and pituitary levels.

Other, Less Common Etiologies of Cushing Syndrome

- *Cyclic CS:* A phenomenon of intermittent hypercortisolism that is often missed clinically, leading to delays in intervention. In between the episodes of hypercortisolism, cortisol concentrations may range from mildly high to normal to low. In cyclical CS, testing may need to be coordinated with the occurrence of symptoms [2, 3].
- *Pseudo-CS:* This refers to the presence of clinical symptoms of CS, such as weight gain, fatigue, acne, hirsutism, menstrual disorders, as well as some biochemical findings compatible with CS, in the absence of endogenous pathologic hypercortisolism. This may be seen in cases of extreme stress (illness or emotional stress), obesity, anorexia nervosa (not associated with weight gain), excessive exercise (not associated with weight gain), alcoholism or alcohol withdrawal, depression, panic disorders, and psychotic conditions [3, 10, 11].
- *Familial CS:* CS is usually not genetically inherited except in some syndromic cases such as Multiple Endocrine Neoplasia type 1 (MEN 1) and Carney complex/syndrome. The former is a genetic condition that predisposes individuals to develop hormone-secreting

tumors of the parathyroid, pancreas, and pituitary gland. CS in MEN 1 may be due to a tumor in either the pituitary, adrenals, or an ectopic site [12]. The latter is an autosomal dominant neoplastic syndrome, characterized by abnormal spotty pigmentation on the face, neck, and trunk, including the lips, conjunctivae, sclera, cardiac myxomas, and PPNAD (median age at diagnosis is 20 years) [13].

Signs and Symptoms

The clinical presentation of cortisol excess is variable (Table 50.1). A primary sign of pediatric CS is growth deceleration or arrest despite significant weight gain. The child or teen typically exhibits accelerated weight gain relative to linear growth velocity. The typical features of a dorsocervical fat pad and central adiposity are observed only in chronic hypercortisolism. Clinicians should consult with an endocrinologist when signs and symptoms of CS are marked and/or progress over time. Signs that can more reliably distinguish CS from other causes of weight gain are proximal muscle weakness, easy bruising, and violaceous striae >1 cm wide [24]. Diagnosis and treatment is similar in pediatric and adult CS [3, 5, 6, 8].

Circadian Rhythm Misalignment in Cushing Syndrome and Weight Gain

Cortisol secretion typically follows a diurnal pattern. Serum cortisol peaks soon after morning awakening and gradually decreases to a nadir after a person falls asleep, close to midnight. In CD (with high pituitary ACTH secretion), mean ACTH pulse amplitude increases, while pulse frequency remains unchanged. This results in an inability of plasma cortisol concentrations to decline at night. Moreover, ACTH-secreting adenomas display partial resistance to cortisol negative feedback [18, 19]. Circadian desynchrony is also seen in states of obesity, long-term shift workers, and with social jet lag, regardless of age [20, 21]. Circadian disruption has been linked to weight gain, although the exact mechanism by which this disruption leads to obesity is still not fully established. Decreased secretion of melatonin (a hormone important for maintaining optimal energy balance) from disruption in the circadian rhythm of ACTH secretion in night-shift workers and with social jet lag may be a potential mechanism [22]. Because disruption in the circadian rhythm can both lead to weight gain and result in challenges in cortisol testing, sleeping patterns should be thoroughly investigated, especially in adolescents who have physiologic circadian dysregulation.

Table 50.1 Signs and symptoms of Cushing syndrome

Physical traits	Growth failure in children: linear growth deceleration with simultaneous weight gain (truncal/central obesity) Moon facies Dorsocervical fat pad (buffalo hump) and supra-clavicular fat pad
Dermatological changes	Facial plethora Acne (steroid-induced) Violaceous striae Bruising Acanthosis nigricans (insulin resistance) Hyperpigmentation (depends on duration and degree of exposure to ACTH) [2, 3]
Hyperandrogenism signs	Hirsutism, alopecia, male-pattern balding in females Acne [14]
Metabolic profile	Obesity Insulin resistance Hypertension *Following long-standing hypercortisolism:* Increasing insulin resistance, glucose intolerance, and frank type 2 diabetes Dyslipidemia: increased low-density lipoprotein, decreased high-density lipoprotein (45–70%) Hypokalemic alkalosis Hepatic steatosis Nephrolithiasis [2, 3, 14]
Cardiovascular diseases (leading cause of death in CS, particularly in adults)	Atherosclerosis EKG abnormalities Myocardial infarction Stroke Pulmonary embolism Coagulopathy [14, 15]
Gonadal problems	Females: amenorrhea, hirsutism, virilization Males: delayed sexual development, gynecomastia, decreased libido
Psychiatric and cognitive dysfunction	Energy/activity decline Mood swings, irritability, depression Cerebral atrophy, short-term memory loss, cognitive dysfunction Sleep disorders (troubled sleep-onset, sleep-maintaining insomnia, morning awakening) Anxiety, mania, psychoses (70–85%) [14, 16, 17]
Non-specific manifestations	Proximal muscle weakness/atrophy (predominantly pelvic girdle musculature) Low bone density, osteoporosis, fractures (50–80%) (seen mainly in adults) Headache, backache Cataracts, glaucoma Abdominal pain [2, 3, 14, 17]

Diagnosis

The first step in the detection of CS is clinical suspicion, followed by documentation of hypercortisolism, and then evaluation of the etiology of CS, as illustrated in the flowchart (Fig. 50.2) [2, 3, 14]. It is important to differentiate between pathological hypercortisolemia and physiologic hypercortisolism seen in pregnancy and pseudo-CS states (e.g., alcoholism, depression, severe obesity, anorexia nervosa, intense chronic exercise, polycystic ovary syndrome (PCOS), and bulimia [11]). Some foods like licorice can inhibit 11 β-hydroxysteroid dehydrogenase type 2, which normally converts cortisol into cortisone and elevate the cortisol levels [31].

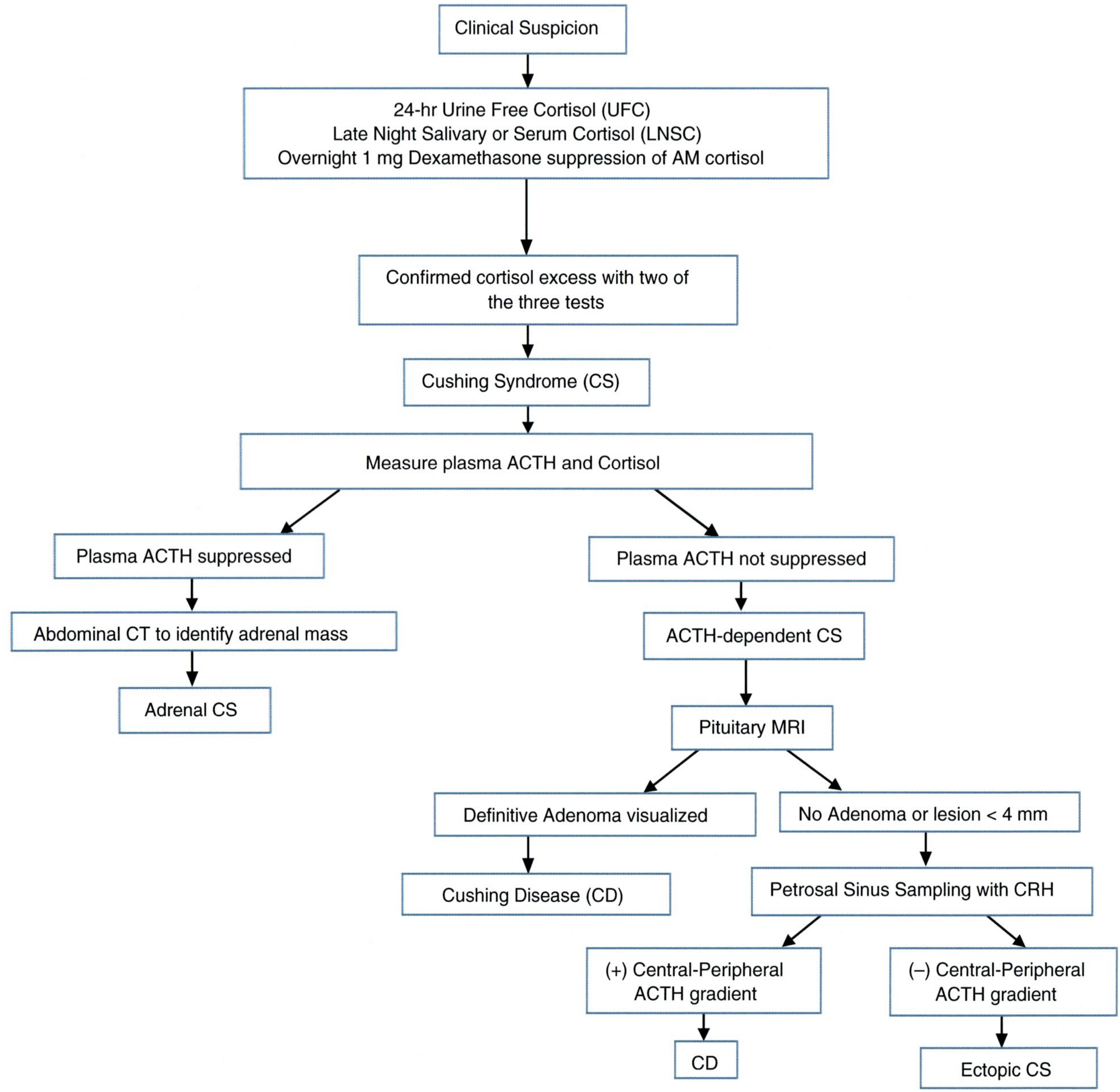

Fig. 50.2 A flowchart for Cushing syndrome diagnostics (Adapted from Cushing Syndrome in Pediatrics by Stratakis et al. [2, 3]). CS Cushing syndrome, ACTH adrenocorticotropic hormone, CT computed tomography, MRI magnetic resonance imaging, CRH corticotropin-releasing hormone, CD Cushing disease

Candidates for Screening

1. Prepubertal and early- to mid-pubertal children with growth deceleration or cessation of linear growth, especially in the setting of weight gain (older adolescents without CS may show this pattern if they have completed puberty and growth from physiological reasons).
2. Patients with clinical characteristics not consistent with their age (e.g., hypertension and glucose intolerance in young patients).
3. Patients with adrenal incidentaloma [26].

The Endocrine Society's Clinical Practice Guideline for the diagnosis of CS suggests excluding exogenous CS prior to performing screening tests. They recommend using two out of three screening tests to establish the diagnosis and highlight the importance of personalizing the choice of tests based on circadian rhythm, medications, and other diseases [14].

Cortisol testing should be deferred in individuals who:

- Recently traveled across time zones (wait for 2–3 weeks for testing) [23].
- Are working night shifts [23].
- Just recovered from an acute illness [24].
- Are taking certain medications: for example, glucocorticoids via any route and oral contraceptive pills. Oral contraceptive pills cause an increase in corticosteroid-binding globulin (CBG) levels; therefore, serum cortisol (which includes free and bound cortisol) will be elevated (may need discontinuation before certain tests) [25].

Diagnostic Tests

- *Twenty-four-hour urine free cortisol (UFC) (sensitivity 80–98%; specificity 45–98%* [21]*):*
  - Reveals integrated tissue exposure to free cortisol over a day and offers an aggregate view on cortisol excretion [26]
  - Measures both creatinine and volume to guarantee completeness of collection [27]
  - Is interpreted as increased if more than twice the upper limit of normal (ULN)
  - Can be done on an outpatient basis
- *Limitations:*
  - If collection is contaminated with blood (from menses) or incomplete.
  - In those with renal insufficiency.
  - May be falsely elevated when urine volume is more than 5 L [28].
  - May be falsely attenuated when glomerular filtration rate is low [27, 29].
  - A urinary tract infection can decrease the measured UFC excretion secondary to metabolism by bacteria in the urine [23].
- *Late-night salivary cortisol (LNSC) (sensitivity 92–100%; specificity 93–100%* [21]*):*
  - Demonstrates an inability of cortisol levels to reach their normal nadir after falling asleep [30]. Patients with CS lose the biologically timed trough and exhibit higher late-night salivary cortisol levels compared with those without CS and those with obesity or other pseudo-Cushing states [11, 18, 19]. Late-night serum cortisol is an alternative if feasible, especially in individuals who have inadequate saliva (like Sjögren's syndrome).
- *Limitations:*
  - Circadian rhythm–governed cortisol secretory pattern is perturbed when the time of sleep initiation changes (i.e., for night shift workers, those traveling across different time zones, teenagers going to bed very late at night) [14]. It usually takes 2–3 weeks of returning to normal sleeping patterns to normalize cortisol secretory dynamics.
  - Improper collection/storage.
  - Use of chewing tobacco [23].
  - Forceful tooth brushing (contamination with blood can falsely elevate the salivary cortisol level).
  - Cannot be performed in patients with gingivitis or Sjögren's syndrome (insufficient saliva) [29, 32, 33].
- *1 mg overnight dexamethasone suppression test (ONDST) (sensitivity 91–97%; specificity 85–90%* [21]*):*
  - Can be done in an outpatient setting
  - Determines intactness of the negative feedback loop of cortisol
  - Involves administration of 1 mg of dexamethasone, orally, between 11 PM and midnight, followed by measurement of serum cortisol between 8 and 9 AM the following morning

    Morning serum cortisol level <1.8 ug/dl (50 nmol/L) → normal

    Morning serum cortisol level >1.8 ug/dl (50 nmol/L) → CS [14]
- *Limitations:*
  - Any condition or medication that increases corticosteroid binding globulin (CBG) levels can result in a false-positive ONDST. Such medications include oral contraceptive pills and mitotane and states like pregnancy.
  - Any condition associated with low CBG levels could result in a false-negative ONDST (nephrotic syndrome/liver cirrhosis).

- Decreased dexamethasone metabolism/clearance (seen with concomitant use of drugs such as cimetidine and fluoxetine, and in renal insufficiency).
- Increased dexamethasone metabolism/clearance (seen with concomitant use of drugs such as phenytoin, rifampin and carbamazepine) [29].

In the case of mild or cyclical CS, a single normal result obtained from either UFC or LNSC may not be enough to detect CS. Hence, CS diagnosis may require obtaining multiple samples (urine, saliva) and a dexamethasone suppression test (DST) [18]. If the results of these tests are definitive or suspicious, then the patient should be referred to a specialist for determination of the etiology of CS.

Treatment

- Treatment of CS is dependent on the cause and should be undertaken by a pediatric endocrinologist (Tables 50.2 and 50.3).

Table 50.2 Cushing syndrome treatment options based on etiology

	Treatment	Details
Iatrogenic Cushing syndrome	Gradual tapering of glucocorticoid or dose adjustment (if this is possible without causing exacerbation of the condition for which glucocorticoids are being administered)	In consultation with the physician treating the underlying condition
Cushing disease	First line → trans-sphenoidal surgery (TSS) (may be repeated) Second line → radiation therapy (single or multiple fraction depending on the size of the lesion and its location) Third line → medical therapy Fourth line → bilateral adrenalectomy	When performed by a neurosurgeon with significant expertise in pituitary surgery: Microadenoma remission rate: 72.8–91% Macroadenoma remission rate 42.9–65% 10-year recurrence rate of CD: About 12% in adults About 42% in pediatric patients [34–49]
Ectopic Cushing syndrome	Surgical resection of the primary tumor (if feasible)	If primary tumor is resected, hypercortisolism is reversed. If ACTH source is not localized medical treatment/bilateral adrenalectomy may be needed [7].
Primary adrenal hyper-cortisolism	Resection of adrenal mass/adrenalectomy	Approach depends on the anatomy of the mass and the laterality of the lesion.

Post-Surgical Monitoring

Effectiveness of treatment is typically evaluated by monitoring urinary free cortisol levels (UFC) or LNSC. After successful TSS, many patients with CD experience a state of symptomatic ACTH deficit that could last up to 1 year (due to suppression of endogenous corticotropes from prolonged autonomous ACTH production from the pituitary adenoma). These symptoms generally get resolved with low-dose glucocorticoid replacement, to compensate for cortisol withdrawal symptoms (fatigue, nausea, dry skin, arthralgia). In the initial weeks following surgery, some patients require higher-than-normal replacement dosing to feel well. This can be slowly tapered under the supervision of a specialist [14]. If surgery does not result in complete remission, radiation or medical therapy is used as an adjunct.

Guidelines for Cushing Syndrome Management

According to the Endocrine Society's Clinical Practice Guideline, once a diagnosis of CS is established, the therapeutic management plan bifurcates based on etiology: ACTH-dependent CS versus ACTH-independent CS [50].

- *ACTH-dependent CS (Ectopic CS or CD):* First-line treatment is tumor localization and resection. Patients in remission should be monitored for disease recurrence. For patients with failed surgery, inoperable tumor, or disease recurrence, the next steps may include:
  - Repeat TSS, radiotherapy, or pituitary-directed pharmacotherapy (CD)
  - Medical therapy (steroidogenesis inhibitors, glucocorticoid receptor antagonists) or bilateral adrenalectomy (Ectopic CS) [50]
- *ACTH-independent CS (adrenal CS):* First-line treatment is unilateral or bilateral adrenalectomy. Patients in remission should be monitored for disease recurrence, while those with residual disease should be managed similarly to those with residual ectopic CS to target the state of hypercortisolism by medical therapy (steroidogenesis inhibitors, glucocorticoid receptor antagonists) or bilateral adrenalectomy [50].

Long-Term Follow-Up

Even after postoperative remission, long-term endocrine follow-up is essential due to the significant rate of late relapse (biochemical recurrence can occur in 1 out of 20 patients). The characteristic hormonal deficiencies seen in CD postoperatively (hypogonadism, hypothyroidism, decreased growth hormone secretion) usually improve over a period of a year. A recent (2019) systematic review and meta-analysis determined that treating CS, regardless of etiology, only partially

Table 50.3 Cushing syndrome pharmacological treatment options and radiation therapy

	Steroidogenesis inhibitors	Corticotroph-directed agents	Glucocorticoid receptor antagonists	Radiation therapy (RT)
Examples	Mitotane Ketoconazole Metyrapone [12, 17]	Neuromodulatory drugs: dopamine agonists (Cabergoline); somatostatin analogs (Pasireotide) [51] Nuclear receptor ligands, which indirectly influence the HPA axis, because they target different nuclear receptors involved in the regulation of the HPA axis, such as the PPAR-γ agonists and retinoic acid receptor agonists (still investigational) [52–65]	Mifepristone [12, 17]	Fractionated RT Stereotactic radiosurgery (SRS) [12, 17]
Mechanism of action	Inhibit ≥1 step of adrenal steroidogenesis [12, 17]	Neuromodulatory drugs: directly influence HPA Nuclear receptor ligands: indirectly influence the HPA axis by targeting different nuclear receptors involved in its regulation [52–65]	Blocks peripheral effects of ↑cortisol. Does not decrease cortisol levels [12, 17]	DNA damage to tumor cells Optimal dose determined by the location and size of the tumor [12, 17]
Details	*Mitotane:* not first-line drug *Ketoconazole:* variable response [12, 17]	Effective in about 30–50% of the patients [12, 17]	↑ACTH and cortisol by peripheral glucocorticoid receptor inhibition → dose adequacy is determined based on improvement in symptomatology [12, 17]	Need medical bridge therapy after RT to control hypercortisolism in latency period [12, 17]
Side effects	Adrenal insufficiency Gastrointestinal symptoms Teratogenesis (Mitotane) Liver dysfunction (Ketoconazole) Worsening of hypertension and hirsutism (Metyrapone) [12, 17]	Hypotension, headaches, and cardiac valvular defects when used in very high doses (Cabergoline) Gastrointestinal symptoms, gallstones, hyperglycemia (Pasireotide) [12, 17]	Nausea, fatigue, headache, hypokalemia, anti-ovulatory and abortive (caution in women of child-bearing age) [12, 17]	↑ Risk of new neoplasms iatrogenic hypopituitarism (net effect of surgery + RT) in 20–40% of patients at 10 years post RT and ↑ subsequently [66]

improves cognitive function and quality of life, without completely normalizing these endpoints [67]. Furthermore, the risk of multisystem comorbidities after CS remains high and needs constant monitoring [26, 68].

Conclusion

Diagnosis of CS requires a high index of suspicion by the primary care provider, a good history, complete examination, appropriate testing, and finally, consultation with specialists for detailed care. A multidisciplinary team and long-term follow-up are necessary to optimize the health of these patients.

References

1. Dinsen S, Baslund B, Klose M, et al. Why glucocorticoid withdrawal may sometimes be as dangerous as the treatment itself. Eur J Intern Med. 2013;24:714–20.
2. Stratakis CA. Cushing syndrome in pediatrics. Endocrinol Metab Clin N Am. 2012;41:793–803.
3. Stratakis CA. An update on Cushing syndrome in pediatrics. Ann Endocrinol (Paris). 2018;79:125–31.
4. Ambrogio AG, De Martin M, Ascoli P, et al. Gender-dependent changes in haematological parameters in patients with Cushing's disease before and after remission. Eur J Endocrinol. 2014;170:393–400.
5. Chrousos GP, Kino T, Charmandari E. Evaluation of the hypothalamic-pituitary-adrenal axis function in childhood and adolescence. Neuroimmunomodulation. 2009;16:272–83.

6. Nieman LK, Biller BM, Findling JW, et al. The diagnosis of Cushing's syndrome: an endocrine society clinical practice guideline. J Clin Endocrinol Metab. 2008;93:1526–40.
7. Karageorgiadis AS, Papadakis GZ, Biro J, et al. Ectopic adrenocorticotropic hormone and corticotropin-releasing hormone co-secreting tumors in children and adolescents causing Cushing syndrome: a diagnostic dilemma and how to solve it. J Clin Endocrinol Metab. 2015;100:141–8.
8. More J, Young J, Reznik Y, et al. Ectopic ACTH syndrome in children and adolescents. J Clin Endocrinol Metab. 2011;96: 1213–22.
9. Morin E, Mete O, Wasserman JD, et al. Carney complex with adrenal cortical carcinoma. J Clin Endocrinol Metab. 2012;97:E202–6.
10. Savage MO, Storr HL, Chan LF, Grossman AB. Diagnosis and treatment of pediatric Cushing's disease. Pituitary. 2007;10: 365–71.
11. Lindholm J. Cushing's disease, pseudo-Cushing states and the dexamethasone test: a historical and critical review. Pituitary. 2014;17:374–80.
12. Lacroix A, Feelders RA, Stratakis CA, Nieman LK. Cushing's syndrome. Lancet. 2015;386:913–27.
13. Bonnet-Serrano F, Bertherat J. Genetics of tumors of the adrenal cortex. Endocr Relat Cancer. 2018;25:R131–52.
14. Nieman LK. Cushing's syndrome: update on signs, symptoms and biochemical screening. Eur J Endocrinol. 2015;173:M33–8.
15. Suarez MG, Stack M, Hinojosa-Amaya JM, et al. Hypercoagulability in Cushing syndrome, prevalence of thrombotic events: a large, single-center, retrospective study. J Endocrinol Soc. 2020;4:bvz033.
16. Andela CD, van Haalen FM, Ragnarsson O, et al. Mechanisms in endocrinology: Cushing's syndrome causes irreversible effects on the human brain: a systematic review of structural and functional magnetic resonance imaging studies. Eur J Endocrinol. 2015;173:R1–14.
17. Sharma ST, Nieman LK, Feelders RA. Cushing's syndrome: epidemiology and developments in disease management. Clin Epidemiol. 2015;7:281–93.
18. Kidambi S, Raff H, Findling JW. Limitations of nocturnal salivary cortisol and urine free cortisol in the diagnosis of mild Cushing's syndrome. Eur J Endocrinol. 2007;157:725–31.
19. Putignano P, Toja P, Dubini A, et al. Midnight salivary cortisol versus urinary free and midnight serum cortisol as screening tests for Cushing's syndrome. J Clin Endocrinol Metab. 2003;88:4153–7.
20. Burgess JR, Shepherd JJ, Parameswaran V, et al. Spectrum of pituitary disease in multiple endocrine neoplasia type 1 (MEN 1): clinical, biochemical, and radiological features of pituitary disease in a large MEN 1 kindred. J Clin Endocrinol Metab. 1996;81:2642–6.
21. Elamin MB, Murad MH, Mullan R, et al. Accuracy of diagnostic tests for Cushing's syndrome: a systematic review and metaanalyses. J Clin Endocrinol Metab. 2008;93:1553–62.
22. Arendt J. Shift work: coping with the biological clock. Occup Med (Lond). 2010;60:10–20.
23. Bansal V, El Asmar N, Selman WR, Arafah BM. Pitfalls in the diagnosis and management of Cushing's syndrome. Neurosurg Focus. 2015;38:E4.
24. Arafah BM. Hypothalamic pituitary adrenal function during critical illness: limitations of current assessment methods. J Clin Endocrinol Metab. 2006;91:3725–45.
25. Coe CL, Murai JT, Wiener SG, et al. Rapid cortisol and corticosteroid-binding globulin responses during pregnancy and after estrogen administration in the squirrel monkey. Endocrinology. 1986;118:435–40.
26. Melmed S. Pathogenesis of pituitary tumors. Nat Rev Endocrinol. 2011;7:257–66.
27. Chan KC, Lit LC, Law EL, et al. Diminished urinary free cortisol excretion in patients with moderate and severe renal impairment. Clin Chem. 2004;50:757–9.
28. Mericq MV, Cutler GB Jr. High fluid intake increases urine free cortisol excretion in normal subjects. J Clin Endocrinol Metab. 1998;83:682–4.
29. Yilmaz N, Tazegul G, Bozoglan H, et al. Diagnostic value of the late-night salivary cortisol in the diagnosis of clinical and subclinical Cushing's syndrome: results of a single-center 7-year experience. J Investig Med. 2019;67:28–33.
30. Krieger DT, Allen W, Rizzo F, Krieger HP. Characterization of the normal temporal pattern of plasma corticosteroid levels. J Clin Endocrinol Metab. 1971;32:266–84.
31. Ploeger B, Mensinga T, Sips A, et al. The pharmacokinetics of glycyrrhizic acid evaluated by physiologically based pharmacokinetic modeling. Drug Metab Rev. 2001;33:125–47.
32. Yaneva M, Mosnier-Pudar H, Dugue MA, et al. Midnight salivary cortisol for the initial diagnosis of Cushing's syndrome of various causes. J Clin Endocrinol Metab. 2004;89:3345–51.
33. Chiodini I, Ramos-Rivera A, Marcus AO, Yau H. Adrenal hypercortisolism: a closer look at screening, diagnosis, and important considerations of different testing modalities. J Endocrinol Soc. 2019;3:1097–109.
34. Swearingen B, Biller BM, Barker FG 2nd, et al. Long-term mortality after transsphenoidal surgery for Cushing disease. Ann Intern Med. 1999;130:821–4.
35. Ludecke D, Kautzky R, Saeger W, Schrader D. Selective removal of hypersecreting pituitary adenomas? An analysis of endocrine function, operative and microscopical findings in 101 cases. Acta Neurochir. 1976;35:27–42.
36. Carmalt MH, Dalton GA, Fletcher RF, Smith WT. The treatment of Cushing's disease by trans-sphenoidal hypophysectomy. Q J Med. 1977;46:119–34.
37. Salassa RM, Laws ER Jr, Carpenter PC, Northcutt RC. Transsphenoidal removal of pituitary microadenoma in Cushing's disease. Mayo Clin Proc. 1978;53:24–8.
38. Tyrrell JB, Brooks RM, Fitzgerald PA, et al. Cushing's disease. Selective trans-sphenoidal resection of pituitary microadenomas. N Engl J Med. 1978;298:753–8.
39. Wajchenberg BL, Silveira AA, Goldman J, et al. Evaluation of resection of pituitary microadenoma for the treatment of Cushing's disease in patients with radiologically normal sella turcica. Clin Endocrinol. 1979;11:323–31.
40. Guthrie FW Jr, Ciric I, Hayashida S, et al. Pituitary Cushing's syndrome and Nelson's syndrome: diagnostic criteria, surgical therapy, and results. Surg Neurol. 1981;16:316–23.
41. Boggan JE, Tyrrell JB, Wilson CB. Transsphenoidal microsurgical management of Cushing's disease. Report of 100 cases. J Neurosurg. 1983;59:195–200.
42. Burch WM. Cushing's disease. A review. Arch Intern Med. 1985;145:1106–11.
43. Brand IR, Dalton GA, Fletcher RF. Long-term follow up of transsphenoidal hypophysectomy for Cushing's disease. J R Soc Med. 1985;78:291–3.
44. Nakane T, Kuwayama A, Watanabe M, et al. Long term results of transsphenoidal adenomectomy in patients with Cushing's disease. Neurosurgery. 1987;21:218–22.
45. Mampalam TJ, Tyrrell JB, Wilson CB. Transsphenoidal microsurgery for Cushing disease. A report of 216 cases. Ann Intern Med. 1988;109:487–93.
46. Pieters GF, Hermus AR, Meijer E, et al. Predictive factors for initial cure and relapse rate after pituitary surgery for Cushing's disease. J Clin Endocrinol Metab. 1989;69:1122–6.
47. McCance DR, Gordon DS, Fannin TF, et al. Assessment of endocrine function after transsphenoidal surgery for Cushing's disease. Clin Endocrinol. 1993;38:79–86.
48. Blevins LS Jr, Christy JH, Khajavi M, Tindall GT. Outcomes of therapy for Cushing's disease due to adrenocorticotropin-secreting pituitary macroadenomas. J Clin Endocrinol Metab. 1998;83:63–7.

49. Semple PL, Laws ER Jr. Complications in a contemporary series of patients who underwent transsphenoidal surgery for Cushing's disease. J Neurosurg. 1999;91:175–9.
50. Nieman LK, Biller BM, Findling JW, et al. Treatment of Cushing's syndrome: an endocrine society clinical practice guideline. J Clin Endocrinol Metab. 2015;100:2807–31.
51. Simeoli C, Ferrigno R, De Martino MC, et al. The treatment with pasireotide in Cushing's disease: effect of long-term treatment on clinical picture and metabolic profile and management of adverse events in the experience of a single center. J Endocrinol Investig. 2020;43:57–73.
52. Miller JW, Crapo L. The medical treatment of Cushing's syndrome. Endocr Rev. 1993;14:443–58.
53. Findling JW, Raff H. Cushing's syndrome: important issues in diagnosis and management. J Clin Endocrinol Metab. 2006;91:3746–53.
54. Tritos NA, Biller BMK. Medical management of Cushing disease. Neurosurg Clin N Am. 2019;30:499–508.
55. Schteingart DE. Drugs in the medical treatment of Cushing's syndrome–an update on mifepristone and pasireotide. Expert Opin Emerg Drugs. 2012;17:279–83.
56. Alexandraki KI, Grossman AB. Medical therapy of Cushing's disease: where are we now? Front Horm Res. 2010;38:165–73.
57. Fleseriu M. Medical management of persistent and recurrent Cushing disease. Neurosurg Clin N Am. 2012;23:653–68.
58. Fleseriu M, Petersenn S. Medical management of Cushing's disease: what is the future? Pituitary. 2012;15:330–41.
59. van der Pas R, de Herder WW, Hofland LJ, Feelders RA. New developments in the medical treatment of Cushing's syndrome. Endocr Relat Cancer. 2012;19:R205–23.
60. Cuevas-Ramos D, Fleseriu M. Medical treatment of Cushing's disease. Minerva Endocrinol. 2016;41:324–40.
61. Feelders RA, Hofland LJ. Medical treatment of Cushing's disease. J Clin Endocrinol Metab. 2013;98:425–38.
62. Nieman LK. Update in the medical therapy of Cushing's disease. Curr Opin Endocrinol Diabetes Obes. 2013;20:330–4.
63. Gadelha MR, Vieira Neto L. Efficacy of medical treatment in Cushing's disease: a systematic review. Clin Endocrinol. 2014;80:1–12.
64. Tritos NA, Biller BM. Medical management of Cushing's disease. J Neuro-Oncol. 2014;117:407–14.
65. Fleseriu M. Recent advances in the medical treatment of Cushing's disease. F1000Prime Rep. 2014;6:18.
66. Tritos NA, Biller BM. Update on radiation therapy in patients with Cushing's disease. Pituitary. 2015;18:263–8.
67. Broersen LHA, Andela CD, Dekkers OM, et al. Improvement but no normalization of quality of life and cognitive functioning after treatment of cushing syndrome. J Clin Endocrinol Metab. 2019;104:5325–37.
68. Dekkers OM, Horvath-Puho E, Jorgensen JO, et al. Multisystem morbidity and mortality in Cushing's syndrome: a cohort study. J Clin Endocrinol Metab. 2013;98:2277–84.

51 Persistent or Recurrent Hypoglycemia in Infants and Todlers

Charlene Lai and Diva D. De León

Introduction

Glucose is an essential source of energy for the brain, and inadequate glucose delivery, particularly in infancy and early childhood, can lead to brain damage and lifelong developmental delays [1, 2]. Therefore, the prompt recognition, diagnosis, and management of a child with hypoglycemia is critical to prevent poor outcomes. A systematic and comprehensive approach for evaluating the integrity of the fasting systems is key for determining the underlying cause of hypoglycemia. This chapter reviews the normal physiology of glucose regulation with a focus on pathophysiology, diagnosis, and management of disorders resulting in persistent hypoglycemia in infants and children.

Normal Fasting Adaptation

The maintenance of an adequate supply of glucose for brain functioning during fasting is dependent on three fasting systems: hepatic gluconeogenesis, hepatic glycogenolysis, and hepatic ketogenesis. In the first 12–16 hours of fasting, plasma glucose levels are maintained largely by hepatic glycogenolysis, with a smaller contribution from gluconeogenesis. Hepatic ketogenesis provides ketones as fuel sources for the brain after the hepatic stores of glycogen are exhausted [3] (Fig. 51.1).

The fourth fasting system is the counter-regulatory hormone response to fasting, which controls these processes.

C. Lai
The Division of Endocrinology and Diabetes, The Children's Hospital of Philadelphia, Philadelphia, PA, USA
e-mail: LAICW@EMAIL.CHOP.EDU

D. D. De León (✉)
The Division of Endocrinology and Diabetes, The Children's Hospital of Philadelphia, Philadelphia, PA, USA

Department of Pediatrics, The Perelman School of Medicine at the University of Pennsylvania, Philadelphia, PA, USA
e-mail: deleon@email.chop.edu

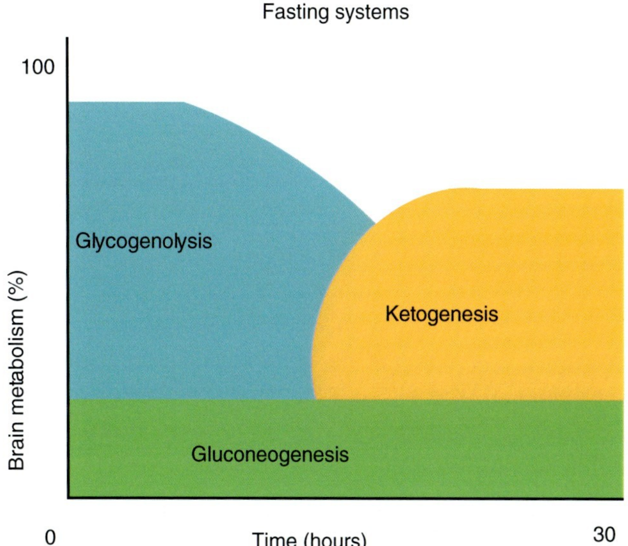

Fig. 51.1 Normal fasting adaptation: Maintenance of a normal plasma glucose during fasting is dependent on hepatic gluconeogenesis, hepatic glycogenolysis, and hepatic ketogenesis. In the first 12–16 hours of fasting, plasma glucose levels are maintained mostly by hepatic glycogenolysis, with a smaller percentage from gluconeogenesis. After liver glycogen stores are exhausted, hepatic ketogenesis provides ketones as fuel sources for the brain. (Adapted from: De León et al. [37])

Insulin suppresses glycogenolysis, gluconeogenesis, and ketogenesis while stimulating the storage of glucose as glycogen. Epinephrine stimulates glycogenolysis, gluconeogenesis, and ketogenesis while suppressing insulin. Glucagon stimulates glycogenolysis and gluconeogenesis. Cortisol stimulates gluconeogenesis, and growth hormone increases lipolysis, providing substrate for ketogenesis [2]. All of these counter-regulatory hormones play a major role in the body's defense against hypoglycemia. When plasma glucose falls below 85 mg/dL, insulin secretion is suppressed, a key step for allowing the activation of the fasting systems. Once plasma glucose reaches 65–70 mg/dL, glucagon and epinephrine are upregulated. At plasma glucose <65 mg/dL, cortisol and growth hormone levels increase [1] (Fig. 51.2).

T. Stanley, M. Misra (eds.), *Endocrine Conditions in Pediatrics*, https://doi.org/10.1007/978-3-030-52215-5_51

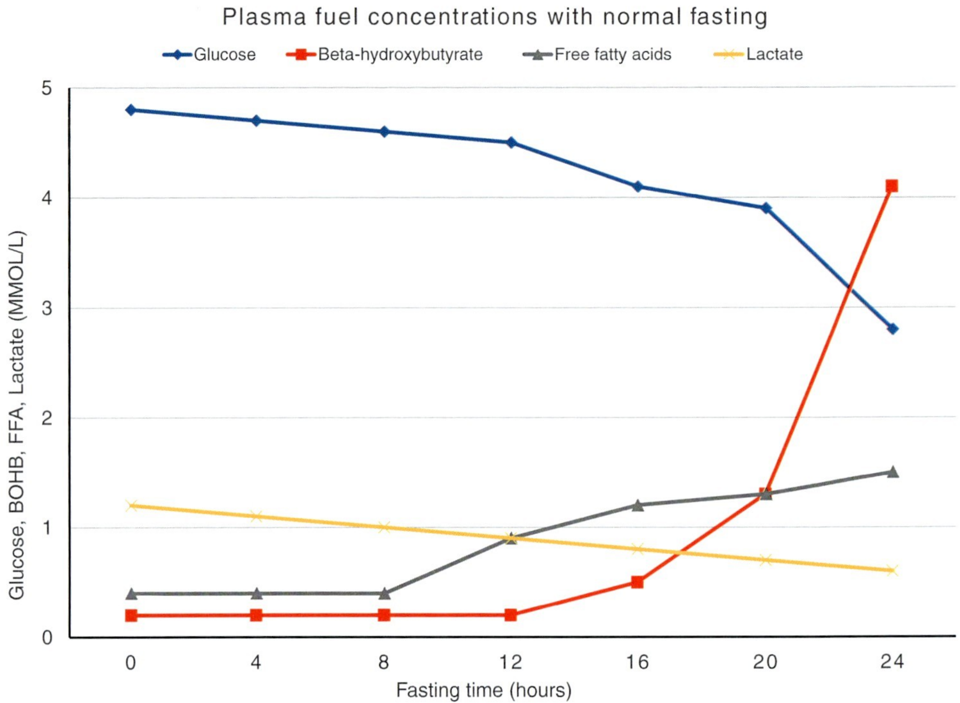

Fig. 51.2 Plasma fuel concentrations with normal fasting: During normal fasting, as plasma glucose levels fall, beta-hydroxybutyrate and free fatty acids increase to be used as alternative fuel sources. Lactate levels in normal fasting stay relatively constant. (Adapted from: De León et al. [37])

The thresholds for activation of the above counter-regulatory processes do not differ between neonates and older children after 3 days of life. During the intra- to extra-uterine transition, plasma glucose decreases to 55–60 mg/dL within the first 2 hours of life. However, after the first 3 days of life, the normal range for plasma glucose in neonates is the same as in older children and adults [1, 4].

When to Suspect a Hypoglycemia Disorder

Because the signs and symptoms of hypoglycemia can be subtle in young children, a high degree of suspicion is necessary for the prompt recognition of a hypoglycemia disorder. In neonates, this is based on the identification and screening for hypoglycemia of at-risk neonates. In older children, as in adults, initial hypoglycemia symptoms are the result of activation of the autonomic nervous system. These symptoms include: palpitations, tremors, anxiety, sweating, hunger, and paresthesias. If hypoglycemia is not corrected, confusion, coma, and seizures are the end result of deficient glucose supply to the brain. Older children should be evaluated if Whipple's triad is met: signs/symptoms suggestive of hypoglycemia, a low plasma glucose, and resolution of symptoms when plasma glucose returns to normal. In neonates and younger children who cannot communicate these symptoms, hypoglycemia should be evaluated if plasma glucose is <60 mg/dL, as measured by a laboratory-quality assay. Neonates at high risk for a persistent hypoglycemia disorder should be evaluated at ≥48 hours of age, after the transitional glucose regulation period has passed [4]. While point-of-care glucose meters may be used as screening tools, confirmatory measurement with a serum glucose sent to the laboratory should always be used for critical steps in the medical decision-making process. Please see Chap. 31 for assay considerations in the measurement of glucose.

Evaluation

The diagnosis of the specific cause of hypoglycemia relies on the measurement of metabolic fuels and counter-regulatory hormones during a spontaneous or provoked episode of hypoglycemia. In a normal infant and child fasted until a plasma glucose of 50 mg/dL: (1) glycogen stores are exhausted, and there will be no glycemic response to glucagon; (2) gluconeogenic substrates have declined (lactate <1.5 mmol/L); (3) free fatty acids (FFA) have tripled (1.5–2 mmol/L); (4) beta-hydroxybutyrate (BOHB) has risen 50–100-fold (2–5 mmol/L); (5) insulin is suppressed (<2uU/mL); and (6) cortisol and growth hormone are increased [5] (Fig. 51.2).

Specific Etiologies

The concentration of these metabolic fuels (beta-hydroxybutyrate [BOHB], free fatty acids [FFA], and lactate) measured in the "critical sample" obtained when plasma glucose is <50 mg/dL can be used to classify hypoglycemic disorders into four main categories: hypoketotic hypoglycemia with decreased FFA, hypoketotic hypoglycemia with increased FFA, hypoglycemia with increased lactate, and hyperketotic hypoglycemia (Tables 51.1 and 51.2, and Fig. 51.3).

Hypoketotic Hypoglycemia with Decreased FFA

The disorders that should be considered if a critical sample has low BOHB (≤1.8 mmol/L) and FFA (<1.7 mmol/L) are neonatal hypopituitarism and insulin-mediated hypoglycemic disorders: hyperinsulinism (HI), insulinoma, exogenous insulin administration, and post-prandial hypoglycemia.

Neonatal Hypopituitarism

Hypoglycemia from growth hormone and cortisol deficiency presents most often in children as hyperketotic hypoglycemia. However, in the neonate, the deficiency of these two hormones can present similar to hyperinsulinism—as hypoketotic hypoglycemia with low FFA and a positive glycemic response to glucagon administration. A direct hyperbilirubinemia is often seen [2, 6, 7].

Table 51.1 Critical sample

Laboratory	Expected value during hypoglycemia (<50 mg/dL)
Plasma insulin	Below the level of detection (<2 uU/mL)
Plasma beta-hydroxybutyrate	≥2 mmol/L
Plasma free fatty acids	≥1.7 mmol/L
Growth hormone	≥7 ng/mL
Cortisol	≥10 mcg/dL
Lactate	≤1.5 mmol/L

Insulin-Mediated Hypoglycemia

Insulin suppresses glycogenolysis, gluconeogenesis, and ketogenesis while stimulating the storage of glucose as glycogen. Thus, in insulin-mediated hypoglycemia, BOHB and FFA are inappropriately low and there is a glycemic response to glucagon.

Hyperinsulinism

Hyperinsulinism is the most common cause of persistent hypoglycemia in infants and children [2, 8]. Hyperinsulinism is a heterogenous disorder that can be genetic or secondary to perinatal factors, transient or persistent. Children with hyperinsulinism usually present soon after birth with severe, recurrent hypoglycemia and a need for exogenous glucose to maintain plasma glucose in the normal range [2, 5].

Table 51.2 Causes of hypoglycemic in children

Hypoketotic with decreased free fatty acids
Neonatal hypopituitarism
Insulin-mediated
Hyperinsulinism
Syndromic hyperinsulinism
Beckwith-Wiedemann syndrome
Kabuki syndrome
Turner syndrome
Insulinoma
Exogenous insulin administration
Post-prandial hypoglycemia
Hypoketotic hypoglycemia with increased free fatty acids
Fatty acid oxidation disorders
Hyperketotic hypoglycemia
Idiopathic ketotic hypoglycemia
Hormone deficiencies
Cortisol deficiency
Growth hormone deficiency
Glycogen storage disorders
Hypoglycemia with lactate elevation
Glycogen storage disease I
Ingestion

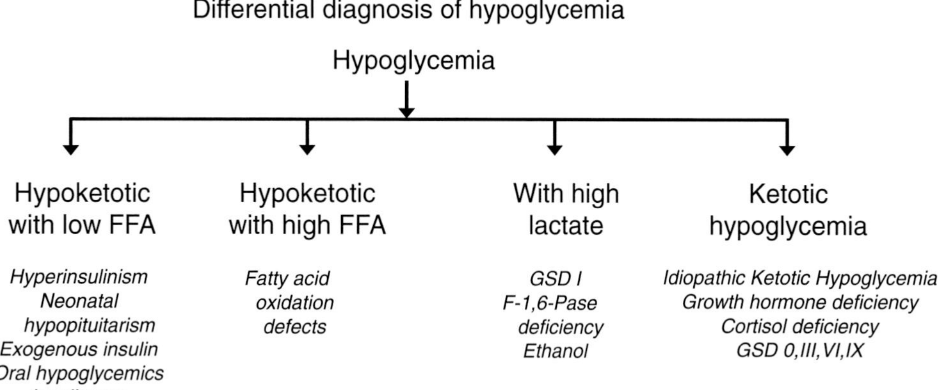

Fig. 51.3 Hypoglycemic disorders can be categorized into four main categories: Hypoketotic hypoglycemia with decreased free fatty acids, hypoketotic hypoglycemia with increased free fatty acids, hypoglycemic with increased lactate, and hyperketotic hypoglycemia

Transient hyperinsulinism is more commonly the result of maternal or perinatal factors, including maternal diabetes and perinatal stress. While hyperinsulinemic hypoglycemia due to poorly controlled maternal diabetes resolves within the first few days of life, perinatal stress-induced hyperinsulinism may persist for several weeks. Perinatal stressors associated with hyperinsulinism include low birth weight, hypoxia, maternal preeclampsia, congenital heart disease, meconium aspiration syndrome, and prematurity. These stressors may impact the process of beta-cell maturation after birth, resulting in dysregulated insulin secretion. Perinatal stress-induced hyperinsulinism typically resolves within the first 2–6 months of life [9, 10].

Persistent hyperinsulinism can be monogenic (known as congenital hyperinsulinism) or can be part of an underlying syndrome. There are currently at least ten identified genes associated with congenital hyperinsulinism. The inheritance pattern can be dominant or recessive. Depending on the gene mutation, these infants may or may not be responsive to diazoxide, the only FDA-approved treatment for HI [5]. The most common type of congenital hyperinsulinism is caused by inactivating mutations in the beta-cell K_{ATP} channels. This form of hyperinsulinism is more frequently unresponsive to treatment with diazoxide. Histologically, hyperinsulinism due to K_{ATP} channel mutations can be diffuse, affecting the whole pancreas, or focal, affecting only a small portion of the pancreas. Focal hyperinsulinism accounts for 40–60% of diazoxide unresponsive hyperinsulinism cases and is due to a combination of a paternally inherited recessive K_{ATP} channel mutation and focal loss of heterozygosity for maternal 11p. These cases are unique because, with perioperative localization of the lesion by 18-F DOPA PET and subsequent resection of the lesion, the hyperinsulinism can be cured [11–14].

Syndromic Hyperinsulinism

Hyperinsulinism can be seen in children with Beckwith-Wiedemann syndrome, Turner syndrome, Kabuki syndrome, Sotos syndrome, and congenital disorders of glycosylation, among others [15–21].

Insulinoma

Insulinomas are rare in the pediatric population and are typically benign. Resection of the tumor is curative [22, 23]. All children with an insulinoma should be tested for multiple endocrine neoplasia type 1.

Exogenous Insulin Administration

Exogenous insulin through deliberate or accidental administration should be considered in the differential of hyperinsulinemic hypoglycemia. The finding of a critical sample with an elevated plasma insulin concentration and a low C-peptide concentration at the time of hypoglycemia confirms the diagnosis. However, if an insulin secretagogue like a sulfonylurea was ingested, both insulin and C-peptide will be elevated. Munchausen by proxy in these situations can be difficult to detect, and a high level of suspicion should be maintained if an otherwise healthy child develops new hypoglycemia with an unpredictable pattern.

Post-prandial Hypoglycemia

Post-prandial hypoglycemia, or "late dumping syndrome," is a common complication of Nissen fundoplication in pediatric patients. The severity of presentation varies from mild, asymptomatic hypoglycemia to seizures. The mechanism is thought to be due to a combination of asynchronous nutrient absorption and insulin secretion, as well as increased secretion of glucagon like peptide 1 (GLP-1). After Nissen fundoplication, food moves more rapidly from the stomach into the small intestine, causing early hyperglycemia which triggers an exaggerated insulin surge and subsequent hypoglycemia 1–2 hours after a meal. In addition, increased secretion of GLP-1 by the small bowel after a meal may contribute to exaggerated insulin secretion [24–26].

Hypoketotic Hypoglycemia with Increased FFA

The finding of low BOHB plasma concentration and high FFA plasma concentration is pathognomonic of a fatty acid oxidation defect (FAO). Deficiency of one of the enzymes in the cascade of fatty acid oxidation leads to accumulation of acylcarnitine precursors. With the advent of universal newborn screening in the United States, most cases of FAO are detected on newborn screening before clinical manifestations. Acute metabolic decompensation, provoked by prolonged fasting or illness, manifests with hypoketotic hypoglycemia, transaminitis, uric acidemia, and elevated levels of ammonia [2].

Hyperketotic Hypoglycemia

A pattern of hyperketotic hypoglycemia is the normal response to starvation. However, in a child with repeated episodes, a pathologic cause of hypoglycemia should be considered, including the disorders outlined below.

Idiopathic Ketotic Hypoglycemia

Idiopathic ketotic hypoglycemia is most commonly seen in children 1–4 years old during an illness that results in prolonged fasting. The resulting hypoglycemia is accompanied by appropriate hormonal and metabolic responses to hypoglycemia, including elevation in BOHB plasma concentration. In most cases, after other endocrine or metabolic disorders have been ruled out, these children may represent the lower end of normal distribution of fasting tolerance. It is important to remember that this is a diagnosis of exclusion, and glycogen storage diseases or ketone utilization defects may present in a similar manner [1, 27, 28].

Hormone Deficiencies

During the newborn period, cortisol and growth hormone deficiencies may present with a hypoketotic hypoglycemia pattern. However, in older infants and children, these hormonal deficiencies present with ketotic hypoglycemia. Cortisol deficiency may be central or primary, including congenital adrenal hyperplasia. Isolated growth hormone deficiency typically does not present with hypoglycemia outside of the newborn period [2, 7] .

Glycogen Storage Disorders

Glycogen storage disorders (GSD) are genetic disorders that result in enzymatic defects affecting the synthesis or breakdown of glycogen. They are a heterogeneous group of disorders that present with varying severity of fasting hypoglycemia with ketosis and hepatomegaly. Children with GSD type III, the most severe, usually present in infancy with failure to thrive, hepatomegaly, hypertriglyceridemia, transaminitis, and cardiomyopathy. GSD 0, VI, and IX typically present in early childhood with milder hypoglycemia and transaminitis. GSD I affects, in addition to glycogenolysis, gluconeogenesis and, unlike the other GSDs, presents with an elevated lactate [29, 30].

Hypoglycemia with Lactate Elevation

Disorders of gluconeogenesis result in hypoglycemia with an accumulation of gluconeogenic substrates, including lactate. These disorders are rare, but the most common is GSD I, glucose-6-phosphatase deficiency [30].

Ingestion

There are many ingestions which can cause hypoglycemia. The more common substances include: oral hypoglycemics, beta-blockers, ethanol, and salicylates.

Urgent or Emergent Considerations and Initial Management

The immediate goal of treatment in children with hypoglycemia is to restore plasma glucose to the normal range (≥70 mg/dL). This is accomplished through administration of glucose by mouth, by enteral tube, or intravenously (IV).

Management in the Outpatient Office

Because point-of-care glucose meters are inaccurate, a low measurement should at least be repeated for confirmation and, ideally, be confirmed by a laboratory-quality measurement before embarking on an investigation for a hypoglycemia disorder. In a child with suspected or confirmed hypoglycemia, plasma glucose should be promptly restored to the normal range by offering 15 grams of carbohydrates by mouth (juice or formula). Plasma glucose should be repeated in 15 minutes to assure that the intervention has been effective. This patient should be referred to an endocrinologist for an expedited appointment or sent to the Emergency Department for further workup.

Management in the Hospital

In the hospital, if plasma glucose cannot be maintained ≥70 mg/dL with feeding alone, IV dextrose should be used for glucose management. The concentration and/or rate of dextrose can be increased as long as access and fluid status is not a concern. If an insulin-mediated process is suspected, a continuous glucagon infusion can be trialed via a peripheral or central line at 1 mg/24 hours in addition to IV dextrose if access or fluid status is a concern. Glucagon may also be given as an intramuscular or subcutaneous injection as a temporizing measure. However, the effects of a single dose will only last for 20–30 minutes [1].

Chronic Management and Considerations for Referral

A child with a suspected or confirmed hypoglycemia disorder should be referred to a pediatric endocrinologist for evaluation and treatment. considerations for referral to a pediatric endocrinologist include

1. Neonates unable to maintain normal plasma glucose concentration after the first 3 days of life
2. A child with a symptomatic episode of hypoglycemia (i.e., presentation with Whipple's triad)
3. Persistent or recurrent hypoglycemia at any age
4. Hypoglycemia or symptoms of hypoglycemia in a child with a family history of a hypoglycemia disorder
5. A child with hypoglycemia or symptoms of hypoglycemia and other characteristics suggesting an underlying hypoglycemia disorder: features of Beckwith-Wiedemann syndrome, short stature, hepatomegaly, etc.
6. A confirmed diagnosis of a hypoglycemia disorder

Chronic Management of Hypoglycemic Disorders

The determination of the specific cause of the hypoglycemia is important to establish specific treatments and prevent further episodes of hypoglycemia. The treatment may include limitation of fasting time, hormonal replacement if the cause is cortisol or growth hormone deficiency, dietary changes, or medications.

Hyperinsulinism

Diazoxide is first-line therapy for hyperinsulinism. For cases that are unresponsive, the priority should be to screen for the possibility of focal hyperinsulinism, because in those cases surgery is curative. If the hyperinsulinism is unresponsive to diazoxide and is determined to not be focal, other treatments include continuous dextrose (D20%) through a gastrostomy, or somatostatin analogues, such as octreotide and lanreotide [5, 7, 31, 32]. Patients should be followed every 3–6 months on therapy to monitor for effectiveness and side effects [33, 34].

Post-prandial Hypoglycemia

Post-prandial hypoglycemia can be treated by multiple methods. First-line therapies are nutritional modifications targeted at slowing the rate of movement of food or formula from the stomach to the small intestine. This can be accomplished by redistributing feeds to run more slowly and/or changing the formula to a thicker formula. If these solutions do not ameliorate hypoglycemia, medium-chain triglyceride (MCT) oil or acarbose may be added [35].

Idiopathic Ketotic Hypoglycemia

Idiopathic ketotic hypoglycemia is usually managed by ensuring that patients eat a well-balanced meal for dinner and a nighttime snack. However, if hypoglycemia persists overnight or in the morning, up to 1 g/kg of uncooked cornstarch can be trialed at bedtime.

Hormonal Deficiencies

Treatment of cortisol deficiency with 8–10 mg/m^2/day of hydrocortisone and/or growth hormone deficiency with 0.3 mg/kg/week of growth hormone should resolve hypoglycemia.

Glycogen Storage Diseases

GSDs are treated with uncooked cornstarch up to 1–2 g/kg from one to multiple times a day and by ensuring that there is no prolonged fasting [29, 36].

References

1. Thornton PS, Stanley CA, De Leon DD, Harris D, Haymond MW, Hussain K, et al. Recommendations from the Pediatric Endocrine Society for Evaluation and Management of Persistent Hypoglycemia in Neonates, Infants, and Children. J Pediatr. 2015;167(2):238–45.
2. Langdon DR, Stanley CA, Sperling MA. Hypoglycemia in the toddler and child. In: Sperling MA, editor. Pediatric endocrinology. 4th ed. Philadelphia: Elsevier/Saunders; 2014. p. 920–55.
3. Stanley CABL. Hypoglycemia. In: Kaye ROF, Barness LA, editors. Core textbook of pediatrics. Philadelphia: Lippinoctt; 1978. p. 280–305.
4. Stanley CA, Rozance PJ, Thornton PS, De Leon DD, Harris D, Haymond MW, et al. Re-evaluating "transitional neonatal hypoglycemia": mechanism and implications for management. J Pediatr. 2015;166(6):1520–5 e1.
5. Lord K, De Leon DD. Hyperinsulinism in the neonate. Clin Perinatol. 2018;45(1):61–74.
6. Choo-Kang LR, Sun CC, Counts DR. Cholestasis and hypoglycemia: manifestations of congenital anterior hypopituitarism. J Clin Endocrinol Metab. 1996;81(8):2786–9.
7. Lord K, De Leon DD, Stanley CA. Hypoglycemia. In: Radovick S, Misra M, editors. Pediatric endocrinology a practical clinical guide. 3rd ed: Springer; 2018. p. 702–13.
8. De Leon DD, Stanley CA. Mechanisms of disease: advances in diagnosis and treatment of hyperinsulinism in neonates. Nat Clin Pract Endocrinol Metab. 2007;3(1):57–68.
9. Collins JE, Leonard JV. Hyperinsulinism in asphyxiated and small-for-dates infants with hypoglycaemia. Lancet (London, England). 1984;2(8398):311–3.
10. Hoe FM, Thornton PS, Wanner LA, Steinkrauss L, Simmons RA, Stanley CA. Clinical features and insulin regulation in infants with a syndrome of prolonged neonatal hyperinsulinism. J Pediatr. 2006;148(2):207–12.
11. Christiansen CD, Petersen H, Nielsen AL, Detlefsen S, Brusgaard K, Rasmussen L, et al. 18F-DOPA PET/CT and 68Ga-DOTANOC PET/CT scans as diagnostic tools in focal congenital hyperinsulinism: a blinded evaluation. Eur J Nucl Med Mol Imaging. 2018;45(2):250–61.
12. Ribeiro MJ, De Lonlay P, Delzescaux T, Boddaert N, Jaubert F, Bourgeois S, et al. Characterization of hyperinsulinism in infancy assessed with PET and 18F-fluoro-L-DOPA. J Nucl Med. 2005;46(4):560–6.
13. Otonkoski T, Nanto-Salonen K, Seppanen M, et al. Noninvasive diagnosis of focal hyperinsulinism of infancy with [18F]-DOPA positron emission tomography. Diabetes Metab. 2006;55:13–8.
14. Adzick NS, De Leon DD, States LJ, Lord K, Bhatti TR, Becker SA, et al. Surgical treatment of congenital hyperinsulinism: results from 500 pancreatectomies in neonates and children. J Pediatr Surg. 2018;
15. Gibson CE, Boodhansingh KE, Li C, Conlin L, Chen P, Becker SA, et al. Congenital hyperinsulinism in infants with turner syndrome: possible association with monosomy X and KDM6A haploinsufficiency. Horm Res Paediatr. 2018;89(6):413–22.
16. Vajravelu ME, De Leon DD. Genetic characteristics of patients with congenital hyperinsulinism. Curr Opin Pediatr. 2018;30(4):568–75.
17. Bogershausen N, Gatinois V, Riehmer V, Kayserili H, Becker J, Thoenes M, et al. Mutation update for kabuki syndrome genes KMT2D and KDM6A and further delineation of X-linked kabuki syndrome subtype 2. Hum Mutat. 2016;37(9):847–64.

18. Alkhayyat H, Christesen HB, Steer J, Stewart H, Brusgaard K, Hussain K. Mosaic Turner syndrome and hyperinsulinaemic hypoglycaemia. J Pediatr Endocrinol Metab. 2006;19(12):1451–7.
19. Hussain K, Cosgrove KE, Shepherd RM, Luharia A, Smith VV, Kassem S, et al. Hyperinsulinemic hypoglycemia in Beckwith-Wiedemann syndrome due to defects in the function of pancreatic beta-cell adenosine triphosphate-sensitive potassium channels. J Clin Endocrinol Metab. 2005;90(7):4376–82.
20. Kalish JM, Boodhansingh KE, Bhatti TR, Ganguly A, Conlin LK, Becker SA, et al. Congenital hyperinsulinism in children with paternal 11p uniparental isodisomy and Beckwith-Wiedemann syndrome. J Med Genet. 2016;53(1):53–61.
21. Grand K, Gonzalez-Gandolfi C, Ackermann AM, Aljeaid D, Bedoukian E, Bird LM, et al. Hyperinsulinemic hypoglycemia in seven patients with de novo NSD1 mutations. Am J Med Genet A. 2019;179(4):542–51.
22. Peranteau WH, Palladino AA, Bhatti TR, Becker SA, States LJ, Stanley CA, et al. The surgical management of insulinomas in children. J Pediatr Surg. 2013;48(12):2517–24.
23. Padidela R, Fiest M, Arya V, Smith VV, Ashworth M, Rampling D, et al. Insulinoma in childhood: clinical, radiological, molecular and histological aspects of nine patients. Eur J Endocrinol. 2014;170(5):741–7.
24. Palladino AA, Sayed S, Levitt Katz LE, Gallagher PR, De Leon DD. Increased glucagon-like peptide-1 secretion and postprandial hypoglycemia in children after Nissen fundoplication. J Clin Endocrinol Metab. 2009;94(1):39–44.
25. Samuk I, Afriat R, Horne T, Bistritzer T, Barr J, Vinograd I. Dumping syndrome following Nissen fundoplication, diagnosis, and treatment. J Pediatr Gastroenterol Nutr. 1996;23(3):235–40.
26. Calabria AC, Charles L, Givler S, De Leon DD. Postprandial hypoglycemia in children after gastric surgery: clinical characterization and pathophysiology. Horm Res Paediatr. 2016;85(2):140–6.
27. White K, Truong L, Aaron K, Mushtaq N, Thornton PS. The incidence and etiology of previously undiagnosed hypoglycemic disorders in the emergency department. Pediatr Emerg Care. 2018;
28. Pershad J, Monroe K, Atchison J. Childhood hypoglycemia in an urban emergency department: epidemiology and a diagnostic approach to the problem. Pediatr Emerg Care. 1998;14(4):268–71.
29. Wolfsdorf JI, Weinstein DA. Glycogen storage diseases. Rev Endocr Metab Disord. 2003;4(1):95–102.
30. Rake JP, Visser G, Labrune P, Leonard JV, Ullrich K, Smit GP. Glycogen storage disease type I: diagnosis, management, clinical course and outcome. Results of the European Study on Glycogen Storage Disease Type I (ESGSD I). Eur J Pediatr. 2002;161 Suppl 1:S20–34.
31. Herrera A, Vajravelu ME, Givler S, Mitteer L, Avitabile CM, Lord K, et al. Prevalence of adverse events in children with congenital hyperinsulinism treated with diazoxide. J Clin Endocrinol Metab. 2018;103(12):4365–72.
32. Vajravelu ME, Congdon M, Mitteer L, Koh J, Givler S, Shults J, et al. Continuous intragastric dextrose: a therapeutic option for refractory hypoglycemia in congenital hyperinsulinism. Horm Res Paediatr. 2018:1–7.
33. Le Quan Sang KH, Arnoux JB, Mamoune A, Saint-Martin C, Bellanne-Chantelot C, Valayannopoulos V, et al. Successful treatment of congenital hyperinsulinism with long-acting release octreotide. Eur J Endocrinol. 2012;166(2):333–9.
34. McMahon AW, Wharton GT, Thornton P, De Leon DD. Octreotide use and safety in infants with hyperinsulinism. Pharmacoepidemiol Drug Saf. 2017;26(1):26–31.
35. Ng DD, Ferry RJ Jr, Kelly A, Weinzimer SA, Stanley CA, Katz LE. Acarbose treatment of postprandial hypoglycemia in children after Nissen fundoplication. J Pediatr. 2001;139(6):877–9.
36. Wolfsdorf JI, Keller RJ, Landy H, Crigler JF Jr. Glucose therapy for glycogenosis type 1 in infants: comparison of intermittent uncooked cornstarch and continuous overnight glucose feedings. J Pediatr. 1990;117(3):384–91.
37. De León DD, Thornton PS, Stanley CA, Sperling MA. Hypoglycemia in the Newborn and Infant. In: Sperling MA, editor. Pediatric endocrinology. 4th ed: Elsevier; 2014.

Type 1 Diabetes Mellitus

52

Ambreen Sonawalla and Rabab Jafri

Overview

Type 1 diabetes mellitus (T1DM) is a disorder of glucose homeostasis that affects millions of children across the United States. For unknown reasons, the prevalence of type 1 diabetes may be increasing: a 21.1% increase in the prevalence of T1DM was detected over 8 years, from 2001 to 2009 [1]. In 2015, 1.25 million American children and adults were known to have T1DM. An estimated 40,000 people are diagnosed with T1DM each year. Among people under the age of 20, *non-Hispanic whites* had the highest rates of new diagnosis of type 1 diabetes [2].

Type 1 diabetes refers to near-complete insulin deficiency, that is, inability of the pancreas to synthesize and/or secrete insulin, whereas type 2 diabetes refers to a state of relative insulin deficiency in the setting of insulin resistance. This nomenclature is somewhat misleading in the sense that some individuals with long-standing type 2 diabetes may also have near-complete insulin deficiency. T1DM is typically autoimmune in nature, with autoimmune destruction of pancreatic beta-cells resulting in impaired insulin synthesis and secretion. Much more rarely, T1DM can be idiopathic (also known as type 1b). The steps to progression of diabetes are listed below.

Key Pathophysiology of Type 1 Diabetes

- Autoimmune diabetes develops in the presence of a genetic predisposition (often characterized by certain variants of HLA-DQA1, HLA-DQB1, and HLA-DRB1).
- An environmental trigger such as an acute illness is thought to provide a "second hit."
- Type 1 diabetes progresses in stages, as described below. It is estimated that about 70% of pancreatic beta-cell mass must be destroyed before T1DM manifests.
- Stage 1: Autoantibodies to pancreatic islet cell antigens develop without dysglycemia.
- Stage 2: The autoimmune destruction of the insulin-producing pancreatic β islet cells eventually leads to insufficient amount of insulin production to meet metabolic needs ➔ Dysglycemia develops without symptoms of diabetes.
- Stage 3: Hyperglycemia further impairs the ability of the pancreas to secrete insulin (glucotoxicity), and symptoms of diabetes ensue from constantly and significantly elevated blood sugars.

Diagnosis

Clinical presentation at home, school or the primary care setting is described below along with the diagnostic criteria (Table 52.1) for diabetes mellitus.

Clinical Presentation in the Primary Care Setting

Type 1 diabetes usually presents with the classic triad of "polys" (polyuria, polydipsia, and polyphagia), along with some degree of weight loss. Less commonly, the presentation may be more subtle, and early, asymptomatic diabetes (stage 2) may be diagnosed through incidental findings such as glucosuria. Any suspicion of T1DM should prompt a fingerstick point of care glucose test and urinalysis (see Chap. 9) with subsequent considerations as below. A few specific scenarios in which keeping a high suspicion of T1DM can expedite diagnosis should be noted.

1. Children presenting with vomiting and weight loss during gastroenteritis epidemics: Vomiting is a symptom of keto-

A. Sonawalla
Arkansas Children's Hospital, Little Rock, AR, USA

R. Jafri (✉)
Massachusetts General Hospital, Boston, MA, USA
e-mail: jafrir@uthscsa.edu

T. Stanley, M. Misra (eds.), *Endocrine Conditions in Pediatrics*, https://doi.org/10.1007/978-3-030-52215-5_52

Table 52.1 Items required for diagnosis

Diagnostic criteria for diabetes mellitus (DM) [3]:
1. In a patient with classic symptoms of hyperglycemia Chap. 9, or hyperglycemic crisis (DKA or HHS), a random plasma glucose ≥200 mg/dL (11.1 mmol/L)
OR
2. HbA1c ≥6.5% (48 mmol/mol)
OR
3. Two-hour plasma glucose ≥200 mg/dL (11.1 mmol/L) during an OGTT (using a glucose load of 1.75 g/kg, up to a maximum of 75 g glucose)
OR
4. Fasting plasma glucose ≥126 mg/dL (7.0 mmol/L) (where fasting is defined as no caloric intake for at least 8 hours).
In the absence of unequivocal hyperglycemia, criteria 2–4 should be confirmed by repeat testing.
The distinction between type 1 and type 2 DM is made based on clinical and laboratory evaluation by an endocrinologist (see also Chaps. 30 and 53).

Abbreviations: *DKA* diabetic ketoacidosis, *HHS* hyperglycemic hyperosmolar syndrome, *HbA1C* hemoglobin A1c, *OGTT* oral glucose tolerance test, *DM* diabetes mellitus

sis, and intercurrent illness can prompt presentation of developing T1DM. In children who also have polyuria and polydipsia, T1DM should be considered.

2. Children presenting with polydipsia and polyuria around the time of potty training: Although these symptoms may be attributed to behavioral changes and/or desire for rewards associated with potty training, these may also be the presenting symptoms of T1DM.
3. Infants and very young children: T1DM can present as early as 6 months of age, and the presentation is usually less "classic" in very young children. Having a low threshold to check a fingerstick glucose in an older infant or toddler with failure to gain weight and any changes in drinking or urination patterns can expedite diagnosis and potentially prevent severe DKA.

Initial Management of Newly Presenting Diabetes

Hyperglycemia (≥200 mg/dL) in a child whose presentation includes polyuria, polydipsia, and/or weight loss is almost always indicative of diabetes mellitus. However, significant illness and/or certain medication use may cause hyperglycemia in the absence of DM. Further testing to differentiate the various causes of hyperglycemia is discussed in Chap. 9.

The first consideration in a child with newly presenting DM is whether or not emergency care is required. Any of the following *warrants immediate emergency department referral, deferring any additional testing to the emergency setting:*

1. Kussmaul respirations
2. Dehydration with inability to tolerate oral intake
3. Vomiting and/or severe headache
4. Altered mental status

These can indicate the presence of diabetic ketoacidosis (DKA) and/or hyperosmolar hyperglycemic state (HHS), and the patient requires urgent evaluation and management in an emergency room or pediatric intensive care unit (PICU). If the patient is able to tolerate oral intake, encourage hydration with sugar-free liquids while awaiting emergency transport.

Key Pathophysiology of Diabetic Ketoacidosis (DKA)

- *Hyperglycemia:*
  - Insulin suppresses counter-regulatory hormone secretion in the normal euglycemic state. In the insulinopenic state, glucagon, epinephrine, cortisol, and growth hormone are increased, leading to:
    Increased glycogenolysis
    Increased gluconeogenesis
    Further increases in lipolysis, exacerbating ketone formation
  - Hyperglycemia results from increased glucose production from the liver and decreased glucose utilization from insulinopenia
- *Ketosis/Ketoacidosis:*
  - Insulin suppresses systemic lipolysis in the normal euglycemic state. In the insulinopenic state, lipolysis is not suppressed, causing ketone body formation.
  - Excess circulating ketone bodies cause a state of metabolic acidosis.
- *Dehydration:*
  - Hyperglycemia that exceeds the renal threshold for reabsorption (approximately 180 mg/dL) causes polyuria/osmotic diuresis.
  - Osmotic diuresis leads to dehydration, as well as obligate losses of electrolytes.
- *Electrolyte Abnormalities:*
  - Osmotic diuresis leads to total body depletion of potassium and phosphate.

At the time of presentation, serum potassium may be normal or high because of insulinopenia (insulin facilitates intracellular potassium transport).

The second consideration in a child with newly presenting DM is whether ketones are present, suggesting possible DKA. Whereas urine ketones from urinalysis are adequate for assessment of ketosis, serum beta-hydroxybutyrate levels and a venous blood gas are very helpful if blood is being drawn to determine the presence of ketoacidosis. Although not all children with ketones will also have acidosis, all children with ketones should be emergently evaluated by a pediatric endocrinologist. Even well-appearing children can have DKA, and assessment of ketone status should be done as soon as hyperglycemia is diagnosed and diabetes suspected.

In a child with newly presenting T1DM who does not have urine or serum ketones, initiation of insulin therapy prevents the development of ketosis and DKA. Institutional protocols differ with regard to whether well-appearing children without ketones who have newly diagnosed T1DM require hospital admission or outpatient treatment, but same-day insulin should be initiated in nearly all circumstances, the only exception being children who appear to have been diagnosed at stage 2 and have only intermittent mild hyperglycemia.

Tips for Communicating a Probable New Diagnosis of T1DM

- Although it is appropriate for the pediatric endocrinologist to communicate a *definitive* diagnosis of T1DM, it can be very helpful if parents have heard of the possibility of T1DM from their primary care provider before the interaction with the pediatric endocrinologist.
- T1DM is managed by a multidisciplinary team. Parents can be reassured that they will be comprehensively cared for and guided in helping their child manage this new diagnosis.
- Standard of care for T1DM is *not* to impose abundant dietary restrictions, but rather to match insulin dosing to the normal healthy diet that the child eats. Children with T1DM can still eat what their peers are eating, have dessert, etc.
- New technologies and innovations for T1DM are developing quickly, such that T1DM should be more easily managed and potentially even cured in the upcoming several years.

With appropriate diabetes management, we expect children with T1DM to live healthy, fulfilling lives without activity restrictions and without subsequent hospitalizations.

Chronic Management

The goal of T1DM management is to: (1) maintain euglycemia; (2) facilitate normal growth and development; and (3) prevent the microvascular and macrovascular complications of chronic hyperglycemia.

Pediatric patients with T1DM are ideally managed by a diabetes management team consisting of a pediatric endocrinologist, nutritionist, nurse educator, social worker, child life specialist and mental health professional [4]. Long-term management requires frequent blood sugar monitoring, which may be achieved via SMBG (self-monitored blood glucose) readings or by the use of a continuous glucose monitor (CGM) worn on the body, and subcutaneous insulin. Insulin may be injected multiple times a day as MDIs (multiple daily injections) consisting of long and rapid-acting insulin preparations or via an insulin pump, which is also worn on the body and delivers insulin via a subcutaneous canula. The estimated total insulin dose (at initial diagnosis) is based on the patient's age, pubertal status, and weight. An insulin pump administers a steady basal dose of insulin throughout the day and night, and bolus doses timed with meals cover carbohydrates consumed during the meal and prevent hyperglycemic excursions from the carbohydrate load. In addition to covering carbohydrates, the mealtime insulin bolus corrects for hyperglycemia at these times. While insulin boluses for carbohydrate coverage may be administered every time the child eats, correction for hyperglycemia should not be repeated any more frequently than every 3 hours or so to avoid hypoglycemia from "stacking" of insulin. The basal rate and insulin boluses are typically adjusted at times of exercise and illness, to account for varying insulin needs at such times. Newer technology allows readings from a continuous glucose monitor to communicate with insulin pumps and allow semi or full automation of blood sugar control.

Management is tailored to a child's developmental level, and the patient and family are empowered to manage aspects of the patient's diabetes independently, early in the course of the diagnosis.

Patients are usually followed by the diabetes team. HbA1c is checked about every 3 months as an indicator of glycemic control. With the widespread use of CGMs, "time in range" (i.e., the percentage of the day that blood glucose is within a specific range, such as 80–180 mg/dL) is another important metric for control. The recommended HbA1c target for the pediatric population was recently raised from <7.0% to <7.5%, though this can vary depending on the individual medical and social factors of the patient [5]. Different types of insulin analogs typically used in the management of pediatric T1DM are listed in Table 52.1.

Long-term management also includes the following:

1. Monitoring for signs, symptoms, and laboratory evidence of comorbid conditions, of which hypertension, hyperlipidemia, thyroid disease, and celiac disease are the most common.
2. Assessment for mental health issues and ability to cope with a chronic medical diagnosis. These patients may require ongoing support in learning to adapt to their disease.
3. Screening for development of complications of hyperglycemia, such as retinopathy, nephropathy, neuropathy, and foot problems.

Table 52.2 Types of insulin typically used in inpatient and out-patient management of T1DM; generic name (brand)

Insulin	Onset of action	Peak action	Duration of action
Ultra-fast acting (Fiasp)	8–10 minutes	~1 hour	3–5 hours
Rapid-acting analogs: lispro (Humalog), Aspart (Novolog), Admelog (Humalog)	15–20 minutes	1–2 hours	3–6 hours
Short-acting insulin: Regular insulin	30–60 minutes	2–4 hours	6–10 hours
Intermediate-acting analogs: NPH	2–4 hours	4–8 hours	10–18 hours
Long-acting analogs: glargine, detemir, degludec	1–2 hours	"Peakless" to minimal peak (detemir)	12–24 hours 42–48 hours (degludec)

Primary care providers can play a valuable role in ensuring that patients with long-standing T1DM receive required annual care, including dilated eye examinations, measurement of microalbuminuria, annual influenza vaccine, and other vaccines recommended specifically for those with diabetes (e.g., 23-valent pneumococcal vaccine).

Several resources exist that allow patients to meet others with type 1 diabetes via organizations such as the Juvenile Diabetes Research Foundation (JDRF), American Diabetes Association (ADA), College Diabetes Network (CDN), and TrialNet. These organizations allow patients to engage in various local and regional activities, learn more about their diabetes management, and prepare for college and transitioning to adult life. Most pediatric diabetes centers are also associated with a local annual diabetes summer camp that patients can participate in. Table 52.2 presents an overview of the most commonly used types of insulins in the management of type 1 diabetes.

Primary care providers can also play an important role in reminding patients and families that diabetes management generally needs to be adjusted when children with T1DM are sick. We often refer to these as "Sick day rules."

Sick day rules:

- Insulin requirements may change during periods of illness leading to risk of hypoglycemia, hyperglycemia, and diabetic ketoacidosis.
- During illness, patients are recommended to check their blood glucose more frequently than usual and give correction doses of rapid-acting insulin as needed [6], but usually not more frequently than every 2–3 hours.
- If blood glucose remains elevated over 250–300 mg/dL for 4–6 hours, urine or blood ketones should also be checked (blood ketones can be checked with a blood ketone meter, or urine ketone strips can be used), and additional units of insulin administered per instructions for moderate to large ketones.
- Adequate hydration throughout the day is essential. Approximately 1 oz per year of age per hour, with a maximum of 8–12 oz per hour, is recommended, ideally of liquids with electrolytes or broth.

Children with T1DM who use insulin pumps and have unexplained hyperglycemia are recommended to change their pump infusion site if they are having difficulty adequately controlling their blood glucose using boluses delivered via the pump, as pump site malfunctions may also lead to inadequate insulin delivery and subsequent hyperglycemia. The patient may need to switch to injections of basal and bolus insulin if issues persist after changing the pump infusion site until new pump supplies arrive.

Patients who are unable to tolerate oral intake, have concern for dehydration, or are unable to correct hyperglycemia or ketonuria at home should urgently visit the nearest emergency room and their endocrinology team should be notified.

Hypoglycemia Management

Hypoglycemia is defined as blood glucose <70 mg/dL (3.88 mmol/l). Some patients have symptomatic hypoglycemia, whereas others may be asymptomatic and have hypoglycemia unawareness. If the patient is awake and able to eat, hypoglycemia is treated with 15 g of oral carbohydrates (for example, 1/2 cup juice or regular soda, 1 tablespoon sugar, 3–4 glucose tablets). Blood glucose should be rechecked in 15 minutes, and the process is repeated until blood glucose is >70 mg/dL. After immediate correction of the hypoglycemia, the patient is recommended to eat a meal or snack containing complex carbohydrates, as well as protein and/or fat, to maintain euglycemia. All patients on insulin should wear a medical alert bracelet and carry an emergency form of glucagon with them at all times in the event that they suffer from severe hypoglycemia that renders them unconscious or unable to take adequate oral carbohydrates. Emergency glucagon was traditionally available in the form of a rescue kit that involved reconstituting powdered glucagon, measuring the appropriate dose and administering as an IM injection. Newer forms of glucagon include premixed and premeasured liquid glucagon injections, as well as nasal glucagon.

References

1. Dabelea D, Mayer-Davis EJ, Saydah S, Imperatore G, Linder B, Divers J, et al. Prevalence of type 1 and type 2 diabetes among children and adolescents from 2001 to 2009. JAMA [Internet]. 2014 [cited 2019 Aug 25];311(17):1778–86. Available from: http://www.ncbi.nlm.nih.gov/pubmed/24794371
2. Centers for Disease Control and Prevention. National Diabetes Statistics Report, 2017. Atlanta, GA: Centers for Disease Control and Prevention, U.S.Dept of Health and Human Services; 2017.
3. Insel RA, Dunne JL, Atkinson MA, Chiang JL, Dabelea D, Gottlieb PA, et al. Staging presymptomatic type 1 diabetes: a scientific state-

ment of JDRF, the Endocrine Society, and the American Diabetes Association. Diabetes Care [Internet]. 2015 [cited 2019 Oct 12];38(10):1964–74. Available from: http://care.diabetesjournals.org/lookup/doi/10.2337/dc15-1419
4. American Diabetes Association. Standards of medical care in diabetes-2019 abridged for primary care providers. Clin Diabetes [Internet]. 2019 [cited 2019 Oct 14];37(1):11–34. Available from: http://clinical.diabetesjournals.org/lookup/doi/10.2337/cd18-0105
5. Chiang JL, Maahs DM, Garvey KC, Hood KK, Laffel LM, Weinzimer SA, et al. Type 1 diabetes in children and adolescents: a position statement by the American Diabetes Association. Diabetes Care [Internet]. 2018 [cited 2019 Aug 25];41(9):2026–44. Available from: http://www.ncbi.nlm.nih.gov/pubmed/30093549
6. Gregory JM, Moore DJ, Simmons JH. Type 1 diabetes mellitus. Pediatr Rev [Internet]. 2013 [cited 2019 Aug 26];34(5):203–15. Available from: http://www.ncbi.nlm.nih.gov/pubmed/23637249

Overview and Initial Management of Type 2 Diabetes in Youth

53

Hannah Chesser and Shylaja Srinivasan

Epidemiology and Etiology

Type 2 diabetes is a serious and growing disease among younger populations. All pediatricians, regardless of specialty, will increasingly be confronted with youth-onset type 2 diabetes and should be familiar with its presentation, diagnosis, and management.

The development of type 2 diabetes in youth has sharply increased over the past 20 years. In 2017, the Center for Disease Control (CDC) documented an incidence of about 5000 new cases per year in the United States [2]. Assuming a 2.3% annual increase, the prevalence of type 2 diabetes in youth less than 20 years of age is expected to quadruple in the next 40 years [3]. Furthermore, about 1 in 5 adolescents have prediabetes and are at increased risk of developing type 2 diabetes, chronic kidney disease, and cardiovascular disease [4].

Type 2 diabetes in youth is different from type 1 diabetes but is also distinct from type 2 diabetes in adults. Unique features include the role of puberty, a more rapidly progressive decline in β-cell function and accelerated development of diabetes complications [5]. Additionally, type 2 diabetes disproportionally affects minority racial and ethnic groups, who tend to have more financial and psychosocial challenges, which may make access to care and treatment more difficult [2].

Type 2 diabetes is a complex disease, influenced by genetic susceptibility and environmental factors conducive to obesity. Obesity is overwhelmingly the most important risk factor for developing type 2 diabetes, especially for children [6]. Childhood obesity, however, is increasing at a more rapid rate than youth-onset type 2 diabetes, likely because of a substantial latency period between the onset of obesity and the related risk for type 2 diabetes [7]. Furthermore, not all obese children go on to develop type 2 diabetes, and some children may develop type 2 diabetes at a relatively lower body mass index percentile. This speaks to the role of genetics in the development of type 2 diabetes [8].

Type 2 diabetes is a heritable condition. The Framingham Offspring Study, a cohort study of primarily Caucasians with low risk for diabetes, suggests that the risk for type 2 diabetes among offspring with a single diabetic parent is 3.5 times higher than the risk in the general population. Those with two parents with type 2 diabetes are six times more likely to develop type 2 diabetes compared with offspring without parental diabetes [9]. Genome-wide association studies in adults have identified over 300 genetic variants associated with type 2 diabetes in adults [10]. While there have been a few candidate gene studies of type 2 diabetes in youth [11, 12], the genetic architecture of type 2 diabetes in youth remains largely unexplored. Recently, the Progress in Diabetes Genetics in Youth (ProDiGY) Consortium was formed to address this gap. ProDiGY is a collaboration of the TODAY and SEARCH for Diabetes in Youth studies along with T2D-GENES, a large adult diabetes consortium. We expect that work from this collaboration will shed additional light on the genetics of type 2 diabetes in youth.

Pathophysiology

The pathophysiology of type 2 diabetes in youth is similar to that in adults with type 2 diabetes, but distinct from that of type 1 diabetes. While type 1 diabetes is characterized by insulin deficiency, type 2 diabetes is characterized primarily by insulin resistance with relative insulin deficiency. Deterioration in both insulin sensitivity and β-cell function is a key step in the natural course of the disease (Fig. 53.1).

Insulin Resistance The first phase of developing type 2 diabetes is a the stage of insulin resistance accompanied by a compensatory increased rate of insulin secretion [13]. Youth secrete proportionally more insulin than adults, and

H. Chesser · S. Srinivasan (✉)
Division of Pediatric Endocrinology and Diabetes, University of California at San Francisco, San Francisco, CA, USA
e-mail: Hannah.chesser@ucsf.edu; shylaja.srinivasan@ucsf.edu

T. Stanley, M. Misra (eds.), *Endocrine Conditions in Pediatrics*, https://doi.org/10.1007/978-3-030-52215-5_53

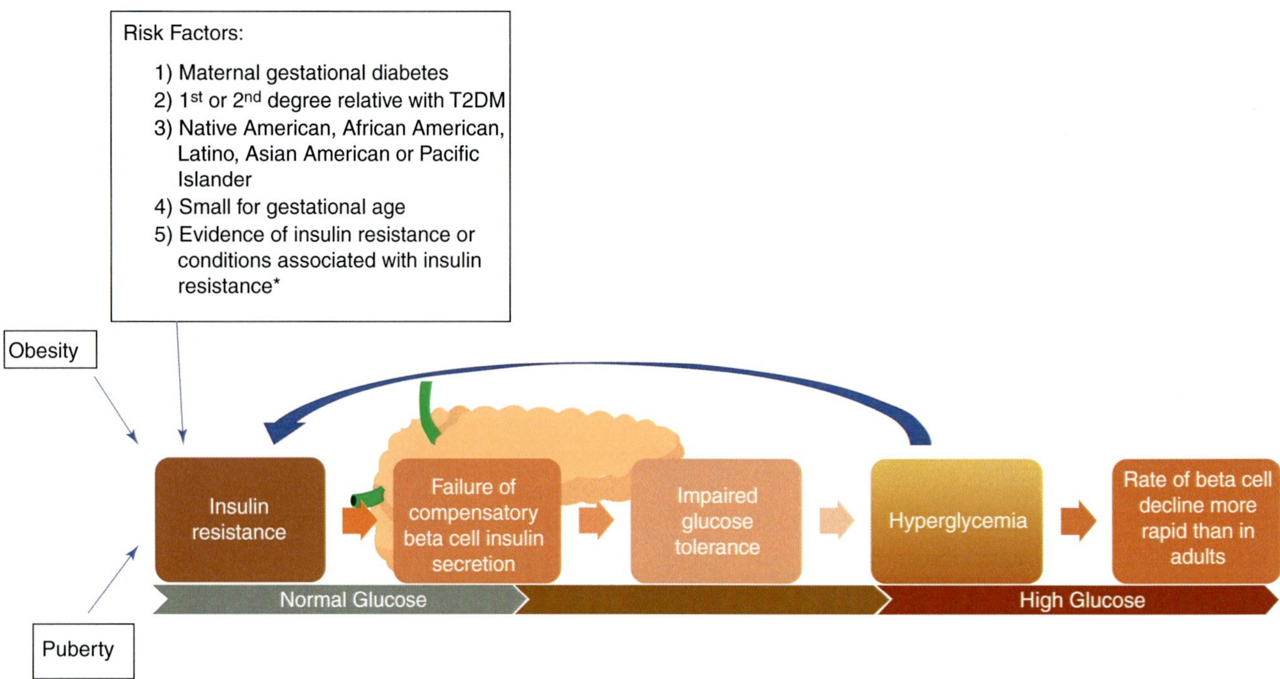

Fig. 53.1 Key pathophysiology of type 2 diabetes

this β-cell hypersecretion is a fundamental difference in the physiology of dysglycemia between youth and adults [14].

Obesity causes increased peripheral resistance to insulin-mediated glucose uptake, which sets the stage for type 2 diabetes. Puberty can increase insulin resistance by up to 50% [15], due to a transient and physiologic increase in growth hormone levels leading to a compensatory increase in insulin secretion. For this reason, type 2 diabetes commonly presents during active puberty. In adolescent girls, polycystic ovary syndrome (PCOS) is also associated with insulin resistance, and girls with PCOS are at increased risk for the developing type 2 diabetes [16]. Finally, hyperglycemia itself, occurring later in the process, can further exacerbate insulin resistance [17].

Impaired Glucose Tolerance The second stage occurs when β cells no longer fully compensate for the increased insulin resistance, leading to impaired glucose tolerance. Impaired glucose tolerance, also called prediabetes, is an independent predictor of the risk of developing type 2 diabetes and cardiovascular disease. Little is known about the natural history of impaired glucose tolerance in children although available literature suggests that the rate of β-cell decline is more rapid than in adults [14, 18], with clinicians often missing the impaired glucose tolerance phase. This more rapid loss of insulin secretory function is irrespective of treatment and may be explained by the relative insulin hypersecretion, meaning increased demand on β cells, seen in youth [14] .

Clinical Presentation

Screening The American Diabetes Association (ADA) recommends targeted screening for children and adolescents at higher risk for type 2 diabetes. Screening should be considered after the onset of puberty or ≥10 years of age, whichever occurs earlier, in children who are overweight (BMI ≥ 85th %) or obese (BMI ≥ 95th %) and have at least one additional risk factor. These risk factors include the following: (1) family history of type 2 diabetes in a first- or second-degree relative, (2) native American, African American, Latino, Asian American, or Pacific Islander race/ethnicities, (3) evidence of insulin resistance or conditions associated with insulin resistance (acanthosis nigricans, hypertension, dyslipidemia, polycystic ovary syndrome, or small-for-gestational age birth weight), and (4) maternal history of diabetes or gestational diabetes mellitus during the child's gestation.

Screening tests include a hemoglobin A1c (HbA1c), a fasting plasma glucose, or a 2-hour plasma glucose during a 75-g oral glucose tolerance test. While HbA1c is not validated in a pediatric population, in practice, it is the most practical screening test because it does not require fasting. If the screening tests are normal, the tests should be repeated at least every 3 years or sooner if BMI is increasing [19]. While uncommon, even if a child is prepubertal and under the age of 10 years old, the diagnosis of type 2 diabetes should be considered with suggestive symptoms [20].

Presentation Most children with type 2 diabetes are, at the time of diagnosis, in mid-to-late puberty and overweight or obese. But the clinical presentation can vary widely: from asymptomatic and incidental diagnosis during routine laboratory testing to a severe presentation with symptomatic hyperglycemia, weight loss and metabolic decompensation, and possibly with diabetic ketoacidosis (DKA) or hyperglycemic hyperosmolar state (HHS). About 40% of children and adolescents with type 2 diabetes have no symptoms on presentation, but are discovered on screening based on risk factors or glycosuria, usually without ketonuria, detected during other medical evaluation [21]. However, about 6% of youth aged 10–19 years with type 2 diabetes may have a severe clinical presentation of polyuria, polydipsia, weight loss and fatigue, and dehydration with ketoacidosis [19].

Table 53.1 Items required for diagnosis and items supporting diagnosis of type 2 diabetes

Required for diagnosis: Presence of one or more of the following:
Type 2 diabetes:
1) Fasting plasma glucose (FPG) ≥ 126 mg/dl (7.0 mmol/l)
2) 2-hour plasma glucose ≥200 mg/dl (11.1 mmol/l) with a 75-g oral glucose tolerance test (OGTT)
3) Serum HbA1C ≥ 6.5%
4) A random plasma glucose ≥200 mg/dl in a patient with classic symptoms of hyperglycemia or hyperglycemic crisis
Prediabetes:
1) FPG 100 mg/dl (5.6 mmol/l) to 125 mg/dl (6.9 mmol/l)
2) 2-hour plasma glucose 140 mg/dl (7.8 mmol/l) to 199 mg/dl (11.0 mmol/l) with a 75-g OGTT
3) Serum HbA1C 5.7–6.4%
Unless symptoms of hyperglycemia (polyuria or polydipsia are present), the diagnosis should be confirmed by repeat testing on a different day
Supporting diagnosis:
Obese or overweight
After onset of puberty (≥10 years old)
Acanthosis nigricans
PCOS
Hypertension or dyslipidemia
Immediate family history of type 2 diabetes
Minority racial and ethnic group
Higher fasting C-peptide levels
Absence of ketones makes type 2 diabetes more likely
Excludes diagnosis:
Serum pancreatic autoantibodies suggest type1 diabetes

Diagnosis of Type 2 Diabetes in Youth

Refer to Table 53.1 for diagnostic criteria of youth-onset type 2 diabetes. The presence of anemia and hemoglobinopathies should be considered when interpreting an HbA1C, as abnormal hemoglobin or rapid destruction of red blood cells may influence the value obtained. It is important to remember that for all three tests, the risk is continuous, extending below the lower limit of the range and becoming disproportionately greater at the higher end of the reference range [22]. Hyperglycemia that is associated with acute stress such as postoperatively or during illness may be transient, and should be treated, but is not diagnostic of diabetes.

It is critical to correctly distinguish between a diagnosis of type 1 and type 2 diabetes because treatment regimens, educational approaches, dietary advice, and outcomes differ greatly between the two. Our current obesity epidemic can make this distinction difficult, as overweight and obesity are common in children with type 1 diabetes as well.

Initial Evaluation During initial laboratory evaluation, pancreatic autoantibodies should always be sent to evaluate for the possibility of type 1 diabetes. The presence of serum pancreatic autoantibodies is suggestive of type 1 diabetes. The antibodies most commonly measured are glutamic acid decarboxylase 65 autoantibodies (GAD), tyrosine phosphatase-like insulinoma antigen 2 (IA2), insulin autoantibodies (IAA), and β-cell-specific zinc transporter 8 autoantibodies (ZnT8). Insulin autoantibodies are useful up to 2 weeks after initiation of insulin therapy [23].

More rapid laboratory markers include serum ketones or urine ketones, which are less specific and not frequently associated with type 2 diabetes. C-peptide levels, drawn before exposure to exogenous insulin, may be used as a measure of insulin secretion and are generally higher in patients with type 2 diabetes compared to patients with type 1 diabetes. However, C-peptide levels decrease during states of acute metabolic decompensation. Therefore, there is overlap in C-peptide levels during acute presentation of both type 1 and type 2 diabetes [24].

As many of these laboratory values take days to result and may not be conclusive, the clinical characteristics at presentation are used to distinguish type 2 diabetes from type 1 diabetes. Youth with type 2 diabetes are generally obese or overweight, typically present during puberty and show clinical evidence of insulin resistance in the form of acanthosis nigricans. Acanthosis nigricans is present in as many as 90% of children with type 2 diabetes [25] but is not necessary for diagnosis. Children with type 2 diabetes usually also have an immediate family history of type 2 diabetes, and many belong to minority racial and ethnic groups.

Emergent Considerations

Diabetic ketoacidosis (DKA) and hyperosmolar hyperglycemic state (HHS) are severe presentations of marked hyperglycemia due to uncontrolled or new-onset type 2 diabetes. Early symptoms may be polyuria, polydipsia, and weight loss. As the degree and duration of hyperglycemia progresses, dehydration worsens, metabolic derangements occur, and neurologic obtundation can develop. The clinical features of DKA in type 2 diabetes are similar to those seen in children with type 1 diabetes.

Hyperosmolar hyperglycemic state (HHS) is even less common than presentation in DKA and involves more severe hyperglycemia (typically serum blood glucose >600 mg/dl) and hyperosmolality with severe dehydration in the absence of significant ketosis. HHS has high morbidity and mortality if not treated appropriately [26]. The treatment of DKA and HHS is similar, including hospitalization for correction of electrolyte abnormalities, rehydration, and the administration of IV insulin.

Initial Management

Unless in hyperglycemic crisis, initial management for new-onset type 2 diabetes can usually be initiated in an outpatient setting with intensive lifestyle modification, diabetes education, and pharmacologic intervention. The American Diabetes Association (ADA) offers guidelines and decision trees on the management of new-onset diabetes in overweight youth based on HbA1c, presence of ketosis or acidosis, and presence of pancreatic autoantibodies [19].

In asymptomatic and metabolically stable (without ketosis or acidosis) patients with HbA1c < 8.5%, metformin monotherapy may be started and titrated up to 2000 mg per day as tolerated. Metformin is given twice daily, whereas extended release formulations can be given once daily and may have fewer gastrointestinal symptoms.

Patients with more marked hyperglycemia, with serum blood glucose ≥250 mg/dL or HbA1c ≥ 8.5%, with symptoms of hyperglycemia such as polyuria and polydipsia but not ketoacidosis, should be started on basal subcutaneous insulin while metformin is initiated and titrated. Insulin therapy allows for quicker restoration of glycemic control. Many patients can be weaned gradually from insulin therapy and subsequently managed for some period of time with metformin and lifestyle modification.

Clinical Key
In asymptomatic patients with type 2 diabetes and HbA1c < 8.5%, metformin monotherapy may be started and titrated up to 2000 mg daily, with close follow-up and HbA1c assessment every 3 months. Patients with HbA1c ≥ 8.5% or serum blood glucose ≥250 mg/dL should be referred urgently to a pediatric endocrinologist for initiation of insulin. Patients with new-onset type 2 diabetes who have hyperglycemia and ketones should be referred emergently to an emergency department given the risk of DKA.

Whether a patient has type 1 or type 2 diabetes is often unclear in the first few weeks of treatment, as presentation can be similar. For the percentage of youth with type 2 diabetes that present with ketoacidosis, the initial therapy should include IV insulin with management of associated metabolic derangements, followed by a transition to subcutaneous insulin, irrespective of ultimate diabetes type. Once pancreatic autoantibody results become available, and a diagnosis of type 2 diabetes is likely, then metformin can be added to the therapy regimen [19].

Lifestyle Modification Intensive lifestyle intervention aimed at weight loss is the backbone of type 2 diabetes management regardless of the pharmacological agents used. The goal weight reduction for youth with prediabetes and type 2 diabetes is 7–10% of their body weight and, ideally, aiming for a BMI less than or equal to the 85th percentile for age and gender. In children who are still actively growing, maintenance of weight without further weight gain will lead to a reduction in BMI over time. A family-centered approach to dietary modification and increased physical activity is most effective [19, 27]. In addition to lifestyle modification counseling and more frequent follow-up visits, providers should consider referral to a dietician or structured weight loss program [28].

Providers should encourage healthy eating behaviors including regular snacks and meals and avoiding eating while watching television or using electronics. Other dietary recommendations include choosing sugar-free beverages, except for milk, reducing portion sizes, and reducing fast food and simple carbohydrate consumption [29]. Foods commonly mistaken as healthy, such as meal replacement bars, granola bars, and sugary cereals, should be discouraged. Lower carbohydrate diets have been suggested for adults with type 2 diabetes [30] and presumably may be beneficial in youth as well.

Youth with type 2 diabetes should engage in moderate-to-vigorous exercise for at least 60 minutes per day [27] and should limit nonacademic screen time to less than 2 hours per day. More frequent follow-up can help families stay motivated to maintain lifestyle modification. Strategies to enhance mental health should be considered key features of lifestyle modification in order to promote habits of healthy living [28].

Treatment Monitoring

The frequency of finger stick blood glucose monitoring for youth with type 2 diabetes should be individualized [29]. Children who are on insulin, have changes in diabetes treatment regimen, have not met treatment goals, or have intercurrent illness may need more frequent finger stick blood glucoses. For other patients, a fasting and 2-hour postprandial finger stick blood glucose a few times a week can provide valuable information on the range of glycemic excursion.

Diabetes technology has changed the landscape of care for patients with type 1 diabetes and continues to shape care for patients with youth-onset type 2 diabetes. Continuous glucose monitoring (CGM) is replacing fingerstick blood glucose checks due to reduced disease burden and has become part of standard care in children with type 1 diabetes. There are ongoing studies to look at the feasibility of CGM use in youth with type 2 diabetes.

HbA1c should be monitored every 3 months. The ADA recommends a HbA1c target of <7%, but a more stringent HbA1c target of <6.5% may be appropriate in youth without significant hypoglycemia or other adverse effects of treatment. Providers may consider a temporary higher HbA1c goal to help motivate patients. Overall, the treatment goal is to maintain near-normal glycemia and prevent and reduce the risk of long-term vascular complications, as well the appropriate management of comorbidities. The treatment regimen should be intensified if treatment goals are not being met.

Long-Term Management

Both immediate management and long-term management of youth with type 2 diabetes entail lifestyle modification aimed at weight loss along with pharmacotherapy, including metformin, basal/bolus insulin, and possibly other antihyperglycemic agents as treatment regimens intensify. Whereas other aspects of pediatric care involve a more conservative, "wait and watch" approach, the case of youth-onset type 2 diabetes requires aggressively intensified therapy when patients are not meeting treatment goals. Many youth with type 2 diabetes are likely to require combination treatment within a few years of diagnosis [15]. Clinicians should consider a consult to a diabetes subspecialist and then referral to a multidisciplinary diabetes team, including a physician, diabetes nurse educator, registered dietitian, and psychologist or social worker [27].

Pharmacologic Agents

Metformin Metformin should be initiated along with lifestyle intervention in all children with type 2 diabetes, due to the low success rate of lifestyle intervention alone in pediatric patients. Metformin is a biguanide that decreases hepatic glucose production by inhibiting gluconeogenesis and increases insulin sensitivity via increased glucose utilization in the peripheral tissues. The main gastrointestinal adverse effects (abdominal pain, bloating, loose stools) that present at initiation of metformin are often transient. To minimize gastrointestinal side effects, the dose should be started at 500 mg once a day and increased by 500 mg every week to reach a maximum daily dose of 2000 mg a day in divided doses. The medication is generally better tolerated when taken with meals.

However, the evidence to routinely prescribe metformin to youth with prediabetes is lacking. Metformin alone or basal insulin followed by metformin does not halt the deterioration of β-cell function in youth at risk for type 2 diabetes [31]. Metformin can cause some weight loss on initiation of treatment, but overall, it is considered a weight neutral drug.

Though considered a safe medication, metformin is contraindicated in children with liver disease, impaired renal function, or in cases of cardiopulmonary dysfunction because of the small risk of lactic acidosis [32]. For this reason, metformin should be discontinued during acute illness or before imaging studies requiring a contrast agent.

In the TODAY study, metformin alone provided durable glycemic control in approximately only half of the subjects (13). For youth who remain above glycemic targets on monotherapy with metformin, either basal insulin or liraglutide should be added to the treatment regimen.

GLP-1 Receptor Agonists ("-tides") At the time of this writing, liraglutide, a long-acting analog of glucagon-like peptide 1, is the only other antihyperglycemic agent for children with type 2 diabetes that has obtained regulatory

Table 53.2 Select classes of diabetes drugs considered in youth

Drug class	Examples of drugs in this class	Mechanism of action	Significant adverse effects
Biguanides (oral)	Metformin	Reduces hepatic glucose production, increases peripheral glucose uptake, decreases insulin resistance	Gastrointestinal Lactic acidosis (very rare)
GLP-1 receptor agonists (injectable)	"-tides" Liraglutide Exenatide	Decreases inappropriate glucagon secretion, enhances postprandial insulin biosynthesis, improves β-cell function, slows gastric emptying, decreases appetite	Acute pancreatitis C-cell hyperplasia/medullary thyroid carcinoma Gastrointestinal Hypoglycemia Headache
DPP-4 inhibitors (oral)	"-gliptins" Saxagliptin Sitagliptin	Inhibits DPP-4 enzyme, reducing endogenous GLP-1 breakdown	Acute pancreatitis URI UTI Nasopharyngitis Headache
Thiazolidinediones (oral)	"-glitazone" Rosiglitazone Pioglitazone	PPAR-ϒ inhibitor; increases insulin sensitivity in liver, muscle, and adipose tissue; decreases hepatic glucose output	Edema Weight gain Anemia Elevated liver enzymes Bone fractures
SGLT-2 inhibitors (oral)	"-flozin" Empagliflozin Dapagliflozin	Blocks glucose reuptake at renal proximal tubule, leading to increased urinary glucose excretion	Euglycemic DKA Urinary tract infection Candidal vulvovaginitis
Sulfonylureas (oral)	"-ride", "-zide" Glipizide Glyburide	Stimulates secretion of insulin from the β cell	Hypoglycemia Weight gain

GLP-1 glucagon-like peptide-1, *DPP-4* dipeptidyl peptidase-4, *SGLT-2* sodium glucose cotransporter-2

approval from the United States Food and Drug Administration. Liraglutide is a long-acting analog of human glucagon-like peptide-1 and acts by increasing glucose-dependent insulin secretion, decreasing glucagon secretion, slowing gastric emptying, and increasing satiety. Liraglutide is a daily injectable medication and may promote weight loss [33]. Dose should be started at 0.6 mg daily and titrated to a maximum dose of 1.8 mg daily over several weeks based on fasting glucose targets. Gastrointestinal side effects, including nausea, vomiting, and diarrhea, are the most bothersome.

Liraglutide is contraindicated in patients with a history of pancreatitis and should be discontinued permanently if a child develops pancreatitis on the medication. Dose-dependent and treatment duration-dependent thyroid C-cell tumors have developed in animal studies with liraglutide therapy. Use is therefore contraindicated in patients with a personal or a family history of medullary thyroid carcinoma and in patients with multiple endocrine neoplasia syndrome type 2. Patients should be informed of symptoms of thyroid tumors such a neck mass, dysphagia, dyspnea, and persistent hoarseness [34].

Other antihyperglycemic agents used in adults do not currently have regulatory approval in the pediatric population, partially because clinical research trials are challenging among this patient population [5]. There are over 10 classes of drugs used in adults with type 2 diabetes. We highlight several of the more commonly considered classes, some of which are off-label use, in youth with type 2 diabetes (Table 53.2). Providers should remain acquainted with the current literature as there are many ongoing pediatric trials of type 2 diabetes medications.

Insulin In certain acute presentations of type 2 diabetes as described earlier, or in cases when glycemic control remains above target, patients may require insulin therapy. The form of insulin therapy should be individualized to the patient, severity of disease, the ability to perform self-blood glucose monitoring, and the risk of hypoglycemia. Long-acting agents, or basal insulin, include insulin glargine, insulin detemir, and insulin degludec. Required doses are typically much higher than used in children with type 1 diabetes because of insulin resistance. The ADA recommends starting basal insulin at 0.5 units/kg/day and escalating the dose every 2–3 days based on fingerstick glucoses [19] . Rapid-acting insulin may also be used for meals and acute correction of high blood glucose. Rapid-acting agents include insulin lispro and insulin aspart. Insulin pump therapy may also be considered.

Bariatric Surgery Select adolescents who are markedly obese (BMI > 35 kg/m^2) with type 2 diabetes may be candidates for bariatric surgery. Bariatric surgery should especially be considered if additional comorbidities are present, such as obstructive sleep apnea and nonalcoholic steatohepatitis [29]. Bariatric surgeries are typically Roux-en-Y procedures or sleeve gastrostomies, with the latter increasingly favored due to a lower risk of complications.

In a comparison of adolescents who received bariatric surgery compared to participants in the TODAY trial, where participants received metformin alone or in combination with rosiglitazone or intensive lifestyle intervention, the surgical group had significant weight loss, better glycemic control, and reduced cardiovascular risk markers [35]. Improvement in metabolic control is often evident within days to weeks following bariatric surgery, likely due to an alteration in metabolism independent of weight loss [36]. Adolescents who undergo bariatric surgery earlier in the course of diabetes have a higher remission rate of diabetes despite similar weight loss [37].

These significant benefits should be balanced with risk of requiring further surgical interventions as well as longer term risk of certain micronutrient deficiencies and possible detrimental effects on bone health [38]. Bariatric surgery should be performed only by an experienced surgeon working as part of a multidisciplinary team, including surgeon, endocrinologist, nutritionist, behavioral health specialist, and nurse.

Comorbidities and Other Considerations for Referral

Recent research has found that young adults who have youth-onset type 2 diabetes have alarming and accelerated rates of severe complications affecting the kidneys, eyes, liver, heart, nerves, and adversely affecting pregnancies [1]. In addition to microvascular and macrovascular complications from diabetes, youth with type 2 diabetes are at increased risk for other obesity related comorbidities, including hypertension, dyslipidemia, and nonalcoholic fatty liver disease. In many cases, these may be present at the time of diagnosis. Screening for these comorbidities and complications should occur at diagnosis and on a regular basis (Table 53.3).

Table 53.3 Screening for type 2 diabetes complications and indications for treatment and referral

Diabetes complications/ comorbidities	At diagnosis	Every visit	Yearly	Initial management and referral
Hypertension	Blood pressure (BP)	Blood pressure	Blood pressure	• If BP > 95th percentile for age, sex, and height, then recommend lifestyle modifications aimed at weight loss • If BP remains >95th percentile after 6 months, then start ACE inhibitor or ARB and refer to nephrology
Nephropathy	Urine albumin/ creatinine ratio (UACR) eGFR calculation		Urine albumin/ creatinine ratio (UACR) eGFR calculation	• Confirm elevated UACR (>30 mg/g creatinine) on two of three samples • If hypertensive and: ◆ UACR 30–299 mg/g creatinine, consider starting ACE inhibitor or ARB ◆ UACR > 300 mg/g creatinine and/or eGFR <60 mL/min/1.73 m^2, strongly consider starting ACE inhibitor or ARB ◆ Refer to nephrology if worsening UACR, eGFR, or uncertain etiology
Nonalcoholic fatty liver disease (NAFLD)	Serum aminotransferases (AST, ALT) Abdominal exam		Serum aminotransferases (AST, ALT) Abdominal exam	• If elevated, recommend lifestyle changes focused on weight reduction • Referral to gastroenterology for worsening or persistent elevation of aminotransferases
Dyslipidemia	Fasting lipid panel after initial glycemic control		Fasting lipid panel	• Optimal cholesterol: LDL < 100 mg/dl (2.6 mmol/L) HDL > 35 mg/dl (0.905 mmol/L) Triglycerides <150 mg/dl (1.7 mmol/L) • If LDL > 130 mg/dl, change diet and optimize glycemic control • If LDL > 130 mg/dl for 6 months, start statin with goal LDL < 100 mg/dl • If TG > 400 mg/dl fasting or >1000 mg/dl nonfasting, optimize glycemic control and begin fibrate with goal of <400 mg/dl fasting

(continued)

Table 53.3 (continued)

Diabetes complications/ comorbidities	At diagnosis	Every visit	Yearly	Initial management and referral
Retinopathy	Dilated fundoscopy or retinal photography		Dilated fundoscopy or retinal photography*	• Referral to ophthalmologist at diagnosis • If abnormal retinal exam, then optimize glycemic control *Can space to every 2 years if normal eye exam and glycemic control
Obstructive sleep apnea	Screen for symptoms	Screen for symptoms	Screen for symptoms	• If symptoms, refer to pediatric sleep specialist for polysomnogram
Depression	Depression screening		Depression screening	• If positive, refer to a mental health provider
PCOS	Evaluate adolescents with suggestive symptoms as needed			• Oral contraceptive pills, metformin, and spironolactone as appropriate
Neuropathy	Foot examination		Foot examination	• Referral to neurology if abnormal

eGFR = Estimated Glomerular Filtration Rate, ACE = Angiotensin-Converting Enzyme, ARB = Angiotensin II Receptor Blocker, AST = aspartate aminotransferase, ALT = alanine aminotransferase, LDL = low-density lipoprotein cholesterol, HDL = high-density lipoprotein cholesterol, TG = triglyceride. Adapted from ADA recommendations [29] and our practices

Conclusion

Youth-onset type 2 diabetes is on the rise secondary to the obesity epidemic in children. While some aspects of the pathophysiology are shared with adult-onset type 2 diabetes, youth-onset type 2 diabetes is tightly linked to puberty and has a more rapid decline in β-cell function. This β-cell dysfunction progresses despite currently approved therapies. Due to the risk of wide-ranging complications that can occur as early as in late adolescence or young adulthood, clinicians need to aggressively manage type 2 diabetes and its associated comorbidities. More research is needed to identify effective approaches to therapy.

References

1. TODAY2 results: tracking type 2 diabetes in youth. Beyond Type 2 2019. https://beyondtype2.org/today2-results-tracking-type-2-diabetes-in-youth/. Accessed 5 Dec 2019.
2. Mayer-Davis EJ, Lawrence JM, Dabelea D, Divers J, Isom S, Dolan L, et al. Incidence trends of type 1 and type 2 diabetes among youths, 2002-2012. N Engl J Med. 2017;376:1419–29. https://doi.org/10.1056/NEJMoa1610187.
3. Imperatore G, Boyle JP, Thompson TJ, Case D, Dabelea D, Hamman RF, et al. Projections of type 1 and type 2 diabetes burden in the U.S. population aged <20 years through 2050. Diabetes Care. 2012;35:2515–20. https://doi.org/10.2337/dc12-0669.
4. Andes LJ, Cheng YJ, Rolka DB, Gregg EW, Imperatore G. Prevalence of prediabetes among adolescents and young adults in the United States, 2005-2016. JAMA Pediatr. 2019:e194498–8. https://doi.org/10.1001/jamapediatrics.2019.4498.
5. Nadeau KJ, Anderson BJ, Berg EG, Chiang JL, Chou H, Copeland KC, et al. Youth-onset type 2 diabetes consensus report: current status, challenges, and priorities. Diabetes Care. 2016;39:1635–42. https://doi.org/10.2337/dc16-1066.
6. Awa WL, Fach E, Krakow D, Welp R, Kunder J, Voll A, et al. Type 2 diabetes from pediatric to geriatric age: analysis of gender and obesity among 120 183 patients from the German/Austrian DPV database. Eur J Endocrinol. 2012;167:245–54. https://doi.org/10.1530/EJE-12-0143.
7. Lee JM. Why young adults hold the key to assessing the obesity epidemic in children. Arch Pediatr Adolesc Med. 2008;162:682–7. https://doi.org/10.1001/archpedi.162.7.682.
8. Abbasi A, Juszczyk D, van Jaarsveld CHM, Gulliford MC. Body mass index and incident type 1 and type 2 diabetes in children and young adults: a retrospective cohort study. J Endocr Soc. 2017;1:524–37. https://doi.org/10.1210/js.2017-00044.
9. Meigs JB, Cupples LA, Wilson PW. Parental transmission of type 2 diabetes: the Framingham offspring study. Diabetes. 2000;49:2201–7. https://doi.org/10.2337/diabetes.49.12.2201.
10. Mahajan A, Taliun D, Thurner M, Robertson NR, Torres JM, Rayner NW, et al. Fine-mapping type 2 diabetes loci to single-variant resolution using high-density imputation and islet-specific epigenome maps. Nat Genet. 2018;50:1505–13. https://doi.org/10.1038/s41588-018-0241-6.
11. Sartorius T, Staiger H, Ketterer C, Heni M, Machicao F, Guilherme A, et al. Association of common genetic variants in the MAP4K4 locus with prediabetic traits in humans. PLoS One. 2012;7 https://doi.org/10.1371/journal.pone.0047647.
12. Ali O. Genetics of type 2 diabetes. World J Diabetes. 2013;4:114–23. https://doi.org/10.4239/wjd.v4.i4.114.
13. Tabák AG, Herder C, Rathmann W, Brunner EJ, Kivimäki M. Prediabetes: a high-risk state for developing diabetes. Lancet. 2012;379:2279–90. https://doi.org/10.1016/S0140-6736(12)60283-9.
14. Consortium TR. Metabolic contrasts between youth and adults with impaired glucose tolerance or recently diagnosed type 2 diabetes: I. observations using the hyperglycemic clamp. Diabetes Care. 2018;41:1696–706. https://doi.org/10.2337/dc18-0244.
15. Hannon TS, Janosky J, Arslanian SA. Longitudinal study of physiologic insulin resistance and metabolic changes of puberty. Pediatr Res. 2006;60:759–63. https://doi.org/10.1203/01.pdr.0000246097.73031.27.
16. Ciaraldi TP, Aroda V, Mudaliar S, Chang RJ, Henry RR. Polycystic ovary syndrome is associated with tissue-specific differences in insulin resistance. J Clin Endocrinol Metab. 2009;94:157–63. https://doi.org/10.1210/jc.2008-1492.
17. Tomás E, Lin Y-S, Dagher Z, Saha A, Luo Z, Ido Y, et al. Hyperglycemia and insulin resistance: possible mechanisms. Ann N Y Acad Sci. 2002;967:43–51. https://doi.org/10.1111/j.1749-6632.2002.tb04262.x.

18. A clinical trial to maintain glycemic control in youth with type 2 diabetes. N Engl J Med. 2012;366:2247–56. https://doi.org/10.1056/NEJMoa1109333.
19. 13. Children and adolescents: standards of medical care in diabetes—2019. Diabetes Care. 2019;42:S148. https://doi.org/10.2337/dc19-S013.
20. Hutchins J, Barajas RA, Hale D, Escaname E, Lynch J. Type 2 diabetes in a 5-year-old and single center experience of type 2 diabetes in youth under 10. Pediatr Diabetes. 2017;18:674–7. https://doi.org/10.1111/pedi.12463.
21. Pinhas-Hamiel O, Dolan LM, Daniels SR, Standiford D, Khoury PR, Zeitler P. Increased incidence of non-insulin-dependent diabetes mellitus among adolescents. J Pediatr. 1996;128:608–15. https://doi.org/10.1016/S0022-3476(96)80124-7.
22. Association AD. 2. Classification and diagnosis of diabetes. Diabetes Care. 2016;39:S13–22. https://doi.org/10.2337/dc16-S005.
23. Mayer-Davis EJ, Kahkoska AR, Jefferies C, Dabelea D, Balde N, Gong CX, et al. ISPAD clinical practice consensus guidelines 2018: definition, epidemiology, and classification of diabetes in children and adolescents. Pediatr Diabetes. 2018;19:7–19. https://doi.org/10.1111/pedi.12773.
24. Katz LEL, Jawad AF, Ganesh J, Abraham M, Murphy K, Lipman TH. Fasting c-peptide and insulin-like growth factor-binding protein-1 levels help to distinguish childhood type 1 and type 2 diabetes at diagnosis. Pediatr Diabetes. 2007;8:53–9. https://doi.org/10.1111/j.1399-5448.2007.00236.x.
25. Fagot-Campagna A, Pettitt DJ, Engelgau MM, Burrows NR, Geiss LS, Valdez R, et al. Type 2 diabetes among north adolescents: an epidemiologic health perspective. J Pediatr. 2000;136:664–72. https://doi.org/10.1067/mpd.2000.105141.
26. Zeitler P, Haqq A, Rosenbloom A, Glaser N. Hyperglycemic hyperosmolar syndrome in children: pathophysiological considerations and suggested guidelines for treatment. J Pediatr. 2011;158:9–14.e2. https://doi.org/10.1016/j.jpeds.2010.09.048.
27. Copeland KC, Silverstein J, Moore KR, Prazar GE, Raymer T, Shiffman RN, et al. Management of Newly Diagnosed Type 2 Diabetes Mellitus (T2DM) in children and adolescents. Pediatrics. 2013;131:364–82. https://doi.org/10.1542/peds.2012-3494.
28. McGavock J, Dart A, Wicklow B. Lifestyle therapy for the treatment of youth with type 2 diabetes. Curr Diab Rep. 2015;15 https://doi.org/10.1007/s11892-014-0568-z.
29. Arslanian S, Bacha F, Grey M, Marcus MD, White NH, Zeitler P. Evaluation and management of youth-onset type 2 diabetes: a position statement by the American Diabetes Association. Diabetes Care. 2018;41:2648–68. https://doi.org/10.2337/dci18-0052.
30. Association AD. 5. Lifestyle management: standards of medical care in diabetes—2019. Diabetes Care. 2019;42:S46–60. https://doi.org/10.2337/dc19-S005.
31. Consortium TR. Impact of insulin and metformin versus metformin alone on β-cell function in youth with impaired glucose tolerance or recently diagnosed type 2 diabetes. Diabetes Care. 2018;41:1717–25. https://doi.org/10.2337/dc18-0787.
32. Stang M, Wysowski DK, Butler-Jones D. Incidence of lactic acidosis in metformin users. Diabetes Care. 1999;22:925–7. https://doi.org/10.2337/diacare.22.6.925.
33. Singh S, Wright EE, Kwan AYM, Thompson JC, Syed IA, Korol EE, et al. Glucagon-like peptide-1 receptor agonists compared with basal insulins for the treatment of type 2 diabetes mellitus: a systematic review and meta-analysis. Diabetes Obes Metab. 2017;19:228–38. https://doi.org/10.1111/dom.12805.
34. Tamborlane WV, Barrientos-Pérez M, Fainberg U, Frimer-Larsen H, Hafez M, Hale PM, et al. Liraglutide in children and adolescents with type 2 diabetes. N Engl J Med. 2019;381:637–46. https://doi.org/10.1056/NEJMoa1903822.
35. Inge TH, Laffel LM, Jenkins TM, Marcus MD, Leibel NI, Brandt ML, et al. Comparison of surgical and medical therapy for type 2 diabetes in severely obese adolescents. JAMA Pediatr. 2018;172:452–60. https://doi.org/10.1001/jamapediatrics.2017.5763.
36. Courcoulas AP, Goodpaster BH, Eagleton JK, Belle SH, Kalarchian MA, Lang W, et al. A randomized trial to compare surgical and medical treatments for type 2 diabetes: the triabetes study. JAMA Surg. 2014;149:707–15. https://doi.org/10.1001/jamasurg.2014.467.
37. Beamish AJ, D'Alessio DA, Inge TH. Controversial issues: when the drugs don't work, can surgery provide a different outcome for diabetic adolescents? Surg Obes Relat Dis. 2015;11:946–8. https://doi.org/10.1016/j.soard.2015.03.006.
38. Shah AS, D'Alessio D, Ford-Adams ME, Desai AP, Inge TH. Bariatric surgery: a potential treatment for type 2 diabetes in youth. Diabetes Care. 2016;39:934–40. https://doi.org/10.2337/dc16-0067.

Vitamin D Deficiency

54

Rebecca J. Gordon

Introduction

Vitamin D plays many diverse roles in the body. It has long been recognized as critical to maintaining calcium and phosphate balance, as well as bone health. Vitamin D that is synthesized from the skin or obtained from the diet is biologically inert and requires its first hydroxylation in the liver by vitamin D 25-hydroxylase to 25-hydroxyvitamin D (25-OH vitamin D). It subsequently requires a further hydroxylation in the kidney by the 25-OH vitamin D 1 alpha-hydroxylase to form the biologically active form of vitamin D $1{,}25(OH)_2$ vitamin D. $1{,}25(OH)_2$ vitamin D interacts with its vitamin D nuclear receptor, which is found in the small intestine, kidneys, bone, and other tissues (Fig. 54.1).

$1{,}25(OH)_2$ vitamin D is essential for optimizing calcium absorption from the gastrointestinal tract and the kidney. Without vitamin D, only 10–15% of dietary calcium and about 60% of phosphorus are absorbed. Vitamin D sufficiency enhances calcium and phosphorus absorption by 30–40% and 80%, respectively [1, 2]. In the kidney, $1{,}25(OH)_2$ vitamin D stimulates calcium reabsorption from the glomerular filtrate. Additionally, $1{,}25(OH)_2$ vitamin D interacts with bone intermediaries including osteoblasts, receptor activator of nuclear factor kappa B ligand, and the subsequently increased number of osteoclasts, resulting in the breakdown of the skeletal matrix and mobilization of calcium from the skeleton. Also, there is emerging evidence that vitamin D has additional roles in promoting immune system maturation and homeostasis, anti-inflammatory, and anti-carcinogenic functions [3].

R. J. Gordon (✉)
Division of Endocrinology, Boston Children's Hospital, Harvard Medical School, Boston, MA, USA
e-mail: Rebecca.Gordon@childrens.harvard.edu

Vitamin D Deficiency

Vitamin D deficiency is common, affecting between 42% and over 50% of children and adolescents [4, 5]. There are similarly high rates of vitamin D deficiency and insufficiency among children and adults, and equally high rates worldwide. The main source of vitamin D is exposure to natural sunlight [1]. Consequently, the major cause of vitamin D deficiency is inadequate sunlight exposure. Wearing a sunscreen with sun protection factor of 30 reduces the synthesis of vitamin D in the skin by more than 95% [6]. People with naturally dark skin tones require at least three to five times longer sun exposure to make the same amount of vitamin D compared to people with light skin tones [7, 8]. *Risk factors for vitamin D deficiency include darker skin tones, obesity, fat malabsorption syndromes, history of bariatric surgery in adolescents, other underlying conditions, such as severe hypoalbuminemia, which can result in low vitamin D binding protein or a dermatologic condition requiring avoidance of all sunlight, and inadequate dietary intake.*

Very few foods naturally contain vitamin D, and a small number of foods are fortified with vitamin D. In the United States and Canada, milk is fortified with vitamin D, as are some orange juices, cereals, yogurts, cheeses, and bread products, while in Europe most countries do not fortify milk. The American Academy of Pediatrics recommends minimal sun exposure due to the increased risk of skin cancer with ultraviolet exposure and has endorsed the 2011 recommendations on vitamin D supplementation from the Institute of Medicine. *The recommended daily allowance (RDA) for vitamin D is 400 IU for infants 0–12 months, then starting at 1 year old, 600 IU for children, adolescents, and young adults* [9].

Many children and most healthy adolescents do not achieve the RDA of vitamin D from dietary sources and sun exposure. *Children at risk for vitamin D deficiency due to inadequate dietary intake include those who do not eat any dairy products such as milk protein allergy or an exclusive vegan diet; those with conditions that decrease one's ability to absorb fat-soluble vitamins such as cystic fibrosis and biliary atresia; and*

T. Stanley, M. Misra (eds.), *Endocrine Conditions in Pediatrics*, https://doi.org/10.1007/978-3-030-52215-5_54

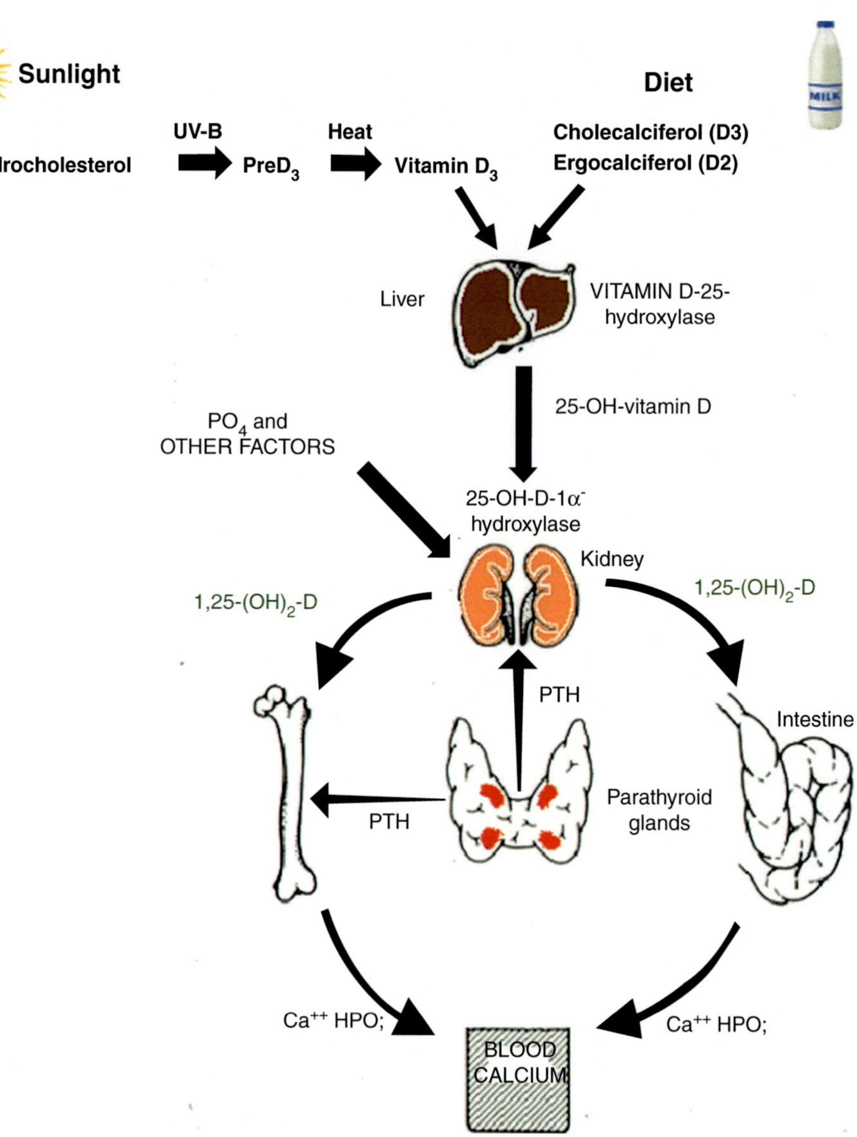

Fig. 54.1 Vitamin D, calcium, and phosphate regulation

those prescribed and taking certain medications including anti-epileptic medications, glucocorticoids, and medications to treat tuberculosis and HIV/AIDS (Table 54.1).

A serum 25-OH vitamin D measurement reflects bodily stores of vitamin D. There has been controversy regarding the definition of vitamin D deficiency. The Institute of Medicine defined vitamin D deficiency as having a serum level of less than 20 ng/mL, reflecting a level that meets the needs of the majority of the general population [9]. In contract, the Endocrine Society defined vitamin D deficiency as having a serum level of less than 20 ng/mL, and notably insufficiency as a serum level between 21 and 29 ng/mL [10]. In healthy children, with no risk factors for vitamin D deficiency or poor bone health, a 25-OH vitamin D level above 20 ng/mL is likely sufficient. However, in children with any of the above-mentioned risk factors for vitamin D deficiency, or in children with known threats to bone health (e.g., non-weight bearing or history of multiple fractures), it is advisable for their 25-OH vitamin D levels to be between 30 and 50 ng/mL as this can be beneficial to maximize calcium absorption and ensure normal range parathyroid

Table 54.1 Medications that may decrease 25-hydroxyvitamin D

Antiepileptic medications
Phenobarbital
Phenytoin
Carbamazepine
Oxcarbazepine
Glucocorticoids
Prednisone
Antituberculosis medications
Rifampin
Isoniazid
HIV/AIDS medications
Ritonavir
Tenofovir
Efavirenz

hormone (PTH) [10, 11]. Additionally, vitamin D may have immunomodulatory effects; therefore, aiming for this slightly higher target may be helpful in controlling exacerbations in patients with certain inflammatory diseases.

Evaluation

It is recommended to screen for vitamin D deficiency in patients at risk for deficiency [10]. If screening for vitamin D deficiency, it is usually sufficient to just evaluate a 25-OH vitamin D level (Table 54.2). Alternatively, it is also reasonable to empirically treat children with risk factors or suspected vitamin D deficiency with 1000–2000 IU daily of cholecalciferol, and then evaluate their 25-OH vitamin D level after 6–8 weeks of supplementation. Measurement of the active metabolite of vitamin D, 1,25$(OH)_2$ vitamin D, is generally reserved for situations where genetic and/or metabolic bone disease is suspected. If there is clinical concern that vitamin D deficiency has resulted in rickets or hypocalcemia, additional workup would include evaluating calcium, magnesium, phosphorus, alkaline phosphatase, PTH, and X-rays (Table 54.2).

Vitamin D deficiency results in abnormalities in calcium, phosphorus, and bone and mineral metabolism. It causes a decrease in the efficiency of intestinal calcium and phosphorus absorption of dietary intake of these minerals, resulting in an increase in PTH [1, 2]. Secondary hyperparathyroidism maintains serum calcium in the normal range at the expense of mobilizing calcium from the skeleton and increasing phosphorus wasting in the kidneys. The PTH-mediated increase in osteoclastic activity causes a generalized decrease in bone mineral density and creates local foci of bone weakness. The secondary hyperparathyroidism results in phosphaturia and low normal or low serum phosphorus. This results in an inadequate calcium-phosphorus product, which causes a mineralization defect in the skeleton. In young children who have little mineral in their skeleton and open epiphyseal growth plates, this defect results in a variety of skeletal deformities collectively known as rickets.

Table 54.2 Diagnosing vitamin D deficiency and associated sequelae

Required for diagnosis
Low 25-hydroxyvitamin D (i.e., <20 ng/mL)
Items supporting diagnosis
Elevated parathyroid hormone
Elevated alkaline phosphatase
Normal or low calcium (if low albumin, suggest albumin-corrected calcium)
Low or low normal phosphorus
Normal or elevated 1,25$(OH)_2$ vitamin D
X-rays to evaluate for rickets

Management and Treatment

Initial management once vitamin D deficiency has been identified includes treatment with either 2000–4000 IU per day or with 50,000 IU weekly for 6 weeks, recognizing that dosing may be dependent on the 25-OH vitamin D level, with higher daily doses typically used to treat more significant vitamin D deficiency [10]. Cholecalciferol (vitamin D3) is preferable to ergocalciferol (vitamin D2) as it is more potent and results in greater and longer lasting increases in serum 25-OH vitamin D level [12]. There are many different over-the-counter and prescription formulations, including liquid, chewable, and pills. Vitamin D can be administered daily, weekly, monthly, or intermittently with high-dose vitamin D (i.e., stoss therapy). Liquid preparations are available in a wide variety of concentrations. Patients should be carefully counseled about the correct volume of administration for the desired dose and cautioned against switching preparations without verifying concentration in order to assure that patients receive the correct dosage.

Of note, when initiating treatment of significant vitamin D deficiency, for example, 25-OH vitamin D less than 10–15 ng/mL and an elevated PTH, it is advisable to ensure adequate calcium intake, as repletion can precipitate hungry bone syndrome (severe hypocalcemia due to rapid mineralization of large amounts of unmineralized osteoid). It is advisable to ensure that patients are receiving the RDA for age of calcium, and frequently additional supplementation with 500–1000 mg per day of calcium when initiating vitamin D repletion, with higher doses if they have an elevated PTH and/or hypocalcemia. *The RDA of calcium is 700 mg/day in 1–3 years old, 1000 mg/day in 4–8 years old, 1300 mg/day in 9–18 years old, and 1000 mg/day in 19–50 years old* [9]. This target is best achieved by dietary intake of calcium-rich foods, such as dairy products. However, if a child or adolescent is unable to consume dietary sources, supplements are an option, ideally divided over multiple doses to optimize absorption, with a maximum dose of 500 mg per dose (as calcium carbonate with a meal), as above that absorption is exceeded.

Once repleted, almost all patients require some maintenance vitamin D, between 400 and 2000 IU daily, to maintain sufficient vitamin D levels [10]. In patients with malabsorption syndromes, patients on medications that affect vitamin D metabolism (Table 54.1), and in patients with obesity, they frequently require a higher dose of vitamin D. They often need two to three times higher dosage, at least 6000–10,000 IU per day, to treat their deficiency. To maintain a 25-OH vitamin D level above 30 ng/mL, they require a higher maintenance therapy of between 3000 and 6000 IU per day [10].

Prior studies have demonstrated that vitamin D toxicity is rare but has been reported with doses exceeding 10,000 IU daily and vitamin D toxicity with hypercalcemia involved daily doses exceeding 40,000 IU or a single dose greater than 300,000 IU [13–16]. There is frequently poor compliance with patients taking their vitamin D supplementation. Stoss therapy of between 200,000 IU and 800,000 IU has been well tolerated, and it should be considered in poorly compliant patients [17, 18]. There is emerging evidence that extremely high levels of 25-OH vitamin D, exceeding 100 ng/mL, may be detrimental [10, 19].

It is very important to monitor 25-OH vitamin D levels after 6–8 weeks on high dose repletion, and after 4 weeks or sooner if there are co-morbidities associated with vitamin D deficiency such as rickets or hypocalcemia. 25-OH vitamin D levels should also be assessed once on a maintenance vitamin D regimen for 2–3 months to determine if that is the optimal regimen for long-term supplementation.

Summary

Vitamin D is essential to maintaining calcium and phosphate homeostasis and bone health. Many children do not achieve the RDA of vitamin D from sun exposure and dietary sources. Consequently, vitamin D deficiency is common, affecting approximately 50% of children and adolescents. It is recommended to screen for vitamin D deficiency in patients at risk for deficiency, such as those who have no dietary intake of vitamin D rich or fortified foods, conditions that decrease one's ability to absorb fat-soluble vitamins, and certain medications. Cholecalciferol (vitamin D3) is preferable to ergocalciferol (vitamin D2) as it is more potent. Initial vitamin D supplementation can be daily, weekly, monthly, or with stoss therapy, with dosage and frequency of administration dependent upon the 25-OH vitamin D level and what will maximize medication compliance. If significant vitamin D deficiency, it is advisable to ensure that patients are receiving the RDA of calcium for age, and frequently benefit from short-term calcium supplementation. Once replete, almost all patients require some maintenance vitamin D to maintain sufficient vitamin D levels.

Reasons to refer to a pediatric endocrinologist include concern for sequelae of vitamin D deficiency, such as rickets or hypocalcemia, and the inability to increase the 25-OH vitamin D level into the sufficient range in compliant patients and following dose escalation.

References

1. Holick MF. Vitamin D deficiency. N Engl J Med. 2007;357(3):266–81.
2. Heaney RP. Functional indices of vitamin D status and ramifications of vitamin D deficiency. Am J Clin Nutr. 2004;80(6 Suppl):1706s–9s.
3. Aranow C. Vitamin D and the immune system. J Investig Med. 2011;59(6):881–6.
4. Gordon CM, DePeter KC, Feldman HA, Grace E, Emans SJ. Prevalence of vitamin D deficiency among healthy adolescents. Arch Pediatr Adolesc Med. 2004;158(6):531–7.
5. Sullivan SS, Rosen CJ, Halteman WA, Chen TC, Holick MF. Adolescent girls in Maine are at risk for vitamin D insufficiency. J Am Diet Assoc. 2005;105(6):971–4.
6. Matsuoka LY, Ide L, Wortsman J, MacLaughlin JA, Holick MF. Sunscreens suppress cutaneous vitamin D3 synthesis. J Clin Endocrinol Metab. 1987;64(6):1165–8.
7. Clemens TL, Adams JS, Henderson SL, Holick MF. Increased skin pigment reduces the capacity of skin to synthesise vitamin D3. Lancet (London, England). 1982;1(8263):74–6.
8. Hintzpeter B, Scheidt-Nave C, Muller MJ, Schenk L, Mensink GB. Higher prevalence of vitamin D deficiency is associated with immigrant background among children and adolescents in Germany. J Nutr. 2008;138(8):1482–90.
9. Ross CA, Manson JE, Abrams SA, et al. The 2011 report on dietary reference intakes for calcium and vitamin D from the Institute of Medicine: what clinicians need to know. J Clin Endocrinol Metabol. 2011;96(1):53–8.
10. Holick MF, Binkley NC, Bischoff-Ferrari HA, et al. Evaluation, treatment, and prevention of vitamin D deficiency: an Endocrine Society clinical practice guideline. J Clin Endocrinol Metab. 2011;96(7):1911–30.
11. Ma NS, Gordon CM. Pediatric osteoporosis: where are we now? J Pediatr. 2012;161(6):983–90.
12. Heaney RP, Recker RR, Grote J, Horst RL, Armas LA. Vitamin D(3) is more potent than vitamin D(2) in humans. J Clin Endocrinol Metab. 2011;96(3):E447–52.
13. Jacobus CH, Holick MF, Shao Q, et al. Hypervitaminosis D associated with drinking milk. N Engl J Med. 1992;326(18):1173–7.
14. Koutkia P, Chen TC, Holick MF. Vitamin D intoxication associated with an over-the-counter supplement. N Engl J Med. 2001;345(1):66–7.
15. Vieth R. Vitamin D supplementation, 25-hydroxyvitamin D concentrations, and safety. Am J Clin Nutr. 1999;69(5):842–56.
16. Cesur Y, Caksen H, Gundem A, Kirimi E, Odabas D. Comparison of low and high dose of vitamin D treatment in nutritional vitamin D deficiency rickets. J Pediatr Endocrinol Metab. 2003;16(8):1105–9.
17. Shepherd D, Day AS, Leach ST, et al. Single high-dose oral vitamin D3 therapy (Stoss): a solution to vitamin D deficiency in children with inflammatory bowel disease? J Pediatr Gastroenterol Nutr. 2015;61(4):411–4.
18. Martin NG, Rigterink T, Adamji M, Wall CL, Day AS. Single high-dose oral vitamin D3 treatment in New Zealand children with inflammatory bowel disease. Transl Pediatr. 2019;8(1):35–41.
19. Vogiatzi MG, Jacobson-Dickman E, DeBoer MD. Vitamin D supplementation and risk of toxicity in pediatrics: a review of current literature. J Clin Endocrinol Metab. 2014;99(4):1132–41.

Central Diabetes Insipidus (Etiology, Epidemiology, and Management)

55

Nourah Almutlaq and Erica A. Eugster

Introduction

Diabetes insipidus (DI) is a heterogeneous disorder that is characterized by the lack of ability to conserve free water and concentrate urine. This results in polyuria and polydipsia, which are the main manifestations of the disease [1].

DI is classified broadly according to its etiology as central or nephrogenic. Central diabetes insipidus (CDI) is due to a deficiency of arginine vasopressin (AVP), which is also called antidiuretic hormone (ADH), whereas nephrogenic DI is due to resistance to ADH action at the collecting tubules of the kidney [2].

AVP is produced and secreted from the neurons of the supraoptic and paraventricular nuclei that are located in the hypothalamus and transported caudally via their axons to the posterior pituitary where it is stored in secretory granules and released. The main stimulus for the release of ADH is serum osmolality, which is detected by the body through delicately sensitive osmoreceptors located within the subfornical organ and the organum vasculosum lamina terminalis, whose neurons transmit signals to supraoptic neurons that respond to variations in osmotic pressure as low as two mOsm/L. ADH is also regulated by hypovolemia, which is sensed through baroreceptors located in the carotid artery, aortic arch, and left atrium that transmit information to the vagus nerve, directly stimulating the secretion of ADH. When AVP is released into the circulation, it acts on the distal convoluted tubule (DCT) and the collecting duct (CD) to absorb free water by stimulating the insertion of Aquaporin-2 channels in the apical membrane of the DCT and CD cells, allowing water to move down its concentration gradient back into the vasculature. A secondary response to a rising serum osmolality is thirst, which is a powerful physiologic mechanism designed to increase water intake. Thus, under normal circumstances, ADH and thirst act in concert to ensure that salt and water balance remains normal [3–5].

In the absence of AVP, free water is lost through the renal collecting system resulting in extreme polyuria, polydipsia, and dilute urine. In a child with an intact thirst mechanism and free access to water, serum sodium and osmolality remain normal at the expense of excessive drinking. Therefore, the body must be challenged through a "water deprivation test" in order to confirm a diagnosis of DI (see Chaps. 17 and 28).

Etiology

Any impairment in ADH production or secretion can result in CDI, which can be congenital or acquired (Fig. 55.1). A number of known genetic etiologies of CDI also exist, which may be transmitted according to a variety of inheritance patterns or arise de novo [6].

Epidemiology

CDI is rare in the pediatric population. According to a large Danish study, the incidence is 3–4 per 100,000 with a higher ratio in boys than in girls [7, 8]. Complaints of polydipsia and polyuria are extremely common in pediatric patients, particularly during the toddler years, but the majority of children with polydipsia and polyuria do not have CDI. Important elements of the history include the quantity of fluid intake, what the preferred beverage is, and whether the excessive drinking and urination also occur at night. Findings that increase the likelihood of CDI include older age, higher baseline serum sodium and osmolality, and a propensity for inappropriate water-seeking behavior such as

N. Almutlaq (✉) · E. A. Eugster
Division of Pediatric Endocrinology, Department of Pediatrics, Riley Hospital for Children at Indiana University Health, Indiana University School of Medicine, Indianapolis, IN, USA
e-mail: nalmutla@iu.edu; eeugster@iu.edu

T. Stanley, M. Misra (eds.), *Endocrine Conditions in Pediatrics*, https://doi.org/10.1007/978-3-030-52215-5_55

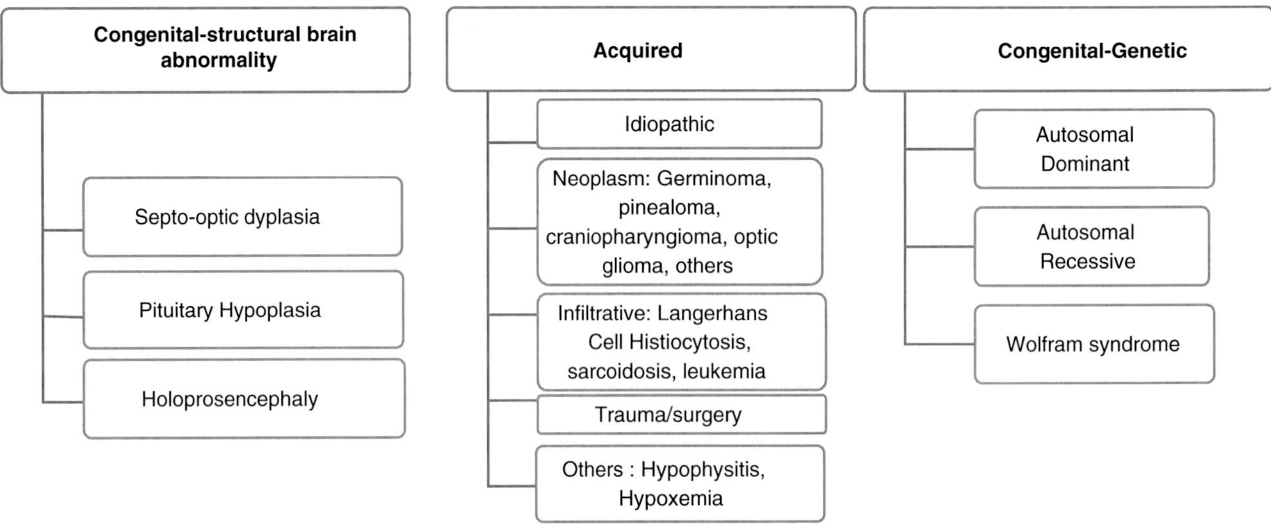

Fig. 55.1 Etiologic categories of CDI along with their differential diagnoses

drinking out of faucets, birdbaths, fountains, and flower vases [9]. Table 55.1 summarizes clinical features consistent with a diagnosis of CDI.

> **Reference Box: Key Pathophysiology**
> - Central diabetes insipidus results from injury to or absence of the AVP-secreting neurons located in the paraventricular and supraoptic nuclei of the hypothalamus, resulting in decreased AVP production.
> - The consequence of inadequate AVP production or secretion is the inability to concentrate urine.
> - Increased polyuria and polydipsia lead to hypernatremia, high serum osmolality, and inappropriately low urine osmolality and specific gravity when water is withheld.

Urgent or Emergent Considerations and Initial Management

DI can be a life-threatening condition when the body's compensatory mechanisms are inadequate such as in children without an intact thirst or in those with no access to water. Particularly vulnerable patients include infants and neurologically impaired children.

The initial management of CDI depends on the severity of the biochemical abnormalities and the clinical situation. In patients presenting with significant hypernatremia, hospitalization in an intensive care unit is required. The free water

Table 55.1 Items required for diagnosis and items supporting diagnosis

	For diagnosis	Supporting diagnosis
History	Polyuria Polydipsia	New-onset enuresis Irritability Dehydration Symptoms of underlying etiology, such as growth deceleration, fatigue, visual changes, headache, and vomiting Family history of CDI Known diagnosis of hypopituitarism
Examination		Visual field deficits Signs of dehydration Failure to thrive
Laboratory tests	Inappropriately dilute urine in the setting of increased serum osmolality	Tests for hypopituitarism
Imaging		Brain MRI: Thickened pituitary stalk Absence of the posterior pituitary bright spot[a] Ectopic posterior pituitary Structural abnormality or intracranial tumor
Genetic		Confirmed mutation in the gene encoding for AVP or its carrier protein, neurophysin II or in genes implicated in Wolfram syndrome

[a]Lack of a posterior pituitary bright spot can be seen a subset of normal individuals and may also be seen in nephrogenic diabetes insipidus

deficit can be calculated using the following formula: [desired decrease in serum sodium (mEq/L) × weight in kg × 4]. It is always safer to aim for a higher serum sodium due to concerns of rapid correction of hypernatremia, which can lead to cerebral edema and cause permanent brain damage. Therefore, targeting serum sodium to the mid-140s is appropriate. The rate of correction of serum sodium depends on the chronicity of the hypernatremia. When this is unknown, a very slow rate of 0.5 mEq/L per hour drop in serum sodium is recommended (no more than 12 mEq/L/day). When laboratory data are consistent with DI, a test dose of AVP or DDAVP is administered. If this is followed by decreased urine output and an increase in urine osmolality and specific gravity, the diagnosis of CDI is confirmed. In children presenting with CDI without a known CNS abnormality, a brain MRI scan is mandatory due to concerns about an intracranial neoplasm or Langerhans cell histiocytosis (see Fig. 55.1).

Chronic Management and Considerations for Referral

All patients with CDI should be referred to a pediatric endocrinologist for ongoing management and follow-up regardless of the etiology. In neurologically normal children, the therapeutic aims of treatment are mainly to decrease polyuria and thirst in order to improve the quality of life and allow for normal growth. The mainstay of treatment in CDI is DDAVP, which is a synthetic analog of endogenous AVP that has a 2000- to 3000-fold lower vasopressor effect. It is available in oral, intranasal, and parenteral forms that differ in potency by a factor of 10. For example, 1 mcg of SQ DDAVP is equal to 10 mcg of intranasal DDAVP, which is equal to 100 mcg of oral DDAVP. Thus, exquisite care must be taken by prescribers and pharmacists to ensure that inadvertent errors in dosing do not occur. The vast majority of children with CDI are treated with DDAVP tablets which come in a 0.1 mg and 0.2 mg strength. However, there is extensive individual variation in DDAVP dose requirements among patients with CDI. At our center, we have observed that children with acquired etiologies of CDI are more likely to require higher doses of DDAVP (≥1 mg per day) than those with congenital causes. The greatest concern with the use of DDAVP is the potential for hyponatremia [10]. This is related to the fact that DDAVP exerts its effect through an "all or none" phenomenon. Once onboard, essentially all water ingested will be conserved by the body until the drug has been metabolized. Therefore, parents are counseled about the importance of waiting until they observe "breakthrough," i.e., diuresis and increased thirst in their child, prior to each dose. A concern for inadvertent hyponatremia also underlies concerns around prescribing DDAVP for nocturnal enuresis in otherwise healthy children. Indeed, this practice has been linked to several tragic cases of brain herniation and death due to excessive fluid intake following the administration of DDAVP [10].

Management of CDI in Special Situations

Infants with CDI

The treatment in this age group is very challenging as they are entirely dependent on administered fluid such as breast milk or formula. Therefore, frequent measurement of serum sodium, especially when starting therapy, is essential in order to minimize the risk of hyponatremia. Thiazide diuretics are preferred by some clinicians as an alternative to DDAVP, although studies have not found these to be more effective [11, 12]. Some endocrinologists have moved toward using intranasal DDAVP preparations in infants with CDI, with the dose administered orally rather than intranasally.

Children with CDI and Lack of an Intact Thirst Mechanism

Effective treatment can be achieved via a fixed daily fluid intake with DDAVP given at doses that allow for appropriate urine output. However, serum sodium tends to fluctuate significantly in children without an intact thirst mechanism. Therefore, they require ongoing monitoring of serum sodium, urine output, and urine specific gravity. Treatment should be initiated in a hospital setting and titrated in order to maintain serum sodium in a "safe" range which is generally from the low 130s to the mid 150s .In neurologically impaired children, free water boluses can be administered per G-tube as needed [13].

Status Postoperative Intracranial Surgery Patients

The management of postoperative CDI can be challenging and fluid balance needs to be closely monitored in an intensive care setting through the assessment of urine output, serum sodium, and urine specific gravity. IV fluids consisting of normal saline along with a continuous intravenous infusion of vasopressin is preferred in the acute setting due to its short duration of action. Children can be transitioned to oral or intranasal DDAVP once they are tolerating a normal PO intake and are otherwise clinically stable [14, 15].

Management of CDI During Chemotherapy

Children who undergo chemotherapy often require excessive fluid therapy, especially when they are administered nephrotoxic chemotherapeutic agents. Hence, it is recommended to hold DDAVP during these periods to avoid the risk of severe hyponatremia. Close monitoring of fluid intake and output, weight, urine specific gravity, and serum sodium levels is required. A vasopressin drip can be started if needed at a very low dose with an initial rate of 0.08–0.10 mU/kg per hour during hydration therapy where it will permit flexible regulation of fluid and electrolyte balance while simultaneously avoiding the risk of giving or holding the DDAVP [16].

Conclusion

CDI is a heterogeneous disorder with a broad differential diagnosis. Its management ranges from the relatively straightforward outpatient care of an otherwise healthy child with an intact thirst mechanism to that of a critically ill child in the intensive care setting, who requires hourly monitoring. An understanding of normal physiology and the mechanism of action of DDAVP will result in optimal outcomes in most cases. Regardless of the clinical setting, a pediatric endocrinologist is an essential part of the treatment team.

References

1. Dabrowski E, Kadakia R, Zimmerman D. Diabetes insipidus in infants and children. Best Pract Res Clin Endocrinol Metab. 2016;30(2):317–28.
2. Cheetham T, Baylis PH. Diabetes insipidus in children: pathophysiology, diagnosis and management. Paediatr Drugs. 2002;4(12):785–96.
3. Davies AG. Antidiuretic and growth hormones. Br Med J. 1972;2(5808):282–4.
4. Tokinaga K, Terano T, Yoshida S. Vasopressin (anti-diuretic hormone: ADH). Nihon Rinsho. 1995;53(Su Pt 2):304–7.
5. Bourque CW, Richard D. Axonal projections from the organum vasculosum lamina terminalis to the supraoptic nucleus: functional analysis and presynaptic modulation. Clin Exp Pharmacol Physiol. 2001;28(7):570–4.
6. Di Iorgi N, et al. Diabetes insipidus--diagnosis and management. Horm Res Paediatr. 2012;77(2):69–84.
7. Blotner H. Primary or idiopathic diabetes insipidus: a system disease. Metabolism. 1958;7(3):191–200.
8. Werny D, et al. Pediatric central diabetes insipidus: brain malformations are common and few patients have idiopathic disease. J Clin Endocrinol Metab. 2015;100(8):3074–80.
9. Haddad NG, Nabhan ZM, Eugster EA. Incidence of central diabetes insipidus in children presenting with polydipsia and polyuria. Endocr Pract. 2016;22(12):1383–6.
10. Hossain T, et al. Desmopressin-induced severe hyponatremia with central Pontine myelinolysis: a case report. Drug Saf Case Rep. 2018;5(1):19.
11. Al Nofal A, Lteif A. Thiazide Diuretics in the management of young children with central diabetes insipidus. J Pediatr. 2015;167(3):658–61.
12. Rivkees SA, Dunbar N, Wilson TA. The management of central diabetes insipidus in infancy: desmopressin, low renal solute load formula, thiazide diuretics. J Pediatr Endocrinol Metab. 2007;20(4):459–69.
13. Di Iorgi N, et al. Management of diabetes insipidus and adipsia in the child. Best Pract Res Clin Endocrinol Metab. 2015;29(3):415–36.
14. Ghirardello S, et al. Diabetes insipidus in craniopharyngioma: postoperative management of water and electrolyte disorders. J Pediatr Endocrinol Metab. 2006;19(Suppl 1):413–21.
15. Wise-Faberowski L, et al. Perioperative management of diabetes insipidus in children. J Neurosurg Anesthesiol. 2004;16(3):220–5.
16. Bryant WP, et al. Aqueous vasopressin infusion during chemotherapy in patients with diabetes insipidus. Cancer. 1994;74(9):2589–92.

Pituitary or Suprasellar Lesions

56

Shilpa Mehta and Brenda Kohn

Introduction

In children, pituitary tumors (Table 56.1) can be benign or malignant. The suprasellar tumors can be developmental in origin, inflammatory, immunologic, and vascular in nature. The intrasellar tumors are mostly represented by pituitary adenomas [3]. (Please refer to Chap. 37 for definitions of terms describing pituitary anatomy.)

Although pituitary tumors are not generally managed in the primary care setting, an understanding of the differential diagnosis of sellar and suprasellar lesions can help greatly in communicating with families and coordinating care. This chapter does not discuss further management in the primary care setting. All of the conditions below should be referred to a pediatric endocrinologist. With the exception of pituitary hyperplasia, most Rathke's cleft cysts, and many pituitary microadenomas, most of these referrals should be urgent or emergent. (See also Chap. 37.)

Clinical Presentation of Pituitary and Suprasellar Tumors

An expanding pituitary mass may alter the size and shape of the sella through bony erosion and remodeling. Although the exact time course of this process is unknown, it appears to be slowly progressive over years or decades [4]. Both suprasellar and parasellar compression and invasion may occur with enlarging tumor with resultant clinical manifestation (Table 56.2).

Table 56.1 Differential diagnosis of pituitary and suprasellar tumors in childhood

Benign tumors
Craniopharyngioma
Pituitary adenomas: functioning or nonfunctioning adenomas
Optic pathway glioma (e.g., pilocytic astrocytoma)
Hypothalamic hamartoma
Pituitary stalk thickening
Pituitary hyperplasia
Pituitary hemorrhage or pituitary apoplexy
Other rare tumors: CNS lipoma, xanthogranulomas, granular cell tumors, gangliogliomas and medulloepitheliomas, heterotopic cerebellar tissue, pediatric subependymomas
Malignant tumors
Germ cell tumor (e.g., germinoma)
Langerhans cell histiocytosis (LCH)
Metastatic disease
Cysts
Rathke's cleft cyst
Arachnoid cyst
Epidermoid cyst/dermoid cyst
Inflammatory/infectious lesions
Hypophysitis
Infectious: abscess, tuberculosis, cysticercosis, toxoplasmosis, sarcoidosis
Vascular lesions:
Aneurysm
Carotid cavernous fistula

Pituitary and Suprasellar Tumors in Childhood

Craniopharyngioma

Craniopharyngiomas (Fig. 56.1) account for 30–50% of sellar and suprasellar tumors occurring in childhood and adolescence [5]. Though histologically benign tumors, their growth pattern may be very aggressive and can cause damage to the optic nerves, pituitary gland, and hypothalamus. The incidence is bimodal with a peak in the pediatric population between 5 and 14 years and then again in the adult population between 50 and 74 years [6]. Craniopharyngiomas are known to originate from squamous epithelium of Rathke's

S. Mehta (✉)
Department of Pediatrics, Division of Pediatric Endocrinology, New York Medical College, Valhalla, NY, USA

B. Kohn
Division of Pediatric Endocrinology and Diabetes, New York University-Langone Medical Center, Hassenfeld Children's Hospital, New York, NY, USA
e-mail: Brenda.kohn@nyulangone.org

T. Stanley, M. Misra (eds.), *Endocrine Conditions in Pediatrics*, https://doi.org/10.1007/978-3-030-52215-5_56

Table 56.2 Local effects of expanding pituitary and suprasellar tumors

Pituitary	Growth failure, multiple pituitary hormone deficiencies
Optic tract	Loss of red perception, bitemporal hemianopia, superior or bitemporal field defects, scotomas, and blindness
Hypothalamus	Temperature dysregulation, obesity, disturbances in sleep, behavioral and autonomic nervous system dysfunction
Cavernous sinus	Ptosis, diplopia, ophthalmoplegia, facial numbness
Temporal lobe	Uncinate seizures
Frontal lobe	Personality disorder, anosmia
Central	Headache, hydrocephalus, psychosis, dementia, laughing seizures
Neuro-ophthalmologic tract	Field defects: Bitemporal hemianopia Acuity loss Pupillary abnormality Optic atrophy

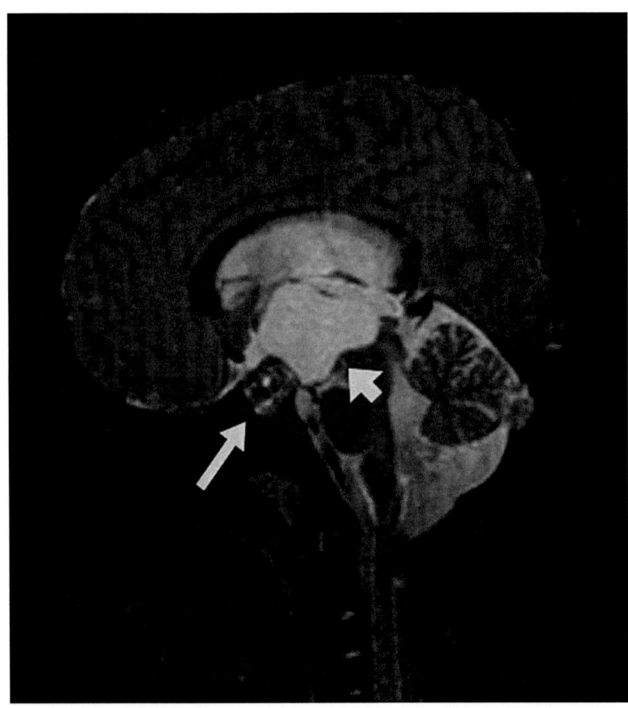

Fig. 56.1 Craniopharyngioma: sagittal T2-weighted image without contrast with mixed solid (long arrow) and cystic (short arrow) sellar/suprasellar mass

pouch or craniopharyngeal duct remnants. Histologically craniopharyngiomas are two different types: adamantinomatous and papillary. In childhood, these tumors are almost always the adamantinomatous type [6]. Craniopharyngiomas may present with neurologic symptoms, visual impairment (62–84%), and endocrine deficits (52–87%). Endocrine deficits due to involvement of the hypothalamic–pituitary axis include GHD (75%), gonadotropin deficiency (40%), ACTH deficiency (25%), and TSH deficiency (25%). At diagnosis, 40–87% of patients present with at least one endocrinopathy [5, 7, 8]. DI is reported in 17–27% of patients preoperatively and 70% of patients postoperatively [7, 8]. Surgical resection is the treatment of choice for craniopharyngiomas. Because the recurrence rate is higher than in all other pituitary tumors, adjunctive radiotherapy is often indicated [9].

Pituitary Adenomas

Pituitary adenomas are rare in early childhood, and their frequency increases during adolescence. Approximately 3% of all diagnosed intracranial tumors in childhood are pituitary adenomas [9]. Pituitary adenomas could be functioning or nonfunctioning tumors [10]. Functioning tumors (Table 56.3) can cause a variety of signs and symptoms depending on the hormone they produce [1]. Nonfunctioning pituitary adenomas may present with GH deficiency (up to 75%), LH/FSH deficiency (~40%), or ACTH and TSH deficiency (~25%) [9].

Optic Pathway Glioma (OPG)

OPGs (Fig. 56.2) are low-grade pilocytic astrocytomas accounting for 2–5% of intracranial brain tumors in children [11]. OPGs develop along the structures of the visual pathways including the optic nerves and chiasm, and along the optic tracts. Over 65% of OPGs are diagnosed in children under the age of 6 years, with the majority of remaining cases diagnosed between 6 and 15 years [11]. Approximately, 50–60% of OPGs are known to occur in patients with neurofibromatosis type 1 (NF1); the remaining are sporadic OPGs [11]. Fifteen to 20% of children with NF1 will develop an OPG; however, only 30–50% are symptomatic [12]. NF1-associated OPGs have a female preponderance while sporadic OPGs have an equal gender distribution. The presence of bilateral OPGs is almost pathognomonic for NF1 and is present in approximately 35% of NF1-associated OPGs [11]. Precocious puberty (25–30%) is the most common initial presentation in children with an NF-1 associated OPG [13]. In contrast, patients with sporadic OPGs present with visual disturbances (63%) [13].

NF1-associated OPGs have a variable course. Many remain indolent and do not progress [11, 13]. Approximately 15% of NF1-associated OPGs show minimal tumor enlargement, another 15% demonstrate significant enlargement, and the remaining 51% are stable on long-term follow-up [14]. Sporadic OPGs have a less benign course, a greater propensity to present with vision loss, and a worse visual outcome [13].

Table 56.3 Pituitary adenomas

Pituitary adenomas	Signs and symptoms	Diagnosis-MRI	Treatment
Prolactin-secreting tumors or prolactinomas [9] Most common (50%) F > M: 3:1	Female: pubertal delay, irregular menstrual periods, amenorrhea, galactorrhea Male: ophthalmological and neurological findings, growth or pubertal arrest and other pituitary dysfunctions (galactorrhea uncommon)	Elevated serum prolactin levels in combination with adenoma identification magnetic resonance (MR)-imaging typically confirm a diagnosis of prolactinoma	Medical therapy with dopamine-agonist therapy (e.g., bromocriptine, pergolide, or cabergoline) is first-line treatment Surgical resection in a small proportion who are refractory to medical therapy or will be intolerant of medication side effects or in emergent situation (acute threat to vision)
Growth hormone secreting tumors: (5–15%) [1, 9] Overproduction of Growth hormone (GH) M > F: 3:2	Gigantism: rapid growth; tall stature Acromegaly: coarsened facial features, enlarged hands and feet, high blood sugar, joint pain, heart diseases, excess sweating, misaligned teeth, increased body hair	Elevated serum insulin-like growth factor-1 (IGF-1)/GH confirms If equivocal IGF-1 levels, an oral glucose tolerance test (OGTT) may be performed, and lack of GH suppression to <1 μg /L is diagnostic of acromegaly MR imaging of the pituitary gland is used to assess the size and location of the adenoma	First-line therapy for GH-secreting adenomas is transsphenoidal resection Medical therapy with somatostatin analogues or pegvisomant, a GH-receptor antagonist may be used if resection fails to provide biochemical remission
ACTH-secreting tumors: [1, 9] Cushing's disease Overproduction of ACTH stimulates adrenal gland to produce excess of cortisol resulting in signs and symptoms of Cushing's disease 4.8%–10% F:M: 3:1	Linear growth arrest with unexplained excessive weight gain, particularly around neck and midsection, moon facies, striae, thinning of the arms and legs, muscle weakness hypertension, elevated blood glucose, acne, bone weakening and fractures, easy bruising, stretch marks, anxiety, irritability and depression, insomnia and poor concentration	Elevated basal and stimulated levels of cortisol and ACTH, Elevated 24-h urinary free cortisol, Circadian cortisol profile: Salivary cortisol at midnight and 8 am showed blunted circadian rhythm Low-dose dexamethasone suppression at midnight does not induce suppression of morning serum cortisol concentrations Suppression of cortisol by more than 50% after high-dose dexamethasone confirms MR imaging confirmation may be complicated by lack of a visible tumor; inferior petrosal sinus sampling may be used to localize ACTH hypersecretion	Transsphenoidal surgical resection Radiation therapy should be considered in patients with persistent hypercortisolism after surgical management or known residual disease that cannot be resected
Thyroid-stimulating hormone secreting tumors (Rare) [1] 1–2%	Symptoms of hyperthyroidism: Weight loss, rapid and irregular heartbeat, palpitation, nervousness or irritability, diarrhea, excessive sweating	TSH may be normal, and a combination of thyrotropin-releasing hormone stimulation test (lack of response of TSH), serum α-subunit (elevated), and the α-subunit/TSH molar ratio (elevated) may be needed to make a diagnosis	Surgical resection is typically the first-line therapy

On follow-up of OPGs, GH deficiency (GHD) was most common (40.3%), followed by central precocious puberty (CPP, 26.0%), gonadotropin deficiency (20.4%), TSH (13.3%), and ACTH (13.3%) deficiencies [15].

The NF1 Optic Pathway Glioma Task Force (1997) and American Academy of Pediatrics Committee on Genetics (2008) have recommended yearly ophthalmologic evaluation until 8 years of age and then every 2 years until 18 years of age in children with NF1 [16]. Neuroimaging is not routinely recommended as part of surveillance for patients with NF1 in the absence of clinical signs and symptoms [17].

Management decisions must be individualized depending on the patient's age, the presence or absence of NF1, and the location of the tumor. The goal of all treatment strategies is to preserve vision for as long as possible. Many patients with OPGs, particularly those with NF1, may maintain stable visual function without deterioration, so observation is the initial preferred treatment especially when the tumor is

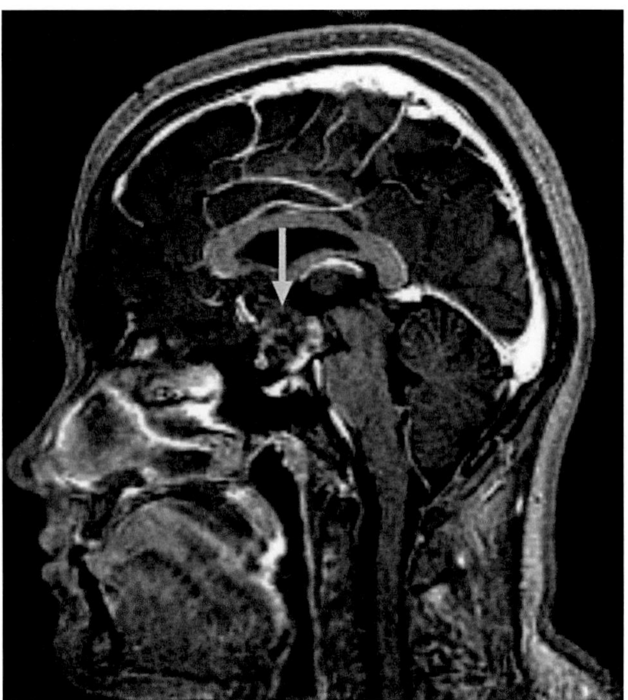

Fig. 56.2 Optic pathway glioma: sagittal T1-weighted image with contrast exhibits a heterogeneously enhancing chiasmatic/hypothalamic mass

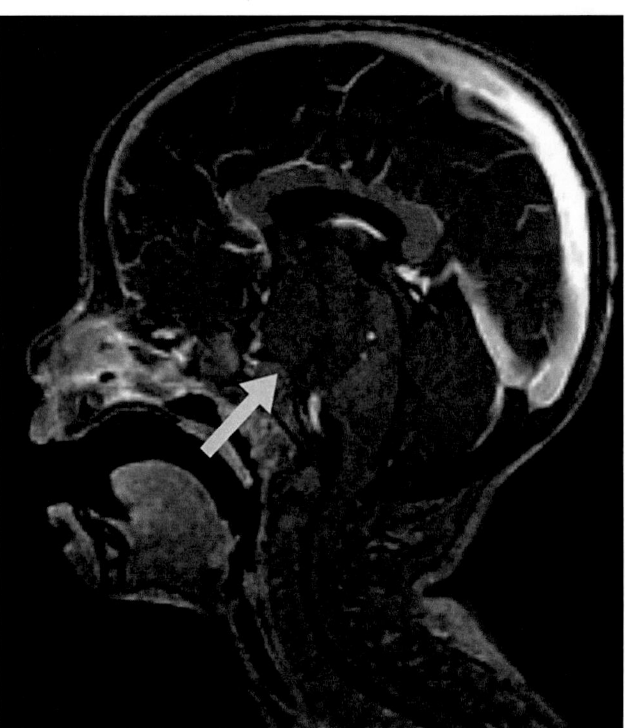

Fig. 56.3 Hypothalamic hamartoma: sagittal T1-weighted image with contrast exhibits large nonenhancing mass isointense to gray matter

confined to the optic nerve [18]. Treatment of OPGs is based upon clinical and radiographic progression [19]. Surgery is very rarely performed, and then only as a last resort for lesions causing significant visual compromise [19]. Although both chemotherapy and radiotherapy can stabilize growth or even decrease the size of tumors, chemotherapy has fewer side effects than radiation therapy (such as secondary tumors, radiation necrosis, and Moyomoya disease) and is generally considered the first-line treatment for progressive lesions in younger patients [20].

Hypothalamic Hamartomas (HH)

HH (Fig. 56.3) are rare congenital malformations consisting of gray matter heterotopia arising from the tuber cinereum and inferior hypothalamus. HH presents with gelastic seizures and/or central precocious puberty (CPP) [21]. The hallmark endocrine feature of HH is central precocious puberty (14–36%) [21]. The average age of presentation of CPP in HH is younger (females: 2.5 years, males: 3.7 years) than occurs in idiopathic CPP (5 years) [22]. The occurrence of other associated endocrine abnormalities is rare with central hypothyroidism (2.4%), growth hormone deficiency (0.8%), ACTH deficiency (0.8%), and panhypopituitarism (0.8%) [22].

Pharmacotherapy with GnRH agonists is the first-line treatment for CPP in HH. Surgical treatment is warranted in instances with intractable epilepsy [23].

Pituitary Stalk Thickening (PST)

Pituitary stalk thickening (Fig. 56.4) can be an incidental finding or discovered as part of the evaluation in a child presenting with central diabetes insipidus (CDI) (33%) [24], visual impairment, or other endocrine dysfunction. One-third of children with central DI with PST are ultimately diagnosed to have either an occult CNS germinoma or LCH or lymphocytic hypophysitis. Enlargement of the pituitary stalk to greater than approximately 2.6 mm is considered pathologic in children [25]. Among patients with DI, progressive stalk thickening over time may be predictive of neoplasia or infiltrative disorder. Notwithstanding, a normal MRI in the presence of CDI does not preclude a germinoma or other pathologic process and warrants 3–6 monthly surveillance and imaging [25].

Germ Cell Tumors (GCTs)

CNS germ cell tumors (Fig. 56.5) account for approximately 3% of primary pediatric brain tumors [26]. GCTs are commonly located in the pineal region (60%), and less commonly, in the suprasellar region (30%) or both (10%) [26]. There is a peak incidence in adolescence and young adulthood with approximately 90% of cases occurring before age 20 years [27]. Intracranial germ cell tumors may present with endocrine abnormalities, signs of increased intracranial

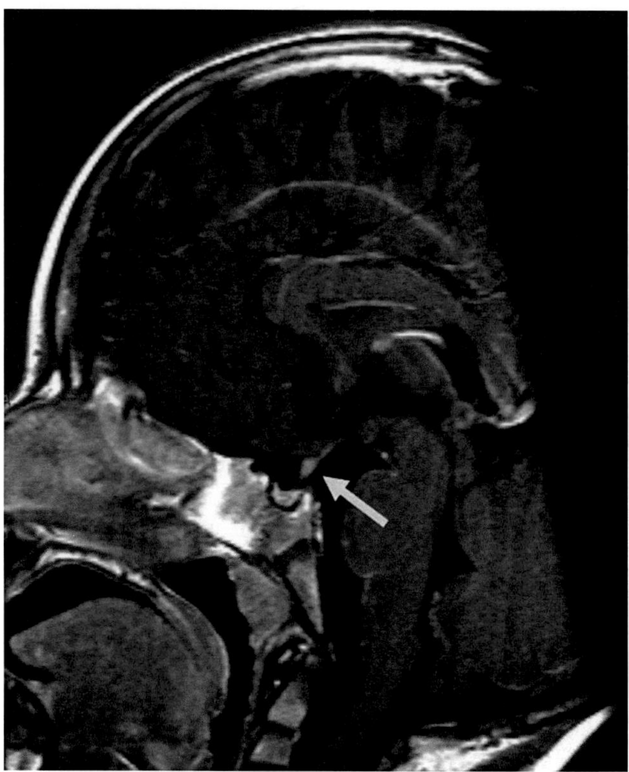

Fig. 56.4 Pituitary stalk thickening: sagittal T1-weighted image with contrast demonstrates nonvisualization of the normal posterior bright spot, as well as abnormal thickening of the superior infundibulum

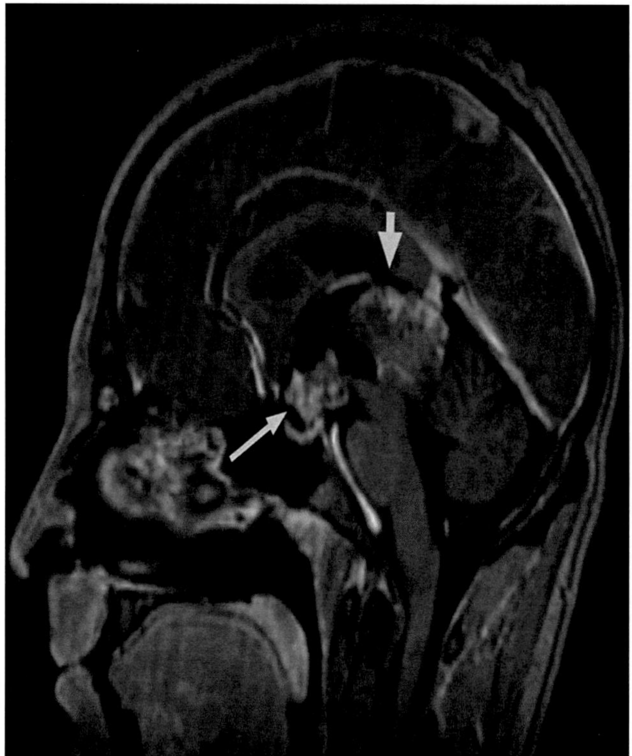

Fig. 56.5 Germ cell tumor: sagittal T1-weighted image with contrast shows heterogeneously enhancing masses in the pineal region (short arrow) and suprasellar cistern (long arrow)

pressure, and/or visual changes, depending on tumor location and size.

Suprasellar germ cell tumors most often present with CDI, and eventually other hypothalamic–pituitary deficiencies emerge such as pubertal delay or precocious puberty, growth hormone deficiency, hypothyroidism, adrenal insufficiency, or panhypopituitarism [26]. Patients may present with visual disturbances and rarely with signs of increased intracranial pressure. Pineal region tumors often present with signs of increased intracranial pressure, and 50% of patients have Parinaud syndrome, characterized by vertical gaze palsy, nystagmus on convergence, and pupillary dilation with poor reactiveness to light [26].

All patients with a suspected GCT warrant a thorough metastatic evaluation including MRI of the brain and spine with gadolinium, measurement of Alpha Feto Protein (AFP) and β-hCG levels in both serum and CSF, and evaluation of pituitary/hypothalamic function [2, 26].

Radiation therapy is extremely effective in treating germinomas, and a complete response is often achieved with craniospinal radiation alone [2, 26].

Langerhans Cell Histiocytosis (LCH)

LCH (Fig. 56.6) occurs in the central nervous system in approximately 4% of pediatric cases; with the hypothalamus–pituitary being the most common location followed by the cerebellum [28]. LCH is a rare disease with a median age at diagnosis of 2–3.8 years [29–32]. The classic triad of

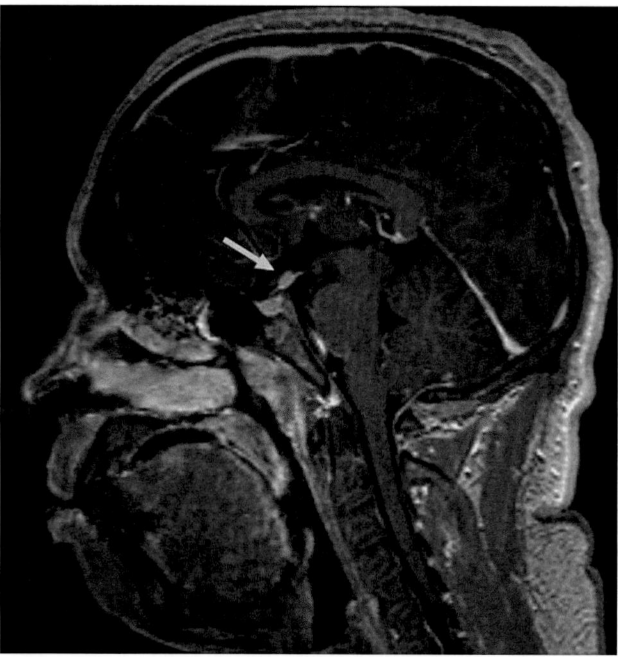

Fig. 56.6 Langerhans cell histiocytosis: sagittal T1-weighted image with contrast demonstrates abnormal thickening of the superior infundibulum

exophthalmos, lytic lesion of the membranous bones, and CDI occurs primarily in the disseminated form of the disease. Involvement of the hypothalamus–pituitary invariably leads to DI [33]. Commonly associated radiologic findings include thickening of the pituitary stalk and absence of the posterior pituitary bright spot, with further progression to space-occupying tumors [28]. Growth hormone deficiency (GHD) resulting from hypothalamic dysfunction affects approximately 50% of LCH patients [34].

Current therapeutic modalities with prolonged low-dose systemic chemotherapy are aimed at preventing disease progression and limiting endocrinopathy [28, 35].

Pituitary Hyperplasia

The most common physiologic cause of pituitary hyperplasia (Fig. 56.7) is puberty [36]. Nevertheless, hyperplasia of the pituitary gland can also occur pathologically in conditions such as long- standing untreated primary hypothyroidism or hemorrhage into the pituitary gland [37]. In hypothyroidism, treatment with L-thyroxine results in the resolution of pituitary hyperplasia with normalization of TSH and prolactin levels.

Pituitary hemorrhage or pituitary apoplexy is another cause of pituitary hyperplasia, which is rare in the pediatric population and typically occurs with an underlying pituitary adenoma [38] but has been reported to occur with no underlying pituitary abnormalities [39]. In cases of an underlying pituitary adenoma, an acute or severe headache warrants urgent neurosurgery evaluation.

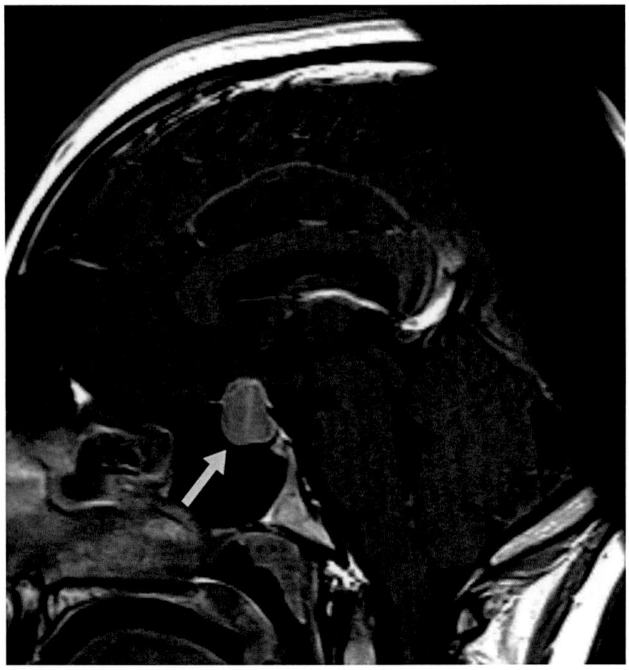

Fig. 56.7 Pituitary hyperplasia: sagittal T1-weighted image with prominent pituitary gland

Rathke's Cleft Cysts (RCCs)

RCCs are congenital cystic remnants of Rathke's pouch arising between the anterior and intermediate lobes of the pituitary gland in the region of the pars intermedia [40]. Although RCCs are often incidental, symptomatic cystic growth can rarely lead to visual deficits and endocrinopathies, requiring surgical resection [41]. The most frequent endocrinopathies associated with RCCs are diabetes insipidus and precocious puberty [42]. RCCs may also commonly present with growth delay in children with evidence of GHD [42].

Arachnoid Cysts

Arachnoid cysts are smoothly marginated CSF-containing lesions with the prevalence between 0.9% and 2.6% among the pediatric population [43]. The majority of arachnoid cysts remain stable and asymptomatic. Rarely, enlargement of the cyst results in symptoms [44]. Suprasellar arachnoid cysts, due to their location, are a known cause of hypothalamic–pituitary dysfunction and may cause precocious puberty, growth hormone (GH) deficiency, hypogonadotropic hypogonadism, adrenocorticotropic hormone (ACTH) deficiency, and hypothyroidism [45].

Epidermoid and Dermoid Cysts

Intracranial epidermoid and dermoid cysts are rare congenital conditions that account for 0.1–1.8% of all intracranial tumors [46]. Dermoid cysts occur midline and can mimic a craniopharyngioma [47]. Intracranial epidermoid cysts are more common than dermoid cysts. They generally are not midline but can be seen in the suprasellar region [48].

Lymphocytic Hypophysitis (LYH)

LYH is common in adults and has become increasingly recognized in children and adolescents. Fifty percent of affected children have the involvement of both the adenohypophysis and neurohypophysis, with anterior pituitary dysfunction and central diabetes insipidus [49]. Anterior pituitary hormone deficiency includes GHD in 76% of children compared with 36–54% in adults, gonadal dysfunction in 32% of children compared with 40–52% in adults, and hypothyroidism in 30% of children in contrast to 49–60% in adults [50]. Central adrenal insufficiency is also less common in affected children, with central adrenal insufficiency reported in 21% in comparison to 57–65% in adults [50]. CDI is more frequent in children (85%) than adults (14–20%) [50]. The clinical course of LYH is highly variable and includes gradual spontaneous remission with or without sequelae or rapid deterioration resulting in panhypopituitarism.

Autoimmune Hypophysitis (AH) Associated with Cancer Chemotherapy

Recent studies have defined a cause of autoimmune hypophysitis that is induced by the use of immune checkpoint inhibitors in cancer chemotherapy. Ipilimumab is a monoclonal antibody (MAB), which can induce acute hypophysitis [51]. Acute ACTH/cortisol deficiency and hypopituitarism along with DI are frequently associated clinical findings. High-dose steroids may be helpful in treating the inflammatory response [52].

Acknowledgment We acknowledge Dr. Benjamin Cohen from Division of Radiology, NYU Langone Health for his contribution to MRI images.

References

1. Calao AM. Pituitary adenomas in childhood. In: Feingold KR, Anawalt B, Boyce A, Chrousos G, Dungan K, Grossman A, et al., editors. Endotext. South Dartmouth: MDText.com, Inc.; 2000.
2. McCrea HJ, George E, Settler A, Schwartz TH, Greenfield JP. Pediatric Suprasellar tumors. J Child Neurol. 2016;31(12): 1367–76.
3. Mehta S, Cohen B, Kohn B. Nonpituitary sellar masses and infiltrative disorders. In: Kohn B, editor. Pituitary disorders of childhood: diagnosis and clinical management. Cham: Springer International Publishing; 2019. p. 173–97.
4. Melmed S, Kleinberg D. Chapter 9 - Pituitary masses and tumors. In: Melmed S, Polonsky KS, Larsen PR, Kronenberg HM, editors. Williams textbook of endocrinology. 13th ed. Philadelphia: Content Repository Only! 2016. p. 232–99.
5. Muller HL. Craniopharyngioma. In: Handbook of clinical neurology, vol. 124; 2014. p. 235–53.
6. Muller HL. Craniopharyngioma. Endocr Rev. 2014;35(3): 513–43.
7. Elliott RE, Wisoff JH. Surgical management of giant pediatric craniopharyngiomas. J Neurosurg Pediatr. 2010;6(5):403–16.
8. Hoffman HJ, De Silva M, Humphreys RP, Drake JM, Smith ML, Blaser SI. Aggressive surgical management of craniopharyngiomas in children. J Neurosurg. 1992;76(1):47–52.
9. Keil MF, Stratakis CA. Pituitary tumors in childhood: update of diagnosis, treatment and molecular genetics. Expert Rev Neurother. 2008;8(4):563–74.
10. Pandey P, Ojha BK, Mahapatra AK. Pediatric pituitary adenoma: a series of 42 patients. J Clin Neurosci. 2005;12(2):124–7.
11. Czyzyk E, Jozwiak S, Roszkowski M, Schwartz RA. Optic pathway gliomas in children with and without neurofibromatosis 1. J Child Neurol. 2003;18(7):471–8.
12. Listernick R, Charrow J, Greenwald M, Mets M. Natural history of optic pathway tumors in children with neurofibromatosis type 1: a longitudinal study. J Pediatr. 1994;125(1):63–6.
13. Listernick R, Darling C, Greenwald M, Strauss L, Charrow J. Optic pathway tumors in children: the effect of neurofibromatosis type 1 on clinical manifestations and natural history. J Pediatr. 1995;127(5):718–22.
14. Kornreich L, Blaser S, Schwarz M, Shuper A, Vishne TH, Cohen IJ, et al. Optic pathway glioma: correlation of imaging findings with the presence of neurofibromatosis. Am J Neuroradiol. 2001;22(10):1963–9.
15. Gan HW, Phipps K, Aquilina K, Gaze MN, Hayward R, Spoudeas HA. Neuroendocrine morbidity after pediatric optic gliomas: a longitudinal analysis of 166 children over 30 years. J Clin Endocrinol Metab. 2015;100(10):3787–99.
16. Hersh JH. Health supervision for children with neurofibromatosis. Pediatrics. 2008;121(3):633–42.
17. King A, Listernick R, Charrow J, Piersall L, Gutmann DH. Optic pathway gliomas in neurofibromatosis type 1: the effect of presenting symptoms on outcome. Am J Med Genet A. 2003;122a(2):95–9.
18. Shapey J, Danesh-Meyer HV, Kaye AH. Diagnosis and management of optic nerve glioma. J Clin Neurosci. 2011;18(12):1585–91.
19. Rasool N, Odel JG, Kazim M. Optic pathway glioma of childhood. Curr Opin Ophthalmol. 2017;28(3):289–95.
20. Lee AG. Neuroophthalmological management of optic pathway gliomas. Neurosurg Focus. 2007;23(5):E1.
21. Maixner W. Hypothalamic hamartomas—clinical, neuropathological and surgical aspects. Childs Nerv Syst. 2006;22(8):867–73.
22. Harrison VS, Oatman O, Kerrigan JF. Hypothalamic hamartoma with epilepsy: review of endocrine comorbidity. Epilepsia. 2017;58(Suppl 2):50–9.
23. Li CD, Luo SQ, Gong J, Ma ZY, Jia G, Zhang YQ, et al. Surgical treatment of hypothalamic hamartoma causing central precocious puberty: long-term follow-up. J Neurosurg Pediatr. 2013;12(2):151–4.
24. Alter CA, Bilaniuk LT. Utility of magnetic resonance imaging in the evaluation of the child with central diabetes insipidus. J Pediatr Endocrinol Metab. 2002;15(Suppl 2):681–7.
25. Raybaud C, Barkovich AJ. Intracranial, orbital, and neck masses of childhood in pediatric neuroimaging. In: Barkovich AJ, Raybaud C, editors. Pediatric neuroimaging. Philadelphia: Lippincott Williams & Wilkins/Wolters Kluwer Health; 2012.
26. Echevarria ME, Fangusaro J, Goldman S. Pediatric central nervous system germ cell tumors: a review. Oncologist. 2008;13(6):690–9.
27. Board PDQPTE. Childhood central nervous system germ cell tumors treatment (PDQ(R)): health professional version. PDQ Cancer information summaries. Bethesda: National Cancer Institute (US); 2002.
28. Grois N, Fahrner B, Arceci RJ, Henter JI, McClain K, Lassmann H, et al. Central nervous system disease in Langerhans cell histiocytosis. J Pediatr. 2010;156(6):873–81, 81.e1.
29. Alston RD, Tatevossian RG, McNally RJ, Kelsey A, Birch JM, Eden TO. Incidence and survival of childhood Langerhans cell histiocytosis in Northwest England from 1954 to 1998. Pediatr Blood Cancer. 2007;48(5):555–60.
30. Guyot-Goubin A, Donadieu J, Barkaoui M, Bellec S, Thomas C, Clavel J. Descriptive epidemiology of childhood Langerhans cell histiocytosis in France, 2000-2004. Pediatr Blood Cancer. 2008;51(1):71–5.
31. Salotti JA, Nanduri V, Pearce MS, Parker L, Lynn R, Windebank KP. Incidence and clinical features of Langerhans cell histiocytosis in the UK and Ireland. Arch Dis Child. 2009;94(5):376–80.
32. Stalemark H, Laurencikas E, Karis J, Gavhed D, Fadeel B, Henter JI. Incidence of Langerhans cell histiocytosis in children: a population-based study. Pediatr Blood Cancer. 2008;51(1):76–81.
33. Grois N, Potschger U, Prosch H, Minkov M, Arico M, Braier J, et al. Risk factors for diabetes insipidus in langerhans cell histiocytosis. Pediatr Blood Cancer. 2006;46(2):228–33.
34. Nanduri VR, Bareille P, Pritchard J, Stanhope R. Growth and endocrine disorders in multisystem Langerhans' cell histiocytosis. Clin Endocrinol. 2000;53(4):509–15.
35. Abla O, Egeler RM, Weitzman S. Langerhans cell histiocytosis: current concepts and treatments. Cancer Treat Rev. 2010;36(4):354–9.

36. Aquilina K, Boop FA. Nonneoplastic enlargement of the pituitary gland in children. J Neurosurg Pediatr. 2011;7(5):510–5.
37. Kocova M, Zdraveska N, Kacarska R, Kochova E. Diagnostic approach in children with unusual symptoms of acquired hypothyroidism. When to look for pituitary hyperplasia. J Pediatr Endocrinol Metab. 2016;29(3):297–303.
38. Satyarthee GD, Sharma BS. Repeated headache as presentation of pituitary apoplexy in the adolescent population: unusual entity with review of literature. J Neurosci Rural Pract. 2017;8(Suppl 1):S143–s6.
39. Chao CC, Lin CJ. Pituitary apoplexy in a teenager--case report. Pediatr Neurol. 2014;50(6):648–51.
40. Spampinato MV, Castillo M. Congenital pathology of the pituitary gland and parasellar region. Top Magn Reson Imaging. 2005;16(4):269–76.
41. Han SJ, Rolston JD, Jahangiri A, Aghi MK. Rathke's cleft cysts: review of natural history and surgical outcomes. J Neuro-Oncol. 2014;117(2):197–203.
42. Evliyaoglu O, Evliyaoglu C, Ayva S. Rathke cleft cyst in seven-year-old girl presenting with central diabetes insipidus and review of literature. J Pediatr Endocrinol Metab. 2010;23(5): 525–9.
43. Al-Holou WN, Yew AY, Boomsaad ZE, Garton HJ, Muraszko KM, Maher CO. Prevalence and natural history of arachnoid cysts in children. J Neurosurg Pediatr. 2010;5(6):578–85.
44. Invergo D, Tomita T. De novo suprasellar arachnoid cyst: case report and review of the literature. Pediatr Neurosurg. 2012;48(3):199–203.
45. Lee JY, Lee YA, Jung HW, Chong S, Phi JH, Kim SK, et al. Long-term endocrine outcome of suprasellar arachnoid cysts. J Neurosurg Pediatr. 2017;19(6):696–702.
46. Caldarelli M, Massimi L, Kondageski C, Di Rocco C. Intracranial midline dermoid and epidermoid cysts in children. J Neurosurg. 2004;100(5 Suppl Pediatrics):473–80.
47. Amelot A, Borha A, Calmon R, Barbet P, Puget S. Child dermoid cyst mimicking a craniopharyngioma: the benefit of MRI T2-weighted diffusion sequence. Childs Nerv Syst. 2017;34:359.
48. Zada G, Lopes MBS, Mukundan S, Laws E. Sellar region epidermoid and dermoid cysts. In: Zada G, Lopes M, Mukundan Jr S, Laws Jr E, editors. Atlas of Sellar and Parasellar lesions. Cham: Springer; 2016.
49. Gellner V, Kurschel S, Scarpatetti M, Mokry M. Lymphocytic hypophysitis in the pediatric population. Childs Nerv Syst. 2008;24(7):785–92.
50. Kalra AA, Riel-Romero RM, Gonzalez-Toledo E. Lymphocytic hypophysitis in children: a novel presentation and literature review. J Child Neurol. 2011;26(1):87–94.
51. Blansfield JA, Beck KE, Tran K, Yang JC, Hughes MS, Kammula US, et al. Cytotoxic T-lymphocyte-associated antigen-4 blockage can induce autoimmune hypophysitis in patients with metastatic melanoma and renal cancer. J Immunother (Hagerstown, Md : 1997). 2005;28(6):593–8.
52. Chodakiewitz Y, Brown S, Boxerman JL, Brody JM, Rogg JM. Ipilimumab treatment associated pituitary hypophysitis: clinical presentation and imaging diagnosis. Clin Neurol Neurosurg. 2014;125:125–30.

Dyslipidemia in the Pediatric Population

57

Bhuvana Sunil and Ambika P. Ashraf

Abbreviations

apoB	Apolipoprotein B
FCH	Familial combined hyperlipidemia
HDL	High-density lipoprotein cholesterol
HeFH	Heterozygous familial hypercholesterolemia
HoFH	Homozygous familial hypercholesterolemia
IDL	Intermediate-density lipoprotein cholesterol
LDL	Low-density lipoprotein cholesterol
Lp (a)	Lipoprotein (a)
TC	Total cholesterol
TG	Triglycerides
VLDL	Very-low-density lipoprotein cholesterol

Introduction

Dyslipidemia, defined as an abnormality in any of the following: increased levels of total cholesterol (TC), low-density lipoprotein cholesterol (LDL), and/or triglycerides (TG), and/or decreased levels of high-density lipoprotein cholesterol (HDL), can be clinically silent but have serious consequences including cardiovascular disease and pancreatitis. Genetic dyslipidemia is very common but often unrecognized. The integration of universal and selective screening guidelines as outlined in Section II outlines the conditions to obtain a lipid profile and preliminary interpretation, while this chapter provides a further in-depth explanation of some of the common dyslipidemias seen in the pediatric population.

B. Sunil · A. P. Ashraf (✉)
Department of Pediatrics, Division of Endocrinology and Diabetes, University of Alabama at Birmingham, Birmingham, AL, USA
e-mail: bsunil@uabmc.edu; aashraf@peds.uab.edu

Epidemiology

Age-appropriate values are illustrated in Table 32.1 (Chap. 32). Analysis of data from the National Health and Nutrition Examination Survey (NHANES) showed that about 20% of children between 6 and 19 years had at least one abnormality in the lipid profile. TC was elevated in ~7.1%, LDL in 6.4%, non-HDL (TC-HDL) in about 6.4%, TG in about 10.2%, and low HDL in about 12.1% [1].

Etiology and Key Pathophysiology

A brief summary of lipid metabolism is presented in this section. Dyslipidemias in children can be monogenic, polygenic, or secondary in nature. The plasma lipoproteins have a lipid (TGs and/or cholesterol esters), and a protein component (apolipoprotein). ApoB-100 is produced in the liver and is the protein component of the VLDL, intermediate-density lipoprotein cholesterol (IDL), and LDL. ApoB-48 is produced in the intestine and serves as the apolipoprotein of chylomicrons. ApoA-1 is the apolipoprotein of HDL.

Fat in the diet is mainly in the form of triacylglycerol, which is broken down by lipases, emulsified by bile salts and phospholipids to form micelles [2], and absorbed through the apical membrane of the enterocytes. Cholesterol is absorbed into the intestinal mucosal cell via the Niemann-Pick C1-like 1 protein (NPC1L1 Transporter protein). Bile acids rich in cholesterol are reabsorbed in the ileum via the Ileal Bile Acid Transport protein (IBAT) [3–6]. Within the small intestinal enterocytes, the microsomal TG transfer protein (MTP) conjugates apoB-48 with the cholesterol ester, phospholipids, and TG-rich lipoproteins (TRLs) to form a mature chylomicron [7, 8]. The chylomicrons enter the systemic venous circulation through the thoracic duct (lymphatic system) where they are metabolized by lipoprotein lipase (LPL) to release free fatty acids (FFA) to tissues [9]. LPL, an enzyme present on the vascular endothelium, most abundantly in the muscle and adipose tissue, hydrolyzes the TG content of the chylo-

T. Stanley, M. Misra (eds.), *Endocrine Conditions in Pediatrics*, https://doi.org/10.1007/978-3-030-52215-5_57

microns [10]. When about 80% of the TG is hydrolyzed from the chylomicron, the chylomicron remnants enter the hepatocytes [11].

VLDL is synthesized in the liver from chylomicron remnants, cholesterol, and FFA along with the apoB-100. Increased carbohydrate/fat intake and insulin resistance states result in increased FFA production and thus, increased levels of VLDL. VLDL is subsequently hydrolyzed by LPL to release FFA. IDL is formed when about ~80% of the TG within the VLDL is hydrolyzed [12]. Half of the IDL can then be taken up by LDL receptor (LDL-R), and the rest is converted to LDL through further hydrolysis by lipases. LDL particles bind to the LDL-R with the association of the LDL-R adaptor protein and are internalized into the cell via endocytosis. Once inside, this complex is acidified, the LDL-R is recycled for further reuptake of LDL, or the entire receptor LDL complex is taken up by the proprotein convertase subtilisin/kexin type 9 (PCSK9) and degraded [13]. The cholesterol is primarily synthesized in the hepatocytes under the regulation of the enzyme HMG CoA reductase and gets incorporated into VLDL, IDL, LDL, and HDL [14–16]. Cholesteryl ester transfer protein (CETP) assists in the exchange of cholesteryl ester from HDL and LDL for TG derived from VLDL, which leads to cholesterol-enriched VLDL, and TG-enriched LDL and HDL. Subsequent hydrolysis by the lipases results in lipid-depleted, atherogenic, small dense LDL particles. Similarly, hydrolysis by lipases results in dissociation of apo A-I, which leads to low HDL levels.

Preβ-HDL particles are synthesized in the liver and intestine, which, with the action of ATP-binding cassette transporter-A1 (ABCA1) transporter, are able to mediate the efflux of intracellular free cholesterol and phospholipids back from circulation and atheroma [17]. The apo-A1 with lipid forms nascent HDL particles, which are later transformed into mature HDL by esterification of free cholesterol into cholesterol ester by lecithin cholesterol acyl transferase (LCAT) [18]. As the HDL increases in size, the enzyme cholesteryl ester transfer protein (CETP) helps to exchange the esterified cholesterol within HDL for TG and thereby promotes reverse cholesterol transport from tissues back to the liver [18].

Table 57.1 elaborates on the main genetic dyslipidemias, the key gene defect, and the affected lipid and lipoprotein lev-

Table 57.1 Genetic dyslipidemias

Name	Genetic defect	Incidence	Lipid abnormality	Lipoprotein abnormality
Autosomal dominant disorders with high LDL				
Familial homozygous hypercholesterolemia	*LDL-R* mutation Gain of function *PCSK9* Familial defective *apo B-100*	1:1000000	TC ↑↑↑	LDL ↑↑↑ HDL normal or ↓
Familial heterozygous hypercholesterolemia	*Same as above* (gene dosing effect)	1:300–400	TC ↑	LDL ↑
Familial combined hyperlipidemia	Unknown	1:100–200	TC ↑ or TG ↑ or both ↑	Variable ↑ in LDL, VLDL, IDL, HDL↓
Autosomal recessive disorders with high LDL				
Lysosomal acid lipase deficiency	*LIPA* gene defect	1: 40,000 to 300,000	TC ↑	LDL ↑, VLDL↑, HDL ↓
Autosomal recessive hypercholesterolemia	*LDL-R* *Adaptor protein*	<1:1000000	TC ↑	LDL ↑
Cholesterol 7α-Hydroxylase deficiency	*CYP7A1* gene	<1: 1000000	TC ↑ or TG ↑	LDL ↑
Sitosterolemia	*ABCG5* *ABCG8*	<1:1000000	TC ↑	LDL ↑ Campesterol ↑ and sitosterol ↑
Dysbetalipoproteinemia	*apoE*	1:5000	TC ↑ and TG ↑	B-VLDL ↑
Autosomal dominant disorders with high TG				
Familial hypertriglyceridemia	Unknown	1: 500	TG ↑	VLDL ↑
Autosomal recessive disorders with elevated TG				
Familial chylomicronemia	*LPL deficiency* *apoC-II deficiency* *apoA5 and GPIHBP1 loss-of-function*	1:1000000	TC ↑ and TG ↑	VLDL normal LDL ↓ and HDL ↓
Autosomal recessive disorders with low HDL				
Tangier disease	*ABCA1*	<1:1000000	TC normal or ↑	HDL↓
Lecithin cholesterol acyl transferase deficiency	*LCAT* (16q22.1)	<1:1000000	TC normal or ↑	HDL↓

Abbreviations: *TC* total cholesterol, *LDL* low-density lipoprotein cholesterol, *HDL* high-density lipoprotein cholesterol, *TG* triglyceride, *AD* autosomal dominant, *AR* autosomal recessive, *LDL-R* LDL receptor, *PCSK9* proprotein convertase subtilisin/kexin type 9, *apoB* apolipoprotein, *ABCG* ATP-binding cassette sub-family G member, *LIPA* lysosomal acid lipase type A, *LPL* lipoprotein lipase, *GPIHBP1* glycosylphosphatidylinositol anchored high-density lipoprotein binding protein 1, *LCAT* lecithin cholesterol acyl transferase

Table 57.2 Causes of secondary dyslipidemia

Cause	Additional supportive labs	Proposed mechanisms	Pattern
Diabetes mellitus	Hemoglobin A1C	Insulinogenic or insulin resistance Lipid abnormalities are related to mostly severity of insulin resistance [68]	LDL↑ HDL↓ TG↑
Hypothyroidism	Free T4, TSH	Decreased LDL-R activity, decreased catabolism of LDL and IDL, decrease in LPL activity, decrease in HDL catabolism, decreased activity of the CETP, insulin resistance [69]	TC↑ LDL↑ TG↑ HDL↑
Cushing's syndrome	24 hour urinary free cortisol/midnight salivary cortisol	Direct and indirect cortisol action on lipolysis, free fatty acid production and turnover, VLDL synthesis and fatty accumulation in the liver, steroid-induced insulin resistance [70]	TC↑ TG↑ variable HDL levels
Nephrotic syndrome	Urinalysis, serum and urine protein measurements, serum albumin levels	Impaired IDL and ↑LDL clearance, decreased lipoprotein lipase activity, decreased hepatic lipase activity, increased levels of the enzyme PCSK9 leading to LDL receptor degradation [71]	TC↑ VLDL↑ IDL↑ TG↑ HDL↑
Chronic kidney disease	Glomerular filtration rate, urinalysis, renal function	Impaired TG lipolysis, increased apolipoprotein C-III (an inhibitor of lipoprotein lipase), reduced insulin sensitivity, impaired HDL maturation, impaired hepatic non-HDL clearance [72, 73]	TC↑ TG↑ HDL↓
Cholestatic liver disease, Primary biliary cirrhosis, Acute or chronic hepatitis	Liver function panel, Gamma glutamyl transpeptidase levels	Steatosis, increased free fatty acid delivery to the liver, increased de-novo lipogenesis, decreased oxidation of lipids, decreased TG export, reduced functional LDL-R, increased abnormal Lipoprotein-X, net effect of virus-host interaction - impaired bile acid uptake, increased bile acid synthesis and bile acid conversion to cholesterol [74–76]	Depending on the stage, varies from TG↑ in stage 1 to HDL↓ in stage 4
Primary metabolic disorders	Genetics +/– metabolic testing	Varying mechanisms: Gaucher's disease – abnormal cellular glycolipids Niemann-Pick disease – abnormal sphingomyelin and cholesterol storage Tay-Sachs disease – abnormal lysosomal storage Glycogen storage disorders [77]	Varied
Post-transplantation	History and medication review	Weight gain, higher risk of diabetes in selective patients +/– use of immunosuppressant medications Corticosteroid use + hyperinsulinsim [78]	Varied
Medications	Thorough history and medication review	*Mechanism varies by drug:* *LDL increasing medications:* Corticosteroids, progestin, danazol, anabolic steroids Cardiometabolic medications: thiazides, amiodarone Others: isotretinoin, sodium glucose co – transporter 2 inhibitors, amiodarone *Medications increasing TG levels:* Hormones: some estrogens and oral contraceptives Cardiometabolic medications: nonselective beta blockers, thiazides Chemo-/immunotherapeutic agents: L-asparaginase, cyclophosphamide, cyclosporine, interferons Some first- and second-generation antipsychotics Drugs: alcohol [79]	Varied

Abbreviations: TC total cholesterol, *LDL* low-density lipoprotein cholesterol, *HDL* high-density lipoprotein cholesterol, *TG* triglyceride, *LDL-R* low-density lipoprotein cholesterol receptor, *IDL* intermediate-density lipoprotein cholesterol, *PCSK9* proprotein convertase subtilisin/kexin type 9, *VLDL* very low-density lipoprotein cholesterol

els. Table 57.2 illustrates common secondary dyslipidemias with the mechanisms contributory to altered lipid levels.

Monogenic dyslipidemias are single gene disorders of production, transport, storage, or clearance of lipoproteins. Polygenic/idiopathic dyslipidemias do not yet have an identified single genetic defect. Secondary dyslipidemias are due to a distinct underlying disease (e.g., hypothyroidism, nephrotic syndrome). Defects involving any of the above steps of production, transport, storage, or clearance of lipoproteins can result in dyslipidemia.

Diagnostic Considerations

As mentioned in Section II, a serum lipid profile is the first step in making a diagnosis of dyslipidemia. A non-fasting lipid profile obtained in the office at any time of the day has reliable screening value and practical convenience. Figure 32.1 in Section II (Chap. 32) illustrates the current screening and approach recommendations adapted from the 2011 Expert Panel on Integrated Guidelines for Cardiovascular Health and Risk Reduction in Children and Adolescents.

Table 32.1 in Section II (Chap. 32) outlines lipid values as expected by age. A workup for secondary dyslipidemia should be undertaken based on clinical presentation. Some considerations include liver function testing, serum albumin, blood glucose level or hemoglobin A1C (HbA1C), renal function tests, serum thyroid-stimulating hormone, and a pregnancy screen. It is useful to obtain serum creatinine kinase (CK) levels at baseline if considering pharmaceutical treatment.

Initial Management

Children with LDL ≥ 250 mg/dL are best referred to a lipid specialist. The same is true of fasting TG level of ≥500 mg/dL, due to the high risk of complications including pancreatitis.

Diet and Lifestyle Modifications

Medical providers are encouraged to familiarize themselves with the Expert panel on integrated guidelines for cardiovascular health and risk reduction in children and adolescents for age-stratified in-depth nutrition recommendations [19]. In summary, fat intake should not be restricted in infants younger than 12 months of age without medical need and supervision. Breastfed infants tend to have sustained cardiovascular benefits. Reduced intake of sugar-sweetened beverages has a positive effect on preventing obesity and the ensuing dyslipidemia. Six months of diet and lifestyle modifications can be instituted either consecutively with pharmacotherapy when warranted or as first-line therapy. The first dietary modification is the Cardiovascular Health Integrated Lifestyle Diet (CHILD)-1 diet, that is, total fat (25–30% of total daily calories), saturated fat (8–10% of daily kcal/estimated energy requirements), avoiding trans-fat, <300 mg/day from cholesterol, dietary fiber (14 g/1000 kcal), fat-free unflavored milk, limiting sodium intake, and sweetened juice (no added sugar) <120 mL/day. Polyunsaturated fatty acid intake of up to 10% of daily calories and monounsaturated fatty acid intake of 10–15% of daily caloric intake are recommended [19].

If the CHILD-1 modifications do not show the desired effects within 3 months of initiation, escalation to the CHILD-2 diet can be made. The CHILD-2 diet consists of 25–30% of total calories from fat, <7% from saturated fat, <10% from monounsaturated fat, and avoiding trans-fat. The CHILD-2-LDL also recommends plant sterol and stanol esters up to 2 g/day, and water-soluble fiber psyllium, dose of 6 g/day (2–12 years) or 12 g/day (>12 years).

For hypertriglyceridemia, the CHILD-2-TG recommends decreasing sugar and sugar-sweetened beverages, replacing simple with complex carbohydrates, and increasing dietary fish to increase omega-3 fatty acid intake [19].

The NCEP also recommends at least 1 hour of moderate-to-vigorous physical activity every day of the week, with vigorous, intense physical activity on at least 3 of these days in agreement with the 2008 Physical Activity Guidelines for Americans [19]. It is important to remember that dietary changes and exercise can only lower LDL levels by about 10–15% for most primary and some secondary dyslipidemias [20]. Plant sterol ester supplementation [21] and water-soluble fiber [22] and psyllium [23] addition can each further provide 5–10% reduction in LDL levels. In high-risk children with very elevated levels, even the maximum effect of diet and exercise may only minimally reduce the LDL, underlining the importance of concomitant pharmacotherapy.

Pharmacological Management

Adapted from the Expert panel on integrated guidelines for cardiovascular health and risk reduction in children and adolescents, Fig. 57.1 is a helpful algorithm for deciding upon the first-line pharmaceutical therapy for elevated LDL and/or TG levels.

Statins Statins are competitive inhibitors of the enzyme 3-hydroxy-3-methylglutaryl–coenzyme A (HMG-CoA) reductase, a key enzyme in cholesterol biosynthesis in the liver. They also have additional effects in reducing apoB and VLDL synthesis, as well as pleiotropic and immunomodulatory effects [24–26]. They are the preferred first-line agents for dyslipidemia with elevated LDL levels. The indications for initiation and follow-up of statin therapy are outlined in Fig. 57.1. In short, indications for statins in children include the following:

In children <10 years of age:

- Homozygous familial hypercholesterolemia (HoFH) with LDL typically above 400 mg/dL – at detection
- Cardiovascular disease within the first two decades of life/post-cardiac transplantation
- LDL ≥ 190 mg/dL + positive family history, OR 1 high risk factor/condition, OR 2 moderate risk factors/conditions (please see Chap. 32 for definition of high and moderate risk factors and conditions)

In children ≥10 years:

- LDL ≥ 190 mg/dL
- LDL ≥ 160 mg/dL + positive family history, OR 1 high risk factor/condition, OR 2 moderate risk factors/conditions

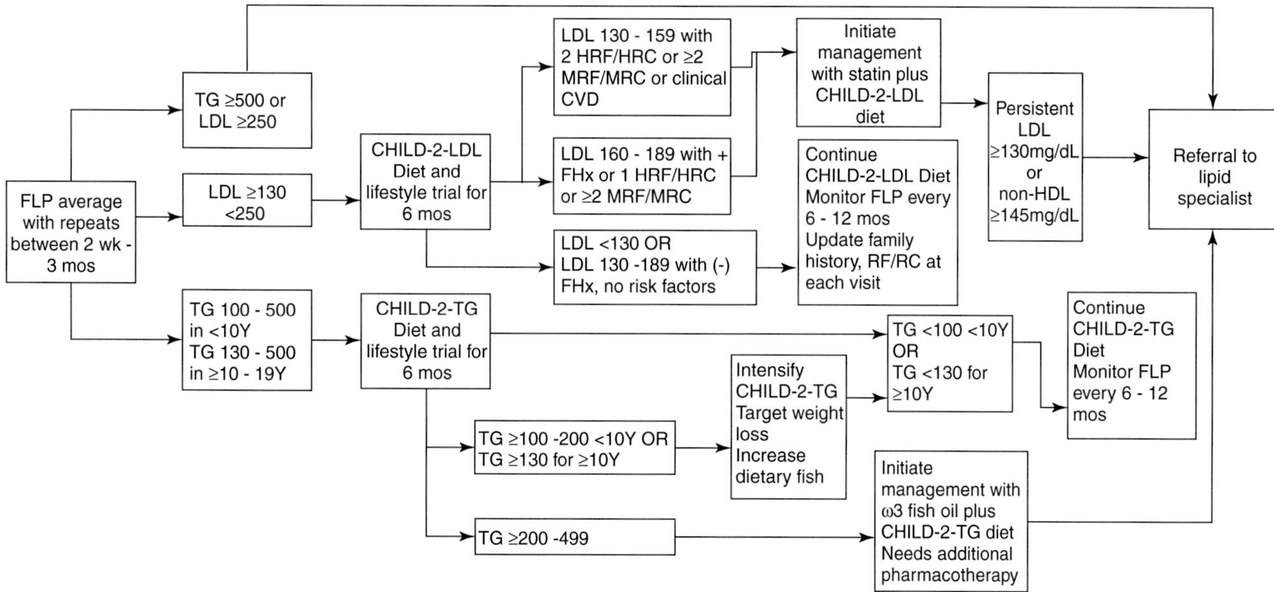

Fig. 57.1 Management algorithm for pediatric dyslipidemia
All values on a fasting lipid panel in mg/dL. To convert to SI units, divide total cholesterol, LDL, HDL, and non-HDL by 38.6; for TG, divide by 88.6.

Positive family history: Parent, grantparent, aunt, uncle, sibling with any of these before the age 55 Y in a male or 65 Y in a female: myocardial infarction, stroke, angina, coronary artery bypass, stent, angioplasty, sudden cardiac death, parent with total cholesterol >240 mg/dL

High-risk condition: Type 1 or 2 diabetes, chronic renal disease/end-stage renal disease/post-renal transplant, post-orthotopic heart transplant, Kawasaki disease with current aneurysms

High risk factor: Hypertension requiring drug therapy (BP ≥ 99th percentile + 5 mmHg), current smoking, BMI ≥ 97th percentile

Moderate risk condition: Kawasaki disease with regressed coronary aneurysms, systemic lupus erythematosus, juvenile rheumatoid arthritis, Human immunodeficiency virus (HIV) infection, nephrotic syndrome

Moderate risk factor: Hypertension not requiring drug therapy, BMI ≥ 95th percentile but <97th percentile, HDL < 40 mg/dL

Abbreviations: LDL low-density lipoprotein cholesterol, HDL high-density lipoprotein cholesterol, FLP fasting lipid panel, TG triglyceride, CHILD-2 Cardiovascular Health Integrated Lifestyle Diet-2, FHx family history, HRF high risk factor, MRF moderate risk factor, HRC high risk condition, MRC moderate risk condition

Adapted from: Integrated Guidelines for Cardiovascular Health and Risk Reduction in Children and Adolescents. Reports of the Expert Panel 2011

- LDL ≥ 130 mg/dL + 2 high risk factors/conditions, OR 1 high risk factor/condition and 2 moderate risk factors/conditions, OR clinical CVD

In addition, when the fasting TG concentration is less than 500 mg/dL, if the non-HDL is above 145 mg/dl, statin treatment is recommended.

The expected effects of statin therapy on TC and LDL levels are dependent on their potency and dosing [27, 28]. Current FDA-approved statins for treatment in children are atorvastatin, simvastatin, rosuvastatin, pravastatin, lovastatin, and fluvastatin. Pravastatin has FDA approval for children age ≥8 years with HeFH. Lovastatin, simvastatin, fluvastatin, atorvastatin, and rosuvastatin have been approved for children ≥10 years with HeFH. Starting doses depend upon the chosen product. Most statins also have a mild effect on increasing HDL by 2–5% and on decreasing TG levels by up to 40%. The general principle behind statin therapy is to use the lowest effective dose and attempt to administer at bedtime, as cholesterol is maximally synthesized during nighttime [19]. Currently, the maximum daily dose studied in pediatrics is 40 mg for lovastatin, pravastatin, and simvastatin; 20 mg for atorvastatin and rosuvastatin; and 80 mg for fluvastatin.

It is important to recognize that most of the safety, efficacy, and tolerability data for statins in pediatrics are derived from children with familial hypercholesterolemia [29–34]. Long-term safety data on statin use in children are generally lacking. The most important adverse effects include myopathy/myolysis, type 2 diabetes mellitus, and hepatic enzyme elevation [35]. Due to a concern for teratogenicity, use of birth control should be concomitantly encouraged in adolescent girls who are on statin therapy, with the understanding that the use of oral contraception itself may elevate lipid levels and need statin dose adjustment [36].

Goals of Management and Monitoring

The goal of statin therapy is to decrease LDL level to <130 mg/dL in moderate risk and <100 mg/dL in high-risk children [19]. Once on stable therapy, lipid levels can be monitored every 6 months. Routine measurements of liver enzymes, HbA1C, or CK levels are to be considered on a case-by-case basis based on clinical presentation or with combination drug therapy.

Special Considerations

As the combination of diabetes and dyslipidemia can be increasingly atherogenic, intensive lipid management is suggested for these patients. After optimizing medical nutrition therapy and diabetes management, the American Diabetes Association (ADA) recommends starting treatment with a statin for LDL > 160 mg/dL or LDL > 130 mg/dL with one or more cardiovascular risk factors (e.g., hypertension, positive family history of premature CVD, smoking status) after age 10, in children with type 1 diabetes. In children and adolescents with type 2 diabetes, statin therapy is indicated if LDL is >130 mg/dl after 6 months of dietary intervention. Treatment goal in both type 1 and type 2 diabetes is achieving LDL concentration <100 mg/dL [37]. In nephrotic syndrome, and conditions of increased insulin resistance including metabolic syndrome and polycystic ovary syndrome, LDL ≥ 160 mg/dL may be a threshold for initiating statin treatment in addition to adequate mediation therapy for the underlying condition, lifestyle, and diet therapy.

Fibric Acid Derivatives These are peroxisome proliferator-activated receptor alpha (PPAR-α) agonists that increase lipoprotein lipase activity and hydrolysis of TGs. They can also upregulate apoA-1 production and increase HDL levels. Although gemfibrozil and fenofibrate have been used in the management of hypertriglyceridemia, there are limited data on their safety in children [56, 57]. Children with average fasting levels of TG ≥ 500 mg/dL or any single measurement ≥1000 mg/ dL should be treated in consultation with a lipid specialist; the CHILD 2-TG diet should be started and use of fibrate should be considered [19]. Adverse effects include dyspepsia, diarrhea, increase in transaminases, and cholelithiasis [58]. They should be used cautiously in children with renal dysfunction and gall bladder disease. When concomitantly used with statins, they have been associated with a higher risk of rhabdomyolysis in adults [59]. When used, they are dosed orally at up to 1200 mg daily gemfibrozil and 40–200 mg daily fenofibrate, but safety and maximum tolerability data in children are lacking.

Second-Line Therapies

Ezetimibe Ezetimibe helps reduce the absorption of dietary cholesterol and plant sterols [38]. Pediatric data on its use comes from studies in children with FH, FCH, polygenic hypercholesterolemia, and sitosterolemia [39–45]. It is FDA approved in boys and post-menarchal girls 10–17 years of age with heterozygous familial hypercholesterolemia (HeFH) in combination with dietary interventions and statins. Ezetimibe can be considered monotherapy for patients intolerant to statins. It has also been used as monotherapy in primary hypercholesterolemia, sitosterolemia, and HoFH; but for these indications, it has only been approved in adults at the time of this writing. Recommended dosing is 10 mg oral dosing once daily, preferably administered ≥2 hours before or ≥4 hours after bile acid sequestrants.

Bile Acid Sequestrants These act by increasing cholesterol excretion and catabolism and enhancing hepatic LDL-R activity, thus increasing LDL clearance. Although they are not systemically absorbed and are considered safe, the compliance is poor due to a high incidence of side effects including bloating, diarrhea, fat-soluble vitamin deficiencies, and elevation in TG levels [46]. When used, concomitant therapy with vitamin supplementation should be considered. Of these, colesevelam has been approved for use in children >10 years of age. Cholestyramine and colestipol are not approved for pediatric use. The recommended dosing of colesevelam is 3.75 g oral dosing once daily or in divided doses twice daily. Due to the large tablet size, oral packets and chewable bars of colesevelam are available for use in children.

PCSK9 Inhibitors Evolucumab and alirocumab are monoclonal antibodies against PCSK9 that help reduce LDL-R degradation and improve uptake of LDL into the hepatocytes from systemic circulation. These are potent and can reduce LDL levels by ~50–60% [47]. Limited studies are available testing PCSK9 inhibitors in pediatrics [48–50]. Dosing derived from these studies including the TESLA part B [48] and HAUSER-RCT [50] are subcutaneous injections of 140 mg every 2 weeks or 420 mg once monthly of evolucumab. They are used off label, concomitantly with statins for HoFH, but do not have FDA approval yet in pediatrics. These are only available as injectable preparations.

Mipomersan This is an antisense oligonucleotide that inhibits apoB synthesis, lowering VLDL and LDL levels. It is not approved for pediatric use and is only available as an injectable medication [51–53]. It has limited data and no FDA approval for use in children. In adults, it is dosed as 200 mg once weekly subcutaneous injection, and 160 mg once weekly dosing has been suggested for bodyweight <50 kg [51]. It carries a boxed warning for hepatotoxicity, and other adverse effects include hypersensitivity, flu-like symptoms, nausea, and headaches.

Lomitapide This is an oral agent that causes selective microsomal TG transfer protein inhibition. It reduces lipoprotein assembly and secretion, VLDL synthesis, and lowers plasma cholesterol levels by over 50%. It has been used in adults with HoFH [54]. Its adverse effects include nausea, bloating, and diarrhea, as well as a risk of hepatotoxicity. Limited pediatric dosing information is available: a pediatric case series in children used escalating doses starting at 2.5 mg and 5 mg oral daily dosing [55]. This medication is not approved for pediatric use yet.

Niacin/Nicotinic Acid Niacin works by inhibition of hormone-sensitive lipase in adipose tissue, which reduces the breakdown of TGs to free fatty acids, thus decreasing the flux of free fatty acids to the liver. It can also directly inhibit hepatocyte diacylglycerol acyltransferase-2, a key enzyme for TG synthesis [60]. It can inhibit HDL degradation and has been shown to increase HDL levels. In the only pediatric study by Coletti et al., in which 21 children aged 4–14 years were treated with oral niacin 500–2250 mg daily, 76% had adverse events and 38% discontinued the medication [61]. Due to its adverse risk profile and low tolerability, niacin is rarely used in pediatrics.

Fish Oils The TG-lowering effect of fish oil is dependent on ω-3 fatty acid content including eicosapentanoic acid (EPA) and docosahexanoic acid (DHA). The proposed mechanism of action is interference of FFA incorporation into TGs, thus inhibiting synthesis. Fish oil can be administered either as a combination therapy with fibrates or as a monotherapy if fibrates are not tolerated to reduce pancreatitis risk in hypertriglyceridemia with fasting TG levels ≥500 mg/dL. For lower but elevated TG levels <500 mg/dL, therapies targeting non-HDL cholesterol are preferred. In pediatrics, two small studies with varying doses of fish oil did not find significant differences in changes in TG levels in adolescents with hypertriglyceridemia [62, 63]. In adults, four prescription strength capsules daily (465 mg/375 mg of EPA/DHA per capsule) have been found to lower TG levels by 20–50% [64–67]. It is important to recognize that fish oils that are available over the counter have lower EPA and DHA content (about 180 mg/120 mg of EPA/DHA per capsule). Therefore, a dose equivalency of up to 10–11 capsules daily of over-the-counter fish oil preparation is needed for comparable prescription strength dosing of high-dose fish oil 2 g twice a day. Prescription strength fish oil is not FDA recommended for pediatric use.

Other Treatments In children with HoFH, to reduce LDL levels, scheduled apheresis is recommended especially if unresponsive to well-monitored combination therapy. Liver transplantation has also been successful in children with HoFH.

Conclusion

Early recognition and management of pediatric dyslipidemia is a vital step in reducing atherosclerotic risk and cardiovascular disease burden in adulthood, especially in recognized genetic dyslipidemias. All children with dyslipidemia will benefit from diet and lifestyle modifications. Pharmacotherapeutic management is based on age, severity, family history of hypercholesterolemia or premature atherosclerotic disease, and the concomitant presence of risk factors and conditions. Statins are the preferred first-line agents for the treatment of disorders with elevated LDL. Several second-line agents are preferably managed in consultation with a pediatric lipid specialist. The mainstay of TG management remains strict dietary changes and weight loss, with modest effect of medications on TG levels. Long-term studies are needed to address long-term effects of current principles of management.

References

1. Perak AM, Ning H, Kit BK, de Ferranti SD, Van Horn LV, Wilkins JT, et al. Trends in levels of lipids and Apolipoprotein B in US youths aged 6 to 19 years, 1999–2016. JAMA. 2019;321(19):1895–905.
2. Cohn JS, Kamili A, Wat E, Chung RWS, Tandy S. Dietary phospholipids and intestinal cholesterol absorption. Nutrients. 2010;2(2):116–27.
3. Park YM. CD36, a scavenger receptor implicated in atherosclerosis. Exp Mol Med. 2014;46(6):e99–e.
4. Valacchi G, Sticozzi C, Lim Y, Pecorelli A. Scavenger receptor class B type I: a multifunctional receptor. Ann N Y Acad Sci. 2011;1229(1):E1–7.
5. Hubacek JA, Berge KE, Cohen JC, Hobbs HH. Mutations in ATP-cassette binding proteins G5 (ABCG5) and G8 (ABCG8) causing sitosterolemia. Hum Mutat. 2001;18(4):359–60.
6. Graf GA, Yu L, Li W-P, Gerard R, Tuma PL, Cohen JC, et al. ABCG5 and ABCG8 are obligate heterodimers for protein trafficking and biliary cholesterol excretion. J Biol Chem. 2003;278(48):48275–82.
7. Narcisi TM, Shoulders CC, Chester SA, Read J, Brett DJ, Harrison GB, et al. Mutations of the microsomal triglyceride-transfer–protein gene in abetalipoproteinemia. Am J Hum Genet. 1995;57(6):1298.
8. Packard C, Demant T, Stewart J, Bedford D, Caslake M, Schwertfeger G, et al. Apolipoprotein B metabolism and the distribution of VLDL and LDL subfractions. J Lipid Res. 2000;41(2):305–17.
9. Lewis GF, Rader DJ. New insights into the regulation of HDL metabolism and reverse cholesterol transport. Circ Res. 2005;96(12):1221–32.
10. Eckel RH. Lipoprotein lipase. N Engl J Med. 1989;320(16):1060–8.
11. Cooper AD. Hepatic uptake of chylomicron remnants. J Lipid Res. 1997;38(11):2173–92.
12. Ginsberg HN, Zhang Y-L, Hernandez-Ono A. Regulation of plasma triglycerides in insulin resistance and diabetes. Arch Med Res. 2005;36(3):232–40.
13. McKenney JM. Understanding PCSK9 and anti-PCSK9 therapies. J Clin Lipidol. 2015;9(2):170–86.
14. Watanabe M, Houten SM, Wang L, Moschetta A, Mangelsdorf DJ, Heyman RA, et al. Bile acids lower triglyceride levels via a pathway involving FXR, SHP, and SREBP-1c. J Clin Invest. 2004;113(10):1408–18.

15. Bengoechea-Alonso MT, Ericsson J. SREBP in signal transduction: cholesterol metabolism and beyond. Curr Opin Cell Biol. 2007;19(2):215–22.
16. Krimbou L, Marcil M, Genest J. New insights into the biogenesis of human high-density lipoproteins. Curr Opin Lipidol. 2006;17(3):258–67.
17. Rothblat GH, Phillips MC. High-density lipoprotein heterogeneity and function in reverse cholesterol transport. Curr Opin Lipidol. 2010;21(3):229.
18. Kuivenhoven J, Pritchard H, Hill J, Frohlich J, Assmann G, Kastelein J. The molecular pathology of lecithin: cholesterol acyltransferase (LCAT) deficiency syndromes. J Lipid Res. 1997;38(2):191–205.
19. Expert panel on integrated guidelines for cardiovascular health and risk reduction in children and adolescents: summary report. Pediatrics. 2011;128(Suppl 5):S213.
20. Yu-Poth S, Zhao G, Etherton T, Naglak M, Jonnalagadda S, Kris-Etherton PM. Effects of the National Cholesterol Education Program's step I and step II dietary intervention programs on cardiovascular disease risk factors: a meta-analysis. Am J Clin Nutr. 1999;69(4):632–46.
21. Kwiterovich PO Jr. The role of fiber in the treatment of hypercholesterolemia in children and adolescents. Pediatrics. 1995;96(5 Pt 2):1005–9.
22. Williams CL, Bollella M, Spark A, Puder D. Soluble fiber enhances the hypocholesterolemic effect of the step I diet in childhood. J Am Coll Nutr. 1995;14(3):251–7.
23. Dennison BA, Levine DM. Randomized, double-blind, placebo-controlled, two-period crossover clinical trial of psyllium fiber in children with hypercholesterolemia. J Pediatr. 1993;123(1):24–9.
24. Davignon J, Mabile L, editors. Mechanisms of action of statins and their pleiotropic effects. Annales d'endocrinologie; 2001.
25. Jasiñska M, Owczarek J, Orszulak-Michalak D. Statins: a new insight into their mechanisms of action and consequent pleiotropic effects. Pharmacol Rep. 2007;59(5):483.
26. Stancu C, Sima A. Statins: mechanism of action and effects. J Cell Mol Med. 2001;5(4):378–87.
27. Wagner J, Abdel-Rahman SM. Pediatric statin administration: navigating a frontier with limited data. J Pediatr Pharmacol Ther. 2016;21(5):380–403.
28. Eiland LS, Luttrell PK. Use of statins for dyslipidemia in the pediatric population. J Pediatr Pharmacol Ther. 2010;15(3):160–72.
29. McCrindle BW, Ose L, Marais AD. Efficacy and safety of atorvastatin in children and adolescents with familial hypercholesterolemia or severe hyperlipidemia: a multicenter, randomized, placebo-controlled trial. J Pediatr. 2003;143(1):74–80.
30. van der Graaf A, Nierman MC, Firth JC, Wolmarans KH, Marais AD, de Groot E. Efficacy and safety of fluvastatin in children and adolescents with heterozygous familial hypercholesterolaemia. Acta Paediatr. 2006;95(11):1461–6.
31. Stein EA, Illingworth DR, Kwiterovich PO Jr, Liacouras CA, Siimes MA, Jacobson MS, et al. Efficacy and safety of lovastatin in adolescent males with heterozygous familial hypercholesterolemia: a randomized controlled trial. JAMA. 1999;281(2):137–44.
32. Knipscheer HC, Boelen CC, Kastelein JJ, van Diermen DE, Groenemeijer BE, van den Ende A, et al. Short-term efficacy and safety of pravastatin in 72 children with familial hypercholesterolemia. Pediatr Res. 1996;39(5):867–71.
33. Lambert M, Lupien PJ, Gagne C, Levy E, Blaichman S, Langlois S, et al. Treatment of familial hypercholesterolemia in children and adolescents: effect of lovastatin. Canadian Lovastatin in Children Study Group. Pediatrics. 1996;97(5):619–28.
34. Braamskamp MJ, Kusters DM, Avis HJ, Smets EM, Wijburg FA, Kastelein JJ, et al. Long-term statin treatment in children with familial hypercholesterolemia: more insight into tolerability and adherence. Paediatr Drugs. 2015;17(2):159–66.
35. Vuorio A, Kuoppala J, Kovanen PT, Humphries SE, Tonstad S, Wiegman A, et al. Statins for children with familial hypercholesterolemia. Cochrane Database Syst Rev. 2017;7:Cd006401.
36. Knopp RH, LaRosa JC, Burkman RT Jr. Contraception and dyslipidemia. Am J Obstet Gynecol. 1993;168(6 Pt 2):1994–2005.
37. Association AD. 12. Children and adolescents: standards of medical care in diabetes—2018. Diabetes Care. 2018;41(Supplement 1):S126–S36.
38. Phan BAP, Dayspring TD, Toth PP. Ezetimibe therapy: mechanism of action and clinical update. Vasc Health Risk Manag. 2012;8:415–27.
39. Yeste D, Chacón P, Clemente M, Albisu MA, Gussinyé M, Carrascosa A. Ezetimibe as monotherapy in the treatment of hypercholesterolemia in children and adolescents. J Pediatr Endocrinol Metab. 2009;22(6):487–92.
40. Clauss S, Wai KM, Kavey RE, Kuehl K. Ezetimibe treatment of pediatric patients with hypercholesterolemia. J Pediatr. 2009;154(6):869–72.
41. Araujo MB, Pacce MS. A 10-year experience using combined lipid-lowering pharmacotherapy in children and adolescents. J Pediatr Endocrinol Metab. 2016;29(11):1285–91.
42. Othman RA, Myrie SB, Mymin D, Merkens LS, Roullet JB, Steiner RD, et al. Ezetimibe reduces plant sterol accumulation and favorably increases platelet count in sitosterolemia. J Pediatr. 2015;166(1):125–31.
43. Othman RA, Myrie SB, Mymin D, Roullet JB, DeBarber AE, Steiner RD, et al. Thyroid hormone status in Sitosterolemia is modified by Ezetimibe. J Pediatr. 2017;188:198–204.e1.
44. van der Graaf A, Cuffie-Jackson C, Vissers MN, Trip MD, Gagne C, Shi G, et al. Efficacy and safety of coadministration of ezetimibe and simvastatin in adolescents with heterozygous familial hypercholesterolemia. J Am Coll Cardiol. 2008;52(17):1421–9.
45. Kusters DM, Caceres M, Coll M, Cuffie C, Gagne C, Jacobson MS, et al. Efficacy and safety of ezetimibe monotherapy in children with heterozygous familial or nonfamilial hypercholesterolemia. J Pediatr. 2015;166(6):1377–84.e1-3.
46. Davidson MH. A systematic review of bile acid sequestrant therapy in children with familial hypercholesterolemia. J Clin Lipidol. 2011;5(2):76–81.
47. Dadu RT, Ballantyne CM. Lipid lowering with PCSK9 inhibitors. Nat Rev Cardiol. 2014;11(10):563.
48. Raal FJ, Honarpour N, Blom DJ, Hovingh GK, Xu F, Scott R, et al. Inhibition of PCSK9 with evolocumab in homozygous familial hypercholesterolaemia (TESLA part B): a randomised, double-blind, placebo-controlled trial. Lancet. 2015;385(9965):341–50.
49. Raal FJ, Hovingh GK, Blom D, Santos RD, Harada-Shiba M, Bruckert E, et al. Long-term treatment with evolocumab added to conventional drug therapy, with or without apheresis, in patients with homozygous familial hypercholesterolaemia: an interim subset analysis of the open-label TAUSSIG study. Lancet Diabetes Endocrinol. 2017;5(4):280–90.
50. Gaudet D, Langslet G, Gidding SS, Luirink IK, Ruzza A, Kurtz C, et al. Efficacy, safety, and tolerability of evolocumab in pediatric patients with heterozygous familial hypercholesterolemia: rationale and design of the HAUSER-RCT study. J Clin Lipidol. 2018;12(5):1199–207.
51. Raal FJ, Braamskamp MJ, Selvey SL, Sensinger CH, Kastelein JJ. Pediatric experience with mipomersen as adjunctive therapy for homozygous familial hypercholesterolemia. J Clin Lipidol. 2016;10(4):860–9.
52. Stein EA, Dufour R, Gagne C, Gaudet D, East C, Donovan JM, et al. Apolipoprotein B synthesis inhibition with mipomersen in heterozygous familial hypercholesterolemia: results of a randomized, double-blind, placebo-controlled trial to assess efficacy and safety as add-on therapy in patients with coronary artery disease. Circulation. 2012;126(19):2283–92.

53. Raal FJ, Santos RD, Blom DJ, Marais AD, Charng M-J, Cromwell WC, et al. Mipomersen, an apolipoprotein B synthesis inhibitor, for lowering of LDL cholesterol concentrations in patients with homozygous familial hypercholesterolaemia: a randomised, double-blind, placebo-controlled trial. Lancet. 2010;375(9719):998–1006.
54. Davis KA, Miyares MA. Lomitapide: a novel agent for the treatment of homozygous familial hypercholesterolemia. Am J Health Syst Pharm. 2014;71(12):1001–8.
55. Ben-Omran T, Masana L, Kolovou G, Ariceta G, Nóvoa FJ, Lund AM, et al. Real-world outcomes with Lomitapide use in paediatric patients with homozygous familial hypercholesterolaemia. Adv Ther. 2019;36(7):1786–811.
56. Wheeler KA, West RJ, Lloyd JK, Barley J. Double blind trial of bezafibrate in familial hypercholesterolaemia. Arch Dis Child. 1985;60(1):34–7.
57. Manlhiot C, Larsson P, Gurofsky RC, Smith RW, Fillingham C, Clarizia NA, et al. Spectrum and management of hypertriglyceridemia among children in clinical practice. Pediatrics. 2009;123(2):458–65.
58. Prasad A. Biochemistry and molecular biology of mechanisms of action of fibrates–an overview. Int J Biochem Res Rev. 2019:26(2):1–12.
59. Bellosta S, Corsini A. Statin drug interactions and related adverse reactions: an update. Expert Opin Drug Saf. 2018;17(1):25–37.
60. Kamanna VS, Kashyap ML. Mechanism of action of niacin. Am J Cardiol. 2008;101(8a):20b–6b.
61. Colletti RB, Roff NK, Neufeld EJ, Baker AL, Newburger JW, McAuliffe TL. Niacin treatment of hypercholesterolemia in children. Pediatrics. 1993;92(1):78–82.
62. de Ferranti SD, Milliren CE, Denhoff ER, Steltz SK, Selamet Tierney ES, Feldman HA, et al. Using high-dose omega-3 fatty acid supplements to lower triglyceride levels in 10- to 19-year-olds. Clin Pediatr (Phila). 2014;53(5):428–38.
63. Gidding SS, Prospero C, Hossain J, Zappalla F, Balagopal PB, Falkner B, et al. A double-blind randomized trial of fish oil to lower triglycerides and improve cardiometabolic risk in adolescents. J Pediatr. 2014;165(3):497–503.e2.
64. Kastelein JJ, Maki KC, Susekov A, Ezhov M, Nordestgaard BG, Machielse BN, et al. Omega-3 free fatty acids for the treatment of severe hypertriglyceridemia: the EpanoVa fOr lowering very high triglyceridEs (EVOLVE) trial. J Clin Lipidol. 2014;8(1):94–106.
65. Harris WS, Ginsberg HN, Arunakul N, Shachter NS, Windsor SL, Adams M, et al. Safety and efficacy of Omacor in severe hypertriglyceridemia. J Cardiovasc Risk. 1997;4(5-6):385–91.
66. Pownall HJ, Brauchi D, Kilinc C, Osmundsen K, Pao Q, Payton-Ross C, et al. Correlation of serum triglyceride and its reduction by omega-3 fatty acids with lipid transfer activity and the neutral lipid compositions of high-density and low-density lipoproteins. Atherosclerosis. 1999;143(2):285–97.
67. Bays HE, Ballantyne CM, Kastelein JJ, Isaacsohn JL, Braeckman RA, Soni PN. Eicosapentaenoic acid ethyl ester (AMR101) therapy in patients with very high triglyceride levels (from the multicenter, placebo-controlled, randomized, double-blind, 12-week study with an open-label extension [MARINE] trial). Am J Cardiol. 2011;108(5):682–90.
68. Kohen-Avramoglu R, Theriault A, Adeli K. Emergence of the metabolic syndrome in childhood: an epidemiological overview and mechanistic link to dyslipidemia. Clin Biochem. 2003;36(6):413–20.
69. Rizos CV, Elisaf MS, Liberopoulos EN. Effects of thyroid dysfunction on lipid profile. Open Cardiovasc Med J. 2011;5:76–84.
70. Arnaldi G, Scandali VM, Trementino L, Cardinaletti M, Appolloni G, Boscaro M. Pathophysiology of dyslipidemia in Cushing's syndrome. Neuroendocrinology. 2010;92(Suppl 1):86–90.
71. Agrawal S, Zaritsky JJ, Fornoni A, Smoyer WE. Dyslipidaemia in nephrotic syndrome: mechanisms and treatment. Nat Rev Nephrol. 2018;14(1):57–70.
72. Saland JM, Ginsberg HN. Lipoprotein metabolism in chronic renal insufficiency. Pediatr Nephrol. 2007;22(8):1095–112.
73. Khurana M, Silverstein DM. Etiology and management of dyslipidemia in children with chronic kidney disease and end-stage renal disease. Pediatr Nephrol (Berlin, Germany). 2015;30(12):2073–84.
74. Katsiki N, Mikhailidis DP, Mantzoros CS. Non-alcoholic fatty liver disease and dyslipidemia: an update. Metabolism. 2016;65(8):1109–23.
75. Su T-C, Lee Y-T, Cheng T-J, Chien H-P, Wang J-D. Chronic hepatitis B virus infection and dyslipidemia. J Formos Med Assoc. 2004;103(4):286–91.
76. Sorokin A, Brown JL, Thompson PD. Primary biliary cirrhosis, hyperlipidemia, and atherosclerotic risk: a systematic review. Atherosclerosis. 2007;194(2):293–9.
77. Burton BK. Inborn errors of metabolism in infancy: a guide to diagnosis. Pediatrics. 1998;102(6):e69–e.
78. Agarwal A, Prasad GVR. Post-transplant dyslipidemia: mechanisms, diagnosis and management. World J Transplant. 2016;6(1):125–34.
79. Henkin Y, Como JA, Oberman A. Secondary dyslipidemia: inadvertent effects of drugs in clinical practice. JAMA. 1992;267(7):961–8.

Overview and Management of Childhood Obesity

58

Liya Kerem and Vibha Singhal

Definition

Whereas obesity colloquially refers to excess adiposity, the Obesity Medicine Association defines obesity as "chronic, relapsing, multi-factorial, neurobehavioral disease, wherein an increase in body fat promotes adipose tissue dysfunction and abnormal fat mass physical forces, resulting in adverse metabolic, biomechanical, and psychosocial health consequences." In common clinical practice, the body mass index (BMI, [weight in kg]/[height in cm^2]) is used as a surrogate marker to assess the adiposity status of the patient. Of note, BMI can overestimate adiposity in children with short stature or those who have relatively high muscle mass, and it may underestimate adiposity in those who have reduced muscle mass in the setting of low levels of physical activity. A recent extensive meta-analysis showed that 25% of youth who had BMI in the healthy range were found to have increased adiposity as measured by reliable techniques such as dual-energy X-ray absorptiometry, hydrostatic weighing, and bioelectrical impedance analysis [3]. The sensitivity of BMI to detect adiposity was lower in males, and the heterogeneity between studies was explained by race, definition of obesity, and the methods by which adiposity was measured.

Importantly, the BMI–adiposity relationship varies between ethnic groups due to inherent differences in body shape and composition, with Hispanic and Asian youth having higher percent body fat (BF%) for a given BMI compared to other ethnicities [4, 5]. Although BMI should be interpreted carefully, it is shown to have a high degree of correlation with fat mass concentration and obesity complications [6–8].

L. Kerem (✉) · V. Singhal
Division of Pediatric Endocrinology, Massachusetts General Hospital, Harvard Medical School, Boston, MA, USA
e-mail: lkerem@mgh.harvard.edu; vsinghal1@mgh.harvard.edu

In youth between 2 and 20 years of age, weight status is evaluated by determining the BMI-percentile-for-age and sex according to reference standards, published by the Centers of Disease Control and Prevention [9] or the World Health Organization [10]. Overweight is defined as a BMI ≥ 85th and <95th percentile for age and sex, obesity is present when the BMI is ≥95th percentile for age and sex and severe obesity corresponds to a BMI ≥ 99th percentile for age and sex, or BMI at or above 35 kg/m^2 (whichever is lower). A newer classification system, described in more detail in Chap. 19, recognizes BMI ≥ 95th percentile as class I obesity, BMI ≥ 120% of the 95th percentile as class II obesity, and BMI ≥ 140% of the 95th percentile as class III obesity, with class II and III obesity being strongly associated with greater cardiovascular and metabolic risk [11]. When a child is younger than 2 years, weight for length is calculated to determine the weight status and there are no standard definitions of overweight and obesity in this age group.

Epidemiology

The prevalence of obesity among youth aged 2–19 years is increasing substantially, from 13.9% in 1999–2000 to 18.5% in 2015–2016 [12]. The factors affecting the prevalence of childhood obesity can be found in Table 58.1.

Importantly, obesity tracks into adulthood, that is, the presence of obesity during childhood predicts obesity in adulthood, with an increased risk for adult obesity among children with severe obesity [17] especially in the presence of parental obesity [18]. A child with severe obesity at 5 years of age has 1-in-10 chance of having obesity at the age of 35 years [17]. Thus, the old dictum that children "grow out of their obesity" is usually not true. Parents should be advised of this risk and also the increased risk for concurrent and future adverse medical conditions. On the contrary, children who manage to resolve their obesity in childhood do not have any increased risk of major cardiovascular risk as adults [19].

T. Stanley, M. Misra (eds.), *Endocrine Conditions in Pediatrics*, https://doi.org/10.1007/978-3-030-52215-5_58

Table 58.1 Factors affecting prevalence of obesity

Age	Prevalence increases with increasing age [12]
Gender	Gender-specific obesity incidence in the United States varies between studies [13]. Worldwide, the prevalence of obesity differs between countries, with higher prevalence in boys than in girls in high-income countries [14]
Race/ethnicity	Lower prevalence in non-Hispanic white and Asian youth compared with non-Hispanic black and Hispanic youth [12]
Socioeconomic status	As the household income decreases, the percentage of overweight/obesity in youth increases [15]
Family history	Severity of childhood obesity is positively associated with family history of obesity [16]

Etiology

The causes of childhood obesity are numerous and tremendously complex. An intricate interaction between genetic, epigenetic, social, and environmental factors contributes to this condition. Common obesity is a polygenic trait, and the development of childhood obesity increases in the presence of an obesogenic environment [20, 21]. Environmental factors include unhealthy diet, sedentary lifestyle, socioeconomic status causing food insecurity, emotional stress, insufficient sleep, and exposure to environmental chemicals [22]. Certain perinatal factors are also associated with increased risk for obesity such as birth size, weight gain velocity during infancy, and breastfeeding status [23]. During the initial evaluation of the child with obesity, it is important to take into consideration endocrine, syndromic, and monogenic causes of obesity that present with specific signs and symptoms. Please refer to Chap. 19 for additional discussion regarding the etiology and differential diagnosis of childhood obesity.

Comorbidities of Childhood Obesity

Childhood obesity is associated with multiple comorbidities and involves endocrine, gastrointestinal, pulmonary, cardiovascular, musculoskeletal, and psychological manifestations [24]. A careful review of systems and physical examination is critical to screen for associated comorbidities and determine appropriate treatment and monitoring.

Endocrine

Type 2 diabetes mellitus (T2DM) results from an interplay between genetic predisposition, obesity, and lack of physical activity. Childhood obesity is associated with insulin resistance, which could lead to hyperinsulinemia, beta-cell dysfunction, and subsequently overt diabetes [25]. The prevalence of type 2 diabetes mellitus (T2DM) and prediabetes is rising rapidly among youth [26] with disproportionate representation in ethnic minorities [27, 28]. Of note, puberty is a physiological state of insulin resistance and could further increase the risk for diabetes development in susceptible individuals. The onset of T2DM after hyperinsulinemia is more precipitous in adolescents as compared to adults [29].

Polycystic ovary syndrome (PCOS) is another endocrine condition that is associated with obesity. Obesity can exacerbate the pathophysiology and clinical manifestation of PCOS, including metabolic syndrome, T2DM, hirsutism, and acne [30], and obesity in adolescence is associated with self-reported symptoms of PCOS in adulthood [31]. The metabolic complications at a similar BMI are greater in the presence of PCOS [32].

Male hypogonadism has also been recognized as one of the many complications of obesity. Mechanisms include increased peripheral conversion of testosterone to estrone and suppression of the hypothalamic–pituitary–gonadotropin (HPG) axis in the setting of obesity-related inflammation [33]. Hypogonadism in adolescent males may present clinically with delayed development of secondary sexual characteristics or slower pubertal progression.

Premature adrenarche is more prevalent in children with obesity as compared to those with normal weight and may present with pubic hair, axillary hair, acne, and adult body odor before the age of 8 and 9 years in girls and boys, respectively [34]. Importantly, BMI status at adrenarche is an important risk factor for the development of metabolic abnormalities during adolescence [35].

Another endocrine finding which is commonly seen in children with obesity is mild subclinical hypothyroidism [36]. Thyroid-stimulating hormone (TSH) levels are at the upper limit of the normal range or slightly increased and free thyroxine (fT4) may be normal or borderline low. Possible mechanisms for subclinical hypothyroidism in obesity include increased levels of leptinstimulating thyrotropin-releasing hormone (TRH) and consequently increasing TSH. Increased conversion rate of T4 to T3 may be a compensatory mechanism to increase energy expenditure, and adipose tissue-associated inflammation may also affect thyroid function [37]. The subclinical hypothyroidism found in obesity is physiologic and does not require treatment.

Finally, childhood obesity may be associated with altered activity of the hypothalamus–pituitary–adrenal (HPA) axis, with a blunted diurnal cortisol rhythm in youth [38], lower salivary cortisol levels throughout the day [39], and increased levels at night in female adolescents [40]. Of note, some studies have shown a weak positive correlation between cortisol levels and BMI in youth [41]. It can be challenging to distinguish obesity (pseudo-cushingoid state) from endogenous cortisol excess (Cushing syndrome).

Cardiometabolic

Excess adiposity in childhood is a strong risk factor for adult arterial vascular abnormalities [42] and is also associated with increased risk for premature death from coronary artery disease and stroke [43]. Excessive weight gain very early in childhood has been shown to be associated with later central obesity, elevated markers of inflammation, and cardiac and vascular abnormalities such as carotid intima-media thickness at age 8 years [44] and greater arterial stiffness at age 5 years [45]. Additionally, childhood obesity is associated with other cardiometabolic abnormalities such as elevated cholesterol, hypertriglyceridemia, and hypertension [46].

Gastrointestinal

Nonalcoholic fatty liver disease (NAFLD) is currently the most frequent cause of chronic liver disease in children worldwide [47]. This condition reflects a spectrum, ranging from lipid accumulation in liver cells (hepatic steatosis) to inflammatory and necrotic liver lesions (nonalcoholic steatohepatitis) and eventually fibrosis and cirrhosis.

Pulmonary

Youth with overweight/obesity have a significantly greater risk for obstructive sleep apnea (OSA) compared with healthy-weight peers, and a one-unit increase in BMI SDS was found to be associated with an average increase in the Apnea–Hypopnea Index of 35% [48]. This is important: OSA is not only associated with cardiovascular complications, but also with behavioral and neurocognitive dysfunction, excessive daytime sleepiness, and a decrease in quality of life [49]. Additionally, this condition is associated with elevated leptin and ghrelin levels, resulting in increased hunger and low satiety [50].

Childhood obesity is also an independent risk factor for childhood asthma [51], and youth with obesity-related asthma tend to have decreased medication responsiveness as well as poor disease control [52, 53]. Obesity-related asthma may have distinct underlying mechanisms, including mechanical fat load, metabolic dysregulation, and adiposity-mediated inflammation [54]. This is important to consider as the use of steroids in asthma and decreased exercise tolerance may further exacerbate obesity and cause a vicious cycle.

Orthopedic

Excess weight in childhood is associated with musculoskeletal discomfort and impairment of mobility [55], as well as increased susceptibility to skeletal fractures [56]. The most common orthopedic complications seen in the setting of overweight/obesity in youth are slipped capital femoral epiphysis (SCFE) and Blount's disease, the latter characterized by disordered growth of the tibial epiphysis resulting in progressive lower limb deformity [57].

Neurologic

Pseudotumor cerebri syndrome is a rare disorder of increased intracranial pressure that presents with severe headaches and risk of blindness [58]. Diagnosis requires an ophthalmology examination to evaluate papilledema as well as a lumbar puncture to show elevated opening cerebrospinal fluid pressure. In a large prospective survey evaluating the incidence of pseudotumor cerebri syndrome in childhood, in children older than 7 years of age, obesity, and female sex were identified as dominant risk factors with more than 80% of cases occurring at ages 12–15 years attributable to obesity [59].

Psychological

Compared to healthy-weight children and adolescents, children with overweight/obesity have a heightened risk of psychological comorbidities including depression, anxiety, perceived low quality of life, low self-esteem, development of eating disorders, and behavioral disorders [60]. Additionally, youth with obesity frequently report weight-related bullying and stigmatization, with a greater prevalence of weight-related teasing being associated with lower self-esteem, greater body fat dissatisfaction, and greater depressive symptoms in boys [61]. In a longitudinal study, weight-related teasing was found to be associated with a greater BMI and fat mass gain during the follow-up period of the study [62].

Clinical and Laboratory Evaluation of Childhood Obesity

The evaluation of a child with overweight/obesity starts with a careful history, including the family history, height, and weight measurement, vital signs including blood pressure that should be taken with an appropriate size cuff and a thorough physical examination. History and review of systems should be targeted to screen for obesity-related complications. Polyuria and polydipsia, blurry vision, fungal vaginitis, and unexplained weight loss could reflect hyperglycemia. Snoring should raise suspicion for OSA, and severe chronic headaches should be evaluated for pseudotumor cerebri syndrome. Review of medications is important to indicate any weight gain-promoting drugs such as anti-psychotics [63], anti-epileptics [64], antihistamines [65], and systemic steroids [66]. It is important to assess associated psychological problems such as anxiety and depression, eating disorders such as binge eating, night eating, and bulimia and to screen for bullying. Dietary history should be obtained in a non-judgmental way. The medical interview should include an assessment of the physical activity of the child, including the amount of sedentary time and non-academic screen time. On physical examination, special attention should be given to the examination of the skin to look for acanthosis nigricans over the posterior neck and axillary area (a marker of insulin resistance). Tonsillar hypertrophy could increase the risk for OSA. Hirsutism and acne require further evaluation for PCOS in pubertal females, while lack of facial hair and small testicular volume could reflect hypogonadism in pubertal males.

Evaluation of the linear growth is critical in a child with obesity. Youth with exogenous obesity tend to have a steady or accelerated growth, while obesity due to an underlying endocrinopathy or syndromic etiology is characterized by deceleration of linear growth. Importantly, certain monogenic causes of obesity are associated with accelerated linear growth (melanocortin 4 receptor deficiency and leptin deficiency). Please see Chap. 19 for details of features on physical examination that could indicate an underlying endocrinopathy or a syndromic cause of obesity. The recommended laboratory evaluation to assess for comorbidities in a child with overweight or obesity appears in Table 58.2.

Treatment of Childhood Obesity

Stepwise Approach to the Treatment of Obesity

The pediatric care provider has a critical role in the initial management of childhood obesity, which begins with age-appropriate and family-centered counseling to educate and support the patient and their family in implementing lifestyle modifications. While the efficacy of behavioral interventions in youth with severe obesity is unclear and usually involves only a modest BMI reduction [71], it may prevent/delay obesity-related comorbidities [72, 73]. A recent systemic review showed that intensive behavioral intervention is required to achieve weight reduction in youth, with at least 25 hours with a provider needed for a significant weight reduction, and with greater improvement in weight reduction and obesity-associated diseases with >52 hours of contact [74] . While it may be unfeasible to implement such an intensive program at the pediatrician's office, some individuals may benefit from fewer encounters as well. The American Academy of Pediatrics Institute for Healthy Childhood Weight [24] recommends a stepwise approach to the management of childhood obesity (Table 58.3). According to expert opinion, goals for safe weight loss are 1 lb/mo for children between the ages of 2–11 years and up to 2 lb/week in adolescents with severe obesity and obesity-related complications [24].

Pharmacotherapy

Pharmacotherapy is an evolving strategy in the field of childhood obesity, and most medications available to adults are still used off-label in the pediatric population. Obesity pharmacotherapy is always given as an adjunct to lifestyle modifications and may enhance the adherence to them [75]. Currently available medications can be classified according to the mechanism they target: nutrient processing, the neuroendocrine–gut hormonal axis, and central nervous system control of appetite and satiety regulation [76]. See Table 58.4 for the different medications, including mechanism of action, adverse effects, and expected weight loss.

Table 58.2 Recommended laboratory evaluation

Age, BMI and presence of risk factors	Laboratory evaluation
Age > 10 years, overweight (BMI 85th–94th%) no risk factors[a]	Fasting lipid profile[b]
Age > 10 years with overweight and at least one risk factor[a]	Fasting lipid profile[b] Hemoglobin A1c[c] AST, ALT[d]
Age > 2 years with obesity (BMI ≥ 95th%)	Fasting lipid profile[e] Hemoglobin A1c[c] AST, ALT[d]

[a]Risk factors include hypertension, dyslipidemia, tobacco use, and family history of obesity-associated comorbidities (T2DM, dyslipidemia, cardiovascular disease) [67]
[b]Normal lipid profile should be repeated every 3–5 years [67]
[c]Asymptomatic individuals with HbA1c ≥ 6.5% on 2 separate occasions have diabetes (criteria used in adults). HbA1c levels between 5.7% and 6.5% are consistent with prediabetes [68]
[d]If ALT is above the upper limit but <80 U/L, counseling for lifestyle modifications is required. If ALT is ≥52 for boys and ≥44 for girls age ≥ 10, an evaluation for NAFLD is required [69]
[e]Normal lipid profile in a child with obesity should be repeated every 2 years [70]

Table 58.3 Stepwise approach to managing pediatric obesity

Stage 1 – Prevention Plus: Initiated at the pediatrician's office. Includes family-based counseling and education regarding lifestyle modification with specific recommendations regarding diet, physical activity, sleeping habits, and screen time [24]. Counseling could be provided by a multidisciplinary team, including a social worker, a nutritionist, or a physical therapist
Stage 2 – Structured Weight Management: Implementation of stage 1 in frequent appointments occurring every 2–4 weeks at the pediatrician's office. Recommendations should be given for a structured diet and physical activity plans
Stage 3 – Comprehensive Multidisciplinary Intervention: Referral to a Pediatric Weight Management clinic where treatment is provided by specialists with active monitoring of diet and physical activity. Patients with BMI ≥ 95% and obesity-related comorbidities and patients with BMI ≥ 99% who did not experience significant weight reduction are advanced to the next stage
Stage 4 – Tertiary Care Intervention: Pharmacotherapy and bariatric surgery are considered by the Pediatric Weight Management clinic providers in addition to implementing healthy lifestyle modifications

Table 58.4 Pharmacological agents for the treatment of obesity

Generic name (trade name)	Mechanism of action	Side effects and contraindications	Expected weight loss together with lifestyle modification	Comments
Orlistat (Xenical®)	Gastric and pancreatic lipase inhibitor that reduces the absorption of triglycerides by 30% [77]	Steatorrhea, flatulence, fecal urgency, and incontinence, vitamin deficiencies and cholelithiasis [78]	Significant modest BMI reduction (−0.94 to −0.5 in 3 randomized, placebo-controlled pediatric trials) [74]	1. FDA approved for children 12 years and above 2. Prescribed with supplemental fat-soluble vitamins (A, D, E, and K)
Metformin	Effects in T2DM – Reduces hepatic gluconeogenesis and intestinal glucose absorption, improves insulin sensitivity by increasing peripheral glucose uptake [79]. Promotes satiety [80]	Nausea, diarrhea, and abdominal upset – Could be diminished with gradual dose increase. No reported liver or kidney toxicity in children (lactic acidosis in adults is very rare) [81]	Mean BMI reduction of 1.16 Kg/m^2 (systemic review of 14 randomized controlled pediatric clinical trials) [82]	FDA approved for T2DM in children 10 years and older
Phentermine	Norepinephrine reuptake inhibitor. CNS-mediated effects of appetite suppression	Dry mouth, insomnia, dizziness, palpitations, flushing, fatigue, and constipation [83]. Contraindicated in pregnancy, cardiovascular disease, hyperthyroidism, glaucoma, and in patients using recreational drugs [84]	Retrospective chart review showing that phentermine use in children was associated with a BMI reduction of −1.6% at 1 month, −2.9% at 3 months, and −4.1% at 6 months compared to lifestyle modification alone [85]	FDA approved for short-term use (12 weeks) as a treatment for obesity in individuals 16 years and older
Topiramate	Mechanism of action promoting weight loss is unknown. Inhibits GABAergic pathways, inhibition of carbonic anhydrase	Paresthesia, somnolence, reversible memory impairment and decreased concentration [86], teratogenicity, kidney stones, and potential decrease in oral contraceptives' efficacy [87]	Retrospective chart review in adolescents with severe obesity showing BMI reduction of −4.9% [88]	FDA approved as an anti-epileptic medication for children older than 2 years of age, approved for migraine prophylaxis for children older than 12 years of age [84]
Naltrexone/ bupropion (Contrave®)	Bupropion is a dopamine and norepinephrine reuptake inhibitor; it centrally suppresses appetite. Naltrexone is an opioid receptor antagonist that has weight-loss effects with an unclear mechanism	Nausea, vomiting, constipation, headache, dizziness, insomnia, dry mouth, and diarrhea. Contraindications – Uncontrolled hypertension, epilepsy, and substance use disorder. Black-box warning for suicidal thoughts and behavior	No published data describing use in children. In adults, weight reduction compared with placebo ranged between 2.5% and 5.2% of initial body weight [89]	FDA approved for weight loss in adults only
Liraglutide (Saxenda®/ Victoza®)	Glucagon-like peptide-1 (GLP-1) receptor agonist. Increases glucose-dependent insulin release, reduces glucagon secretion and gastric emptying. Promotes satiety via CNS-mediated effects [90]	Nausea, diarrhea, vomiting, dyspepsia, constipation, and pancreatitis. Contraindicated in patients with a personal or family history of medullary thyroid carcinoma and patients with multiple endocrine neoplasia syndrome type 2	Randomized-controlled and open-label pediatric trials with liraglutide and exenatide (another GLP-1 receptor agonist) – BMI reduction between 2.7% and 4.29% [91, 92], no significant effect on weight in another study that did not include lifestyle modification [93]	FDA approved for T2DM in children 10 years and older and FDA approved for T2DM and weight loss in adults
Phentermine/ topiramate ER (Qsymia®)	See above for individual medications	See above for individual medications	No published data describing use in children. In adults, 56 weeks of treatment as compared with placebo, led to significant weight reduction (between 5.1% and 10.6%, depending on the dose) [94]	FDA approved for weight loss in adults

Abbreviations: *5-HT 2C* serotonin receptor 2C, *BMI* body mass index, *CNS* central nervous system, *FDA* United States Food and Drug Administration, *T2DM* type 2 diabetes mellitus

Metabolic and Bariatric Surgery

Metabolic bariatric surgery (MBS) has been performed in adolescents for several decades. The main two types of bariatric surgery include Roux-en-Y gastric bypass (RYGB) and vertical sleeve gastrectomy (VSG). RYGB requires the creation of a small proximal gastric pouch together with an associated roux limb of jejunum, thus effectively excluding the remaining stomach and proximal small bowel from ingested enteral content. This procedure results in restriction of caloric intake as well as food malabsorption. Laparoscopic sleeve gastrectomy involves resection of most of the greater curvature of the stomach creating a narrower tubular stomach. This procedure has a lower risk of malabsorption and micronutrient deficiencies. The most recently updated guidelines from the American Society of Metabolic and Bariatric Surgery (ASMBS) and American Academy of Pediatrics (AAP) recommend considering bariatric surgery in all youth (no minimum age) with severe obesity [95, 96]. According to these evidence-based recommendations, either RYGB or VSG should be considered for adolescents with a BMI $\geq$ 35 Kg/m^2 or$\geq$120% of the 95th percentile and a clinically significant and obesity-associated comorbidity or with a BMI $\geq$ 40 Kg/m^2 or $\geq$140% of the 95th percentile. Importantly, it is stressed that prior weight loss attempts, Tanner stage, and bone age should not be barriers to definitive treatment [95]. Contraindications for pediatric MBS include a medically correctable cause of obesity, an active substance abuse problem, and a medical, psychiatric, psychosocial, or cognitive condition that prevents adherence to postoperative dietary and medication regimens and pregnancy. It is recommended that vitamin levels should be monitored in children before and after MBS with long-term need for vitamin supplementations [95].

Recent data show that 5 years following RYGB, 60% of adolescents maintained a weight reduction of 20% or more, with a decline in the prevalence of T2DM from 14% prior to 2% post-bariatric surgery [97]. A significant improvement was seen in hypertension as well. Among this cohort of 161 patients, 20% required an additional intra-abdominal procedure, the majority requiring cholecystectomy. This recent longitudinal assessment found better metabolic improvement in adolescents compared with adults, suggesting that youth receiving early surgical intervention may have a greater potential for recovery from obesity-associated comorbidities [97]. Future studies should precisely evaluate the consequences of bariatric surgeries on growth and development.

References

1. Ogden CL, Carroll MD, Kit BK, Flegal KM. Prevalence of childhood and adult obesity in the United States, 2011-2012. JAMA. 2014;311(8):806–14.
2. Skinner AC, Skelton JA. Prevalence and trends in obesity and severe obesity among children in the United States, 1999-2012. JAMA Pediatr. 2014;168(6):561–6.
3. Javed A, Jumean M, Murad MH, Okorodudu D, Kumar S, Somers VK, et al. Diagnostic performance of body mass index to identify obesity as defined by body adiposity in children and adolescents: a systematic review and meta-analysis. Pediatr Obes. 2015;10(3):234–44.
4. Dugas LR, Cao G, Luke AH, Durazo-Arvizu RA. Adiposity is not equal in a multi-race/ethnic adolescent population: NHANES 1999-2004. Obesity (Silver Spring). 2011;19(10):2099–101.
5. Deurenberg P, Deurenberg-Yap M, Guricci S. Asians are different from Caucasians and from each other in their body mass index/body fat per cent relationship. Obes Rev. 2002;3(3):141–6.
6. Akindele MO, Phillips JS, Igumbor EU. The relationship between body fat percentage and body mass index in overweight and obese individuals in an urban African setting. J Public Health Afr. 2016;7(1):515.
7. Ranasinghe C, Gamage P, Katulanda P, Andraweera N, Thilakarathne S, Tharanga P. Relationship between Body Mass Index (BMI) and body fat percentage, estimated by bioelectrical impedance, in a group of Sri Lankan adults: a cross sectional study. BMC Public Health. 2013;13:797.
8. Abdelaal M, le Roux CW, Docherty NG. Morbidity and mortality associated with obesity. Ann Transl Med. 2017;5(7):161.
9. Kuczmarski RJ, Ogden CL, Guo SS, Grummer-Strawn LM, Flegal KM, Mei Z, et al. 2000 CDC growth charts for the United States: methods and development. Vital Health Stat. 2002;11(246):1–190.
10. de Onis M, Onyango AW, Borghi E, Siyam A, Nishida C, Siekmann J. Development of a WHO growth reference for school-aged children and adolescents. Bull World Health Organ. 2007;85(9):660–7.
11. Skinner AC, Perrin EM, Moss LA, Skelton JA. Cardiometabolic risks and severity of obesity in children and young adults. N Engl J Med. 2015;373(14):1307–17.
12. Hales CM, Carroll MD, Fryar CD, Ogden CL. Prevalence of obesity among adults and youth: United States. NCHS Data Brief. 2015-2016;2017(288):1–8.
13. Cheung PC, Cunningham SA, Narayan KM, Kramer MR. Childhood obesity incidence in the United States: a systematic review. Child Obes. 2016;12(1):1–11.
14. Di Cesare M, Soric M, Bovet P, Miranda JJ, Bhutta Z, Stevens GA, et al. The epidemiological burden of obesity in childhood: a worldwide epidemic requiring urgent action. BMC Med. 2019;17(1):212.
15. Eagle TF, Sheetz A, Gurm R, Woodward AC, Kline-Rogers E, Leibowitz R, et al. Understanding childhood obesity in America: linkages between household income, community resources, and children's behaviors. Am Heart J. 2012;163(5):836–43.
16. Corica D, Aversa T, Valenzise M, Messina MF, Alibrandi A, De Luca F, et al. Does family history of obesity, cardiovascular, and metabolic diseases influence onset and severity of childhood obesity? Front Endocrinol (Lausanne). 2018;9:187.
17. Ward ZJ, Long MW, Resch SC, Giles CM, Cradock AL, Gortmaker SL. Simulation of growth trajectories of childhood obesity into adulthood. N Engl J Med. 2017;377(22):2145–53.
18. Parsons TJ, Power C, Logan S, Summerbell CD. Childhood predictors of adult obesity: a systematic review. Int J Obes Relat Metab Disord. 1999;23(Suppl 8):S1–107.
19. Juonala M, Magnussen CG, Berenson GS, Venn A, Burns TL, Sabin MA, et al. Childhood adiposity, adult adiposity, and cardiovascular risk factors. N Engl J Med. 2011;365(20):1876–85.
20. Herrera BM, Keildson S, Lindgren CM. Genetics and epigenetics of obesity. Maturitas. 2011;69(1):41–9.
21. Marginean CO, Marginean C, Melit LE. New insights regarding genetic aspects of childhood obesity: a mini review. Front Pediatr. 2018;6:271.

22. Kumar S, Kelly AS. Review of childhood obesity: from epidemiology, etiology, and comorbidities to clinical assessment and treatment. Mayo Clin Proc. 2017;92(2):251–65.
23. von Ehr J, von Versen-Hoynck F. Implications of maternal conditions and pregnancy course on offspring's medical problems in adult life. Arch Gynecol Obstet. 2016;294(4):673–9.
24. Barlow SE, Expert C. Expert committee recommendations regarding the prevention, assessment, and treatment of child and adolescent overweight and obesity: summary report. Pediatrics. 2007;120(Suppl 4):S164–92.
25. Hannon TS, Rao G, Arslanian SA. Childhood obesity and type 2 diabetes mellitus. Pediatrics. 2005;116(2):473–80.
26. Chen L, Magliano DJ, Zimmet PZ. The worldwide epidemiology of type 2 diabetes mellitus--present and future perspectives. Nat Rev Endocrinol. 2011;8(4):228–36.
27. Writing Group for the SfDiYSG, Dabelea D, Bell RA, D'Agostino RB Jr, Imperatore G, Johansen JM, et al. Incidence of diabetes in youth in the United States. JAMA. 2007;297(24):2716–24.
28. Ma RC, Chan JC. Type 2 diabetes in East Asians: similarities and differences with populations in Europe and the United States. Ann N Y Acad Sci. 2013;1281:64–91.
29. Nadeau KJ, Anderson BJ, Berg EG, Chiang JL, Chou H, Copeland KC, et al. Youth-onset type 2 diabetes consensus report: current status, challenges, and priorities. Diabetes Care. 2016;39(9):1635–42.
30. Christensen SB, Black MH, Smith N, Martinez MM, Jacobsen SJ, Porter AH, et al. Prevalence of polycystic ovary syndrome in adolescents. Fertil Steril. 2013;100(2):470–7.
31. Laitinen J, Taponen S, Martikainen H, Pouta A, Millwood I, Hartikainen AL, et al. Body size from birth to adulthood as a predictor of self-reported polycystic ovary syndrome symptoms. Int J Obes Relat Metab Disord. 2003;27(6):710–5.
32. Palomba S, Santagni S, Falbo A, La Sala GB. Complications and challenges associated with polycystic ovary syndrome: current perspectives. Int J Women's Health. 2015;7:745–63.
33. Mushannen T, Cortez P, Stanford FC, Singhal V. Obesity and hypogonadism-A narrative review highlighting the need for high-quality data in adolescents. Children (Basel). 2019;6(5):63.
34. Utriainen P, Laakso S, Liimatta J, Jaaskelainen J, Voutilainen R. Premature adrenarche--a common condition with variable presentation. Horm Res Paediatr. 2015;83(4):221–31.
35. Kaya G, Yavas Abali Z, Bas F, Poyrazoglu S, Darendeliler F. Body mass index at the presentation of premature adrenarche is associated with components of metabolic syndrome at puberty. Eur J Pediatr. 2018;177(11):1593–601.
36. Salerno M, Capalbo D, Cerbone M, De Luca F. Subclinical hypothyroidism in childhood - current knowledge and open issues. Nat Rev Endocrinol. 2016;12(12):734–46.
37. Sanyal D, Raychaudhuri M. Hypothyroidism and obesity: an intriguing link. Indian J Endocrinol Metab. 2016;20(4):554–7.
38. Ruttle PL, Javaras KN, Klein MH, Armstrong JM, Burk LR, Essex MJ. Concurrent and longitudinal associations between diurnal cortisol and body mass index across adolescence. J Adolesc Health. 2013;52(6):731–7.
39. Kjolhede EA, Gustafsson PE, Gustafsson PA, Nelson N. Overweight and obese children have lower cortisol levels than normal weight children. Acta Paediatr. 2014;103(3):295–9.
40. Hillman JB, Dorn LD, Loucks TL, Berga SL. Obesity and the hypothalamic-pituitary-adrenal axis in adolescent girls. Metabolism. 2012;61(3):341–8.
41. Kiess W, Meidert A, Dressendorfer RA, Schriever K, Kessler U, Konig A, et al. Salivary cortisol levels throughout childhood and adolescence: relation with age, pubertal stage, and weight. Pediatr Res. 1995;37(4 Pt 1):502–6.
42. Laitinen TT, Pahkala K, Venn A, Woo JG, Oikonen M, Dwyer T, et al. Childhood lifestyle and clinical determinants of adult ideal cardiovascular health: the cardiovascular risk in Young Finns study, the childhood determinants of adult health study, the Princeton follow-up study. Int J Cardiol. 2013;169(2):126–32.
43. Twig G, Yaniv G, Levine H, Leiba A, Goldberger N, Derazne E, et al. Body-mass index in 2.3 million adolescents and cardiovascular death in adulthood. N Engl J Med. 2016;374(25):2430–40.
44. Skilton MR, Marks GB, Ayer JG, Garden FL, Garnett SP, Harmer JA, et al. Weight gain in infancy and vascular risk factors in later childhood. Pediatrics. 2013;131(6):e1821–8.
45. Evelein AM, Visseren FL, van der Ent CK, Grobbee DE, Uiterwaal CS. Excess early postnatal weight gain leads to thicker and stiffer arteries in young children. J Clin Endocrinol Metab. 2013;98(2):794–801.
46. Chung ST, Onuzuruike AU, Magge SN. Cardiometabolic risk in obese children. Ann N Y Acad Sci. 2018;1411(1):166–83.
47. Nobili V, Alisi A, Newton KP, Schwimmer JB. Comparison of the phenotype and approach to pediatric vs adult patients with nonalcoholic fatty liver disease. Gastroenterology. 2016;150(8):1798–810.
48. Andersen IG, Holm JC, Homoe P. Obstructive sleep apnea in children and adolescents with and without obesity. Eur Arch Otorhinolaryngol. 2019;276(3):871–8.
49. Capdevila OS, Kheirandish-Gozal L, Dayyat E, Gozal D. Pediatric obstructive sleep apnea: complications, management, and long-term outcomes. Proc Am Thorac Soc. 2008;5(2):274–82.
50. Shechter A. Obstructive sleep apnea and energy balance regulation: a systematic review. Sleep Med Rev. 2017;34:59–69.
51. von Mutius E, Schwartz J, Neas LM, Dockery D, Weiss ST. Relation of body mass index to asthma and atopy in children: the National Health and nutrition examination study III. Thorax. 2001;56(11):835–8.
52. Forno E, Lescher R, Strunk R, Weiss S, Fuhlbrigge A, Celedon JC, et al. Decreased response to inhaled steroids in overweight and obese asthmatic children. J Allergy Clin Immunol. 2011;127(3):741–9.
53. Quinto KB, Zuraw BL, Poon KY, Chen W, Schatz M, Christiansen SC. The association of obesity and asthma severity and control in children. J Allergy Clin Immunol. 2011;128(5):964–9.
54. Vijayakanthi N, Greally JM, Rastogi D. Pediatric obesity-related asthma: the role of metabolic dysregulation. Pediatrics. 2016;137(5):e20150812.
55. Taylor ED, Theim KR, Mirch MC, Ghorbani S, Tanofsky-Kraff M, Adler-Wailes DC, et al. Orthopedic complications of overweight in children and adolescents. Pediatrics. 2006;117(6):2167–74.
56. Goulding A, Grant AM, Williams SM. Bone and body composition of children and adolescents with repeated forearm fractures. J Bone Miner Res. 2005;20(12):2090–6.
57. Daniels SR. Complications of obesity in children and adolescents. Int J Obes. 2009;33(Suppl 1):S60–5.
58. Best J, Silvestri G, Burton B, Foot B, Acheson J. The incidence of blindness due to idiopathic intracranial hypertension in the UK. Open Ophthalmol J. 2013;7:26–9.
59. Matthews YY, Dean F, Lim MJ, McLachlan K, Rigby AS, Solanki GA, et al. Pseudotumor cerebri syndrome in childhood: incidence, clinical profile and risk factors in a national prospective population-based cohort study. Arch Dis Child. 2017;102(8):715–21.
60. Rankin J, Matthews L, Cobley S, Han A, Sanders R, Wiltshire HD, et al. Psychological consequences of childhood obesity: psychiatric comorbidity and prevention. Adolesc Health Med Ther. 2016;7:125–46.
61. Lampard AM, MacLehose RF, Eisenberg ME, Neumark-Sztainer D, Davison KK. Weight-related teasing in the school environment: associations with psychosocial health and weight control practices among adolescent boys and girls. J Youth Adolesc. 2014;43(10):1770–80.
62. Schvey NA, Marwitz SE, Mi SJ, Galescu OA, Broadney MM, Young-Hyman D, et al. Weight-based teasing is associated with gain in BMI and fat mass among children and adolescents at-risk for obesity: a longitudinal study. Pediatr Obes. 2019;14:e12538.

63. Reekie J, Hosking SP, Prakash C, Kao KT, Juonala M, Sabin MA. The effect of antidepressants and antipsychotics on weight gain in children and adolescents. Obes Rev. 2015;16(7):566–80.
64. Hamed SA. Antiepileptic drugs influences on body weight in people with epilepsy. Expert Rev Clin Pharmacol. 2015;8(1):103–14.
65. Ratliff JC, Barber JA, Palmese LB, Reutenauer EL, Tek C. Association of prescription H1 antihistamine use with obesity: results from the National Health and Nutrition Examination Survey. Obesity (Silver Spring). 2010;18(12):2398–400.
66. Curtis JR, Westfall AO, Allison J, Bijlsma JW, Freeman A, George V, et al. Population-based assessment of adverse events associated with long-term glucocorticoid use. Arthritis Rheum. 2006;55(3):420–6.
67. Krebs NF, Himes JH, Jacobson D, Nicklas TA, Guilday P, Styne D. Assessment of child and adolescent overweight and obesity. Pediatrics. 2007;120(Suppl 4):S193–228.
68. American Diabetes A. (2) Classification and diagnosis of diabetes. Diabetes Care. 2015;38(Suppl):S8–S16.
69. Vos MB, Abrams SH, Barlow SE, Caprio S, Daniels SR, Kohli R, et al. NASPGHAN clinical practice guideline for the diagnosis and treatment of nonalcoholic fatty liver disease in children: recommendations from the Expert Committee on NAFLD (ECON) and the North American Society of Pediatric Gastroenterology, Hepatology and Nutrition (NASPGHAN). J Pediatr Gastroenterol Nutr. 2017;64(2):319–34.
70. Expert Panel on Integrated Guidelines for Cardiovascular H, Risk Reduction in C, Adolescents, National Heart L, Blood I. Expert panel on integrated guidelines for cardiovascular health and risk reduction in children and adolescents: summary report. Pediatrics. 2011;128(Suppl 5):S213–56.
71. Ryder JR, Fox CK, Kelly AS. Treatment options for severe obesity in the pediatric population: current limitations and future opportunities. Obesity (Silver Spring). 2018;26(6):951–60.
72. Savoye M, Caprio S, Dziura J, Camp A, Germain G, Summers C, et al. Reversal of early abnormalities in glucose metabolism in obese youth: results of an intensive lifestyle randomized controlled trial. Diabetes Care. 2014;37(2):317–24.
73. Ryder JR, Vega-Lopez S, Ortega R, Konopken Y, Shaibi GQ. Lifestyle intervention improves lipoprotein particle size and distribution without weight loss in obese Latino adolescents. Pediatr Obes. 2013;8(5):e59–63.
74. O'Connor EA, Evans CV, Burda BU, Walsh ES, Eder M, Lozano P. Screening for obesity and intervention for weight management in children and adolescents: evidence report and systematic review for the US preventive services task force. JAMA. 2017;317(23):2427–44.
75. Apovian CM, Aronne LJ, Bessesen DH, McDonnell ME, Murad MH, Pagotto U, et al. Pharmacological management of obesity: an endocrine Society clinical practice guideline. J Clin Endocrinol Metab. 2015;100(2):342–62.
76. Coles N, Birken C, Hamilton J. Emerging treatments for severe obesity in children and adolescents. BMJ. 2016;354:i4116.
77. Pilitsi E, Farr OM, Polyzos SA, Perakakis N, Nolen-Doerr E, Papathanasiou AE, et al. Pharmacotherapy of obesity: available medications and drugs under investigation. Metabolism. 2019;92:170–92.
78. Torgerson JS, Hauptman J, Boldrin MN, Sjostrom L. XENical in the prevention of diabetes in obese subjects (XENDOS) study: a randomized study of orlistat as an adjunct to lifestyle changes for the prevention of type 2 diabetes in obese patients. Diabetes Care. 2004;27(1):155–61.
79. Rena G, Hardie DG, Pearson ER. The mechanisms of action of metformin. Diabetologia. 2017;60(9):1577–85.
80. Adeyemo MA, McDuffie JR, Kozlosky M, Krakoff J, Calis KA, Brady SM, et al. Effects of metformin on energy intake and satiety in obese children. Diabetes Obes Metab. 2015;17(4):363–70.
81. Inzucchi SE, Lipska KJ, Mayo H, Bailey CJ, McGuire DK. Metformin in patients with type 2 diabetes and kidney disease: a systematic review. JAMA. 2014;312(24):2668–75.
82. McDonagh MS, Selph S, Ozpinar A, Foley C. Systematic review of the benefits and risks of metformin in treating obesity in children aged 18 years and younger. JAMA Pediatr. 2014;168(2):178–84.
83. Yanovski SZ, Yanovski JA. Long-term drug treatment for obesity: a systematic and clinical review. JAMA. 2014;311(1):74–86.
84. Srivastava G, Fox CK, Kelly AS, Jastreboff AM, Browne AF, Browne NT, et al. Clinical considerations regarding the use of obesity pharmacotherapy in adolescents with obesity. Obesity (Silver Spring). 2019;27(2):190–204.
85. Ryder JR, Kaizer A, Rudser KD, Gross A, Kelly AS, Fox CK. Effect of phentermine on weight reduction in a pediatric weight management clinic. Int J Obes. 2017;41(1):90–3.
86. Coulter AA, Rebello CJ, Greenway FL. Centrally acting agents for obesity: past, present, and future. Drugs. 2018;78(11):1113–32.
87. Rosenfeld WE, Doose DR, Walker SA, Nayak RK. Effect of topiramate on the pharmacokinetics of an oral contraceptive containing norethindrone and ethinyl estradiol in patients with epilepsy. Epilepsia. 1997;38(3):317–23.
88. Fox CK, Marlatt KL, Rudser KD, Kelly AS. Topiramate for weight reduction in adolescents with severe obesity. Clin Pediatr (Phila). 2015;54(1):19–24.
89. Vorsanger MH, Subramanyam P, Weintraub HS, Lamm SH, Underberg JA, Gianos E, et al. Cardiovascular effects of the new weight loss agents. J Am Coll Cardiol. 2016;68(8):849–59.
90. Ladenheim EE. Liraglutide and obesity: a review of the data so far. Drug Des Devel Ther. 2015;9:1867–75.
91. Kelly AS, Rudser KD, Nathan BM, Fox CK, Metzig AM, Coombes BJ, et al. The effect of glucagon-like peptide-1 receptor agonist therapy on body mass index in adolescents with severe obesity: a randomized, placebo-controlled, clinical trial. JAMA Pediatr. 2013;167(4):355–60.
92. Kelly AS, Metzig AM, Rudser KD, Fitch AK, Fox CK, Nathan BM, et al. Exenatide as a weight-loss therapy in extreme pediatric obesity: a randomized, controlled pilot study. Obesity (Silver Spring). 2012;20(2):364–70.
93. Danne T, Biester T, Kapitzke K, Jacobsen SH, Jacobsen LV, Petri KCC, et al. Liraglutide in an adolescent population with obesity: a randomized, double-blind, placebo-controlled 5-week trial to assess safety, tolerability, and pharmacokinetics of Liraglutide in adolescents aged 12-17 years. J Pediatr. 2017;181:146–53 e3.
94. Smith SM, Meyer M, Trinkley KE. Phentermine/topiramate for the treatment of obesity. Ann Pharmacother. 2013;47(3):340–9.
95. Pratt JSA, Browne A, Browne NT, Bruzoni M, Cohen M, Desai A, et al. ASMBS pediatric metabolic and bariatric surgery guidelines, 2018. Surg Obes Relat Dis. 2018;14(7):882–901.
96. Armstrong SC, Bolling CF, Michalsky MP, Reichard KW. Section On Obesity SOS. Pediatric metabolic and bariatric surgery: evidence, barriers, and Best practices. Pediatrics. 2019;144(6):e20193223.
97. Inge TH, Courcoulas AP, Jenkins TM, Michalsky MP, Brandt ML, Xanthakos SA, et al. Five-year outcomes of gastric bypass in adolescents as compared with adults. N Engl J Med. 2019;380(22):2136–45.

Transgender Care

59

Kate Millington and Coleen Williams

Abbreviavtions

DSM – 5	Diagnostic and statistical manual of mental disorders 5
FSH	Follicle-stimulating hormone
GAH	Gender-affirming hormones
GnRH	Gonadotropin releasing hormone
HDL	High-density lipoprotein cholesterol
ICD	International Classification of Diseases
IUD	Intrauterine device
LGBTQ	Lesbian, gay, bisexual, transgender, queer
LH	Luteinizing hormone
PFLAG	Parents and Friends of Lesbians and Gays
TGD	Transgender or gender-diverse

Introduction

In modern primary care practice, it is likely that a provider will encounter a transgender or gender-diverse (TGD) patient, a person who experiences incongruence between the sex that they were assigned at birth and their gender identity. It is important to make a distinction between sex and gender because these terms capture two separate, distinguishable factors, which are often interchanged incorrectly. For the purposes of this chapter, *sex* will refer to the designation at birth (e.g., female, male, intersex), typically based on external genital anatomy and sometimes on other physiologic features such as the sex chromosomes, whereas *gender* will refer to a person's internal sense of self (Box 59.1) [1–3]. Cisgender refers to a person whose gender identity matches the sex that they were assigned at birth. Transgender refers to a person whose gender identity does not match the sex that they were assigned at birth; for example, a transgender patient may be someone who was assigned male sex at birth who has a female gender identity.

Box 59.1: Glossary of Terms[a]

Sex or sex assigned at birth: Physical attributes that signal biologic femaleness or maleness typically assigned at birth typically based on genital appearance

Gender identity: Inner sense of one's gender

Gender expression: Outward manner by which an individual displays their gender (e.g., clothing, hairstyle, speech, and mannerisms)

Transgender: A person whose gender identity differs from their sex assigned at birth

Cisgender: A person whose gender identity is congruent with their sex assigned at birth

Gender-diverse: An individual whose gender identity differs from their sex assigned at birth and may be more complex than male or female

Transmasculine or transfeminine: Terms to describe gender diverse and nonbinary individuals based on the "direction" of their gender identity

Non-binary: A gender identity that is neither male nor female

Sexual orientation: Term to describe an individual's preference for sexual partners and/or romantic attraction, and is not directly related to gender identity

[a]Terminology in transgender health is rapidly evolving. These terms may be out of date, so we recommend asking patients which terms they prefer.

Historically, gender identity has been conceptualized within a binary framework, with only two options: female/woman/girl and male/man/boy. There is now a greater appreciation that gender identity expands far beyond only two options. Outside of the traditional binary are identities

K. Millington (✉) · C. Williams
Division of Endocrinology, Boston Children's Hospital, Boston, MA, USA
e-mail: kate.millington@childrens.harvard.edu; coleen.williams@childrens.harvard.edu

T. Stanley, M. Misra (eds.), *Endocrine Conditions in Pediatrics*, https://doi.org/10.1007/978-3-030-52215-5_59

that reflect an ever-expanding gender diversity; genderqueer, gender fluid, nonbinary, agender, and many more. Gender identity and expression differ depending upon a person's cultural background and their intersecting identities, such as race, ethnicity, and socioeconomic status [1–5]. Language about gender is fluid; it is growing and changing on a regular basis to capture people's rich diversity of experiences. It is less important to memorize the various terms and definitions, such as the ones previously listed, and it is more important to be open to listening to and learning from patients. There are many gender-affirming resources that are reputable to turn to when a patient uses a new term and definition about gender that a physician has not yet encountered including *The World Professional Association for Transgender Health (WPATH), American Psychiatric Association, American Psychological Association, the Human Rights Campaign (HRC), Gender Spectrum, United States Transgender Survey, and the Gay and Lesbian Student Education Network (GLSEN).* It is recommended that primary care physicians be aware of and sensitive to the myriad gender identities and expressions that exist, and ask what they mean to each patient. Doing so will lend to creating a safe and affirming space for TGD youth and their families during their primary care visits.

Primary care physicians have an important role in identifying and supporting TGD youth. They may be among the first medical providers with whom patients feel comfortable disclosing their gender identity to and, in some cases, may be asked to provide gender-affirming medical care. Supporting gender identity and gender transition can improve psychosocial outcomes [6–8]. Gender-affirming care of TGD children and adolescents can encompass a wide range of options from support for social transition, to adjunctive therapies such as voice therapy, to medical and surgical treatments. Treatment should be individualized based on the patient's goals, developmental stage, and the ability to provide fully informed consent for irreversible treatments or procedures. The WPATH Standards of Care and The Endocrine Society Clinical Practice Guidelines provide guidance regarding treatments and monitoring, which are briefly outlined here [9, 10]. This chapter will review the role of primary care providers in transgender health.

Creating a Gender-Inclusive Environment

A crucial step to providing gender-affirming care to TGD patients and reduce the barriers to health care is to create an inclusive and safe office space that is welcoming to all patients. This is particularly important for the TGD community because they face significant discrimination in society as a whole, as well as when seeking medical care. The TGD population suffers from high rates of poverty, homelessness, and mental illness including anxiety, depression, and, most concerning, suicide [8, 11–15]. As many as 20% of TGD adults reported being refused medical care because of their gender identity, and over 25% reported being verbally harassed in a medical setting. Furthermore, 50% of TGD adults have had to teach their medical provider about transgender health in order to receive medical treatment, and one quarter to one third have avoided seeking needed medical care due to discrimination [8, 16]. Thus, primary care providers have an opportunity to create more positive, helpful, and healing experiences for TGD individuals across the lifespan.

To create a gender-affirming space, primary care physicians and their staff can utilize various methods of representation of TGD individuals throughout the office to communicate their awareness of and sensitivity to gender diversity. Medical spaces can display signs familiar to and associated with the lesbian, gay, bisexual, transgender, and queer (LGBTQ) community, such as the rainbow pride and/or transgender pride flag. LGBTQ sensitivity training, often called *Safe Zone* training, can further help office staff to learn the components of creating a safe space, and the display of "safe space" stickers and/or certificates of completion can help LGBTQ youth feel comfortable [8, 17–21].

In addition to signage and symbols of inclusivity, another step to creating a gender-affirming practice is to ensure that physicians and their staff have created forms and documentation that capture patients' gender identity, affirmed name, and pronouns, and that these terms are used during encounters and in documentation [22–24]. Some patients, for a variety of reasons, may not want their affirmed name and pronouns used. Although it may appear to be complicated, it can be as simple as asking, "What name and pronouns would you like to go by during your visit today?" and "What name and pronouns would you like used in the medical notes and in your chart?" Questions such as these not only open a dialogue about gender but also demonstrate that the primary care staff are sensitive to the idea that the patient may have different preferences and concerns that are important to discuss. Physicians and staff will likely make mistakes, most often without any ill intent, when it comes to using a patient's affirmed name and pronouns. It is important to briefly acknowledge the mistake and apologize prior to moving on. For example, a physician may say after making a mistake, "I'm sorry. I didn't use your pronouns correctly. I'm going to try that again." Apologies and correcting statements acknowledge the error, validate the impact it had on the patient, and move the patient–doctor relationship forward [25].

It is important for physicians to be prepared for either parents or children to screen positively for gender diversity, or to "come out" as a TGD youth or parents of a TGD child, and to subsequently seek support. If a child or the parents disclose gender diversity for the child, it is important that physicians respond with openness and take a nonjudgmental stance. The coming out process is often distressing for both children and their parents; therefore, being met with warmth, understanding, and empathy is crucial. It is beneficial when a physician can provide normalization and validation, as well as psychoeducation about gender identity that is accurate, evidence-based, and gender-affirmative. Physicians should be aware of local resources for transgender youth, such as LGBTQ community groups and chapters of PFLAG (Parents and Friends of Lesbians and Gays).

Gender Dysphoria

Some TGD patients, but not all, experience gender dysphoria. The diagnosis and treatment of gender dysphoria should be done by a multidisciplinary team of mental health and medical providers not only to aid in diagnostic interviewing but also to develop treatment recommendations. The *Diagnostic and Statistical Manual of Mental Disorders 5* (DSM-5) defines gender dysphoria in children, adolescents, and adults as incongruence between a person's assigned sex and their experienced/expressed gender [26]. Full diagnostic criteria for both gender dysphoria in children and in adolescents/adults are available for reference through the DSM-5 or the most recent International Classification of Diseases (ICD) [26]. Gender dysphoria typically leads to significant emotional distress and functional impairment for the individual experiencing it, which is one of the main reasons that gender-affirming treatment, both medical and psychosocial, is crucial. A provider skilled in the assessment of readiness should evaluate patients prior to medical and surgical gender-affirming treatments. The WPATH Standards of Care and The Endocrine Society Clinical Practice Guidelines lay out the framework for determining readiness, and their utilization is recommended for medical and mental health providers [9, 10].

Gender-Affirming Medical Treatment

Medical gender transition for TGD youth can include pubertal blockade and/or gender-affirming hormones. Common medications used in medical gender transition are listed in Table 59.1.

Pubertal Blockade

Medical pubertal blockade allows time for TGD children to further explore their gender identity while preventing the development of physical changes that occur during puberty (e.g., voice deepening, development of an "Adam's apple" in birth-assigned males, breast development in birth-assigned females), which may decrease the need for future surgical procedures [6, 27]. Gonadotropin-releasing hormone (GnRH) analogs block the secretion of luteinizing hormone (LH) and follicle-stimulating hormone (FSH) and suspend pubertal development. Studies of central precocious puberty, for which GnRH analogs have been used for decades, have shown no impairment in reproductive endocrine function or fertility after discontinuation [28, 29]. Patients should be counseled that an abrupt decrease in sex steroids can cause hot flashes, but that this symptom abates with time. Bone health should be optimized with adequate vitamin D and calcium intake. Injectable forms of GnRH agonists can cause sterile abscesses [27]. Depending on the patient's insurance coverage, GnRH agonists can carry a significant cost. Progestins can also be used, and although they are not as potent as GnRH analogs, can be a less-expensive alternative.

Gender-Affirming Hormones

Gender-affirming hormones (GAH) (i.e., testosterone for transmasculine patients and estrogen for transfeminine patients) promote irreversible physical changes that bring the body in line with the patient's affirmed gender. GAH reduce gender dysphoria, improve body image, and enhance psychological well-being [6, 7]. Although initiation of GAH has historically been restricted to older adolescents (i.e., after 16 years of age), current best practice is that the timing of initiating GAH therapy should be individualized to every patient based on their readiness, goals, and ability to provide informed consent/assent. Many transgender health specialists advocate earlier initiation of GAH in order to lessen gender dysphoria, optimize adolescent bone-mass accumulation, and allow the patient to experience puberty contemporaneously with his or her peers [30].

GAH therapy in children who have undergone pubertal blockade should be started at a low dose and increased over the course of several years under the guidance of a pediatric endocrinologist. Adolescents who have completed their growth can be treated with adult doses of GAH (Table 59.1).

Feminizing Therapy

The goal of feminizing therapy for transfeminine individuals is to promote feminine secondary sex characteristics while maintaining both estradiol and testosterone levels in the physiologic female range, 30–200 pg/mL and <55 ng/dL, respectively. Estrogen should be given as 17β-estradiol, which has lower thrombosis and cardiovascular risk, and can be administered orally, transdermally, or by intramuscular injection. Transdermal estrogen is preferred given its lower thrombosis risk [31, 32]. It can take up to 3 years for estradiol to exert its full effects, such as breast growth, hair and skin changes, and changes in body composition. Estrogen therapy can also lead to a decrease in erections and libido, decrease in muscle mass, and redistribution of fat mass [10]. In TGD adults, estrogen treatment has been associated with increased risk of venous thromboembolism and ischemic stroke, although many studies included patients on supraphysiologic doses of estrogen and/or using ethinyl estradiol, which is known to have higher thrombotic risk than

Table 59.1 Commonly used medications in gender-affirming care

	Route of administration	Dose range	Comments
Pubertal blockade			
GnRH analogs			May also be used to suppress testosterone production in older patients desiring feminization
Leuprolide acetate	Intramuscular	7.5–15 mg every month; 11.25–30 mg every 3 months	
Triptorelin pamoate	Intramuscular	22.5 mg every 6 months	
Histrelin acetate	Subcutaneous implant	50 mg implant once yearly	May be effective for longer than 1 year.
Progesterone			
Medroxyprogesterone acetate	Oral	20–80 mg daily	Can also be used for suppression of menses
	Intramuscular	150 mg every 3 months	
	Subcutaneous	104 mg every 3 months	
Menstrual suppression			
Norethindrone ("mini-pill")	Oral	0.35 mg daily	Must be taken at the same time every day
Norethindrone acetate	Oral	2.5–15 mg daily	
Micronized progesterone	Oral	100–200 mg daily	Excipient contains peanut oil
Etonogesterol (Implanon)	Subcutaneous implant	One device every 3 years	
Levonorgestrel IUD	Intrauterine	52 mg device every 5 years 19.5 mg device every 5 years 13.5 mg device every 3 years	
Feminization			
17β-Estradiol	Oral	2–6 mg daily	For pubertal induction increase from 5 mcg/kg/day to 1–2 mg/day over the course of 1.5–2 years Postpubertal adolescents can be increased more rapidly over 6–12 months
	Patch	50–200 mcg	For pubertal induction increase from 6.25 mcg/day (1/4 of the 25 mcg patch) to adult dose over the course of 1.5–2 years
Estradiol valerate or cypionate	Intramuscular	5–30 mg every 2 weeks 2–10 mg every week	
Spironolactone	Oral	100–300 mg daily	(anti-androgen)
Bicalutamide	Oral	50 mg daily	(anti-androgen)
Masculinization			
Testosterone enanthate or cypionate	Intramuscular	50–100 mg every week 100–200 mg every 2 weeks	For pubertal induction increase from 25 mg every 2 weeks to 50–100 mg/week over the course of 1.5 to 2 years Post – pubertal adolescents can be increased from 75 mg every 2 weeks to adult dose over 6–12 months
	Subcutaneous	50–100 mg every week	
Testosterone	Patch	4–8 mg daily	May cause skin irritation
	gel	25–100 mg daily	Patients should be counseled regarding the risk of transfer to others
	Axillary gel	60–120 mg daily	
	Pellets	300–450 mg (4–6 pellets) every 3–6 months	

17β-estradiol [31–34]. Studies of the effect of estrogen treatment in transfeminine adolescents have reported a small and likely clinically insignificant increase in high-density lipoprotein cholesterol (HDL) and serum triglycerides [35–37]. A specialist in medical gender transition should be consulted prior to initiating estrogen in patients with a significant personal or family history of thrombosis.

Spironolactone, a potassium-sparing diuretic with antiandrogen properties, can also be used to reduce testosterone production and action in transfeminine patients, particularly if unwanted hair growth is a chief concern [38, 39]. Spironolactone may lead to mild diuresis, so patients should be counseled regarding appropriate hydration. Hyperkalemia, when seen, occurs in the first 6 months of treatment and is unlikely to be clinically significant in patients without other medical comorbidities [40].

Masculinizing Therapy

For transmasculine individuals, the goals of GAH with testosterone are to produce masculine secondary sex characteristics by maintaining serum testosterone levels in the normal male range (i.e., 300–1000 ng/dL). Testosterone esters (enanthate, cypionate) injected either intramuscularly or subcutaneously are favored in pediatric practice for the ease of dose adjustment and ability to titrate small doses for pubertal induction. Transdermal testosterone, administered by patches or gels, may be appropriate for older postpubertal adolescents and adults. Although the effects of testosterone therapy such as increase in muscle mass, decreased fat mass, male-pattern hair growth (as well as male-pattern baldness), deepening of the voice, atrophy of breast tissue, increased libido, clitoromegaly, changes in facial structure, and increased prominence of the laryngeal cartilage (i.e., Adam's apple) begin in the first several months, full effects may not be seen for 2–5 years [10]. Adverse effects of testosterone include polycythemia (though hematocrit typically remains in the normal male range), transaminitis, acne, and hypertension [10, 41, 42]. Concern has been raised about an increase in aggressive behavior from testosterone treatment based on observations of individuals utilizing supraphysiologic doses of testosterone for its anabolic properties; however, physiologic levels of testosterone in transgender men have not been correlated with an increase in aggression [43–45]. If patients report mood changes after injections, smaller, more frequent doses can be utilized. In TGD adolescents, testosterone has been associated with a small decrease in HDL and an increase in systolic blood pressure [35–37].

Menstrual Suppression

For transmasculine individuals, menses can contribute significantly to gender dysphoria. Suppression of menstruation is achieved in greater than 90% of patients with adult-dose testosterone therapy [42, 46–48]. For the remaining 10% of patients and for patients who are not being treated with testosterone, menstrual suppression can be achieved by administration of progesterone or a progestin in the form of oral or injectable medroxyprogesterone, oral norethindrone, or levonorgestrel-releasing intrauterine devices can be used for menstrual suppression (Table 59.1).

Adjunctive Gender-Affirming Therapy Options

Beyond medical gender transition, TGD youth may wish to pursue additional techniques to aid in social transition and to reduce gender dysphoria. Clinicians should ask youth about their use of these techniques, counsel patients on their safe use, and refer to other professionals when necessary (Table 59.2) [49].

Table 59.2 Adjunctive gender-affirming intervention options

Legal name/ gender marker change	Many TGD youth and adults alike wish to pursue legal name changes and legal gender marker changes. This can be a complicated process, but often an affirming and crucial step in a person's transition.
Binding	Chest binding is the use of a specifically designed "binder," tightly fitted bra, or other material to reduce the appearance of the breasts. This may result in breathing restriction, breast pain, or skin irritation or infection. Procurement of specially made "binders" for this purpose, which fit appropriately, can reduce these risks. Also, encouraging TGD youth to take breaks from binding, such as when they are at home and certainly when they are sleeping each night, also assists in reducing discomfort and risks.
Hair removal	Permanent hair removal can be very important for TGD youth of all gender identities. Both laser hair removal and electrolysis can be used, and each method carries specific risks and benefits. Additionally, permanent hair removal is also a necessary step before some gender-affirming surgical procedures.
Packing	The process of packing involves placing a penile prosthesis in the underwear to produce the appearance of male genitalia. Some prostheses also allow the wearer to stand to urinate ("stand-to-pee" or STP devices).
Tucking	Tucking is the process of moving the penis and scrotum posteriorly after shifting the testicles into the inguinal canal in order to provide a smooth contour. This can result in testicular pain, urinary trauma, or urinary infection, as well as skin irritation if tape or other adhesives are used. Encouraging youth to take breaks from tucking and to use the bathroom regularly are important methods of risk reduction.
Voice augmentation	Voice therapy can be pursued to alter a person's voice to better suit the affirmed gender; this is often pursued with a speech therapist. Surgical options may also be pursued depending on the patient's preference and/or satisfaction with other methods of altering the voice that have been tried previously. Typically, transfeminine individuals aim to have a higher, softer sounding voice, whereas transmasculine individuals aim to have a lower, deeper sounding voice.

Fertility Preservation

Many transgender adults, like cisgender adults, desire children [50]. There is no information regarding the possibility of fertility in adolescents who were treated with GnRH analogs followed by GAH [50, 51]. Treatment with GAH may affect fertility. Estrogen treatment can lead to azoospermia. Testosterone treatment causes amenorrhea and effects follicular development in the ovary, yet there are many cases of conception and successful pregnancy in transgender men who have been treated with testosterone [52]. Procedures to aid in conception for transgender men and women exist, but can be costly and may not be successful in all cases. There are several reports of successful births following fertility preservation in transgender men, and the field is changing rapidly [53]. TGD youth should be counseled regarding the potential risk of loss of fertility and fertility preservation options prior to beginning any type of medical gender-affirming therapy. Conversations regarding fertility preservation should include the risks and benefits of currently available techniques such as oocyte retrieval and cryopreservation, embryo cryopreservation, and sperm retrieval and cryopreservation. A reproductive endocrinologist familiar with transgender care can assist in counseling patients regarding their fertility preservation options [9, 50].

Psychotherapy

In addition to gender-affirming medical treatments and adjunctive interventions like voice therapy, psychotherapy may be beneficial. Psychotherapy can address co-occurring mental health concerns such as depression, anxiety, and suicidality [6, 8, 12–15]. Therapy with a TGD client should be practiced through a gender-affirming lens, meaning that it should never be utilized to try to change a person's gender identity and that it should honor gender diversity as part of the human experience. The mental health concerns that the TGD population commonly experience are caused or exacerbated by societal stigma and discrimination and often require treatment independently from gender concerns [2, 5]. Primary care providers play an important role in recommending various behavioral health and psychotherapy interventions. Pediatricians and primary-care staff can discuss with youth how psychotherapy can assist with improving mood, reducing negative symptoms like anxiety, improving coping strategies, and facilitating family communication. Furthermore, psychotherapists who are well versed in gender-affirming care will be able to assist with navigating unique experiences such as coming out, social transition, and preparing for medical intervention.

Conclusion

Primary care providers play an important role in supporting TGD youth and may be the first place that TGD youth turn for help. Although mental health outcomes have been historically poor, gender-affirming care including gender affirmation by providers and office staff can help to improve psychological well-being. Gender-affirming care can have a direct impact on patient psychological outcomes and can be incredibly rewarding for the entire primary care team.

References

1. Defining transgender terms. In: Monit. Psychol. http://www.apa.org/monitor/2018/09/ce-corner-glossary, 2018. Accessed 6 Oct 2019.
2. American Psychological Association. Guidelines for psychological practice with transgender and gender nonconforming people. American Psychologist. 2015;70(9):832–64. https://doi.org/10.1037/a0039906; https://www.apa.org/practice/guidelines/transgender.pdf.
3. Key concepts and terms. www.glsen.org, 2014.s Accessed 6 Oct 2019.
4. Clark BA, Veale JF, Townsend M, Frohard-Dourlent H, Saewyc E. Non-binary youth: access to gender-affirming primary health care. Int J Transgend. 2018;19:158–69.
5. Hidalgo MA, Ehrensaft D, Tishelman AC, Clark LF, Garofalo R, Rosenthal SM, Spack NP, Olson J. The gender affirmative model: what we know and what we aim to learn. Hum Dev. 2013;56:285–90.
6. de Vries ALC, McGuire JK, Steensma TD, Wagenaar ECF, Doreleijers TAH, Cohen-Kettenis PT. Young adult psychological outcome after puberty suppression and gender reassignment. Pediatrics. 2014;134:696–704.
7. Fisher AD, Castellini G, Ristori J, et al. Cross-sex hormone treatment and psychobiological changes in transsexual persons: Two-year follow-up data. J Clin Endocrinol Metab. 2016;101:4260–9.
8. James SE, Herman JL, Rankin S, Keisling M, Mottet L, Anafi M. The 2015 U.S. Transgender Survey. Washington DC; 2016.
9. Hembree WC, Cohen-Kettenis PT, Gooren LJ, Hannema SE, Meyer WJ, Murad MH, Rosenthal SM, Safer JD, Tangpricha V, T'Sjoen GG. Endocrine treatment of gender-dysphoric/gender-incongruent persons: an Endocrine Society Clinical Practice Guideline. J Clin Endocrinol Metab. 2017;102:3869–903.
10. Coleman E, Bockting W, Botzer M, et al. Standards of care for the health of transsexual, transgender, and gender-nonconforming people, Version 7. Int J Transgend. 2012;13:165–232.
11. Toomey RB, Syvertsen AK, Shramko M. Transgender Adolescent Suicide Behavior. Pediatrics. 2018;142:e20174218.
12. Healthy People 2020. Healthy people 2020 transgender health fact sheet, 2010.
13. Equality NC for T. Understanding issues facing transgender Americans, 2017.
14. Downing JM, Przedworski JM. Health of transgender adults in the U.S., 2014–2016. Am J Prev Med. 2018;55:336–44.
15. Stotzer RL. Violence against transgender people: a review of United States data. Aggress Violent Behav. 2009;14:170–9.
16. Grant JM, Mottet LA, Tanis J, Herman JL, Harrison J, Keisling M. National Transgender Discrimination Survey Report on health and health care. Natl Cent Transgend Equal. 2010; https://doi.org/10.1016/S0016-7878(90)80026-2.
17. Safe space kit. www.glsen.org, 2016. Accessed 6 Oct 2019.

18. Kano M, Silva-Ban-Uelos AR, Sturm R, Willging CE. Stakeholders' recommendations to improve patient-centered "lGBTQ" primary care in rural and multicultural practices. J Am Board Fam Med. 2016;29:156–60.
19. Poynter KJ. Safe zones: training allies of LGBTQIA+ young adults. London: Rowman & Littlefield; 2017.
20. Creating a safe and welcoming clinic environment. In: Cent. Excell. Transgender Heal. transhealth.ucsf.edu/trans?page=guidelines-clinic-environment, 2018. Accessed 5 Nov 2019.
21. Black WW, Fedewa AL, Gonzalez KA. Effects of "safe school" programs and policies on the social climate for sexual-minority youth: a review of the literature. J LGBT Youth. 2012;9:321–39.
22. Cahill S, Makadon H. Sexual orientation and gender identity data collection in clinical settings and in electronic health records: a key to ending LGBT health disparities. LGBT Heal. 2014;1:34–41.
23. Deutsch MB, Buchholz D. Electronic health records and transgender patients—practical recommendations for the collection of gender identity data. J Gen Intern Med. 2015;30:843–7.
24. Tate CC, Ledbetter JN, Youssef CP. A two-question method for assessing gender categories in the social and medical sciences. J Sex Res. 2013;50:767–76.
25. Guss CE, Woolverton GA, Borus J, Austin SB, Reisner SL, Katz-Wise SL. Transgender adolescents' experiences in primary care: a qualitative study. J Adolesc Health. 2019;65:344–9.
26. American Psychiatric Association. Diagnostic and statistical manual of mental disorders: diagnostic and statistical manual of mental disorders. 5th ed. Arlington: American Psychiatric Association; 2013.
27. Mahfouda S, Moore JK, Siafarikas A, Zepf FD, Lin A. Puberty suppression in transgender children and adolescents. Lancet Diabetes Endocrinol. 2017;5:816–26.
28. Heger S, Partsch CJ, Sippell WG. Long-term outcome after depot gonadotropin-releasing hormone agonist treatment of central precocious puberty: final height, body proportions, body composition, bone mineral density, and reproductive function. J Clin Endocrinol Metab. 1999;84:4583–90.
29. Jay N, Mansfield MJ, Blizzard RM, Crowley WF, Schoenfeld D, Rhubin L, Boepple PA. Ovulation and menstrual function of adolescent girls with central precocious puberty after therapy with gonadotropin-releasing hormone agonists. J Clin Endocrinol Metab. 1992;75:890–4.
30. Vance SR, Ehrensaft D, Rosenthal SM. Psychological and medical care of gender nonconforming youth. Pediatrics. 2014;134:1184–92.
31. Toorians AWFT, Thomassen MCLGD, Zweegman S, Magdeleyns EJP, Tans G, Gooren LJ, Rosing J. Venous thrombosis and changes of hemostatic variables during cross-sex hormone treatment in transsexual people. J Clin Endocrinol Metab. 2003;88:5723–9.
32. Asscheman H, Giltay EJ, Megens JAJ, De Ronde W, Van Trotsenburg MAA, Gooren LJ. A long-term follow-up study of mortality in transsexuals receiving treatment with cross-sex hormones. Eur J Endocrinol. 2011;164:635–42.
33. Getahun D, Nash R, Flanders WD, et al. Cross-sex hormones and acute cardiovascular events in transgender persons: a cohort study. Ann Intern Med. 2018;169:205–13.
34. van Kesteren PJM, Asscheman H, Megens JAJ, Gooren LJ. Mortality and morbidity in transsexual subjects treated with cross-sex hormones. Clin Endocrinol. 2003;47:337–43.
35. Jarin J, Pine-Twaddell E, Trotman G, Stevens J, Conard LA, Tefera E, Gomez-Lobo V. Cross-sex hormones and metabolic parameters in adolescents with gender dysphoria. Pediatrics. 2017;139:e20163173.
36. Chew D, Anderson J, Williams K, May T, Pang K. Hormonal treatment in young people with gender dysphoria: a systematic review. Pediatrics. 2018;141:e20173742.
37. Olson-Kennedy J, Okonta V, Clark LF, Belzer M. Physiologic response to gender-affirming hormones among transgender youth. J Adolesc Health. 2018;62:397–401.
38. Prior JC, Vigna YM, Watson D. Spironolactone with physiological female steroids for presurgical therapy of male-to-female transsexualism. Arch Sex Behav. 1989;18:49–57.
39. Brown J, Farquhar C, Lee O, Toomath R, Jepson RG. Spironolactone versus placebo or in combination with steroids for hirsutism and/or acne. Cochrane Database Syst Rev. 2009; https://doi.org/10.1002/14651858.CD000194.pub2.
40. Millington K, Liu E, Chan Y-M. The utility of potassium monitoring in gender-diverse adolescents taking spironolactone. J Endocr Soc. 2019;3:1031–8.
41. Shumer DE, Nokoff NJ, Spack NP. Advances in the Care of Transgender Children and Adolescents. Adv Pediatr Infect Dis. 2016;63:79–102.
42. Gava G, Mancini I, Cerpolini S, Baldassarre M, Seracchioli R, Meriggiola MC. Testosterone undecanoate and testosterone enanthate injections are both effective and safe in transmen over 5 years of administration. Clin Endocrinol (Oxf). 2018;89(6):878–86. https://doi.org/10.1111/cen.13821.
43. Trenton AJ, Currier GW. Behavioural manifestations of anabolic steroid use. CNS Drugs. 2005;19:571–95.
44. Defreyne J, Kreukels B, T'Sjoen G, Stahporsius A, Den Heijer M, Heylens G, Elaut E. No correlation between serum testosterone levels and state-level anger intensity in transgender people: results from the European Network for the Investigation of Gender Incongruence. Horm Behav. 2019;110:29–39.
45. Defreyne J, T'Sjoen G, Bouman WP, Brewin N, Arcelus J. Prospective evaluation of self-reported aggression in transgender persons. J Sex Med. 2018;15:768–76.
46. Nakamura A, Watanabe M, Sugimoto M, Sako T, Mahmood S, Kaku H, Nasu Y, Ishii K, Nagai A, Kumon H. Dose-response analysis of testosterone replacement therapy in patients with female to male gender identity disorder. Endocr J. 2012;60:275–81.
47. Spratt DI, Stewart II, Savage C, Craig W, Spack NP, Chandler DW, Spratt LV, Eimicke T, Olshan JS. Subcutaneous injection of testosterone is an effective and preferred alternative to intramuscular injection: demonstration in female-to-male transgender patients. J Clin Endocrinol Metab. 2017;102:2349–55.
48. Carswell JM, Roberts SA. Induction and maintenance of amenorrhea in transmasculine and nonbinary adolescents. Transgend Health. 2017;2:195–201.
49. Deutsch MB. Guidelines for the primary and gender-affirming care of transgender and gender nonbinary people introduction to the guidelines. San Francisco; 2016.
50. Nahata L, Chen D, Moravek MB, Quinn GP, Sutter ME, Taylor J, Tishelman AC, Gomez-Lobo V. Understudied and under-reported: fertility issues in transgender youth—a narrative review. J Pediatr. 2019;205:265–71.
51. Hudson J, Nahata L, Dietz E, Quinn GP. Fertility counseling for transgender AYAs. Clin Pract Pediatr Psychol. 2018;6:84–92.
52. Light AD, Obedin-Maliver J, Sevelius JM, Kerns JL. Transgender men who experienced pregnancy after female-to-male gender transitioning. Obstet Gynecol. 2014;124:1120–7.
53. Maxwell S, Noyes N, Keefe D, Berkeley AS, Goldman KN. Pregnancy outcomes after fertility preservation in transgender men. Obstet Gynecol. 2017;129:1031–4.

Index

T. Stanley, M. Misra (eds.), *Endocrine Conditions in Pediatrics*, https://doi.org/10.1007/978-3-030-52215-5

B

C

H

T